Communication Behavior and Aging

A Sourcebook for Clinicians

Communication Behavior and Aging
A Sourcebook for Clinicians

EDITED BY
Barbara B. Shadden, Ph.D.

Associate Professor
Program in Speech Pathology-Audiology
University of Arkansas
Fayetteville, Arkansas

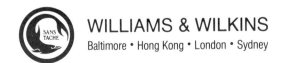

WILLIAMS & WILKINS
Baltimore • Hong Kong • London • Sydney

Editor: John Butler
Associate Editor: Victoria M. Vaughn
Copy Editor: Stephen Siegforth
Design: Saturn Graphics
Illustration Planning: Wayne Hubbel
Production: Raymond E. Reter
Cover Design: Bets Ltd.

Printed in the United States of America

Library of Congress Cataloging-in-Publication Data

Communication behavior and aging.

   Bibliography: p.
   Includes index.
   1. Communicative disorders in the aged.
2. Aged—Communication. I. Shadden, Barbara B. (Barbara Bennett)
[DNLM: 1. Communication—in old age. 2. Communicative Disorders—in old age. WL340 C7339]
RC423.C63 1988   618.97′6855   87-10383
ISBN 0-683-07723-6

                            87 88 89 90 91
10 9 8 7 6 5 4 3 2 1

This book is dedicated to my parents, Louisa and Richard Bennett. For close to 40 years they have trusted and believed in me, encouraged all my efforts, and provided judicious direction when it was needed. As all three of us have aged, we have learned to like as well as love each other, and to communicate as friends as well as parent and child. By their own examples, my parents showed me the meaning of commitment and caring, and taught me that the world can and should be a better place in which to live. That message is what this book is all about.

Preface

This text is intended to serve as a source-book for understanding normal communication changes, communication disorders, and service delivery options from a gerontological perspective. It is dedicated to the concept of understanding and developing strategies for management of age-related communication deficits. Information is presented within the context of a unified model of communicative functioning in the elderly. Introductory chapter abstracts emphasize key issues and topics of particular interest in considering communicative behavior.

The text is divided into four major sections. Section I, "Defining the Problem," is designed to provide the reader with a clear, practical appreciation of the importance of interpersonal communication in aging and of the daily realities of communication breakdown and behavior. The first chapter highlights the fact that communication is both a major tool for adaptation in the elderly and a potential target for age-related decrement. The second chapter contains a summary of the perceptions of older persons and their frequent communication partners concerning the nature and quality of interpersonal communications with and by the elderly. Data are drawn from interviews and are used to focus attention on the diversity of experiences of older persons and on the critical roles of both communication partners in determining and executing strategies for dealing with age-related communication breakdown.

In Section II, "Aspects of Aging Which Impact on Interpersonal Communication," the resources and decrements associated with aging are documented. Five chapters offer basic descriptive information concerning those intrinsic and extrinsic aspects of normal aging that define the status of the older person and that can potentially affect communicative interactions. In addition to coverage of more standard gerontological topics such as sociocultural, cognitive, and physiological changes, separate chapters address the topics of psychiatric problems in the elderly and pharmacology and the

aging system. Each author provides expert and thorough coverage of aging from his or her unique professional perspectives.

Section III, "The Communication Status of Older Persons," presupposes a theoretical model of a continuum of communication processes from normal to disordered. The reader is provided with an overview of normal hearing and speech-language changes that accompany aging. A separate chapter focuses on interpersonal communication processes and interactions, emphasizing the effects of age-related changes identified in Section II as well as current research and theory concerning the communication process and the elderly. A final chapter summarizes the most common communication disorders found in older persons, including dementia as a distinct example of pathological aging. Appropriate prevalence and descriptive data are provided.

Section IV, entitled "Age-Related Concerns in the Management of Communication Disorders," begins with a clinician-oriented chapter which addresses issues of attitude, responses to aging, increased client demands for social/emotional support, and willingness to be flexible in modifications of interventions. The reader is challenged to question his/her own beliefs and expectations. Management issues are then subdivided into concerns related to programming for the individual client and those related to broader based interventions addressing communication needs within the context of environmental, familial, and professional variables. As a result, focus is shared equally with the older person and his world.

The first subgroup of chapters, entitled "Direct Services to the Communicatively Impaired Older Adult," includes primarily those topics related to needed modifications in the assessment and treatment of hearing and speech-language impaired older persons. A separate chapter on management of the dementia patient explores clinical issues in serving this client base.

The second grouping of chapters is entitled,

"Completing the Programming Cycle," consistent with the text's philosophy that the impact of communication deficits extends beyond individuals and individual skills to embrace the entire social network and environment. The first chapter in this section presents a framework for expanding intervention options (including environmental interventions). Subsequent topics include: education, counseling, and support for significant others; group treatment programs for the elderly; a guide to basic agencies providing services and funding to older persons; and strategies for enhancing interdisciplinary service provision. As can be seen, particular attention is paid to the professional's responsibility for active involvement in networking and coordinating services with other service providers and agencies.

Although speech-language pathologists and audiologists are the primary professionals responsible for the assessment and treatment of communication disorders in the elderly, this textbook is designed to be of practical assistance to any professional or student in one of the numerous disciplines with a gerontological emphasis. Several aspects of the book's design increase the likelihood that readers from a variety of professional backgrounds can benefit from the content of various chapters.

First, the book is gerontologically oriented and relates to all communication behaviors and deficits, not simply speech-language-hearing disorders. Clearly, more comprehensive gerontological training is required for all concerned professionals. Professional preparation must include appropriate emphasis upon communication behaviors and disorders. By avoiding detailed discussions of specific therapy techniques for each disorder type and by stressing instead those ways in which assessment and treatment procedures must be accommodated to the needs of older clients, even the management sections of the text become accessible and relevant to readers from other disciplines.

Second, many of the broader-based management strategies addressing environments, significant others, and basic coping or communication skills require the active participation of professionals outside of speech-language pathology and audiology. It is imperative that all members of the aging network understand what other members do—the kinds of deficits treated, the strategies utilized, and the demands placed upon service agencies and providers. Finally, it is becoming increasingly obvious that research concerning communication and aging would benefit from an interdisciplinary perspective.

Acknowledgments

Few activities in life can be as obsessive and potentially destructive as the writing and editing of a book. Thus, there would literally be no book without the total support of my husband Harry. He cooked, shopped, washed clothes, and generally made certain that our home and our daily lives kept going when I abdicated all responsibilities. He also listened when I needed to talk, gave backrubs and hugs when I despaired, and went fishing when I needed to be alone. He did everything in his power to take away all sources of interference and pressure . . . without one complaint.

Harry was not alone, however, in paying the price for my commitment to this project. My debt of gratitude extends to the many friends who were understanding and accepting of my promise to be a real person again . . . soon . . . maybe next year. My thanks also go to my colleagues, who tolerated my stressed-out demeanor at work, and even more so to my students. The graduate students in particular found so many ways to show their caring, respect, and support.

A few individuals deserve particular mention. Our secretary, Helen Bayles, took each new request for assistance in stride, calmly working long hours to get materials typed so I could feel some sense of closure. Deborah Dowdle, graphic artist, unfailingly provided illustrations well ahead of schedule and went out of her way to be understanding and helpful in one particular crisis. My friend Kent Brown was always there to listen and commiserate with my latest tale of woe . . . and to ease the isolation somewhat. He also took time from his own busy schedule to critique several chapter drafts. Phil Trapp is another friend who put up with my litany of complaints. Our lunches together always seemed to restore my perspective on life, however briefly.

Finally, I would like to express my appreciation for the time and efforts of all of the contributors to this text, and to those who assisted them in preparing their chapters. Each contributor became involved because he or she cares about the communication needs of older persons.

Contributors

Jane A. Barr, M.S.W., Specialist in Aging, Ozark Guidance Center, Springdale, Arkansas

Barbaranne J. Benjamin, Ph.D., Distinguished Visiting Lecturer, The University of Toledo, Toledo, Ohio

Mary Ellen Brandell, Ed.S., Coordinator of Clinical Services, Speech-Language Clinic, Central Michigan University, Mt. Pleasant, Michigan

Richard R. Brandell, R.Ph., Registered Pharmacist, Downtown Drugs, Mt. Pleasant, Michigan

Harold G. Cox, Ph.D., Professor and Chair, Department of Sociology and Social Work, Indiana State University, Terre Haute, Indiana

G. Sandra Fisher, M.A.T., Deputy Director, Office of Management and Policy, Administration on Aging, Department of Health and Human Services, Washington, DC

LeeAnn C. Golper, Ph.D., Staff Speech Pathologist and Training Coordinator, Portland Veterans Administration Medical Center, Portland, Oregon
Clinical Assistant Professor, Department of Neurology, Oregon Health Sciences University, Portland, Oregon
Assistant Professor, Speech and Hearing Science Program, Portland State University, Portland, Oregon
Assistant Professor, Department of Special Education, University of Oregon, Eugene, Oregon

Michael E. Groher, Ph.D., Assistant Chief, Audiology and Speech Pathology, Veterans Administration Medical Center, New York, New York
Professional Associate, Department of Rehabilitation Medicine, The New York Hospital, New York, New York
Adjunct Faculty, Adelphi University, Garden City, New York

Richard Hult, Ph.D., Associate Professor, School of Pharmacy, Ferris State College, Bay Rapids, Michigan

Donald H. Kausler, Ph.D., Professor, Department of Psychology, University of Missouri, Columbia, Missouri

Richard A. Kenney, Ph.D., Professor and Chairman, Department of Physiology, George Washington University, Washington, DC

Rosemary Lubinsky, Ed.D., Associate Professor, Department of Communicative Disorders and Sciences, State University of New York at Buffalo, Amherst, New York

James T. Moore, M.D., Medical Director, Halifax Psychiatric Center, Daytona Beach, Florida

Michael A. Nerbonne, Ph.D., Professor and Director, Division of Audiology, Department of Communication Disorders, Central Michigan University, Mt. Pleasant, Michigan

Carolyn A. Raiford, Ph.D., Associate Professor, Program in Speech Pathology-Audiology, University of Arkansas, Fayetteville, Arkansas

Barbara B. Shadden, Ph.D., Associate Professor, Program in Speech Pathology-Audiology, University of Arkansas, Fayetteville, Arkansas
Staff Speech-Language Pathologist, Washington Regional Medical Center, Veterans Administration Medical Center, Fayetteville, Arkansas

Thea Spatz, M.S., Doctoral Candidate, Public Health, University of Arkansas-Fayetteville, Fayetteville, Arkansas

John D. Tonkovich, Ph.D., Director, Speech-Language Pathology Department, Rehabilitation Institute, Inc., Detroit, Michigan

E. Philip Trapp, Ph.D., Professor, Department of Psychology, University of Arkansas-Fayetteville, Fayetteville, Arkansas

Contents

III. The Communication Status of Older Persons

IV. Age-Related Concerns in the Management of Communication Disorders

A. DIRECT SERVICES TO THE COMMUNICATIVELY IMPAIRED ADULT

Defining the Problem

1 Communication and Aging: An Overview

BARBARA B. SHADDEN

Editor's Note

Chapter 1 provides the theoretical foundation for this text by emphasizing the need for an interface of knowledge from many disciplines in order to understand communication behaviors in aging. Several important premises are established. First, the author highlights the fact that communication skills may be affected by the aging process and by others' perceptions of aging and older individuals. This occurs at a time when there is increased risk for specific speech-language or hearing disorders. Ironically, many of the life changes associated with aging can be dealt with most effectively through use of communication as a tool for social interaction and for obtaining necessary services. In effect, interpersonal communication skills may begin to change or show deficits when they are most needed for successful adaptation. This complex interaction has been captured in the Communication and Aging Model presented in this chapter. Possible avenues for communication intervention can be inferred from the various levels of this model. Second, over the next 50 years, caseloads of speech-language pathologists and audiologists will show disproportionate increases of older persons. In order to provide adequate services to this client group, all concerned professionals must understand the effects of aging on communicative behaviors and the ways in which assessment and treatment approaches must be modified and/or expanded to meet the special needs of this group. Again, the Communication and Aging Model provides some guidance in defining these special needs and in suggesting needed areas of gerontological professional preparation.

Few professionals working with older clients have escaped exposure to the litany of the facts of aging. We know that the size of the older population is increasing rapidly, and we have been told repeatedly that service provision to the elderly poses distinct problems and challenges. Unfortunately, this knowledge has not, as yet, propelled us into action. As Achenbaum suggests, "... we have not spent much time thinking about the ramifications of characterizing America as an aging society" (1, p 25).

On a societal level, we have only recently begun to acknowledge and grapple with the fact that the graying of America will result in significant shifts in social and political bases, dramatic demands for resource reallocations (particularly in the area of funding for health services and maintenance income), and a sharp increase in the service requirements of this segment of the population. There is growing uncertainty concerning ways of meeting the needs of the elderly in terms of leisure time activities, support networks, and quality of life.

On a personal level, increasing longevity has begun to blur the distinctions between the traditional life-cycle divisions of middle and old age (31). We are just now considering the implications of increased needs for intrafamily support of older members at a time when the extended family is disappearing in our culture, and when an extended life span means that children of older parents may themselves move into old age while still carrying the burden of responsibility for those parents (28). For the professional, the growing proportion of elderly in this society mandates attention to the implications of the increasing age of our clients.

This book is about aging—from the unique perspective of communication processes and disorders. Although frequently overlooked, the choice of communication as a vantage point for viewing aging is a logical one. Successful communication can be found at the core of social adjustment, integration, adaptation, and life satisfaction—many of the concerns expressed in today's gerontological literature. Communication adequacy further defines the degree to which individuals can seek out and effectively utilize available resources and services. At the mass media level, communication shapes and controls our perceptions and expectations of aging and the elderly. Thus it is not surprising that Carmichael states: "Many of the problems of the aged are directly related to communication" (9, p 121).

What is needed is a unified view of aging. Unfortunately, both communication and gerontology are multidisciplinary areas of study. As such, they benefit from the input of professional expertise across a broad spectrum of interests but suffer from a lack of holistic integration. This textbook seeks to integrate some of these disparate pieces of information within a reasonable organizational framework that will allow the reader to sample the information base and draw conclusions necessary to designing strategies for facilitating communication behaviors and interactions in the elderly. Our task, as Birren suggests,

. . . is something like putting together a giant jigsaw puzzle. The biological, psychological, and social pieces, after all, should be fitted together in a way that makes sense of one's personal experience (5, p 264).

The following pages present a brief overview of the demographics of aging and of communication dysfunction in the elderly. The importance of communication with and to older persons is highlighted further, and a model for the role of the communication process in aging is offered. This model will be used to emphasize our needs as professionals in understanding the interaction between communication and aging and will provide a rationale for the organizational structure of this textbook.

THE DEMOGRAPHICS OF AGING AND COMMUNICATION DISORDERS

What is aging? Clearly the aging process begins at, or before, birth; common usage dictates application of the term to the later years in the life cycle. A more precise definition of aging, however, is elusive. A complex number of physiological, psychological, and social factors define how "old" an individual really is, how he perceives his aging, and how his aging is studied by those in different academic and professional disciplines. The complexity of these age-related life changes and variations in adaptive strategies, coupled with pronounced individual differences in life experiences, lead to greater heterogeneity in the older population than in any other age group.

One solution to the problem of defining aging is to resort to the use of chronological age. Chronological age as a yardstick of old age is convenient in that it allows us to discuss demographic profiles of the older population, particularly in terms of socioeconomic characteristics and projections for the future. If 65 years is used as the demarcation for the beginning of old age, there were 28 million elderly in the United States in 1984, comprising less than 12% of the total population of the country. These figures represent a ninefold increase in numbers and a threefold increase in percentages since 1900 (2). Women outnumbered men by a ratio of 148 women to 100 men, with 50% of the women being widows. Only 5% of the older population was institutionalized, with about 30% of the noninstitutionalized group living alone. Around 90% of the current elderly population are White. Although the percentage of older persons below the poverty level in 1984 was slightly below the rate for persons under the age of 65 years, median incomes for the elderly were lower than for the nonelderly (2, 46).

These facts, and many others, will be covered in greater detail in Chapter 3 in this text. However, several demographic trends must be highlighted here. First, the older population is expected to continue to grow dramatically in the next 50 years. It is projected that there will be close to 65 million elderly in the year 2030, comprising over 21% of the nation's population. Second, the fastest growing segment of the older population has been and continues to be the old-old group (85 + years). The latter growth projection is of considerable interest because the old-old group is most heavily represented in institutions such as nursing homes and is most likely to have chronic health problems and restrictions in independent living activities (2).

These trends are particularly significant when the prevalence of communication problems and disorders in the elderly is considered. It has been estimated that at least 8 million older Americans have a speech, language, or hearing disorder (38). At present, approximately 20% of the total population of speech-language impaired individuals falls in the over-65 category; however, by the year 2050, the elderly will constitute 39% of this speech-language impaired population. Similar proportional increases will be seen within the hearing impaired population. The elderly currently constitute 43% of the hearing impaired population, but this will rise to a projected 59% by 2050 (17). Since older communicatively impaired adults are currently underserved in our caseloads, the implications for future service delivery demands and deficiencies are of considerable concern (18).

THE CONTINUUM OF COMMUNICATION SKILLS IN THE ELDERLY

Statistics concerning the demographics of aging and the prevalence of communication disorders in the elderly do not fully define the communication status of this segment of the population. As Rees (36) has indicated, communication behaviors occur on a continuum—from one extreme that might be considered optimal to another that reflects the clearly disordered. In order to understand the importance of communication to the elderly and the ways in which aging may threaten communicative adequacy, it is first necessary to develop an operational definition of this entity called communication.

A variety of definitions have been offered in the limited gerontological literature concerning aging and communication (40). Berger and Luckman (3) define conversations (and thus communication) as mechanisms by which social realities in the form of shared meanings are created, maintained, modified, and affirmed. Lubinski (27) emphasizes the constructive or destructive social aspects of communication by describing it as providing, "... an error-creating and error-correcting mechanism for the establishment of interpersonal relationships" (p.238). Regardless of one's unique perspective, communication must always entail the sending and receiving of both verbal and nonverbal messages between two or more specific individuals within a specific social and physical context.

There is every reason to believe that communication processes are modified or eroded in some older individuals—either as a function of changes within the individual or of social pressures, attitudes, and isolation. For example, Oyer and Oyer (32) list the following as potential barriers to communication for the elderly: (a) a youth-oriented society; (b) physical isolation; (c) shifting societal values; (d) sensory losses; (e) diminished power or influence; (f) lack of transportation; and (g) retirement in general. To this might be added geographical dispersal of friends and family, gradual erosion of social support networks due to the death of members of those networks, and increased health problems.

Most of these factors produce essentially external barriers—that is, they describe situational or environmental limits on communication frequency and adequacy. In addition, more recent research efforts have begun to focus on internally generated changes in speech, language, or communication behaviors, to be described in Chapters 9 and 10. Ulatowska and her colleagues (45), for example, have identified some dominant areas of communication change that result from causative factors in *addition* to possible differences in underlying cognitive processes. These areas include: (a) linguistic shifts in the semantic and pragmatic domains; (b) changes in social functions actively adopted by older persons as they become removed from the mainstream of social interaction; and (c) sensory impairments and their associated compensatory adjustments. There is renewed interest in the manner in which the communication behaviors of older individuals may reflect compensatory adjustments or adaptations to life changes on all levels.

Thus aging appears to threaten the older adult's ability to use communication as an effective tool. Age-related life changes, external and internal to the individual, can modify and potentially interfere with interpersonal communication. However, the same life changes dictate that the older person can maximize his adjustment to aging through use of social communication. We are faced, therefore, with the proverbial vicious cycle.

The contention that communication is an important coping mechanism is a critical one that deserves further elaboration. Woelfel (49) describes communication as a kind of energy. He suggests that cutting off persons from the receiving of information transmitted through communication effectively isolates those persons from activity. Inactivity in turn breeds major health problems (mental or physical) and can speed the aging process artificially. Similarly, the sending and effective communication of information is a critical ingredient in social interaction. In most social exchanges, partners assist each other in achieving a positive sense of self and self-worth. The older person may be effectively removed from opportunities to engage in this process of self-validation.

Dowd (15) takes this hypothesis one step further in his postulation of exchange theory as a viable explanation for aging. Exchange theory suggests that the lives of the elderly are dependent upon the relative power resources of the social actors involved. Power allows each of us to reach our personal, social, economic, and physical goals. For the elderly, these goals may include life satisfaction, financial security, obtaining needed services, and nourishing social needs. Unfortunately, the older person is disadvantaged with respect to the resources he can bring to bear in social exchanges. Dowd suggests that these resources include personal characteristics, material possessions, relational characteristics, authority, and "generalized reinforcers." It is probable that only generalized reinforcers are left relatively intact by old age.

In practical terms, Dowd suggests that power relationships are worked out in the social arena—more specifically, through conversation in the form of talking and listening (15). The energy that Woelfel (49) refers to, therefore, is in part the energy intrinsic to the ability to act and effect change or meet goals. The individual who is without adequate resources to control the course of his life is a troubled individual.

Nowhere is this more apparent than in the area of social support networks. Although there are many definitions for support networks, Walker's (48) explanation is perhaps the most useful for this text. According to Walker, a person's social network is ". . . that set of personal contacts through which the individual maintains his social identity and receives emotional support, material aid and services, information and new social contacts" (48, p 35). In a sense, therefore, the support network consists of individuals who function as significant others to older persons (4). Britten (7) has stated that an important factor in the adjustment of aged individuals is sociability, including satisfaction with others in personal relationships. For the most part, these social relationships fall under the heading of informal support networks.

Countless researchers have documented the relationship between the presence and adequacy of social supports and such intangibles as happiness, mental health, physical health, coping strategies, and use of available resources (4, 10, 11, 14, 26, 29, 37, 44). Schonfeld et al (39), for example, reported that the need for mental health services appeared to be directly related to social support network adequacy and perceived internal locus of control. In the former instance, it was hypothesized that social support provides an emotional buffer between life events and mental decline, enhancing ability to cope and reducing the effects of stress. This concept is echoed by Caplan (8). Similar findings are repeated in numerous other studies, although Rundall (37) cautions against equating the fact and size of social networks with the concept of a support network. Informal support networks are believed to provide a critical supplement to the formal support networks provided by agencies and professionals at the organizational or bureaucratic level (47).

The point of this discussion is that the central role of communication is implicit in every aspect of the gerontological literature that describes both the impact of aging upon individuals and the ways in which individuals seek to cope with the decrements and changes associated with advanced age. An understanding of this role is predicated upon certain basic tenets about human behavior in general and the behavior of older individuals in particular.

First, all human behavior is directed in part towards an effort to maintain homeostasis or equilibrium, whether it be environmental or internal (19, 23–25). Our physiological systems are designed with preservation of homeostasis in mind, and there is considerable evidence that our mental or emotional states likewise reflect this intrinsic strategy of maintenance of homeostasis. While it has been argued that older individuals may not be subject to or respond negatively to higher than normal levels of stressors (21), it is still commonly accepted that life changes are characteristic of old age. Life changes or crises include events involving loss (or the subjective experience of loss) and situations that disrupt customary modes of behavior, alter circumstances and planning, and impose a need for psychological change (25).

Perhaps it is more helpful to conceive of stress in the terms proposed by Stagner (42). Stress is defined as the external pressure event, which may or may not produce *strain* dependent upon the extent of change inflicted by the event and the individual's perceptions of the degree of stress. *Coping*, therefore, becomes a voluntary activity directed against the external stress, in an effort to protect the internal mechanism. In contrast, *defense* can be viewed as unconscious changes or responses with a similar protective goal.

This discussion forms the framework for understanding the manner in which communication can be both the target for decremental life changes (and thus a potential stressor) and a primary mechanism for coping with these same changes. As we attempt to build a model for the communication process in aging, this basic concept will guide our efforts. Any interventions designed to influence communication behavior positively must be guided by an understanding of its role and vulnerability and must take into consideration the multiple avenues for effecting change.

A MODEL FOR COMMUNICATION AND AGING

The model presented in Figure 1.1 attempts to integrate much of the fact and theory from the preceding discussion. It is admittedly incomplete and biased in perspective, in that aging and the older individual are approached

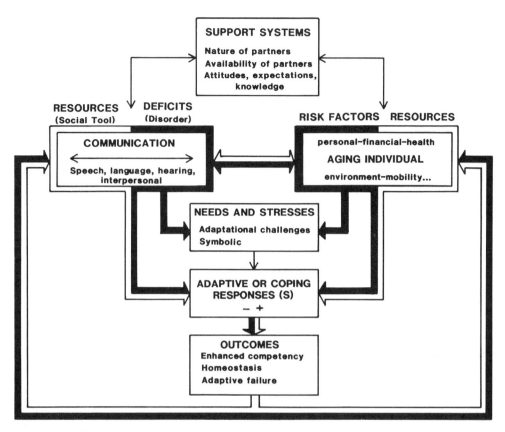

Figure 1.1. The Communication and Aging Model.

strictly from the communication perspective. The model suggests those characteristics and processes that must be considered in assessing communication needs in particular, and in designing comprehensive management programs for a communicatively impaired older client.

The aging individual's status at any point in time can be described in terms of an inventory of personal and situational characteristics that fall either to the debit (risk factor) or credit (resources) side of the resource continuum. A similar inventory can be made of the communication skills of that individual. Speech, language, hearing, and social communication attributes can be assessed and placed along the continuum from specific deficit (a communication disorder) to maximal resource (as a social tool). The individual's personal and situational characteristics influence communicative functioning and vice versa. The presence and adequacy of the social support system also define, in part, the nature of communication and personal resources and in turn are influenced by the individual's relative strengths and deficits in each of these areas.

For the elderly individual, those attributes that fall at the deficit or risk end of continuum can be used to target specific needs or stressors. These may take the form of adaptational challenges (e.g., specific concrete difficulties that must be overcome in the course of daily existence) or symbolic challenges (e.g., the sense of loss and grief experienced with the death of a loved one, the gradual erosion of hearing, the loss of status) (25). Regardless of the nature of the need or stressor, the model assumes that the individual will struggle, consciously or unconsciously, to maintain or reassert homeostasis. This struggle requires some form of adaptive or coping response. The nature, degree, and adequacy of coping responses will be defined by the specific need (its perceived importance, the degree of adaptational or symbolic challenge) and the entire inventory of aging and communication attributes.

This is a highly dynamic model of aging, communication, and adaptation. It assumes that, like individuals of all ages, the elderly will continue to make responses to life changes in order to resolve the resulting strain and/or to reestablish some kind of equilibrium. Once a coping response is emitted, however, the actual outcome results in enhanced competency (an improvement over previous status), homeostasis, or adaptive failure. The response, regardless of its outcome, ultimately becomes a new factor in the inventory of personal and communication attributes.

This model serves three important functions. First, as already noted, an individual's response to a specific need or stressor can be predicted in part by an understanding of the constellation of personal, environmental, and communicative resources available to him. For example, an individual who has suffered a major stroke affecting language functioning is most likely to produce full and adequate coping responses if he has a good support network, a high level of emotional stability, no financial worries, and reasonable health apart from the stroke.

Second, the model emphasizes the fact that we must be cautious in interpreting behavioral and communicative change in the elderly as primary deficits. Instead, it is quite possible that observed changes may reflect adaptive or compensatory strategies employed by the older individual to maintain some degree of homeostasis. For example, stereotypes of the rambling, loquacious, conversationally insensitive older person may have some reality basis that can be explained in adaptive terms. The hearing impaired older person might attempt to overcome confusion in group conversations by dominating the conversation and refusing to relinquish the floor. Similarly, the isolated older individual with a dwindling support network may use excessive verbal behavior as a tool for holding the listener's attention and soliciting the listener's emotional support.

Third, interventions can occur at any stage in this model, depending upon the inventory made of the individual's needs, resources, and current adaptive strategies. One hearing impaired individual may require only a hearing aid fitting and limited aural rehabilitation, while a second may benefit from additional interventions with significant others, and a third may show only limited improvement if modifications in the physical environment are not made.

IMPLICATIONS FOR PROFESSIONALS

An appreciation of the demographics of aging—and the facts of communication changes and disorders in the elderly—should be sufficient to convince professionals that the communication needs of older persons require our attention and intervention. What is less clear is the extent of the knowledge base required in order to insure that these interventions are comprehensive and maximally effective. What do we need to know—and why? Who must be served? How must we serve them? What aspects of aging will influence communication behaviors and service delivery options? The Communication and Aging Model in Figure 1.1 provides a starting point for answering some of these questions.

For example, the model supports the premise that a life span developmental model should govern our understanding of aging and of the elderly. Birren (5) has noted that aging is a counterpoint (in biological, psychological, and sociological terms) of early child development, not in the sense of a mirror image but instead as a complement to the developmental model. We accept unquestioningly the need for a thorough understanding of the characteristics, behaviors, and stages in the normal development of children, as a kind of prerequisite to understanding and managing any breakdown in that normal process. The same argument can and should be made for a comparable understanding of adult development in the later years (30).

Unfortunately, the training of speech-language pathologists and audiologists has been less than adequate concerning developmental processes at the latter end of the life stage continuum (35). Similar concerns were voiced by Peters (33) in discussing the preparation of service providers working within the aging network in Kansas. He noted that " . . . most of the staff interviewed had no understanding of the broader theoretical research and public policy issues of gerontology, although the importance of both was recognized" (33, pp 116–117).

One of the most important tasks facing the clinician is the determination of the extent to which a given behavior reflects the influence of normal aging, pathological aging, or a specific disorder. Normal aging may be defined loosely as the expected and unavoidable " . . . running out of the biological time clock for the individual" (46, p 1). In contrast, pathological aging is defined by Birren (5) as a premature breakdown of an organ system due to disease or trauma. In its most common usage, the term pathological aging refers to disease processes leading to dementias or pseudodementias which accelerate the signs and products of the normal aging process. Both normal and pathological aging may result in changes in communication behaviors and strategies apart from the specific speech-language-hearing disorders. Our assessment and treatment procedures must account for and discriminate among all three of these age concomitants.

Treatment procedures must also take into consideration known age differences in types of speech-language disorders and prognosis. Davis (12) has presented a particularly cogent explanation of the importance of understanding aging in the management of aphasia in particular, noting that test scores should probably be differentiated by age. For example, it has been reported that older aphasic patients perform significantly more poorly than younger aphasic adults on selected test measures and generally evidence greater severity of language deficits (20). There is also evidence more Wernicke's and global aphasics are found in samples of older aphasics as compared with younger patients, and the mean age of the Wernicke's aphasic is significantly greater than Broca's or anomic aphasic individuals. Recovery rate is reportedly slower in older patients (13).

An understanding of aging and of the unique characteristics and life situation of a particular older client is important to the management decision-making process in a variety of more general ways. For example, unique problems can be encountered in simply communicating with an older client—e.g., in history taking or providing information and counseling. In addition to well-documented deficits in hearing and vision (43), it has been suggested that some older individuals may present a variety of behaviors designed to avoid disclosure or to deny health or communication problems (16). Others may appear excessively loquacious, apparently unable to come to closure or to respond directly, possibly as a strategy for maintaining contact and soliciting attention. Professionals from a variety of disciplines have pleaded eloquently for greater attention to the verbal and nonverbal signals that our older clients send us. We are asked to read between the lines of the client's message, in order to obtain clues as to the physical and mental state of the individual (6, 16, 34).

Client-clinician communications may be complicated by major differences in age, interests, language patterns, and life experiences between the communication participants (13). The clinician typically is younger than the client. Whether or not this age difference is evaluated negatively by the older client, it is often a source of discomfort to the clinician and almost always creates potential barriers to assuming a common frame of reference (16). The extent to which these barriers can be overcome depends, in part, upon the clinician's understanding of their existence and awareness of strategies for overcoming their possible negative impact.

Client-clinician age differences may also jeopardize the clinical interaction because of the threat of ageism—of negative attitudes and expectations related to aging and the elderly (41). Kastenbaum (22), for example, contends that the clinical milieu is still poisoned by the ageism that is present at the societal level. Whether the clinician's reaction is simply one of frustration and helplessness (16) or reflects a more serious negative evaluation of client prognosis and rehabilitation potential (13), the problem of ageism among professionals can only be minimized through adequate knowledge of aging.

Treatment considerations reflecting the impact of aging upon behavior and communication also include awareness of the manner in which assessment and treatment procedures must be accommodated to the physiological, psychological, and sociological changes evidenced by the older individual. Modifications may be required in scheduling and timing of sessions, task presentation and practice conditions, testing materials, and visual or acoustic conditions in the test environment. Of particular concern is the content of therapy stimuli and communication tasks. Davis and Holland (13) summarize some of these concerns and advocate completion of a life cycle form, along with a reference historical time line, as a means of determining experientially relevant topics.

The Communication and Aging Model in Figure 1.1 is particularly useful in identifying variables that must be considered and addressed in planning interventions for communication-impaired older individuals. The model suggests that a client's total rehabilitation needs can only be understood after the intrinsic and extrinsic forces acting upon that individual have been identified. These forces include, but are not limited to: emotional status; health and physical status; mobility; support systems; living environments; financial resources; and cognitive functions. In many instances, the older client may require interventions that extend beyond the more traditional one-on-one therapy. The professional must consider ways of providing for the support needs of the client and his/her significant others, the physical and social environmental modifications that will enhance communication, and the identification of and referral for other needed services.

Implicit in this statement is another broader issue pertaining to professional roles. One of the major professional challenges in the next few decades will be the redefinition and clarification of professional roles with respect to the elderly. How can the more basic communication needs of older persons be met—and by whom? What are appropriate settings for service provision to the elderly? What types of interdisciplinary outreach are required, and how can the individual professional interact effectively with the "aging network"—that unique aggregate of agencies and service providers that has mushroomed in the past 20 years since the passage of the Older Americans Act? The answers to these and numerous other questions pertaining to professional roles can be developed only through an understanding of the communication needs and attributes of the elderly.

Last but not least, a thorough gerontological foundation is the only reasonable basis for developing appropriate research questions and methodologies that will allow us eventually to understand the nature of the communicative process in the elderly. The present state of knowledge can be described as fragmented, at best. Unless researchers go beyond their specific disciplines to embrace a more holistic model of the developmental process of aging, new information will continue to add randomly to the knowlege base and will lack practical, clinical significance.

SUMMARY

Chapter 1 has attempted to define the basic conceptual framework for this text on *Communication Behavior and Aging*. The definitions and demographics of aging have been reviewed briefly, and the reader has been introduced to the importance of communication to older persons, with emphasis placed upon the various internal and external barriers to communication that may arise as a product of age-related life changes. It has been suggested that communication serves as an important tool in successful adaptation to aging while simultaneously being vulnerable to alteration and decrement due to the same aging processes.

To illustrate this complex cycle of adaptation and deficit, a Model for communication and aging was proposed. The model emphasizes the fact that older individuals are constantly seeking to achieve homeostasis in the face of a changing world and frequently reduced resources. It was proposed that avenues for intervention can be defined, in part, by an understanding of this model. The model also serves to clarify the information base required by professionals hoping to initiate research or provide clinical interventions addressing the communication needs and behaviors of the elderly. Subsequent chapters in this text will provide the reader with a foundation of gerontological knowledge concerning: aspects of

normal aging; both normal and disordered aspects of communicative functioning in the elderly; and management strategies for the older communicatively impaired adult, his significant others, and his environment.

References

1. Achenbaum WA: The aging of "The First Nation." In Pifer A, Bronte L (eds): *Our Aging Society.* New York, W.W. Norton, 1986, p 15.
2. American Association of Retired Persons: *A Profile of Older Americans: 1985.* Washington, DC, American Association of Retired Persons, 1985.
3. Berger PL, Luckman T: *The Social Construction of Reality.* Garden City, NJ, Doubleday, 1967.
4. Biegel DE, Shore BK, Gordon E: *Building Support Networks for the Elderly: Theory and Applications.* Beverly Hills, CA, Sage, 1984.
5. Birren JE: The process of aging: Growing up and growing old. In Pifer A, Bronte L (eds): *Our Aging Society.* New York, W.W. Norton, 1986, p 262.
6. Blazer D: Techniques for communicating with your elderly patient. *Geriatrics* 33: 79–84, 1978.
7. Britten JH: Dimensions of adjustment of older adults. *J Gerontol* 18:60–65, 1963.
8. Caplan G: *Support Systems and Mutual Help.* New York, Behavioral Publications, 1974.
9. Caporael LR: The paralanguage of caregiving: Baby talk to the institutionalized aged. *J Pers Soc Psychol* 40:876–884, 1981.
10. Coe RM, Wolinsky FD, Miller DK, Prendergast JM: Social network relationships and use of physician services. *Res Aging* 6:243–256, 1984.
11. Cohen CI, Teresi J, Holmes D: Social networks, stress, adaptation, and health. *Res Aging* 7:409–431, 1985.
12. Davis GA: Effects of aging on normal language. In Holland AL (ed): *Language Disorders in Adults: Recent Advances.* San Diego, College-Hill, 1984, p 79.
13. Davis GA, Holland AL: Age in understanding and treating aphasia. In Beasley DS, Davis GA (eds): *Aging: Communication Processes and Disorders.* New York, Grune & Stratton, 1981, p 207.
14. Deimling GT, Harel Z: Social integration and mental health of the aged. *Res Aging* 6:515–527, 1984.
15. Dowd JJ: *Stratification among the Aged.* Monterey, CA, Brooks/Cole, 1980.
16. Epstein L: Issues in geropsychiatry. In Obler LK, Albert ML (eds): *Language and Communication in the Elderly.* Lexington, MA, Lexington Books, 1980, p 139.
17. Fein DJ: The prevalence of speech and language impairments. *ASHA* 25(2):37, 1983.
18. Fein DJ: Projection of speech and hearing impairments to 2050. *ASHA* 25(11):31, 1983.
19. Gaitz CM: *Aging and the Brain.* New York, Plenum Press, 1972.
20. Holland AL: Some differential effects of age on stroke-produced aphasia. In Ulatowska HK (ed): *The Aging Brain: Communication in the Elderly.* San Diego, College-Hill, 1985, p 141.
21. Hyer L, Barry J, Tamkin A, McConatha D: Coping

in later life: An optimistic assessment. *J Appl Gerontol* 3:82–96, 1983.

22. Kastenbaum R: Can the clinical milieu be therapeutic? In Rowles GD, Ohta RJ (eds): *Aging and Milieu: Environmental Perspectives on Growing Old.* New York, Academic Press, 1983, p 3.

23. Koncelik JA: Human factors and environmental design for the aging: Aspects of physiological change and sensory loss as design criteria. In Byerts TO, Howell SC, Pastalan LA (eds): *Environmental Context of Aging.* New York, Garland STPM Press, 1979, p 107.

24. Lawton MP: Sociology and ecology of aging: Environment as communication. In Ulatowska HK (ed): *The Aging Brain: Communication in the Elderly.* San Diego, College-Hill, 1985, p 7.

25. Lieberman MA, Tobin SS: *The Experience of Old Age: Stress, Coping, and Survival.* New York, Basic Books, 1983.

26. Lipman A, Longino CF: Formal and informal support: A conceptual clarification. *J Appl Gerontol* 1:141–146, 1982.

27. Lubinski RB : Why so little interest in whether or not old people talk: A review of recent research on verbal communication among the elderly. *Int J Aging Hum Dev* 9:237–245, 1978-1979.

28. Maddox GG: The social and cultural context of aging. In Usdin G, Hofling K (eds): *Aging: The Process and the People.* New York, Brunner/Mazel, 1978, p 20.

29. Mancini JA, Simon J: Older adults' expectations of support from family and friends. *J Appl Gerontol* 3:150–160, 1984.

30. Maurer JF: Introduction. In Jacobs–Condit, L (ed): *Gerontology and Communication Disorders.* Rockville, MD, American Speech-Language-Hearing Association, 1984, p 9.

31. Neugarten BL: Personality and the aging process. *Gerontologist* 12:9–15, 1972.

32. Oyer HJ, Oyer EJ: Communicating with older people: Basic considerations, In Oyer HJ, Oyer EJ (eds): *Aging and Communication.* Baltimore, University Park Press, 1976, p 1.

33. Peters GR: Interagency relations and the aging network: The state unit on aging and AAA's in Kansas. In Streib GF (ed): *Programs for Older Americans,* Research Series, vol 1. Gainesville, FL, University of Florida Center for Gerontological Studies, 1981, p 96.

34. Pfeiffer E: Handling the distressed older patient. *Geriatrics* 34:24–29, 1979.

35. Raiford CA, Shadden BB: Graduate education in gerontology. *ASHA* 27:37–43, 1985.

36. Rees NS: E pluribus unum. *ASHA,* 23:281–284, 1981.

37. Rundall TG, Evashwick C: Social networks and help-seeking among the elderly. *Res Aging* 4:205–226, 1982.

38. Sayles AH, Adams JK: *Communication problems and Behaviors of Older Americans.* Rockville, MD, American Speech-Language-Hearing Association, 1979.

39. Schonfeld L, Garcia J, Streuber P: Factors contributing to mental health treatment of the elderly. *J Appl Gerontol* 4:30–39, 1985.

40. Sigman SJ: Conversational behavior in two health care institutions for the elderly. *Int J Aging Hum Dev* 21:137–154, 1985.

41. Solomon K: Social antecedents of learned helplessness in the health care setting. *Gerontologist* 22:282–287, 1982.

42. Stagner R: Stress, strain, coping, and defense. *Res Aging* 3:3–32, 1981.

43. Steel RK: A clinical approach to communication with the elderly patient. In Obler LK, Albert ML (eds): *Language and Communication in the Elderly.* Lexington, MA, Lexington Books, 1980, p 133.

44. Strain LA, Chappell NL: Confidants: Do they make a difference in quality of life? *Res Aging* 4:479–502, 1982.

45. Ulatowksa HK, Cannito MP, Hayashi MM, et al: Language abilities in the elderly. In Ulatowska HK (ed): *The Aging Brain: Communication in the Elderly.* San Diego, College-Hill, 1985, p 125.

46. U.S. Bureau of Census: *Demographic and Socioeconomic Aspects of Aging in the United States,* Current Population Reports, Series P-23, No. 138. Washington, DC, U.S. Government Printing Office, 1984.

47. Wagner DL, Keast F: Informal groups and the elderly. *Res Aging* 3:325–331, 1981.

48. Walker KN, McBride A, Vachon MLS: Social support networks and the crisis of bereavement. *Soc Sci Med* 11:35, 1977.

49. Woelfel J: Communication across age levels. In Oyer HJ, Oyer EJ (eds): *Aging Communication.* Baltimore, University Park Press, 1976, p 63.

2 Perceptions of Daily Communicative Interactions with Older Persons

BARBARA B. SHADDEN

Editor's Note

The nature and success of any communicative interaction depends, in part, on the perceptions and expectations of the participants in that interaction. While anecdotal accounts of "typical" communication behaviors are common, there is little formal documentation of the way in which older persons and their frequent communication partners perceive each other's skills and attitudes. Chapter 2 presents the results of an interview study of the perceptions of older persons, children of older parents, and professionals serving the elderly. Each respondent was asked to respond to formal and informal probes concerning: how older persons communicate; how others communicate with older persons; common topics of conversation, as well as who older persons are most likely to communicate with; the frequency of communication contacts; and the nature of and problems created by specific communication disorders. Observations are reported in considerable detail, with attempts made to identify patterns of response (within and across groups) for each of the broad topics of interest. It was suggested that both commonalities and discrepancies in these response patterns can be explained best by considering four variables: (a) the nature and degree of speech accommodation assumed to be necessary: (b) the nature and extent of individual experiences or personal involvements with older persons; (c) the presence and severity of contributing age-related problems; and (d) the respondent's knowledge of aging processes and behaviors. These variables, and each of the commentaries provided by individual respondents, provide the reader with an understanding of the perceived day-to-day realities in the interpersonal interactions of older persons. All subsequent information in this text must be considered in the light of these observations.

I suppose I deserve being talked to that way. I've gotten so old. Most people think that when you get so old, you either freeze to death or you burn up. But you don't. (1, p 19).

This quote from the grandmother in Albee's play *The American Dream* reminds us in a particularly sobering fashion that communication is a real-life phenomenon, one which defines the social and power relationships of the participants and which provides or destroys the nurturance and sense of self-worth upon which all of us depend. Unfortunately, as one pages through the gerontological literature seeking references to communication processes and disorders, it is far too easy to become distracted by theories and isolated facts—and to lose perspective on the daily reality of communication with and by older persons.

Ultimately, communication is a complex, everchanging event, the product of multiple adaptations and compromises on the part of the participants. Much of the success or failure of any communicative interaction results from the perceptions and expectations of the partners. What behaviors, attitudes, strengths, and weaknesses do these participants anticipate when they engage in conversation with older individuals? How do they describe older persons' communication behaviors and the behaviors of those communicating with the elderly? Who talks with older persons? How frequent are these contacts? What do they talk about? How frequent are people's contacts with communicatively impaired older adults, and what problems are created in such interactions?

In order to answer these and other questions, it is necessary to turn to the key players in the communication game—those persons most likely to come into contact with older individuals (13). Presumably this includes (but is not limited to) family members, service providers and, of course, older persons themselves (2, 4, 5, 23). We must ask them what they think, feel, and observe. In doing so, however, we leave behind laboratory conditions of controlled experimentation to enter the domain of perception, belief, and individual experience, a domain wherein there is neither fact nor fiction, right nor wrong. This excursion can be justified by the following arguments.

First, one of the major sources of interference or noise in the communication process is the accumulated perceptions, expectations, and attitudes of both sender and receiver. The form and content of a message are shaped by one's perceptions of the attributes of the receiver of the message (10). Conversely, there is a tendency to conform behaviorally to the expectations of others (9). Even the decision to engage in or avoid interaction is influenced by value judgments concerning both the relative worth of the potential communication partner and the degree to which the anticipated rewards warrant the effort required by the conversation.

Second, given society's prevalent "ageism" (14), investigation of the attitudes of those involved in communication interactions with older persons is of particular concern. In one study examining perceptions of communicative behavior, older persons evaluated themselves as adequate communicators on a number of dimensions but rated other older persons as stereotypically poor in interpersonal communication skills (22). In contrast, a group of health professionals displayed a pronounced positive response bias, as seen in their unwillingness to agree with negatively toned statements, *even if* the statement reflected documented realities. Despite these intriguing findings, the use of an attitude scale was found to be unduly restrictive in terms of the number of potential topics available for participant reaction and the lack of opportunity for response elaboration. Alternate research methodologies were recommended.

Finally, all subsequent portions of this text will be addressing issues of aging, its effects on communication behavior, and its implications for communication interventions. The views of the communication participants, as presented in this chapter, provide a kind of yardstick against which the facts and theories of other contributors can be measured. What these real people believe, and consequently act upon, must be understood as part of the psychosocial milieu within which our interventions take place.

THE PROJECT

The observations reported in this chapter were developed during 1986 through a series of interviews with older persons (over the age of 65 years), children of older (over 65) parents, and professionals providing services to the elderly. Each of these groups was targeted because of their potential involvement as communication partners to the elderly and their presumed differing perspectives on the communication process (due to distinctive role relationships with older persons and varying degrees of personal involvement with the elderly). The purpose of the project was to provide preliminary data reflecting the perceptions of these individuals concerning five aspects of communication with and by older persons:

1. How older persons communicate;
2. How others communicate with older persons;
3. Common topics in daily conversations;
4. Who older persons communicate with, which older persons others communicate with, and the frequency of communication contacts;
5. Hearing and speech-language disorders.

A brief description of the research methodology follows.

Participants

Participants were identified through various contacts in the northwest Arkansas area (both rural and urban settings). No attempt was made to randomize selection of participants or to control formally the many variables that might affect responses. However, samples were selected so as to broadly represent known diversity within each group. Factors taken into consideration (when appropriate to group membership) included: age, sex, residential status, marital status, socioeconomic status, health status, educational level, current or prior occupation and work setting, degree of professional or personal involvement with older persons.

Fifteen children of older parents, 15 professionals, and 20 older individuals agreed to be interviewed for this project. Interviews from two of the older adults were subsequently discarded because of irrelevant responses. An additional six children and five older persons were approached but declined participation. Most of the noncooperating children were experiencing difficulties of varying forms with one or both parents at the time of the proposed interview. Most of the noncooperating older adults expressed distrust of the interview process or a feeling that they had little to offer ("I couldn't help you").

The basic characteristics of the three respondent groups are summarized in Tables 2.1 through 2.3. The older interviewees represented a fairly heterogeneous sample for this region (see Table 2.1). Ages ranged from 68 to 89 years, with a mean of 74.5 years. Although 11 individuals owned their own homes, several of these reported extremely low incomes and the homes were very limited (a one room "shack," in one instance). Income levels ranged from Social Security only to upper middle class incomes derived from generous retirement pensions and investments.

The child respondents (see Table 2.2) ranged in age from 32 to 61 years, with a mean of 42.6 years. Their parents' ages ranged from 65 to 89 years, with a mean of 75.1 years. The professional group (see Table 2.3) ranged in age from 28 to 65 years, with a mean age of 46.1 years.

Table 2.1
Characteristics of Older Respondents

Code	Age	Sex	Race	Mar.[a]	Educ.	Occupation	Residence	Health	Personal Time with Older[b]	Child, w/in 25 miles
1	81	F	Bl.	W	9th	Domestic	Own home (alone)	Fair	GD	No
2	81	F	Wh.	W	BA	Restaurant business	Own home (alone)	Fair	GD	No
3	70	M	Wh.	D	8th	Furn. maker (welfare)	Rent house (alone)	Poor	Some	No
4	68	F	Wh.	M	HS + 1	Homemaker	Own home (w/husband)	Good	GD	No
5	76	M	Wh.	M	HS	Builder	Own home (w/wife)	Good	Some	Yes
6	70	F	Wh.	S	HS + 2	Typist	Apartment (alone)	Good	GD	No
7	89	F	Wh.	W	HS + ?	Homemaker	Lives with diff. family members	Good	Some	Yes
8	73	M	Wh.	M	HS + ?	Construct. engineer	Own home (w/wife)	Good	Some	No
9	72	F	Wh.	M	BA+	Social wk.	Own home (w/husband)	Good	Some	No
10	68	M	Wh.	S	Ed.D.	Univ. Prof.	Own home (alone)	Good	GD	No
11	73	M	Wh.	M	BA	Mech. Eng.	Own home (w/wife)	Good	Some	Yes
12	68	F	Wh.	M	HS	Homemaker	Own home (w/husband)	Fair	Some	No
13	69	F	Wh.	W	8th	Seamstress	Own home (alone)	Fair	GD	Yes
14	77	F	Wh.	W	HS + 2	Ran nursery school	Retirement Community Apt. (alone)	Fair	Some	Yes
15	75	M	Wh.	S	8th	Carpenter	Nursing Home	Fair-to-poor	GD	No
16	72	F	Wh.	S	HS	Odd jobs	Nursing Home	Fair-to-poor	GD	No
17	79	F	Bl.	W	HS	Day care	Own home (alone)	Fair	Some	Yes
18	77	F	Bl.	W	HS	Factory	Retirement Low-Income Hi-rise apt. (alone)	Fair-to-poor	GD	Yes

[a]Marital status: M = married; D = divorced; S = single; W = widowed.
[b]Personal time with older persons: VL = very little; Some; GD = great deal.

Table 2.2
Characteristics of Child Respondents

Code	Age	Sex	Race	Mar.[a]	Educ.	Occupation	Time with Older[b]	Parent(s)
1	44	M	Wh.	W	PhD	University professor	VL	Father (76) lives in CA in retirement hotel—fair health
2	32	F	Wh.	D	HS	Secretary	VL	Father (72) in nurs. home, mother (72) in own home with respondent—fair health
3	37	F	Wh.	M	HS	Custodian	VL	Father (84) lives in own home locally—good health
4	49	F	Wh.	S	PhD	University professor	Some	Father (81) and mother (78) in own home 200 mi. away—poor health
5	44	F	Wh.	D	BSF	Runs own business	VL	Father (76) and mother (68) in own home 150 mi. away—father in fair to poor health, mother good
6	49	F	Wh.	M	MS	Educational examiner	VL	Father (73), mother (72) in own home 100 mi. away—good health
7	41	F	Wh.	M	BA	Runs own Business	GD	Mother (68) lives in own home 40 miles away—good health
8	42	M	Wh.	M	PhD	University professor	GD	Mother (79) lives in FL in apartment—poor health
9	53	M	Wh.	M	BA	Telecommun. specialist	Some	Mother (73) lives with another child, 350 mi. away—good health
10	61	F	Wh.	M	HS	Data entry (unemployed)	VL	Mother (89) in geriatric center—poor health
11	59	M	Wh.	M	9th	Farmer	VL	Mother (88) lives with them—fair to poor health
12	46	F	Wh.	D	HS	Waitress	VL	Mother (75) in hi-rise, low income elderly apartments—fair health at best
13	36	F	Wh.	M	MS	Homemaker	Some	Father (69) and mother (65) in own home in TX—fair health
14	46	F	Bl.	M	HS	Homemaker	Some	Mother (74) lives next door in own home—fair health
15	41	M	Bl.	S	BA	Sales	VL	Father (76) and mother (68) in local apartment in good health

[a]Marital status: M = married; S = single; W = widowed; D = divorced.
[b]Personal time with older persons: VL = very little; some; GD = great deal.

All professionals had worked with the elderly for 3 or more years with a mean contact time of 9.5 years. All but two reported that the majority of their clients were over the age of 65. The two exceptions (a minister and a pharmacist) noted that they spent more time with their elderly clients than with other age groups. Apart from clients, professionals were evenly divided in describing how much time they spent with older persons.

The Interview Instrument

To ensure that a common core of topics and specific questions was addressed in each interview, a Communication Protocol was developed and subsequently modified after pilot use with five individuals. The Communication Protocol consisted of a 6-page form containing specific questions and/or statements requiring

Table 2.3
Characteristics of Professional Respondents

Code	Age	Sex	Race	Mar.[a]	Educ.	Occupation (Setting)	Percentage of Older Clients	Years w/Old. Client	Time with Older[b]	Parent(s)
1	53	F	Wh	D	BA	Soc. work (nurs. home)	75–100	5	Some	Deceased
2	61	F	Wh	M	HS+	Soc. work (hospital)	75	6	VL	Deceased
3	39	F	Wh	M	HS	Nurs. aide (nurs. home)	100	3	Some	Father—65 Mother—60
4	52	M	Wh	M	MD	Doctor (VA hospital)	75	8	GD	Mother—84
5	64	F	Wh	M	HS+	Site director (senior cntr.)	100	10	GD	Mother—84
6	42	F	Wh	W	RN	Nurse (VA hospital)	90	13	Some	Mother—76 Father—79
7	65	F	Wh	S	HS+	Phys. ther. (VA hospital)	80	14	GD	Deceased
8	30	F	Wh	M	BA	Claims rep. (Soc. Security)	50+	7	VL	Father—60 Mother—52
9	26	F	Wh	S	BA+	Director (Adult day cntr.)	100	5	Some	Father—55 Mother—53
10	43	M	Wh	D	BA + 11	Minister	15	15	VL	Father—68 Mother—70
11	53	M	Wh	M	BS	Pharmacist	25	30	Some	Mother—79
12	28	F	Wh	S	MA	Audiologist (ENT office)	60	5	VL	Father—47 Mother—47
13	31	M	Wh	M	HS + 2	Branch mgr. (Med'l rental)	90	3	VL	Mother—59
14	40	F	Wh	M	RN	Nurse (home health)	90	5	GD	Mother—70
15	65	F	Wh	D	BA	Director (Adult cntr., Hi-rise apt.)	100	14	GD	Mother—85

[a]Marital status: M = married; D = divorced; S = single; W = widowed.
[b]Personal time with older persons: VL = very little, some; GD = great deal.

a single response (yes/no, rating, or percentage), followed by a series of possible interview probes to encourage elaboration on a given topic (see Appendix for basic topics). The only portion of the Communication Protocol that differentiated among the three groups of interviewees was a single page relating to communication skills of the older respondent, the older parent, or the professional's older clients.

Procedures

Interviews were conducted at a time and place chosen by the participant and used a low-structure, depth interview technique (20). Questioning proceeded along a continuum from indirect probes (broad topic areas) to direct probes (specific subquestions), with the intent being to elicit as much open-ended discussion

as possible. If opportunities to present specific questions did not arise spontaneously, the Communication Protocol was completed at the end of the interview. The length of the interviews ranged from 35 to 80 minutes, with an overall mean of 48 minutes and group means of 40 minutes (professionals), 48 minutes (children), and 56 minutes (older adults). All interviews were audio tape recorded, with additional handwritten notes maintained during the process. Relevent responses were transcribed (along with interviewer comments on behavior and attitude) and organized under separate headings related to the five communication topic areas of interest. The Communication Protocol responses were totalled, and means, ranges, and modal responses were calculated, as appropriate.

The remainder of this chapter is devoted to a discussion of respondent perceptions concerning how older people communicate and how others communicate with them, what they talk about, who they talk with, and the impact of communication disorders. In view of the amount of data collected, only selected observations are highlighted.

OUTCOMES

At the end of each interview, respondents were asked whether or not they felt older persons experienced more problems in their daily communications than younger persons. Two-thirds of the older respondents, 87% of the child respondents, and 93% of the professional respondents believed this to be true. Thus, the majority of interviewees in all groups believe that the older person experiences difficulties in communication above and beyond those experienced by other age groups.

How Older Persons Communicate

Adequacy of Communication and Changes with Age

A number of specific Communication Protocol items probed impressions of the adequacy of older persons' communications and the presence and nature of changes in communication behavior with aging. Interviewees were asked: "Do most older persons communicate adequately?" Although this very general question created some discomfort, 70% of the older group, 60% of the professional group, and 53% of the child group indicated that most older persons communicate adequately. Child respondents were most likely to express negative opinions on this and subsequent questions concerning the communicative adequacy of the elderly.

Respondents were next asked what percentage of older persons do not communicate well. Mean responses were 38% in the older group, 37% for the professionals, and 46% in the child group. However, when given an opportunity to respond to a similar question concerning younger persons (under 65 years), mean percentages were comparable (older, 34%; professional, 37%; child, 41%). More than two-thirds of the interviewees commented that this raised important concerns about the adequacy of communication among people in general.

The apparent congruence of perceptions concerning the adequacy of communication skills of persons over and under the age of 65 might suggest that the problem of communi-

cation crosses age boundaries. It is important to remember, however, that respondents were uncomfortable about assigning percentages to an essentially negative description of older individuals. The opportunity to demonstrate a lack of bias by providing similar judgments about younger persons might have influenced responses. Casual comments often suggested that younger person inadequacies in communication were not attributed to the same cause as older person inadequacies.

Eighty-seven per cent of the child and professional respondents and 61% of the older respondents reported that people change the way they communicate as they get older. However, only 22% of the older group felt these changes reflected a worsening of communication skills, as compared with 40% of the professional and 60% of the child groups. Indeed, a number of older (17%) and professional (20%) respondents suggested that communication skills became better with increasing age. Responses shifted dramatically when the question was rephrased in terms of persons over 85 years of age. All but four interviewees indicated that they anticipated a worsening of communication skills in this age group. This perception of the impact of advanced age was supported by subsequent comments.

When asked what actual *percentage* of older persons show a worsening of communication skills, almost one-fourth (11) of the interviewees said they could not respond to this question. On the average, child and professional groups reported that more than one-half of all older persons show a worsening of communication skills (54 and 57%, respectively), followed by 46% in the older group.

Descriptions of Communication Behavior

There is a striking contrast between the starkness of yes/no or percentage responses and the elaborative commentaries that emerged when interviewees were asked to reflect on how older people communicate and the nature of changes in communication associated with aging. The range of descriptive comments identified in the informal interview probes is summarized in Table 2.4. Several general response patterns are noteworthy.

Response Patterns. First, a number of respondents in all groups made mention of the heterogeneity in the older population, either through direct reference or by providing specific examples of the dependency of communication skills on other factors. For example:

In terms of conversational give and take, if the older

Table 2.4
How Older Persons Communicate, as Described by Child, Professional, and Older Respondents

Descriptor	Child (N = 15)	Prof. (N = 15)	Old (N = 18)
Communication Characteristics			
Rambling, digressive, sidetracking, take longer to complete thought, go around topic, complex and involuted responses to questions	1	6	2
More talkative	2		2
Repetitive	4	2	
Slower, more labored, deliberate	4		
Slower to respond, don't "track" as fast, don't come to closure conversationally as fast, don't always comprehend, problems with complex information	1	4	1
Confused, disoriented, dislocated, problems with attention and focus on information, or inappropriate fixation on one piece of information	3	3	2
Vocabulary			
Word finding difficulties	1		2
Better/more vocabulary than younger persons	1	1	
Different vocabulary than younger persons		1	1
Listening skills			
Good listening skills, work harder at listening		2	
Poor listening skills, don't pay attention, don't react	1	3	
General conversational skills			
Better, more experienced, more particular in language choices, better training in social and communication skills		2	2
Poorer, cut in on someone else's communication or interrupt, poor turn taking, try to control conversation this way	1	1	
Willingness to engage in conversation			
More willing, more likely to strike up conversation, to send out body language indicating interest, willing to talk with a broader spectrum of people	1	3	1
More discriminating and selective			1
Conversational style			
More direct, sense of "less to lose," not out to make an impression		3	2
Afraid, feel inferior, feel people don't care or don't think older person has anything to communicate	5	1	1
More passive, nonassertive, see selves as victims	1	1	1
Memory factors (topic, previous conversations, previous events or information)	1	3	3
Content factors			
Doesn't work to find common ground, no shared reference or experience, no attempt to find topics that can be understood by others, highly personalized and self-centered in topics	10	6	6
Talk about the past	5		4
Crave information	1		
Other directed and empathetic in topics		1	
Talk mostly about good things and avoid unpleasant	2		
Generally poor communicators (lack of practice)			4
Contributing Problems			
Hearing	7	6	3
Vision	2	2	
Health	7		1
Mobility/motor limitations	5		1

Table 2.4—*continued*

Descriptor	Child (N = 15)	Prof. (N = 15)	Old (N = 18)
Other (vocal change, dentures)		3	
Being alone	1	2	3
Activity or engagement restrictions	1	1	1
Dementia (pathological old age correlates)	7	5	13
Society			
Stereotypes and expectations	2		
Too much TV watching, too little door-to-door visiting anymore			2
Personality and Emotional Attributes			
Rigid, inflexible, set in ways		3	2
Cautious		1	
Respectful, polite, sweet		3	
Abusive, cranky, irritable	1	1	
Withdrawn, passive, introspective, self-concerned	4	3	1
Lonely		2	3
More outgoing			1
Inappropriate social behavior			1
More tolerant			1

person doesn't need attention from others, he will engage in this give and take appropriately. If the older person feels left out, however, or lives by himself and has few contacts, he will try to take over the conversation.

Heterogeneity was also noted in the context of different communication styles for different communication partners.

. . . there are at least two modes. Among their peers, their communications are fuller, more relaxed, show more variety . . . they are more comfortable and have more reference points. In contrast, in communicating with a younger person or people in trade roles and service capacities, they have less in common.

If an older person is talking to another older person, they will communicate very differently than if they are talking to a younger person. When talking to the younger person, they seem to feel as if they have to 'bestow their knowledge.'

Second, respondents differed considerably in terms of whether or not they appeared to be assigning responsibility (or fault) for poor communication to the older person or to others. It was also clear that very similar observations could be interpreted differently.

Older persons are more direct. They have fewer hidden agendas, partly because there is less going on in their lives. They will often state what they're feeling at the time, with nothing to hide and no one to impress.

Most of us use role identities, and this is not available to the older individual. The lack of role identities makes old people feel uncomfortable with revealing what they feel or need.

The third general pattern relates to changes in communication being attributed to intensification of preexisting behavioral and/or personality patterns. The respondents' own comments express this best.

Age seems to bring an exaggeration of previous experiences and behaviors, and along with it a kind of inflexibility.

Changes in communication behaviors seem to reflect an amplification of preexisting communication styles.

The fourth pattern reflects the fact that, without exception, the clearly negative comments outnumbered the clearly positive in all categories. Thus, impressions of older persons' communication skills and changes in communication with aging appear to be skewed towards the negative end of the behavioral continuum.

Communication Attributes. With this general introduction, it is now appropriate to look more closely at individual responses. Problems targeted by one-sixth or more of all respondents, in order of highest to lowest frequency of mention, included: (a) dementia (and related problems of mental deterioration); (b) failure to work at or utilize topics of common interest that might reflect shared reference (high levels of personalized and egocentric responses); (c) hearing loss; (d) rambling, digressive, sidetracked conversational styles; (e) topical focus on the past; (f) confusion, disorientation, and problems with attention and focus; and (g) withdrawal, passivity, introspection.

Arbitrarily, all commentaries are subdivided in Table 2.4 into those pertaining specifically to the following topics: *Communication Characteristics, Contributing Problems,* and *Personality and Emotional Attributes.* There were several unique clusters of times within the *Communication Characteristics* section. One cluster related to the actual manner of communication delivery. Older persons were seen as rambling, digressive, repetitive, slower, and more labored, with good but different vocabularies and occasional word-finding problems.

A second cluster of items related to issues of comprehension, listening skills, attention, and focus. There was specific disagreement concerning listening skills, with two comments noting that older persons listen well and work harder at the listening process, and four others describing the older person as a poor listener.

Older persons are self-centered. They don't listen. They also can't hear but that's different from not listening.

Sometimes older persons don't react if others talk to them. They simply act as if they're not listening or play smug. They just don't want to be bothered with listening.

Other comments in this cluster suggested that older persons become confused, disoriented, or dislocated in conversations and experience problems with appropriate attention to and focus on information. They " . . . fixate on a key piece of information, even if it was a minor point, due in part to the fact that they don't have that much else to talk about." Different terms were used to describe problems in speed and accuracy of comprehension—for example, older persons seem to have "a minimal energy field," " . . . everything seems to take greater effort, including following a conversation." The elderly were described as being slower to respond and to come to closure in a conversation, as well as having trouble "tracking information," particularly complex data.

A third cluster of items was related to what might loosely be termed conversational style and social skills. There appeared to be considerable discrepancy here in the tone and content of responses. For example, some respondents described older persons as being more likely to strike up a conversation, or sending out body language signals indicating a willingness to communicate with a broad spectrum of people. In contrast, one individual suggested that older adults become more discriminating and selective in their choices of conversational partners. Four respondents noted that the elderly are better conversationalists, and are more particular in their language choices, yet others said that

the elderly were generally poor communicators. Poor turn-taking skills and a tendency to cut in on someone else's part of a conversation as a means of controlling the event were noted by two respondents.

The degree of openness or engagement in conversation also appeared to be controversial. Some respondents said older persons were more direct, open, and engaged, whereas others felt many elderly were passive, nonassertive, and adopted the victim role in interactions. ("One characteristic of victims is that they don't communicate wants and needs.") Another group of interviewees focused on the older person's feeling of inferiority and fear of others' responses.

Older persons feel inferior. They feel as if they're not understood and no one has time for them. Consequently, they don't really say what they feel, even though they might talk more.

Most older people are afraid to talk to young persons. They're afraid they'll say the wrong thing and be rejected. The response may be, 'You're old, you don't know.'

A final cluster of responses in the *Communication Characteristics* section relates broadly to conversational content and topic selection. Close to half of the respondents (including two-thirds of the child group) noted that older persons do not seem to have, to find, or to put forth the effort to find a common ground or shared reference and experience for the conversation, perhaps as a function of an apparent increase in egocentricity and self-centered topic selection.

Older persons seem to think people can read their minds. This may be true for someone close to the older person, but it seems that, as people get older, they think everyone can.

The one strong contradiction to this came from a professional who noted:

In general, as people get older, they move from a more self-centered pivot point to a broader scope, and become more empathetic because of their general life experience.

The *Contributing Problems* category of responses in Table 2.4 includes advanced age, mental condition and alertness, activity level and social involvement, and the presence of complicating conditions such as dementia, hearing impairment, and visual impairment. Between one-third and one-half of the respondents in each group noted the importance of these factors as major determiners of communicative adequacy. As one professional indicated: "There are few older people who grow old with a whole package of health and attitude and mental abilities." Many professionals stated clearly that breakdown in communication occurs *only* because of illness, stroke, and disease processes affecting the mind. More than one-half (13 of 18) of the older interviewees indicated that negative change in communication is associated typically or only with much older individuals ("People communicate *better* until they get really old").

The specific importance of maintenance of activity level and social involvement was noted by professional and older interviewees. It was suggested that lack of practice due to either of these factors leads to a decrement in communication skills. Further, isolation was felt to contribute to an unhealthy process of disassociation as the older person approaches death. If the older person is feeling, "Stop the world, I want to get off," one might assume he would be disinterested in making the effort required for productive communicative interactions.

The third category, *Personality and Emotional Attributes*, presents some fairly stereotypical observations of the older person as rigid, inflexible, cautious, abusive/cranky/irritable, with a tendency to be withdrawn, passive, self-centered, and lonely. In contrast, three professionals described older persons as being more respectful, polite, and sweet. There may be no real contradiction here, since all of these attributes can be viewed, in part, as coping strategies. It is interesting to note that some of the more negative attributes have been associated in other research with better stress management (15, 24).

Communication Behaviors of Older Persons Known Best by Respondents

Each group was also given an opportunity to relate their observations concerning the communication behaviors of the older persons they might know best—themselves (for older group), their parents (for child group), or their clients (for professional group). Responses are summarized briefly in the following sections.

Older Respondents' Descriptions of Their Own Communication.   More older interviewees felt they personally communicated adequately (83%) than felt older persons in general communicated adequately (72%). Thirty-nine per cent indicated that their skills had gotten better, and 11% felt they had worsened as they have grown older, a much brighter portrait than provided for the elderly in general. In response to a separate question, 78% reported that their communication skills had changed over time. Typical positive changes noted included: an increase in tactfulness; better accommodation

to people's levels of functioning; and greater awareness of the need for precision (articulation, loudness, rate) and for cueing in to the listener. A worsening of communication skills was associated by one individual with the fact that " . . . everything seemed to fall apart at age 65." She reported that she has difficulty finding the words she wants, particularly descriptive terms like adjectives, and tends to withdraw into herself because of this problem. Another respondent who described a worsening of communication skills said that he was lonesome much of the time and preoccupied with his wife's struggle with Alzheimer's disease. This isolation has made him more talkative and self-centered when he is around others. None of the older respondents with discernible, interfering hearing losses indicated that their communication skills had deteriorated in any way.

Some individuals who reported that their communication skills had stayed essentially the same did note minor changes. One woman indicated that she is now more familiar with life, making her a better communicator. Another admitted that she remembers the past better than the present and cannot think as quickly. Three respondents made reference to changes in their communications being related to the attitudes and responses of younger persons.

Child Respondents' Descriptions of Their Parents' Communication.   Two-thirds of the child respondents indicated their parents communicated adequately, somewhat higher than the 53% who felt older persons in general communicated adequately. Eighty-seven per cent felt their parent(s)' communication had changed as they aged. The nature of changes over time were described as: getting better (27%), staying the same (27%), and getting worse (47%). All of the child respondents were willing and eager to discuss their parent(s)' communications. Only general summary observations are included here.

Positive changes were often described as reflecting the parent and child relating better as adults and as persons. Improved parental openness and honesty about feelings were noted by several respondents. Maintenance of communication skills was attributed by some to their parent(s)' high levels of activity and social involvement.

Worsening of communication skills was attributed partially to stroke or to hearing loss, as well as to an intensification of preexisting patterns (e.g., repeating oneself, increases or decreases in the amount of talking, poor attention, demands for information, and approval seeking). Other described negative communication changes that mirrored comments made about older persons in general, included: personality or emotional changes (cranky, irritable, paranoid); poor listening and attending skills; confusion and memory gaps; egocentrism; and inadequate give and take (turn-taking) in conversation. Most of those who saw a worsening of their parent(s)' communication skills had little contact with older persons apart from parents. All of those who reported a worsening of skills described a similar deterioration for the elderly in general (17).

Professionals' Descriptions of their Clients' Communication. Three-fifths of the professional respondents indicated that their older clients communicated adequately, and the mean percentage of older clients described as *not* communicating adequately was computed to be 40%. These figures are comparable to responses concerning older persons in general. However, 60% of the professional interviewees also indicated that their clients had more communication problems than other elderly individuals. Apparently one can perceive one's clients as having more communication problems than the population at large, yet still describe them as communicating satisfactorily. This may be another instance of reluctance to attribute negative descriptors to the older person.

Those respondents who indicated that their clients had more communication problems than the general population were predictable, in that they worked in institutional settings, programs designed for needy individuals, or directly with hearing impaired or physically unwell patients. The exception to this pattern pertained to four hospital professionals, only one of whom noted special communication problems in her older patients, related to a preoccupation with physical problems and excessive demands for the professional's communication time.

How Others Communicate with Older Persons

All of the child and professional respondents and 89% of the older respondents reported that people communicate differently with older persons than with other age groups. There was less agreement, however, as to the qualitative nature of these differences. Close to half of the older and child respondents (44 and 47%, respectively) and 80% of the professional respondents felt these communications could be described as being worse than with other age groups. Only five interviewees suggested differences were clearly better. Clearly, the professionals appear to assume the most jaundiced view of the behavior of persons communicating with the elderly.

Communication Characteristics

The interviewees' descriptive comments concerning how others communicate with older persons are loosely organized into two categories in Table 2.5—*Modifications in Communication* and *Attitudes towards Communicating with Older Persons*. One-third or more of all respondents noted a patronizing or condescending attitude, simplification of speech, and increased loudness. The next most commonly noted characteristics included: efforts to find topics in common or noncontroversial subjects; a lack of engagement and a superficial, standoffish quality; an attitude of greater sweetness, kindness, or thoughtfulness; and a slowing of the rate of speech. General comments pertaining to attitudes are of interest:

The majority of young persons give the feeling that a person is old and therefore doesn't know better. They seem to be saying something as if trying to pacify the older person.

They think we're not as 'hep' and make allowances for us because we're not up on a lot of things.

People ask questions which require simple answers. This in part eliminates the need to interpret or engage. It acts as a kind of close-out.

Others are more accommodating of differences of opinion in the older person, they're not as argumentative, they're far more polite and attentive.

You find yourself wanting to make the older person feel they're communicating adequately even when they're not.

There's a tendency for younger persons to withdraw from talking to the elderly. They don't really give them a chance, and the older person doesn't know what's going on in the younger person's world.

Some of the discrepancies in Table 2.5 may be explained partially by assuming that similar behaviors are interpreted differently by individual respondents. For example, the same set of behaviors might be interpreted as sweet, kind, and supportive by one individual, and as patronizing and "talking down" by another. This conclusion is supported by comments from respondents indicating that treating an older person in a child-like manner may be viewed by one as necessary and by another as a sign of inappropriate distancing:

There's a kind of selection process, selecting topics and words that may impede conversation. Even if your choices in the selection process are reasonable, it will not be open, full disclosure.

People talk to an older person as if they were talking to a child, instead of someone their own age. There's no real evidence for any kind of respect for age. It's

Table 2.5
How Others Communicate with Older Persons, as Described by Child, Professional, and Older Respondents

Descriptor	Child (N = 15)	Prof. (N = 15)	Old (N = 18)
Modifications in Communication			
Louder	8	3	5
Simpler	10	4	3
Slower	7		2
More repetitive	5	1	1
Increased nonverbal (eye contact, gestures)	1		1
Poor eye contact		1	
Watch language choices	1		
Give older person more time to respond	2		
Listen carefully	7		
Don't listen, don't believe or care about what older person says		2	4
Topical changes			
Work to find topics in common, noncontroversial	9	1	2
Talk around the point carefully			1
Don't pick common topics or frame of reference		1	4
Subject matter is deeper with older person			1
Others don't know how to communicate with older persons		2	1
Attitudes towards Communicating with Older Person			
Pacifying, not explaining, assume older person does not know better, not anticipating good communication	2	3	
Enter conversation with presuppositions about older person (they are "just marking time"), don't want to communicate with them, disgusted by them	2		
Lack of true engagement, standoffish, superficial, nonrelating, tuning out older person	2	5	3
Don't want to talk with hearing-impaired person		2	
Patronizing, treat older person like child, talk as though not there, talk down, condescend	5	12	9
Awkward, stressed, uncomfortable, want to withdraw	1	2	3
Lack of respect or compassion		2	
Sweeter, kinder, more complementary, thoughtful, want to make older person feel good or feel comforted, don't want to embarrass, more patient	2	3	5
Deferential and respectful	2	1	3

more as if, 'You're a nice person but you're not part of my life,' or 'I'm nice because you're old.'

Clearly, one's assumptions about older people are viewed as critical in determining behavior. There are also descrepancies in terms of the degree to which other (younger) persons are seen as wishing to obtain the older person's approval. For example, "There are a lot of people who would be disgusted to hold a conversation with an older person," in contrast with, "there is a kind of ingrained desire for child-adult approval."

People accommodate their speech style and content to more closely approximate that of another person *if* they wish to communicate and interact interpersonally with that other person (11). Issues of accommodation are most directly touched on by respondents in discussing topic selection, as shown in the following two quotes:

Others struggle harder to find common topics.

Younger persons tend to talk about things the older person doesn't want to talk about. Yet communication depends on the two partners. You have to meet half way.

One of the problems encountered is the degree to which accommodation, if made, takes into consideration the real and highly individualized characteristics of the older person, or instead reflects stereotypes (good and bad) of generic elderly. As one older respondent noted,

"Others don't try to find out who the older person really is."

The children of older parents provided almost 50% more specific comments than either of the other two groups, the majority of which were oriented towards modifications in communications made by others. They appeared very sensitive to the difficulties of talking with older persons—the effort that must be expended, and the changes that must be made. As one respondent said, "It's just darn hard to talk to an older person." Another indicated that she found herself switching conversational modes when talking to an older person as if preparing for anticipated difficulty—". . . a kind of silent deep breath, a careful monitoring of the older person in terms of what I think they're understanding."

In contrast, professionals and older persons seemed to place relatively greater emphasis on attitudes, rather than behaviors. In the case of professionals, this may reflect their work emphasis on the older client, his/her behavior, and the effects of others' attitudes on these behaviors. Some support for this can be derived from the observation that professionals who provided few, it any, comments about modifications in communication were also those who reported very little personal contact with older persons outside of the work setting. In essence, these professionals might be considered least involved emotionally and thus most fixated on the attitudes of others, typically within a negative framework.

This negativism is also seen, to a lesser extent, in the wording of comments from older participants. Over two-thirds of the professionals' and one-half of the older persons' responses fell in the clearly negative category, as compared with 18% of the children's responses. As noted above, the children probably most closely identified themselves with the "others" in questions about how others communicate with older persons.

A final pattern of interest was the difficulty experienced by many older persons in separating out their own personal experiences from those of older persons in general. Many of their comments reflect this orientation:

They talk loud, they act as if I'm stupid, and they don't care. In fact, no one cares today.

I don't want anyone to feel sorry for me. Please don't assume that I don't understand. Please explain to me.

Older respondents also tended to blame younger persons and to fixate on teenagers and young adults in responding.

If a younger person hasn't been around older people enough to know, they act very foolishly. . .older persons don't like being around very young persons.

Teenagers know much more than we did when young, but that doesn't mean we can't learn.

Comments about Personal Communications with Older Persons

Within groups, 28% of the older persons, 67% of the professionals, and 100% of the children indicated that they communicated differently when talking with an older person. Older persons generally described changes for the better—more interested, respectful, and polite; more accommodating to hearing loss; generally showing you care. Regardless of the age of the respondent, the frame of reference was always a person older than themselves.

The professionals who indicated that they did not communicate differently invariably qualified this by adding, "I try not to," "not any more," or "not unless the individual requires it." Those who did describe themselves as communicating differently mentioned: providing a great deal of attention; being calmer and sweeter; increasing nonverbal cues; talking louder and slower; increasing explanations and rephrasing comments; and trying to anticipate problem areas in discussion or letting the older person talk and select topics of interest. One respondent even specifically noted, "You need to treat some like a baby." Problems with making sufficient time available were noted by another interviewee:

In the health field, we have so many other pressures that we don't or can't take enough time, and if we spend time, the older person may look forward to and expect it in the future. If we can't provide it, the client is hurt a great deal.

The child respondents tended to indicate that they did most of the things that they had described other people doing. When asked to elaborate, there was considerable consensus that they: (a) talked clearer, simpler, slower, and louder; (b) were careful in selecting topics and phrasing and in monitoring communications; (c) listened better or more carefully; and (d) attempted to show more respect, kindness, understanding and protectiveness.

Topics of Conversation

Topics Initiated by Older Persons

There is much greater consensus concerning the topics that older persons initiate and discuss most frequently (see Table 2.6). Topics related to all aspects of the past were men-

Table 2.6
Common Topics of Conversation Raised by Older Persons, as Described by Child, Professional, and Older Respondents

Topic	Child (N = 15)	Prof. (N = 15)	Old (N = 18)
Past, life experiences, successes, jobs, etc.	7	13	10
Health, ailments, illnesses, dying and death	8	12	5
Family (particularly children and grandchildren)	7	9	6
Religion, the hereafter, spiritual concerns	2	3	3
Topics of everyday interest (general observations)	5	4	2
Gossip/talk about immediate environment and people in that environment, unusual happenings	1	3	4
Gardening	2	4	1
Home		1	
Weather	1	2	2
Youth—the problems with youth	1		
Politics, social concerns, ideas, news	2	1	1
Financial concerns	1	3	1
Food		1	
Advice and judgment of others	2	1	
Younger persons' futures, concerns, successes	1		
Expressions of gratitude			1

tioned by 30 of the 48 interviewees, followed by topics related to health, ailments, death and dying (25 respondents), and to family, particularly children and grandchildren (22 respondents). Religious concerns also were mentioned with some frequency. A few respondents made comments acknowledging the heterogeneity in the older population or relating choice and range of topics to factors such as education, activity level, or degree of social engagement.

The idea of topics of everyday interest was suggested by close to one-fourth of the respondents. In addition, a number of persons mentioned very specific everyday topics such as gardening, weather, or the news. A kind of self-centered, self-absorbed quality was implied by many children or professionals. Even one older respondent commented, "Older folks tend to show a preoccupation with their own concerns and in their own sphere of interest." One must wonder, however, whether topics of personal interest do not, in fact, constitute the core elements in conversations of persons of all ages.

Simply listing common topics does not capture evaluative perceptions. For example, in reference to a preoccupation with the past, one child respondent phrased her response in terms of ". . . boring everybody with their stories about the past." Several other child and professional respondents appeared uncomfortable with mentioning the past, expressing awareness of the "stereotypical" nature of the response and adding general qualifying comments such as "You can't blame them" or "They have a right."

Reasons for frequent discussion of past-related topics were proposed by others:

Older persons discuss their past experiences as a way of providing backgrounds that will validate them with others.

The elderly talk about past successes as a kind of role confirmation.

Older persons talk mostly about things 40 or 50 years before because they are more the same. They are not changing as much as the world is changing. There's not so much foolishness about them.

Topics Initiated by Others in Talking with an Older Person

When respondents were asked to describe topics likely to be initiated by the conversational partners of older persons, some interesting patterns of commentary were noted. There were markedly fewer responses as compared with the earlier question about topics initiated by older persons (see Table 2.7). One-third of the older interviewees could provide no specific topics, and several of them stated that there was no discernible pattern. One-fifth of the professionals had similar difficulties, although all child respondents provided at least one specific topic area. The actual topics mentioned directly parallel those identified for older persons (e.g., the past, health, family, topics of everyday personal interest).

Table 2.7
Common Topics of Conversation Raised by Others Talking with Older Persons, as Described by Child, Professional, and Older Respondents

Topic	Child (N = 15)	Prof. (N = 15)	Old (N = 18)
Past, life experiences, successes, jobs, etc.		3	2
Health of older person	3	4	2
Family (particularly children and grandchildren)	4	4	2
Generic, routine questions ("How are you?", "How was your day?")—topics that are nonsensitive, nontouchy, superficial	5	5	3
Topics of everyday interest or knowledge to older persons (general observations)	1	4	5
News/TV/radio/worldly topics/politics	1	1	2
Friends			2
Weather	2	1	1
Gardening		1	
Other hobbies/leisure activities			1
What younger person is doing	2	1	3
Asking for advice	1		
Topics not interesting to older person			1
"Can I help?"		1	

In addition, one-third of the professional and child respondents focused on the conversational partner's use of generic or routine social questions—"How are you today?" or "How was your day?" Some interviewees felt this reflected a desire to avoid sensitive, touchy topics and to maintain a kind of superficiality associated with distance (e.g., "Younger persons tend to talk about the safe topics within the family").

It was also suggested that younger conversational partners are uncomfortable with aging and thus ". . . . don't want to get too personal about things such as aging and death." Some respondents noted that the use of routine questions specifically reflects lack of interest, a desire to avoid spending time with or getting close to an older persons, a fear of "getting stuck in conversation" with an older person.

Respondents frequently commented on behavioral trends that might explain the kinds of topics selected or the social/communicative stance adopted by the partner. Several related themes were evident. A number of individuals noted that younger persons do not really know what topics are appropriate, safe, or interesting to the elderly, leading to considerable discomfort in the communication situation. This discomfort may stimulate excessive asking of questions (in an attempt to find an appropriate topic) or may result in a fixation on topics commonly believed to be of interest (such as health and family).

Younger persons are more likely to bring up health than the older person—"How are you feeling" or "Can you get around?" They think it concerns the older person and they have no other topic.

Younger people tend to bring up the past and family history because they serve as a kind of bright spot for the older individual.

More commonly, child and professional respondents felt that uncertainty about how to select topics and initiate conversation led to a kind of passivity on the part of the conversational partner.

Younger persons generally let the older persons set the agenda, particularly if the old person is not well known.

If the younger person has had a good relationship with a grandparent, they know how to approach an older person. Otherwise, they become very uncomfortable trying to find a topic, to carry on a conversation, and may in fact be very awkward in initiation.

Younger persons tend to spend a lot of their time answering questions, giving information about their lives, and not initiating.

Each of these comments reveals a perceived lack of shared reference and an unequal balance within the communication exchange between older and younger conversational partners. Regardless of whether the younger partner is seen as desiring to maintain communication but unable to utilize appropriate strategies, or repelled by these problems and avoidant of the elderly, the comments hark back to earlier observations about differences between older persons' communications with age peers and with younger partners.

Table 2.8
Older Persons' Communication Partners, as Described by Child, Professional, and Older Respondents

Communication Partner	Child (N = 15)	Prof. (N = 15)	Old (N = 18)
Family	8	12	4
Other older persons, peers	7	6	9
Neighbors	6	5	2
Health professionals	5	5	2
Other professionals (minister, AAA)		3	1
Church acquaintances	2	3	1
Community service people (merchants, bank, restaurants, etc.)	1	4	2
People at special centers for elderly			1
People who "understand"	1		
Young children		1	

Conversational Partners and Frequency of Contact

Communication patterns can be examined from the perspective of communication partners and the frequency of communication contacts. These measures may also provide an indirect index of support networks (7).

Who Older Persons Talk With

There was considerable agreement across groups that older persons most commonly communicate with other older persons (age peers) and with family (see Table 2.8), although older respondents were less likely to see family as a source of frequent communication contacts. Age peer contacts sometimes occurred in the form of "calling" or "telephone" friends, described as a major interpersonal lifeline, particularly if one is unable to gain ready access to the social community. Other conversational partners mentioned often by all but the older group were various professionals (particularly those involved with health services), then neighbors, followed by community service people (e.g., bankers, grocery store clerks) and acquaintances at church.

Reasons for perceived patterns of communication partners were suggested by a number of respondents. One professional noted that older persons become very possessive of the "fringe people" in their lives, "people the rest of us don't see as being that critical." The postman's arrival or an interaction with a familiar teller at the bank represent critical social and communicative events to be anticipated and prolonged. One child stated that he believed older persons found and related to partners by using criteria involving the least expected rejection and consequently the highest degree of confidence and greatest perceived usefulness.

Whom (Which Older Persons) Do Younger Persons Talk With?

Two-thirds of the child and close to one-half of the professional and older respondents indicated that younger persons communicated most frequently with older persons who were family members. The next most commonly mentioned category was church acquaintances. All other categories, while predictable (e.g., friends of parents, neighbors, former colleagues), received three or fewer mentions (see Table 2.9). Half of the older interviewees stated specifically that they could distinguish no clear pattern and/or had never thought about this issue.

These responses are relatively consistent with the literature in suggesting that the average person under the age of 65 years may have little if any contact beyond the superficial variety with older persons except family members, and that older persons may be similarly restricted in intergenerational contacts (25). If there is validity to these perceptions, they suggest a major source for communication breakdown in the older person's world. Maintenance of communication skills requires experience. Communicative separation or segregation of the older person tends to foster stereotypical expectations and behaviors. Further, as noted earlier, reactions to the elderly in general are frequently colored by limited and highly individualistic contacts with a few specific older persons. If that older person is a family member, subsequent communicative interactions involving the elderly will be influenced by all of the complex dynamics of family structure and role relationships, complicated by the problems and con-

Table 2.9
Older Communication Partners of Younger Persons, as Described by Child, Professional, and Older Respondents

Communication Partner	Child (N = 15)	Prof. (N = 15)	Old (N = 18)
Family	10	7	8
Church acquaintances	3	3	1
Neighbors	1	2	
Job setting or civic organization		3	
Former colleagues	1		
Clients	2		
Friends of parents	1		
Those with common interests		1	
No response or no discernible pattern			9

cerns of caregiving and role reversals involving aging parents (18).

Frequency of Communications Involving Older Persons

The picture painted so far is one of restricted range of communication partners. Interviewees were asked to comment on frequency of communication specifically in two structured questions. First, they were asked whether or not they believed older persons had fewer persons to talk with than other age groups. Ninety-four per cent of the older respondents and 87% of both the child and professional respondents believed this to be true. Several comments were made to qualify the concept of reduced frequency of contact in terms of the particular subcommunity (e.g., the primarily Black community) or the specific town. All child and professional respondents and 89% of the older respondents also stated that younger individuals communicated less frequently with the elderly than with other age groups.

Given this consensus about reduced frequency of communication, respondents were asked why they felt older persons had fewer individuals to talk with. Comments are presented in Table 2.10, categorized loosely into factors related to aging, to the older person's skills and personal attributes, and to the partners who contribute to the communication cycle.

For each respondent group, the majority of the comments fell under the general heading of factors related to aging. The most prevalent single explanation pertained to the fact that friends and family members have died and it becomes increasingly more difficult to make new friends or contacts. In addition, one-half of the older respondents noted geographical dispersal of family and friends. Other factors included: physical or mobility restrictions

(including illness and poor health); removal from the person's social and professional roles; restricted access due to isolation in retirement communities or other age-segregated residential facilities; and specific problems with transportation.

The two dominant themes related to aging, therefore, appear to encompass the gradual erosion of social networks and restrictions in mobility and access. Again, this is consistent with the communication literature (18, 19).

Few factors relating to the older person's skills and attributes were identified. The most commonly offered explanation in this category pertained to the older individual's failure to make an effort to reach out to others, waiting instead for others to come to them. Related comments described the older person as withdrawn, inactive, with a reduced desire to communicate and limited initiative, partly because the elderly ". . . see everything as a hassle." Some responses appeared vaguely accusatory (e.g., "Some older people will want to withdraw, but all the opportunity in the world is out there and they've got to get out of the house to do it"). Other comments referred to the older person's not having much to say or having fewer interests, to generally poor communication skills, and to a fear that others don't care, won't be interested, or might be alienated by something said by the older adult.

They are afraid their conversation won't interest the younger person or they will back off if not understood . . . afraid they didn't phrase it right and not wanting to embarrass.

Comments pertaining to the behaviors and/or attitudes of conversational partners were limited primarily to observations that younger persons do not want, or are unable, to take the time to talk with older individuals. Avoidance of the elderly and dislike of being around older persons were also mentioned.

Table 2.10
Why Older Persons Have Fewer Communication Contacts, as Described by Child, Professional, and Older Respondents

Descriptor	Child (N = 15)	Prof. (N = 15)	Old (N = 18)
Factors Related to Aging			
Friends and family have died, difficult to make new friends	7	8	8
Geographical dispersal of family and friends	1	4	9
Retirement, out of the social or role matrix, not in organizations	3	3	2
Illness, poor health, other physical restrictions, mobility restrictions	14	3	3
Isolation in a restricted, "retirement" environment	3	5	4
Specific problems with transportation	1	4	
Hearing loss (particularly if older person denies)			1
Factors Related to Older Person's Skills and Attributes			
Older persons generally have poor communication skills		2	
Older persons are more discriminating as to whom they interact with		1	
Older person does not make an effort, waits for others to come to him/her, is withdrawn, inactive, has reduced desire to communicate, has limited initiative, sees things "as a hassle"	2	4	2
Older person does not have much to say, fewer interests	2		
Older person afraid others won't care, won't be interested; older person afraid he/she will say the wrong thing and alienate others		2	1
Factors Related to Communication Partners			
Others don't want to talk with older persons, don't take the time to talk with older persons, avoid older person, don't want to be around the elderly	3	3	4
Others don't have the time, tired at the end of a work day		1	1
People don't visit like they used to			1
TV gets in the way of social interactions			1

Communication Disorders

Hearing Loss

All respondents indicated that they had some personal or professional contact with one or more hearing impaired older persons. Estimates of the prevalence of hearing impairment in the elderly ranged from 10 to 90%, with considerable consistency in terms of group means (53 to 59%). It should be noted that these means correspond reasonably well with normative studies in the literature (8, 21).

Respondents also evaluated whether hearing loss in the elderly creates a considerable barrier, a mild barrier, or no barrier to communication. Sixty percent of the children, 78% of the older adults, and 87% of the professionals felt hearing loss created a considerable barrier to communicate. The lower percentage of child respondents may be attributed in part to the reported belief that older persons do not have as much trouble hearing as they do lis-

tening. Several older respondents noted a steady worsening of hearing problems with advanced age.

Ironically, four of the five older individuals with noticeable hearing problems in the interview situation felt that hearing loss was only a mild barrier to communicate. The fifth talked about what a terrible problem hearing impairment created, without once acknowledging his own hearing difficulties.

When asked to describe the problems created by hearing loss, responses fell into two broad categories. The first cluster of responses included statements of the specific problems created in three overlapping arenas: (a) situational; (b) social/interpersonal/communicative; and (c) emotional. The second category of responses dealt with management strategies—for older persons and their conversational partners. Interview comments are summarized in Table 2.11.

Three problem areas were cited by more than one-fourth of the respondents: acceptance or

Table 2.11
Problems Created by Hearing Loss (HL), as Described by Child, Professional, and Older Respondents

Descriptor	Child (N = 15)	Prof. (N = 15)	Old (N = 18)
Problems			
A. *Situational*			
Problems hearing in groups (and associated anxiety and sensitivity)		1	2
Problems with room acoustics, noise	3		2
Problems with hearing environmental noises	1		1
All situations are a problem		1	
B. *Social/Interpersonal/Communicative*			
Misunderstandings, can't follow questions, can't understand conversational topics	5	6	4
Conversational breakdown (inappropriate style, poor turn taking, bizarre responses)	1	1	
Interpersonal relationship breakdown—general	1		
Arguments/family conflicts/spouses badger each other	3	2	
Hearing-impaired person tunes out others	3		
Others shy away from hearing-impaired person		2	3
Hearing-impaired persons uses HL to control others	1		
Constant strain for hearing-impaired person to hear	1		1
Alertness drops, responses become vague	1		
C. *Emotional Reactions*			
Some older persons accept HL and do nothing			2
Denial of hearing loss	3	4	3
Paranoid, blame others	2	3	4
Anger on part of hearing-impaired (with self or others)		2	2
Older person feels left out, isolated, embarassed, withdraws from social contact (world closes in)	3	7	5
Frustration (hearing-impaired person)	2	4	
Frustration, impatience, aggravation (others)	2	5	
Loss of confidence on part of hearing-impaired person		1	
Increased dependence	1		
Management Strategies			
Need a whole new way of talking		2	2
Talk louder	2	3	4
Face the person, get closer	3	1	1
Repeat one's comments	4	2	1
Talk slower		2	
Use shorter, "lighter," simpler comments		2	
Reduce prolonged discussion		2	
Don't want hearing aid, don't realize its benefits, too proud to use, financial problems	2	1	2
Get a hearing aid	1	4	2

denial of the problem; misunderstandings; and isolation. With respect to acceptance/denial, two older respondents noted that some hearing-impaired persons seem to accept the problem and "give in to it," making no effort to improve the situation. Others described elderly individuals as being unwilling to admit that they cannot hear, perhaps because of fear of appearing unwhole, incapable, or even senile. At least one interviewee noted that denial of hearing problems creates more interpersonal difficulties than the hearing loss itself; another commented that some persons adopt a strategy of ".... acting as if they had heard" and become a danger to themselves and others. Some children of older parents suggested that denial of the problem acts as a mechanism for controlling others or as an excuse for tuning out the environmental noises and people: "You don't know if they can't or won't hear."

The second commonly cited problem area was the fact that hearing loss leads to frequent misunderstandings, to an inability to follow a conversation or to answer questions appropriately. Logically, this can be seen as contributing to the third major problem area—the resulting isolation of the hearing impaired older person, as the individual feels left out and begins to withdraw from social settings because of embarrassment or confusion. "The world closes in . . . on the hearing impaired person."

Together, these three factors provide the basis for all other described problems. Certainly, the catalog of emotional responses experienced by hearing impaired elderly (anger, frustration, paranoia, loss of confidence) and of other's reactions (frustration, aggravation, impatience, shying away from the older person) can be related to these difficulties. Basic problems in interpersonal relationships and family conflicts can also be traced to the combined effects of these three factors. Even specific comments about the nature of communication breakdown (inappropriate style and choice of topics, attempts to control by monopolizing, poor turn-taking skills, poor group communication skills) relate to strategies of acceptance, problems in comprehending, and social isolation.

Between one-fourth and one-third of the responses in each group dealt with ways to manage hearing loss, most frequently by speaking louder, repeating oneself, and facing the person at close range. Others noted slowing the rate of speech, using shorter or simpler statements and articulating more clearly, and/or reducing prolonged or extended conversations. As two separate professionals indicated: "You have to learn a whole new way of talking." Only one group of comments pertained to what the hearing impaired person could do—specifically, making use of hearing aids. However, five interviewees commented that older persons (men in particular) do not want hearing aids, are too proud to wear them, or do not realize their benefits. No mention was made of the other assistive listening devices now available to enhance situational listening, and no respondent mentioned listening and communication strategies that could be used by the hearing impaired person.

Speech-Language Disorders

All professionals, 89% of the older respondents, and 60% of the child respondents reported acquaintance with an older person with a specific speech-language disorder. These responses are not surprising. Any professional working closely with the elderly would be expected to have contact with speech-language impaired older persons at some time, in contrast with the child respondents' limited contacts with older persons apart from their parents.

Mean percentage estimates of the prevalence of these disorders were almost identical (23, 25, and 26%); group modal responses were always in the bottom one-third of the response distribution. The few extreme individual responses, in the 75 to 95% range, were associated with interesting speculations about hidden deficits in the elderly:

I suspect many more elderly are speech-language impaired than are diagnosed.

If you include the direct effects of aging on speech and language, and the effects of dementia, close to 90% of the elderly may be affected.

Respondents had less to say about speech-language impairment than about hearing loss. As shown in Table 2.12, types of responses were arbitrarily grouped into three categories: *Communication Characteristics, Consequences of the S-L Disorder,* and *Management Strategies.* Across groups, one fifth or more of the interviewees noted the following: (a) difficulties visiting and conversing with the speech-language impaired person; (b) problems in understanding what the person is trying to communicate; (c) the emotional response(s) of the communication-disordered individual; and (d) the need to show that you care about what the person is trying to communicate. More detail is provided in Table 2.12.

The dominant feeling was a sense of great discomfort about trying to communicate with a speech-language impaired individual, coupled with a sense of helplessness and, occasionally, a desire to curtail the communicative moment because of these feelings. Much of this reported discomfort appeared to revolve around the inability of the speech-language disordered individual to make himself understood, with relatively little attention to the fact that the same person might be having trouble *receiving* information. In effect, respondents appeared distressed by a situation in which they saw themselves as failing to meet the other's needs. There was also a sense of horror about the plight of the speech-language impaired individual ("It would be awful to lose your communication that way")

Few comments were offered by interviewees concerning strategies for communicating with speech-language impaired older adults, with the majority provided by professionals. In addition, all management comments were gen-

Table 2.12
Problems Created by Speech-Language (S-L) Impairment, as Described by Child, Professional, and Older Respondents

Descriptor	Child (N = 15)	Prof. (N = 15)	Old (N = 18)
Communication Characteristics			
Cannot be understood well, cannot explain what they want or need, garbled speech, trouble forming ideas	3	3	8
Cannot receive information well		1	
Word-finding problems	1	3	
Memory problems—general		1	1
Verbal diarrhea		1	
Weak-minded, confused			3
Personality changes		1	
Frail vocal quality, can't be heard on phone	1		
Consequences of the S-L Disorder			
Hard to visit or carry on conversation with person, cannot get into prolonged conversation, uncomfortable and embarassing in conversation, dread of being around S-L-impaired person, desire to cut conversation short because one feels stupid, frustrated and stressed	5	3	8
Takes more time, effort, hard work to communicate with S-L impaired person	3	1	
Emotional responses			
Deep concern about how S-L impaired person feels, concern about hurting his/her feelings	1	2	2
Frustration	1	3	
Violence		1	
Fear		1	
Withdrawal		1	
Depression		1	
Think others believe they are mad		1	
Become stubborn, don't want to try to participate			2
Management Strategies			
Try to show you care, you want to communicate and understand what they are trying to say		7	3
Use sign language, more facial expression and nonverbal		2	1
Use visual aids		1	
Get others to interpret (third party)		1	1
Be more patient	2		1

eral, relating only to showing the person that you care, that you want to understand and are being more patient. Two individuals mentioned using a third person (e.g., family member) as an informant or interpreter (perhaps another sign of helplessness). A sense of ineffectuality was evident.

A similar lack of clarity and specificity was evident in descriptions of the characteristics of speech-language impaired persons. In addition to the fact that such individuals cannot be understood well, word-finding problems were noted by four respondents, and confusion or weak-mindedness was mentioned by three. This

limited reference to specific attributes, coupled with the comments about weak-mindedness, suggests misinformation or lack of information and experience on the part of respondents.

Only the professional interviewees offered any kind of detailed commentary concerning the affected person's emotional experiences and responses, mentioning frustration, fear, depression, withdrawal, and stubbornness, among others. Older and child respondents were more inclined to discuss how *they* felt in trying to interact with the older person—in other words, the problems created for the conversational partner.

CONCLUSIONS

The preceding pages have detailed the observations of older persons, children of older parents, and professionals concerning communicative interactions involving the elderly. These observations act as a kind of collage reflecting the diversity of experiences, perceptions, and expectations that contribute to the real-life communication world of the older individual. Heterogeneity of responses is undoubtedly a dominant theme. However, it appears profitable to conclude this chapter by attempting to summarize participant comments and identify key variables that influence perceptions and, presumably, behavior.

A Synopsis of Participant Observations

Most respondents felt that the majority of older persons communicate adequately. However, there was also considerable consensus that older persons experience more problems in their daily communications than do their younger counterparts, and that older individuals change the way they communicate as they age. Respondents showed less agreement as to the qualitative nature of these changes unless the person was considered to be someone of considerably advanced age (over 85 years). Factors such as advanced age, mental deterioration, sensory loss, and social isolation were believed to be major contributors to communication deterioration.

Perceptions of the general adequacy of older persons' communications were not totally supported by descriptive observations. The majority of comments were negative in tone or content. Most commonly noted difficulties included: dementia; failure to work at or utilize topics of common interest (highly personalized and egocentric behaviors); hearing loss; rambling, digressive conversational styles; overreliance on the past as a topic of conversation; confusion, disorientation, and problems with attention; and withdrawal, passivity, and introspection. Additional observations pertaining to personality and emotional attributes reflected stereotypical extremes—the sweet grandmother type; the crotchety, inflexible grouch; or the withdrawn, passive recluse. Perceptions appeared to reflect in part the nature and frequency of personal experiences with older persons.

Greater consensus was reached concerning the fact that other people communicate differently with the elderly. The types of changes in communication behaviors described by all respondents were similar, although the qualitative judgment of these changes as good/bad or appropriate/inappropriate varied from group to group. For example, most professionals felt communication patterns with the elderly were worse than with other age groups, whereas less than half of the older and child respondents believed this to be true. In fact, most children of older parents focused on the degree of effort involved in changing communication in order to "help" the older adult. The most commonly noted changes in others' communications included: a patronizing or condescending attitude; simplification of speech; increased loudness; efforts to find noncontroversial topics of conversation; a lack of engagement or superficiality; an attitude of greater sweetness and kindness; and a slowing of speech rate.

Greatest consensus was reached concerning common conversational topics, communication partners, and frequency of communication contacts. Conversational topics perceived as initiated by older persons included: the past; health, illness, or death; family; and religion. Topics of everyday interest were noted by a number of respondents. The topics initiated by *others* were comparable, with a number of comments focusing on the younger person's use of generic, social questions. It was clear that many perceived older persons as being given the lead or control in conversations or as being catered to.

Around 90% of the respondents in all groups felt that older persons had a restricted range of communication contacts. It was also agreed that younger persons communicate less with the elderly than with other age groups. Restricted communication networks were attributed to age-related factors associated with erosions of social networks and restrictions in mobility and access. It was also noted that older persons withdraw and do not try to relate, while younger persons avoid the elderly or fail to take the time to reach out. The most commonly described communication partners for older persons were believed to be age peers and family members, although community service persons and professionals were also listed. For younger persons, frequent communication contacts were felt to be only with family members.

Finally, all respondents indicated some contact with hearing-impaired older persons. Mean estimates of the prevalence of hearing loss fell between 53 and 59%, with the majority of respondents noting that hearing loss creates a considerable barrier to communication. The three most commonly cited problems created by hearing impairment included: the older adult's inappropriate acceptance or denial of the problem; the communicative misunderstandings created by hearing loss; and the social isolation and emotional problems created by this isolation. A fair bit of negativism was evident. Almost all of the responses dealing with management strategies emphasized how one must talk with a hearing impaired person. Little mention was made of hearing aids, and no interviewee mentioned communication strategies that could be used by the hearing impaired older individual.

Fewer respondents reported personal contacts with a speech-language impaired older person, although the prevalence of speech-language problems was estimated to be around 25%. Descriptive comments were most notable for their paucity, vagueness, and a strong sense of lack of information and ineffectuality. The most commonly noted problems included: difficulties conversing with a speech-language impaired person; problems in understanding what the person is trying to communicate; the emotional reactions of the impaired individual; and the need to show that you care about what the person is trying to say.

Dominant Variables

Central to the understanding of these intra- and intergroup response patterns are four basic issues: (a) the nature and degree of communication accommodation assumed to be necessary; (b) the nature and extent of individual experiences or personal involvements with older persons; (c) the presence and severity of contributing age-related problems; and (d) the respondent's knowledge of aging and its concomitants. These four variables and their impact on communication partners and communicative interactions are shown schematically in Figure 2.1. Each variable is capable of influencing the perceptions and expectations of the members of the communication dyad, as well as their actual behaviors. In turn, these attitudes and behaviors contribute to the actual communication interaction, influencing dynamics such as: the success or failure of the interaction, the quality of the interaction, its frequency and most common partners, and the strategies used when a communication disorder is present. This same communicative interaction is directly responsible for further

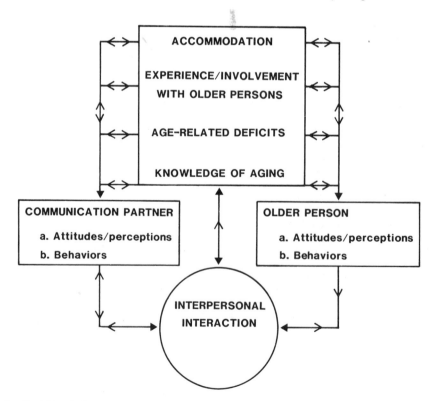

Figure 2.1. Variables influencing perceptions and expectations of members of young-old communication interactions.

modifications in the partners' attitudes and behaviors, and also contributes new input to each of the four contributing variables. In essence, the degree to which communication can be used successfully as a tool for coping with life stresses and for meeting social, physical, or psychological needs is controlled by these dominant influences.

Accommodation

Giles and his colleaques have postulated that the success or failure of any communication interaction is dependent upon the degree to which communicators engage in speech accommodation (10). Speech accommodation refers to modifications in speech style designed to expedite the transmission of a message and to signal willingness to engage in communication interactions. Many of the comments offered by participants reflect some level of awareness of this process. For example, descriptions of inappropriate topic selection (by both older persons and their partners) and of modifications in loudness, rate of speech, articulation, and word selection suggest a breakdown in accommodation existing side by side with apparent attempts to adjust speech style to perceived deficits or needs.

There is little doubt that respondents perceive younger persons as attempting to accommodate, at least in selection of words, message length, and nonverbal characteristics of loudness and clarity. What is less clear, however, is whether or not these accommodations are appropriate—in other words, whether or not individuals are accommodating to their stereotypes of the elderly or to the actual unique characteristics of the individual with whom they are communicating (5, 6). Data from this project suggest that many accommodations are stereotypical, since they are relatively universally applied. In particular, it was noted that people may select topics that they *believe* older people are interested in, based on their past experiences or stereotypical expectations. Many respondents also stated that younger persons may not desire interaction with an elderly individual, presumably leading to the absence of the necessary accommodations for effective communication.

There is less consensus concerning whether or not older persons accommodate appropriately, if at all, in their communicative interactions. The issue of a possible increase in egocentrism in the elderly (11, 12, 16) finds some support in the number of responses suggesting that the older person does not try to accommodate—in choice of topic, vocabulary,

or conversational style. Some interviewees even noted a basic breakdown in social communicative skills, associated with a dominance of the communicative interaction or the opposite extreme, a withdrawal from social intercourse.

The issue of accommodation also touches heavily on the question, "What's at stake for the communication partners?" Dowd's exchange theory would suggest that the stakes are typically unequal when the communication involves a young-old dyad (9). One's perceptions of a communication event may be colored by one's needs, one's role relationship to the other, one's interests, and one's perceptions and stereotypes. Some of these will be touched on in greater detail in subsequent paragraphs.

Individual Experience/Personal Involvement with Older Persons

Much of the response diversity described in this paper can be attributed to the nature and extent of individual experiences or personal involvements with older persons. For example, some responses of children of older parents appeared to be colored by the immediacy of their personal contacts with the parent(s). These child respondents tended to be slightly more negative about the communication skills of older persons, and the most negative were those who saw their parent(s)' communication in a less than favorable light. Child respondents were also more likely to be positive or neutral about changes in other person's communications addressed to the elderly. They were highly aware of the effort involved in communications with older individuals (particularly those with a hearing impairment). Child respondents were likely to reflect extremes of attitude and emotion, from a deep anger at older persons' communicative inadequacies to a kind of distorted picture of the perfect older person who has attained some epitome of aging through life experience.

Older respondents, in contrast, tended to be more favorable in their judgments of the communication skills of the elderly, less inclined to see things as problems, and less inclined to have thought about the nature of others' communications with older individuals. Presumably, older individuals would have a vested interest in seeing the communication situation of the elderly in a relatively positive context—e.g., they might not be able to afford to look too closely at some of the imbalances in communications that may exist. However, there were a wide range of responses in the older interviewee group, from those who saw no problems with communications to those who felt severely "put-upon" by the world.

Finally, professional respondents appeared to reflect somewhat middle-ground positions—more balanced and qualifying in their perspectives, more analytical, more behavioral and management oriented. There was, however, some evidence that professional perceptions of older persons in general were colored by both the respondents' own age (and peer group) and their experiences with a specific client base. Since professionals would be expected to have least personal vested interest and fewer complex role relationships in interactions with the elderly (depending upon the age of the professional), the nature of their communications with older persons would dictate an objective or uninvolved perspective. In addition, factors related to professional knowledge of aging and of ageism may have colored responses, as described later.

The Presence and Severity of Contributing Age-Related Problems

Almost without exception, respondents agreed that considerably advanced age brings with it a deterioration in communication skills. Comments focused on the communication effects of such age-related problems as hearing and vision impairment, memory loss and confusion (with or without dementia), health breakdown, and social isolation. It should be noted that these aging concomitants are easy to blame and irrefutably responsible for some of the changes in communication found in the elderly.

Nevertheless, it is important to remember that such easily identified changes in life status and functioning may also shape perceptions and evaluations of all elderly and of interactions with this age segment of the population. If it is perceived as effortful to talk with a hearing impaired older individual who is also very lonely and a bit confused, communicators are likely to avoid or limit such interactions. Comments to this effect were offered by a number of respondents.

Knowledge of Aging and of Ageism

The degree to which one sees all elderly as experiencing the age decrements noted above, or as possessing the attributes of the few older persons with whom one has had personal contact, is mitigated to some extent by one's knowledge of aging. Respondents with greater

knowledge of aging (frequently professionals) tended to product more qualified responses or to provide age-related explanations for perceived behavioral patterns. In contrast, limited aging information may have been responsible for the frequency of occurrence of many stereotypical descriptors of older persons' communication. For example, a few respondents experienced no discomfort or cognitive dissonance in stating that the majority of elderly were cranky, withdrawn, rambling, or forgetful.

Unfortunately, knowledge of aging often includes knowledge of ageism, of the fact that society has recently demonstrated fairly pronounced and negative biases against aging and the elderly. Professionals, in particular, showed some evidence of a positive response bias, a kind of tendency to avoid making or agreeing with any statement that could be construed as having a negative connotation with respect to the elderly (3, 22). This positive bias could lead to denial of less pleasant realities.

Inadequate information about aging was evident throughout participant responses, particularly in comments about specific communication disorders. Although many respondents produced fairly accurate estimates of the prevalence of such disorders, they repeatedly demonstrated a lack of information or misinformation about the causes and consequences of speech-language or hearing impairment, with almost no knowledge of apropriate management strategies for communicating with the speech-language impaired individual. In addition, awareness of management strategies that could be utilized by the elderly individual was limited.

Final Thoughts

A sample of 48 respondents, further subdivided into three distinct subgroups, clearly does not constitute a large "N" in the traditional research sense, particularly when a number of potentially influential subject variables were considered but not controlled precisely in subject selection. Subsequent research efforts could benefit from sampling in other geographical locations and from inclusion of larger numbers of subjects whose profiles could be documented and analyzed. Nevertheless, data reported in this chapter suggest considerable success in meeting the goal of identifying the range of existing perceptions concerning communication with and by older individuals.

The commonalities observed—and all of the distinctive and contrasting individual and group commentaries—constitute major realities in the day-to-day interpersonal interactions of older persons. As subsequent authors in this text describe aging, changes in communication behavior with aging, and management strategies for working with specific communication disorders, the reader should continue to utilize this chapter as a frame of reference for comparing fact with fiction, and for examining the communication environment of the older client.

References

1. Albee R: *The American Dream*. New York, Coward-McMann, 1961.
2. Biegel DE, Shore BK, Gordon E.: *Building Support Networks for the Elderly: Theory and Applications*. Beverly Hills, CA, Sage, 1984.
3. Butler R: Overview on aging. In Usdin G, Hofling CK (eds): *Aging: The Process and the People*. New York, Brunner/Mazel, 1978, p 1.
4. Cantor MH: Neighbors and friends: An overlooked resource in the informal support system. *Res Aging*. 1:434–463, 1979.
5. Caporael LR: The paralanguage of caregiving: Baby talk to the institutionalized aged. *J Pers Soc Psychol* 40:876–884, 1981.
6. Caporael LR, Lukaszewski MP, Culbertson GH: Secondary baby talk: Judgments by institutionalized elderly and their caregivers. *J Pers Soc Psychol* 44:746–754, 1983.
7. Chappell NL: Informal support networks among the elderly. *Res Aging* 5:77–99, 1983.
8. Darbyshire JO: The hearing loss epidemic: A challenge to gerontology. *Res Aging*. 6:383–394, 1984.
9. Dowd JJ: *Stratification among the Aged*. Monterey, CA, Brooks/Cole, 1980.
10. Giles H: Social psychology and applied linguistics. *ITL: Review of Applied Linguistics* 35:27–40, 1977.
11. Helfrich H: Age markers in speech. In Scherer KR, Giles H (eds): *Social Markers in Speech*. Cambridge, England, Cambridge University Press, 1979, p 63.
12. Hutchinson JM, Jensen M: A pragmatic evalua-

tion of discourse communication in a nursing home. In Obler LK, Albert ML (eds): *Language and Communication in the Elderly*. Lexington, MA, Lexington Books, 1980, p 59.
13. Jones D: Social isolation, interaction and conflict in two nursing homes. *Gerontologist* 12:230–234, 1972.
14. Kogan N: Beliefs, attitudes, and stereotypes about old people: A new look at some old issues. *Res Aging* 1:11–36, 1979.
15. Lieberman MA, Tobin SS: *The Experience of Old Age: Stress, Coping, and Survival*. New York, Basic Books, 1983.
16. Looft WR: Egocentrism and social interaction across the life span. *Psychol Bull* 78:73–92, 1972.
17. Neugarten BL: Personality and the aging process. *Gerontologist* 12:9–15, 1972.
18. Oyer EJ: Exchanging information within the older family. In Oyer HJ, Oyer EJ (eds): *Aging and Communication*. Baltimore, University Park Press, 1976, p 43.
19. Oyer HJ, Oyer EJ: Communicating with older people: Basic considerations.. In Oyer HJ, Oyer EJ (eds): *Aging and Communication*. Baltimore, University Park Press, 1976, p 1.
20. Peters GR: Interagency relations and the aging network: The state unit on aging and AAA's in Kansas. In Streib GF (ed): *Programs for Older Americans*, Research Series, vol 1. Gainesville, University of Florida Center for Gerontological Studies, 1981, p 96.
21. Punch J: The prevalence of hearing impairment. *ASHA* 25(4):27, 1983.
22. Shadden BB: Communication process and aging: Information needs and attitudes of older adults and professionals (grant report). Washington, DC, American Association of Retired Persons, 1982.
23. Strain LA, Chappell NL: Confidants: Do they make a difference in quality of life? *Res Aging* 4:479–502, 1982.
24. West GE, Simons RL: Sex differences in stress, coping resources, and illness among the elderly. *Res Aging*, 5:235–268, 1983.
25. Woelfel J: Communication across age levels. In Oyer HJ, Oyer EJ (eds): *Aging and Communication*. Baltimore, University Park Press, 1976, p 63.

Appendix
Communication Protocol

Would you say older persons experience more problems in their daily communications with other people than younger persons?   Yes   No

HOW OLDER PERSONS COMMUNICATE

1. Do you think most older persons communicate adequately?   Yes   No
2. A. What percentage of older persons do not communicate well?   _____
   B. What percentage of persons below the age of 65 years don't communicate well?   _____

PROBE—perceptions of the communication behaviors of older person

HOW OTHER PERSONS COMMUNICATE WITH OLDER PERSONS

3. Do people communicate differently with older persons than with younger?   Yes   No
4. Do you think people communicate with older persons than they do with younger persons?   Better   the Same   Worse

PROBE—the manner in which people communicate differently with older communication partners (also circumstances and perceived reasons for differences)

5. Do you find yourself communicating differently when talking with an older person?   Yes   No

PROBE—perceptions of differences in one's own communication behaviors.

PROBE—the nature of a typical communication interaction between an older and younger person.

FOR OLDER PERSONS ONLY

6. A. Do you think you communicate adequately?   Yes   No
   B. As you have grown older, do you think your communication skills have . . .   Gotten   Stayed   Gotten
                                                                                   Better   the Same   Worse
   C. Do you think your communication behaviors have changed as you have gotten older?   Yes   No

PROBE—nature of own communication skills and changes over time.

FOR CHILDREN OF OLDER PARENTS ONLY

6. A. Do you think your parent(s) communicate adequately?   Yes   No
   B. As they have grown older, do you think their communication skills have . . .   Gotten   Stayed   Gotten
                                                                                   Better   the Same   Worse
   C. Do you think your parent(s)' communication behaviors have changed as they have gotten older?   Yes   No

PROBE—nature of parent's communication behaviors and changes over time.

FOR PROFESSIONAL RESPONDENTS ONLY

6. A. Do you think your older clients communicate adequately?   Yes   No
   B. What percentage of your older clients don't communicate well?   _____

C. Do you think your older clients have more communication
problems than the population of older persons in general? **Yes** **No**

PROBE—*specific or unique communication problems of your clients,*
including situational difficulties.

COMMUNICATION STEREOTYPES

7. I'm going to give you some statements about older persons in
communication situations. To what percentage of older persons
do you feel these statements apply?
   a. Older persons have trouble hearing what is said in a conversation. _____
   b. Older persons are good story tellers. _____
   c. People listen carefully to what older persons have to say. _____
   d. People are uncomfortable talking to older persons. _____
   e. Older persons tend to ramble in conversations. _____
   f. Older persons have trouble remembering the words they want
   to say. _____
   g. Older persons are concise and clear in their conversations. _____
   h. Older persons listen carefully to what others have to say. _____
   i. People turn to older persons for information and advice. _____
   j. Older persons talk mostly about the past. _____
   k. People tend to "talk down" when talking to an older person. _____
   j. Older persons have pleasant speaking voices. _____

CHANGES IN COMMUNICATION BEHAVIOR WITH AGE

8. Do people change the way in which they communicate as they
get older? **Yes** **No**

9. A. When people reach old age (past age 65), do you think their
   communication skills . . .
   than when they were younger?

   | Get | Stay | Get |
   | Better | the Same | Worse |

   B. Would your answer change if I said specifically people over
   the age of 85? Would you say the communication skills of the
   over 85 person generally . . .

   | Get | Stay | Get |
   | Better | the Same | Worse |

10. What percentage of older persons show a worsening of communication skills as they get older? _____

PROBE—*nature of changes in communication as individuals age.*

WHAT DO OLDER PERSONS TALK ABOUT AND WHY?

PROBE—*topics raised by older persons, by others communicating*
with and older persons, reasons for communication.

HOW OFTEN DO OLDER PERSONS GET A CHANCE TO COMMUNICATE AND WITH WHOM?

11. Do you think older persons in general have fewer people to talk
with than younger persons? **Yes** **No**

PROBE—*reasons, effects.*

12. Do you think people in general communicate with older persons . . .

   _____ **More than with other age groups**
   _____ **With the saame frequency as other age groups**
   _____ **Less than with other age groups**

PROBE—*who are older persons most likely to communicate with*
and which older persons most people are likely to com-
municate with.

COMMUNICATIONS DISORDERS

13. In your opinion, what is the percentage of older persons who have a hearing loss?   _____

14. Do you think hearing loss in older persons creates . . .

    _____ **A Considerable Barrier to Communication**
    _____ **A Mild Barrier to Communication**
    _____ **No Barrier to Communication**

PROBE—*problems created by hearing loss and what can be done about hearing loss in older persons.*

15. Do you know any older persons with a speech or language disorder (for example, as a result of stroke or Parkinson's disease or laryngectomy)?   **Yes   No**

16. What percentage of older person have a specific speech/language disorder as a result of one of these kinds of problems?   _____

PROBE—*problems encountered in trying to communicate with a person with a speech-language disorder.*

Aspects of Aging which Impact on Interpersonal Communication

II

3 Social Realities of Aging

HAROLD COX

Editor's Note

There are a variety of ways to approach examination of the social realities of aging. Clearly, as provided in this chapter, we must consider the basic demographic phenomenon of relatively rapid growth in the size of the older population, with disproportionate contributions to this growth being made by women and by those over 85 years of age. Rather than focus exclusively on demographic phenomena, however, author Cox has chosen instead to target the many theories that have been developed to account for either the social behaviors of older persons or strategies for successful aging. Beginning with a review of the more widely known disengagement and activity theories of aging, the chapter proceeds with a discussion of more recent perspectives. These perspectives include continuity theory, symbolic interaction theory (with its applications in considering breakdown and reconstruction in social interactions), and exchange theory. Dowd's exchange theory is referred to in several other chapters in this text. Of particular interest to practicing professionals, however, are the implications of the symbolic interaction model for social adaptation and maladjustment in the elderly. Symbolic interaction theory postulates that most adult behavior is learned through language communication; as a result, social labeling tends to become an important determinant of an individual's self-concept and behavior. Cox provides a detailed analysis of the significance of this premise for understanding the actions and reactions of older persons in general, and for examining patterns of health services utilization in particular. His discussion should stimulate the reader to reexamine client behaviors from a different perspective and to consider creative solutions to problems of social adjustment in older adults.

The 20th century has brought demographic shifts in the age composition and the overall makeup of the American population. There has been a steady decrease in the size of the typical American family from the large family in 1900 to the small two- and three-children families of the 1980s. The demographic effect has been to see a gradual decrease in the percentage of our total population under the age of 20. Simultaneously an ever advancing medical technology in the 20th century has resulted in a considerable improvement in the doctors' ability to save and prolong life. The result in the United States and other developed nations has been the same—a growing number and percentage of these nations' populations living to age 65 and beyond. Barring any unforeseen demographic changes in the near future, the number of older persons in western Europe and the United States will continue to grow and constitute an ever larger per cent of the population. Moreover, Cowgill (6) points out that

*a*Many of the ideas presented in this chapter were originally developed by the author, Harold Cox, in *Later Life: The Realities of Aging.* Englewood Cliffs, NJ, Prentice Hall, 1984.

the aging of the population is no longer true just for the industrialized nations of the West but rather is becoming a worldwide phenomenon. Cowgill states:

Most of the new nations of Africa and Asia have already doubled the average length of life, as compared with primitive lands and some Asian and Latin American countries are pressing toward the modern standard of 70 years, which has already been surpassed by most European countries. (6, p 19).

DEMOGRAPHICS

The growth of the older population in the United States is typical of what has occurred in the West in the 20th century (see Figure 3.1). In 1900 there were 3 million Americans over age 65, comprising approximately 4% (1 in 25) of the total population. In 1970, 20 million Americans were over the age 65, and more than 10% (1 in 10) of the total population. In 1980 there were 25,544,000 Americans over 65, comprising approximately 11% (1 in 9) of the total population. Demographers estimate that by the year 2000, 36 million Americans will be over

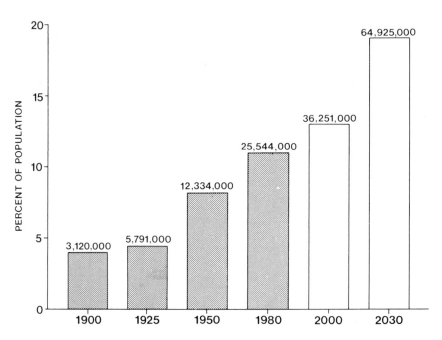

Figure 3.1.   U.S. population age 65 and older 1900 to 2030. Data for 1985 to 2030 are projections. (From U.S. Bureau of the Census, Social Security Administration.)

age 65; they may comprise as much as 13% of the total population (27).

These figures are based on the current birthrate. Should the birthrate suddenly rise, the percentage of the total population over age 65 would drop slightly. The long-range trend in the birthrate has been downward, however, and no one is predicting any dramatic reversals in the next 30 years. Any further drop in the birthrate would make the 65+ group comprise an even larger percentage of the total population.

Population figures for the 65+ age group have grown by 3 to 4 million per decade since 1940. Growth during the 1970s exceeded earlier projections; it climbed at an annual increment of 460,000. Every day approximately 5,000 persons reach their 65th birthday, and 3,600 persons in the same age group die. This means an increase of 1,400 persons in the 65+ group each day. Figure 3.2 reveals how much more rapidly the 65+ group is growing compared to the total population since 1900 (26).

Not only are more people living to age 65, but once they reach that age they live longer (24). In 1900 fewer than 1 million Americans were 75 and older, and 2.3 million persons were 85 and older. While the 65 and older group has increased approximately eightfold since 1900, the population 85 and older has grown 22 times its size in the same period. Moreover, as shown in Figure 3.3, the 85+ group is projected to grow more rapidly than the 65+ age group until

about 2010, when cohorts born in the baby boom of the 1940s and 1950s begin to retire (1). Since it is the 85+ group which makes the greatest demand for services one can easily see the implications of the growth of this age group for the resources of Federal, state, and local governments.

While the proportion of the total population made up of individuals 65 and above has been increasing dramatically, the numbers and percentage of this group comprised of women have increased even more rapidly (21). As Figure 3.4 indicates, the women 65 and above have increased from just under 5% of the total population in 1960 to approximately 6% in 1980. This group is projected to grow to just over 9% in 2050. The men 65 and above made up approximately 4% of the population in 1960, 4.25% of the population in 1980, and are projected to grow to over 7.50% of the population by the year 2050. It is clear that both in numbers and in the percentage of the total population, the increases for women have been more rapid than the increases for men. Moreover, this is also true for the 85 and above age group. Women are contributing disproportionately to the profile of an expanding older population.

Louis Harris and associates (10) believe that there are three basic reasons for the current growth of America's older population. First, the large number of people born when the birthrate was high are now reaching age 65.

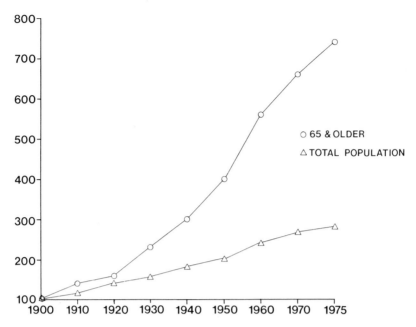

Figure 3.2.   Rate of increase 65 and older vs. that of total U.S. population from 1900 to 1975. (From Bureau of the Census.)

Second, a high rate of immigration of younger adults during World War II further added to the number of people now reaching 65. Finally, improvements in medical technology have created a dramatic increase in life expectancy.

While the number of persons arriving at age 65 is expected to increase for the foreseeable future, the increase should prove gradual rather than dramatic between now and the year 2010. The reason for this is that the 1930s was a peri-

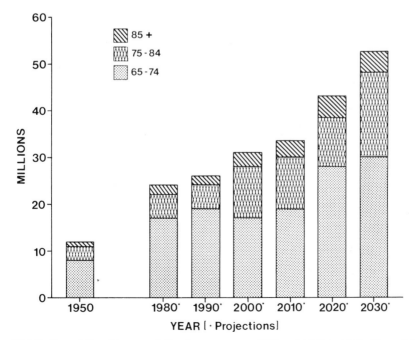

Figure 3.3.   Distribution of the older population by age group, 1950 and 1980 to 2030. (From U.S. Bureau of the Census.)

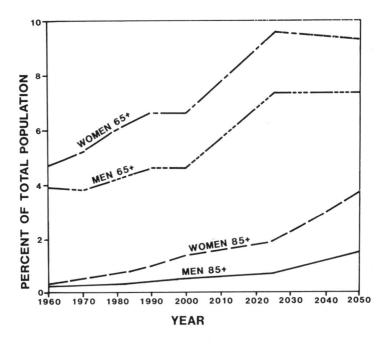

Figure 3.4. Proportion of the population 65 and over and 85 and over by sex 1960 to 2050. (From U.S. Bureau of the Census.)

od of low birthrate. Since these people will be retiring between now and the year 2010, there will be no sudden shifts in demographic characteristics. Also, the *dependency ratio* will probably not change appreciably in the next 30 years (see Fig. 3.5). The dependency ratio is calculated by comparing those in the work force with those out of the work force. Thus most people under 18 and over 65 are out of the work force and depend on those between 19 and 64 to produce the goods and services that they need (25). Since those born in the baby boom

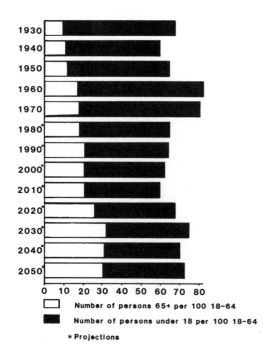

Figure 3.5. Number of persons aged 65 and older and under 18 per 100 persons aged 18 to 64 to 1930 to 1980, and projections to 2050. (From Bureau of the Census.)

following World War II are now entering the labor force, they have the effect of keeping the dependency ratio lower that it would otherwise be.

This high birthrate after 1945 is presently creating difficulties for many because jobs must be found for a large group of younger people. The major problem, however, is expected to come in the year 2010 and thereafter, when the postwar baby boom begins to retire and is followed by fewer people who will be in the working years and must support them (1). The dependency ratio should increase dramatically at that time. One can only imagine what changes may be necessary in production, taxation, and the support system for older Americans. And there is an additional question: Will taxpayers in their working years be willing to be taxed as heavily as will be necessary to support this large group of retirees?

THEORETICAL PERSPECTIVES ON AGING

The goal of any scientific enterprise is to explain some aspect of the natural or social world in a logical and understandable manner. All scientific explanations are grounded in theory and attempt to account for a given set of phenomena with the development of a model that is predictive and that can be empirically demonstrated. A theory is a set of logically interrelated propositions that account for some set of phenomena.

The sequential process that the scientist goes through in developing a theory includes: (a) the establishment of precise definitions for the variables he or she deals with; (b) the framing of propositions which assert that two or more phenomena are logically related; and (c) the development of a theory which is a set of interrelated propositions that account for the phenomena in question. Inductively, the scientist goes from definition of the variables to propositions relating two or more variables to the development of a theory. A theory, a set of logically interconnected propositions, can then be developed to account for the phenomenon in question.

Scientists never entirely prove or disprove a theory. They merely develop a greater or lesser degree of confidence in its predictive power. This is because a theory does not rest on a single proposition but on a series of propositions, any one of which may be partly or entirely in error. The empiricist derives hypotheses from a theory stating that, if the theory is true, we should expect to find certain predicted relationships between the variables. Sometimes the hypotheses are supported by research findings; sometimes they are not supported. Research findings always contribute to the theory by either: (a) supporting the theory when the hypothesized relations are proved valid; (b) reshaping the theory, should part of the hypotheses be proved but other parts disproved; (c) refuting the theory should the hypotheses be all disproved; or (d) initiating a new theory should unanticipated findings lead the research in an entirely new direction.

Some of the earlier theories of aging were as much philosophical explanations of how one ought to age successfully and gracefully as they were theories that explained the behavior of older persons. For example, disengagement and activity theory resemble philosophical recommendations of how to live one's life during the later years as much as they do theories. Propositions and hypotheses, however, have been derived from those theoretical perspectives and have been tested by different researchers. Therefore the disengagement and activity perspectives can be considered theories.

Disengagement Theory

In its simplest form, as originally described by Elaine Cumming and William Henry (7), disengagement theory stated that aging involves an inevitable withdrawal or disengagement from social roles resulting in decreased interaction between the aging person and others in the social milieu to which he or she belongs. The process of withdrawal suggested by the theory is mutually satisfying for the individual and the social system. For the individual, the withdrawal is satisfying since he/she no longer has to compete with younger rivals. For the society, the withdrawal of the older person allows younger and supposedly more energetic and competent individuals to assume the functional roles which must be fulfilled for the survival of the system.

Vern Bengtson (2) argues that the disengagement theory implies a dramatic shift from middle to older age marked by an entirely new balance of forces between the personality and the social systems of the individual. The manner in which the individual has organized the diverse roles that he or she is currently assuming into an organized and consistent view of self is called personality. Social systems refer to the variety of social groups that the individual identifies as his or hers and with whose members he or she regularly interacts (e.g., family, fellow workers, members of the Lions

Club, etc.). The extent to which social norms impinge on the individual would be greatly reduced in older age, and the sources of psychological well-being in older age would be considerably different from those of middle age. Whether in fact this much of a shift in the personality system actually occurs is highly debatable.

Richard Kalish (13) believes that the theory of disengagement must be evaluated on three different levels, each of which should be carefully analyzed in terms of whether it refers to psychological disengagement or social disengagement. The levels of evaluation as he sees them are: (a) disengagement as a process; (b) disengagement as inevitable; and (c) disengagement as adaptive (13).

Disengagement is often viewed as a process, since for most people it does not occur all at once but gradually over a period of time. The last child may leave home when the couple is in their early 50s; parental responsibilities are thereby withdrawn. The wife may decide to give up her job after the expenses of putting children through college are no longer pressing. The husband may decide not to serve another term on the county council. Later, he may decide to take early retirement at age 62 rather than wait until 65. As a process, disengagement is always selective in that the individual chooses to withdraw from some roles and not from others, and the process takes place over a number of years rather than all at once.

Disengagement is presumed to be inevitable since everyone at some point will die. If advancing age brings with it an increasing probability of sickness and death, then disengagement is inevitable. The individual is considered ready to disengage upon recognizing that the length of life or amount of life space available to him or her is shrinking and that his or her energy level is declining. Life space refers to the area of the world, community, neighborhood, and home which the individual considers his or her environment. Sometimes older persons may give up driving, travel out of the neighborhood less frequently, and spend greater amounts of time in their home or apartment. Thus the life space in which they exist and travel begins to shrink as they become less mobile and feel less capable of coping with broader and more diverse environments.

Disengagement is regarded as adaptive from both the individual and the social point of view. Disengagement presumably allows the individual to withdraw from previous work roles and from competition with younger counterparts as his or her energy presumably declines. Thus the individual adapts to aging and to the loss of energy and the capability to compete with

others by withdrawing from the social situation that demands competition. From the societal point of view, disengagement permits younger employees to assume critical positions as the older ones become less efficient, thereby allowing for the smooth transition of power and control from one generation to the next.

The critics of disengagement theory have been numerous, adamant, and persistent. They were quick to challenge the presumed inevitability of the disengagement process. Many gerontologists questioned whether the process was functional for either the individual or the social system. George Maddox (16), for example, pointed out that different personality factors might make the individual more or less amenable to disengagement. Since there is social pressure to disengage, gerontologists who focused on personality factors felt that those who, throughout their lives, had dealt with stress by turning inward and insulating themselves from the world would probably continue to manifest a pattern of withdrawal. On the other hand, those who were inclined to remain engaged had probably been so inclined over the course of their entire lives. For this group, the kind of activities engaged in might change, but they would seek relationships allowing them to resist general disengagement patterns. From the societal perspective many have questioned whether it is functional or desirable to remove from critical social positions some of the most capable, experienced, and reliable workers.

Activity Theory

Robert Havighurst (11) had been one of the leading exponents of activity theory. The activity theorists present a view of successful aging that is exactly the opposite of that presented by the disengagement theorists. The activity theorists basically argue that the individual should remain as active as possible for as long as possible. For every role that is given up in the middle and later years a new role should be found.

Middle class Americans throughout their lives have generally believed that activity is good for the individual and is often an indication of a successful life. Middle class families encourage their children early in life to become involved in as many activities as possible. Boy Scouts, Girl Scouts, Little League baseball, the YMCA, music lessons, and a multitude of other activities quickly consume the spare time of these children. Adult life for middle class Americans is a continuation of this activity pattern with the Rotary, the country club, church, ladies auxiliary, and a host of other activities consuming most, if not all, of the available hours of the day. It is easy to see why this group believes that remaining active in later life is the way to age successfully. These are the values they have endorsed throughout their lives. Similarly, activity theory most fully reflects the values endorsed by the Golden Age Magazines. Many older Americans insist that they would "rather wear out than rust out."

Activity theory assumes that the relationship between the social system and the personality system remains fairly stable as an individual passes from the status of middle age to that of old age. It holds that the norms for old age are the same as those for middle age, and that the older person should be judged in terms of middle age criteria of success (2).

Thus, activity theory emphasizes the stability of personality system orientations as an individual ages and ignores any need for societally structured alternatives to compensate for losses that the individual experiences as part of the aging process. One obvious difficulty of the theory is that it does not seriously consider what happens to the person who cannot maintain the standards of middle age in the later years. If the individual accepts the belief that he or she must remain active while experiencing physiological losses as part of aging, the result could be considerable frustration, anxiety, and guilt about one's inability to handle the behavioral expectations of activity.

Lemon et al. (15) isolated what appear to be two fundamental propositions of activity theory: (a) that there is a positive relation between social activity and life satisfaction in old age; (b) that role losses such as widowhood and retirement are inversely related to life satisfaction. Their findings from a study of people moving to a retirement community did not support these propositions. The more active older persons were not necessarily the most satisfied with their lives. Only social activity with friends was in any way related to life satisfaction. This study therefore raised questions about the validity of the basic propositions of activity theory and cast doubts on the theory itself. On the other hand, studies by Jeffers and Nichols (12), Havighurst (11), and others—to name only two—have repeatedly found positive associations between morale, personal adjustment, and activity levels.

Continuity Theory

Disenchanted with both the disengagement and activity theories of aging, gerontologists began to look for alternative views of the aging process. Building on the well-established sociological concept of continuity in socialization and life-style, continuity theory emerged. The theory assumes and looks for continuity of behavior patterns throughout different phases of the life cycle.

Sociologists often use the term role continuity to describe the process of growth and change throughout the life cycle. Role continuity assumes that the activities one is involved in and the roles he or she is participating in at one stage of life are an adequate preparation for what will be expected of him/her at the next stage. The boy learning to drive his father's tractor, the little girl playing doctor, the young man conducting a chemical experiment as a class exercise, the young woman working as a camp counselor, and the apprentice imitating the master craftsman are all developing skills at one stage of life that can be used in a later stage.

Formally, the parent attempts to socialize children into adult roles by advising, encouraging, and sending them to school to acquire the desired skills. Informally, children learn the proper attitudes and values required for assuming adult responsibilities through the games they are taught to play, the gifts they receive, and the model of adult behavior provided to them by the parent. Thus both formal and informal childrearing practices contribute continuity to the socialization process by which the individual is prepared for the next stage of life. Similarly, there is considerable *anticipatory socialization*, by which a person imagines, so to speak, what it will be like to assume the role and responsibilities of the next period of life.

Each successive grade in school is predicated on what is taught in a previous grade. Education builds knowledge and skills in increments, so that the high school graduate is presumed to be considerably more informed than a fourth-grader, who is herself superior in this respect to those in grades below her. During the life course, movement into adult status in the early 20s presumes successful handling of adjustment problems in the teen years. Life cycles thus have patterns in which there is considerable continuity from one stage to the next, with each succeeding age built on the experiences and skills of the previous period.

While role continuity implies that skills learned now will be useful at the next phase of life, role discontinuity suggests that what the individual is doing now is not a preparation for roles that he/she must assume in the next life stage. Retirement for most individuals involves considerable role discontinuity. Career and occupational skills are no longer needed, and work is not expected to be a vital part of one's life. Leisure is for the first time readily available; the constant drive for achievement and success no longer dominates one's life.

Continuity theory holds that, in the course of growing older, the individual is predisposed toward maintaining stability in the habits, associations, preferences, and life-style that he or she has developed over the years. This theory asserts that the individual's reaction to aging can be understood only by examining the complex interrelationships among biological, psychological, and social changes in the individual's life and the previous behavior patterns. Exponents of the theory believe that a person's habits, preferences, associations, state of health, and actual experiences will in large part determine that person's ability to maintain his/her life-style while retiring from full-time employment and perhaps having to adjust to the death of a loved one. The person's lifelong experiences thus create dispositions to a preferred life-style that he or she will attempt to maintain if at all possible.

Disengagement and activity theory both posit a single direction that they believe is most appropriate for successful adaptation to the aging process. Continuity theory, on the other hand, starts with the single premise that the individual will try to maintain as long as possible his or her preferred life-style, and then holds that adaptation can go in several different directions depending on how the individual perceives his or her changing status and attempts to adjust to this change. Continuity theory does not assert that one must be disengaged or be active in order to be well adjusted in the later years, but rather that the decision regarding which roles are to be discarded and which maintained will in large part be determined by the individual's past history and preferred style of life.

Peterson (19) seems to endorse the continuity perspective when asserting that if disengagement occurs it is very selective, with some roles being discarded and other being maintained in later life. Peterson believes that the individual hangs on to those roles that brought him/her the greatest status and gives up on those which brought less status. Thus, the individual will attempt to maintain as long as possible a positive self-concept by continuing in those activities and roles that are most directly related to this ideal self and by discarding those less directly related. Peterson and the proponents of continuity theory assert that you can predict retirement adjustment patterns only by knowing the individual's past history, as well as by having more understanding of his/her ideal self and the relation of past roles to this ideal.

Thus, continuity theory anticipates a multiplicity of adjustment patterns in later life.

The major disadvantage of continuity theory is that it is most difficult to test empirically. Each individual's pattern of adjustment in retirement must become a case study in which the researcher attempts to determine to what degree the individual was able to continue in his or her preferred life-style.

Symbolic Interaction Theory and Aging

Symbolic interaction theory, developed by Mead (17), Cooley (4), Thomas (23), and other social thinkers, has become one of the basic perspectives of sociologists. This theory maintains that the acquisition of language makes human beings qualitatively different from any other form of life, since no other animal has the ability to speak and communicate symbolically. The symbolic interactionist asserts that through language, humans live in a symbolic environment as well as a physical environment and can be motivated to act by symbols as well as physical stimuli.

Through the use of language man has the capacity to stimulate others in ways that he/she is not stimulated. A young woman may tell a young man that she loves him in order to get a commitment for future dates, presents, etc., when in fact she does not love him and does not intend for the relationship to be a permanent one. Thus, through the use of language, she may stimulate her date in ways that she herself is not stimulated.

The exponents of symbolic interaction theory maintain that the communication of symbols allows human beings to learn huge numbers of meanings and values and, hence, ways of acting from other persons. Thus, it is assumed that most adult behavior is learned specifically in symbolic communication rather then trial-and-error conditioning.

The symbolic interactionists view thinking as a process by which possible solutions and future courses of action are examined and assessed for their relative advantages in term of the values of the individual. One plan is then chosen for action. Thinking is greatly facilitated by the acquisition of language. Thinking is a symbolic process of deductive trial and error.

Stryker (22) outlined what he considered to be the basic assumptions of the theory:

1. Humankind must be studied at its own level. Valid principles of human social psychological behavior cannot be inferred from

the study of nonhuman forms, since humans are qualitatively and quantitatively different from their predecessors in the evolutionary process. Thus, principles derived from other forms of life cannot completely account for human behavior.

2. The most fruitful approach to human social behavior is through the analysis of society. Interaction is the basic building block of society from which both individual and societal patterns of behavior are derived. Utilizing this block, sociology builds in the direction of collective behavior; social psychology builds in the direction of the behavior of individuals.

3. A baby is neither social nor antisocial but rather asocial, with potentialities for social development. A baby has impulses, but these impulses must be channeled in a given direction.

4. In the interaction process, the human being is an actor as well as a reactor, and does not simply respond to external stimuli. What constitutes a stimulus depends on the activity in which a human being is involved. A human's environment is a selected segment of the "real world," the selection having been made in the interest of behavior initiated by that human being. Thus, through the learning of a culture (including specialized cultures found in particular segments of society), we are able to predict each other's behavior most of the time and adjust our own behavior to the predicted behavior of others.

One of the derivations of the symbolic interaction perspective has been the importance of social labeling in determining the individual's behavior. We tend to think of ourselves in terms of how other people define us and react to us. Much of our self-concept is derived from how others categorize and respond to us. From the labeling perspective much of the behavior of older persons is determined by the reaction of significant others in their social milieu. Thus, the behavior of older Americans is in large measure determined by the norms of the social group to which they belong.

The Social Breakdown Syndrome

Using a perspective which is consistent with the assumptions of the symbolic interactionist, Zusman (28) has constructed a model for a social breakdown syndrome. Zusman proposes a multistage cycle of social breakdown that is consistent with Figure 3.6, which can be utilized to examine what happens to older persons in American society at the time of retirement.

First the organism's precondition or susceptibility to psychological breakdown must be considered. For the older person whose self-concept and identity are firmly based in his occupational role, compulsory retirement can produce problems of identity and self-worth. At the point of retirement, the means of carrying out a social role disappear; the man is a doctor without patients, a lawyer without a case, a business manager without a business, and a professor without a class.

Second, at the point of retirement the individual is excluded from former co-workers. As an isolated person he may find himself completely unable to function in his former role. He no longer is a vice-president of a company with secretarial assistance and a group of subordinates to carry out his orders. His role and status among peers are significantly changed.

Third, he begins to find that others perceive

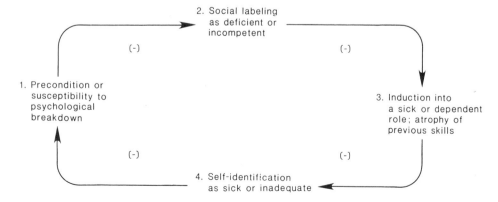

Figure 3.6. The social breakdown syndrome (a vicious cycle of increasing incompetence). (From Bengtson VL: *The Social Psychology of Aging,* p 47. Indianapolis, IN, Bobbs-Merrill, ©1973, The Bobbs-Merrill Company, Inc.

and evaluate him differently as a retired person, rather than as an employed person. He no longer sees respect in the eyes of former subordinates, praise in the faces of former superiors, and approval in the manner of co-workers. In terms of Cooley's (4) looking glass self, the looking glass throws back a changed image; he is done for, an old timer, put on the shelf. The reaction of his co-workers, both subordinates and superiors, is quite different when he occasionally returns to the workplace.

Thus, the individual has arrived at the second point in the Zusman model (Fig. 3.6). The labeling of the individual by those around him as incompetent or deficient is in some respects debilitating. Significant others often begin to treat the older person as through he/she were feeble, sick, or dependent long before he/she really is.

If the individual accepts the definitions of himself that are projected by significant others, he may well be induced to assume the sick role. This is the third step in the downward spiral on the model of social breakdown.

Parsons (18) described what he considered to be the privileges and obligations of the sick role. The privileges of the role include:

1. The patient is exempt from normal social role responsibility. He no longer is expected to work, pay bills, or be responsible for his/her family.
2. The patient is exempt from any sense of personal responsibility, nor is he expected to pull himself together because he is sick. Others will see that he is bathed and fed.

Parsons delineates two obligations of the sick role which are:

1. The patient is obliged to seek professional help.
2. The patient is obliged to want to and try to get well since the sick role is presumed to be a temporary one.

Thus, on the third step of the social breakdown syndrome, the older person is often induced to assume the sick role. This problem is further compounded by the fact that the older person may be granted the privileges of the sick role without the commensurate obligation to get well. He/she arrives, therefore, at point four on the social breakdown syndrome. He/she believes they are feeble, sick, and dependent and begins to permanently assume these elements of the sick role.

Thus, we see the social breakdown syndrome describes a process which is believed to characterize the dynamic relationship between personal susceptibility, negative labeling, and the development of psychological weakness. This could easily be applied to the pattern of personal deterioration of many elderly individuals in American society.

Kuypers and Bengston (14) have developed an alternate model which they call the social reconstruction syndrome. Their model suggests that assistance to the aging individual at various points along the social breakdown syndrome can result in an entirely different outcome. Instead of ending in a sick dependent role, Kuypers and Bengston (14) suggest that the social reconstruction model posits that assistance be provided to individuals in such a way that their sense of independence is increased by the building of their confidence in maintenance and coping skills (Fig. 3.7).

First, efforts can be made to liberate the individual from an age-inappropriate view of his status; the functional ethic which suggests that self-worth is contingent on performance in an economic or productive social position is particularly inappropriate in old age. In counseling, for example, one might urge the older person to adopt a more humanitarian frame of self-judgment and not to judge himself on the basis of productivity alone. Urge the individual to assume family, volunteer, and community roles which may be badly needed but are not rewarded in the form of wages and salaries. Thus, the individual will be encouraged to feel confident and useful.

Second, improved social services to older persons can enhance their adaptive capacity by lessening the debilitation of environmental conditions such as poor housing, poor health and poverty. Providing older adults with a handyman who cleans the gutters, takes care of the yard, and maintains the furnace and other appliances may allow them to remain living independently in their own homes much longer. This would increase confidence in the ability to cope with the environment.

Third, the ability to live independently and (with assistance) manage the home and environment will enable older persons to have an internal locus of control and to define themselves as able. The self-confidence of the elderly in their abilities can be maintained if those who serve them give up some of their own power and control and allow self-determination in the direction of programs serving them. Imagine an old age home whose personnel and decision-making bodies are comprised of the elderly themselves, while the nursing and social service staff might be younger people. Imagine a program of continuing education administered by an elderly council rather than controlled by the extension division of existing colleges.

Cousert (5) utilized the social breakdown

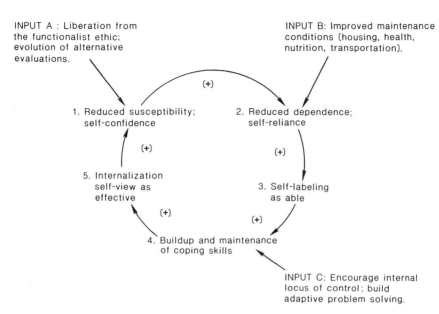

Figure 3.7. The social reconstruction syndrome (a benign cycle of increasing competence through social system inputs). (From Bengtson VL: *The Social Psychology of Aging*, p 48. Indianapolis, IN, Bobbs-Merrill Co., ©1973, The Bobbs-Merrill Company, Inc.)

syndrome and the social reconstruction model to explain the tendencies of older persons to visit medical doctors more frequently and mental health professionals less frequently. This pattern seems unusual when doctors who treat older patients estimate that anywhere from 40–75% of the people they see have psychological and psychosomatic problems rather than physcial ones. Sainsbury (20) conducted an investigation of the mental health of older people which indicated that both psychosis and psychosomatic systems increased after age 65. A study done in New York City found that, among persons with impaired mental health, 34% of those between the ages 20 and 29 had seen a doctor, while only 21% of those between the ages of 50 and 54 had done so (9). The older the patient, the less likely he/she is to see doctors about emotional problems.

Utilizing a labeling perspective, Cousert (5) argues that older persons avoid visits to mental health professionals because such visits could precipitate their being negatively labeled by family and friends, the mental health personnel perhaps, and ultimately themselves. Being labeled mentally ill is problematic at any age in life, but it has particularly dire consequences for older persons, who at best will be treated as though they are senile or at worst could be institutionalized by the doctor or their families. Moreover, the negative labeling may well destroy an already uncertain self-concept on the part of the individual.

Cousert (5) believes that treating an older person as though he/she is feeble and senile may encourage the individual to behave this way, even if he or she is perfectly healthy. The sociological concept of reference groups suggests that, as persons begin to identify with a group such as the elderly, they will take on some of the significant characteristics of the group. Social psychologists believe that a person seeks maximum congruency among the aspects of self-concept, self-behavior toward other persons, and perceptions of the behavior of others toward him or her.

There are a number of reasons why the older person may avoid visiting a mental health professional. First, as noted above, the individual may fear being negatively labeled by significant others following a visit to a psychiatrist. Second, older persons themselves may hold a negative view of psychiatrists and of persons who undergo psychiatric treatment. Their own negative attitudes toward mental health treatment as well as the fear of being labeled as senile or mentally ill are strong deterrents against visiting a psychiatrist.

Figure 3.8 follows Zusman's (28) social breakdown model and explains in more detail why older persons avoid visiting mental health professionals. Once again we begin at the point where the individual's self-confidence is shaken because he is currently experiencing some problems (Fig. 3.8, Step 1). He visits a psychiatrist who does not immediately assure him

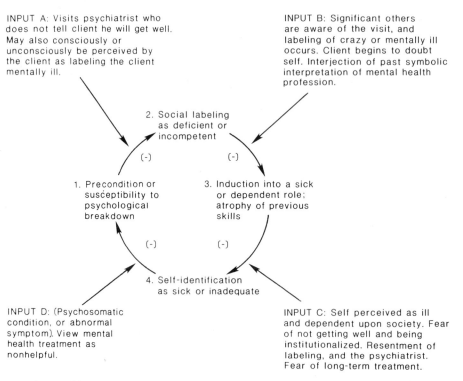

Figure 3.8. The social breakdown syndrome—going to a psychiatrist. (Adapted from Cousert D: The attitude of Older People toward Visiting a Psychiatrist. Unpublished paper, Indiana State University, 1977.)

that he will get well but tells him instead that his problem may require further diagnosis and office visits (Input A). This may be perceived by the client as proof that he is mentally ill and has a serious problem (Step 2). Friends and family come to know that the individual has visited a psychiatrist and is going to have to make other visits. They begin to define the individual as senile or losing his mind, thus labeling him as incompetent (Input B). The person is encouraged by those around him to act sick, and previous interpersonal skills begin to deteriorate. The patient becomes increasingly frightened. He is now afraid of not getting well or of perhaps being institutionalized (Input C). He begins to think and to act as through he were sick. Thus a further deterioration of self-confidence and further changes in behavior occur.

The outcome for the older person that visits a medical doctor, Cousert (5) believes, more nearly approximates the social reconstruction model. In Figure 3.9 we see that the older person with a shaken self-confidence and uncertain identity visits a medical doctor with a health problem (Fig. 3.9, Step 1). The doctor, after examining the patient, tells him that he is not seriously ill and will get well if he follows the doctor's instructions. The doctor often gives

the patient a mild tranquilizer or perhaps something to lower his blood pressure (Input A). The patient's uncertainty is eased, and self-confidence returns (Fig. 3.9, Step 2). The patient feels no further need to visit a doctor for the particular symptom and routinely gets the medicine refilled (Input B). The individual gains confidence in his ability to handle his problem. Significant others, in hearing the doctor's report, now define the older person as having only a minor physical illness. Prognosis for recovery is excellent. The individual is treated as normal by significant others (Input C). This tends to bolster the individual's self-confidence, thus building maintenance and coping skills (Fig. 3.9, step 4). The individual can now internalize a view of himself as capable of dealing with his problems. If the need arises he will return to the doctor who so ably helped him through the first crisis.

Thus Cousert is able to use the social breakdown and social reconstruction models to explain the differential attitudes of older persons toward the psychiatrist versus the medical doctor (5). He believes the older person is likely to receive reassurance and a reduction of his anxiety about his health from the medical doctor but may inadvertently receive information from the psychiatrist that leads to further anx-

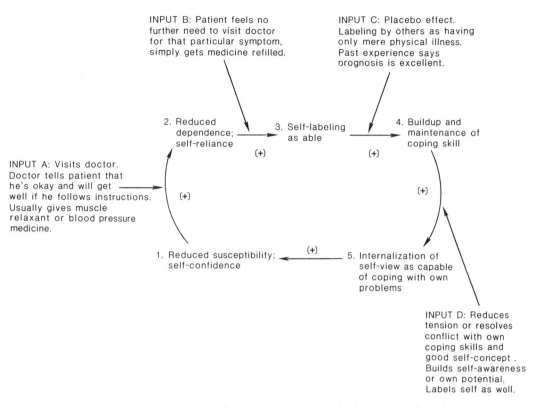

INPUT B: Patient feels no further need to visit doctor for that particular symptom, simply gets medicine refilled.

INPUT C: Placebo effect. Labeling by others as having only mere physical illness. Past experience says prognosis is excellent.

INPUT A: Visits doctor. Doctor tells patient that he's okay and will get well if he follows instructions. Usually gives muscle relaxant or blood pressure medicine.

2. Reduced dependence; self-reliance

3. Self-labeling as able

4. Buildup and maintenance of coping skill

1. Reduced susceptibility; self-confidence

5. Internalization of self-view as capable of coping with own problems

INPUT D: Reduces tension or resolves conflict with own coping skills and good self-concept . Builds self-awareness or own potential. Labels self as well.

Figure 3.9. The social reconstruction syndrome—going to a medical doctor. (Adapted from Cousert D: Symbolic Interactionist Approach to Attitude of Older People toward Psychiatrists versus Medical Doctors. Unpublished paper, Indiana State University, 1977.)

iety and a loss of self-confidence. If Cousert is correct, this would in part explain the very low number of older persons who seek out the services of mental health professionals.

Aging as Exchange

Dowd (8) argues that the weakness of both disengagement and activity theories is that researchers in the past have taken the underlying assumptions of these theories as givens, without ever questioning their validity. Neither theory attempts to adequately answer the question of why social interaction decreases in old age. Instead, this is taken as a given which requires no further explanation. Rather than assuming automatically and without question that social interaction decreases in later life, Dowd argues that we should first determine: does social interaction decrease, and if so, why?

Dowd (8) asserts that the exchange model can perhaps best explain the decreased social interaction patterns of older Americans. This exchange model views the decreased social interaction of older persons as resulting from

an intricate process of exchange between society and its older population, associated with the power-dependent relationships of the elderly. The basic premises on which exchange theory rests are:

1. Society is made up of social actors in pursuit of common goals.
2. Pursuing these goals, actors enter social relations with other actors which entail some cost in the form of time, energy, effort, and wealth.
3. Actors expect to reap as their reward the achievement of desired goals; for this they are willing to assume the necessary costs.
4. Regardless of the nature of the exchange relationship, each actor will attempt to maximize rewards and minimize costs.
5. Exchange processes are more than an economic transaction, since they involve intrinsic psychological satisfaction and need gratification.
6. Only those activities that are economical will be repeated (3).

Power enters the exchange relationship when one of the participants in the exchange values the rewards gained in the relationship more that the other participant. The exchange theorists' view of power is that it is derived from imbalances in the social exchange. Blau (3) argues that much of social life is an intricate exchange in which each participant in the social interaction approaches and withdraws in patterns that add to or subtract from his or her store of power and prestige.

In viewing aging as exchange, Dowd (8) asserts that the decreased social interaction of older persons is the result of a series of exchange relationships, in which the power of older persons relative to their social environment is gradually diminished, until all that remains of their power resources is the humble capacity to comply. Where the worker was once able to exchange skills, knowledge, or expertise for needed wages, the final exchange becomes one of compliance with mandatory retirement in return for sustenance in the form of social security, retirement pensions, and Medicare. Thus from the exchange perspective, the probability of continued engagement in social relationships is principally a function of the already existing relationship between the aging person and society. The skills of many aging workers may rapidly become outmoded, resulting in an unfavorable power balance between the aging worker and the employer. The end result of the unfavorable power balance is that the older worker is forced to retire.

Blau (3) notes that, in any complex work organization, there are limited resources; therefore it is possible for management to balance one exchange relationship only by unbalancing others. As one group gains a relative advantage, another group is threatened. Younger workers exchange their labor for wages and the implicit promise of job security and promotion. The longer the older worker remains on the job, the more he or she is blocking the career path of younger workers.

From the perspective of exchange theory, then, aging workers primarily face the problem of decreasing power resources. As their particular skill becomes outmoded they have little to exchange that is of critical value. One answer, therefore, to the question of why older persons disengage is not that it is mutually satisfying for the individual and society, but rather that in the exchange relationship between older persons and society, society enjoys a distinct advantage (8).

The exchange theory offers a new perspective from which to view the process of aging and the interaction between the individual and the social system. Only future research will be able to determine the value of this approach as an explanation of the aging process.

CONCLUSION

The 20th century has witnessed the gradual but steadily increasing number and percentage of the American population living to age 65 and beyond. Moreover, demographic projections indicate that this trend is likely to continue for the next 40 to 50 years.

While the older population has been increasing, the number and percentage of the population made up of those under the age of 19 has been decreasing. The result has been that there is very little change in the dependency ratio (which is basically a measure of how many in the working years, 19 to 65, are supporting how many of those out of the working years, under 18 and over 65). The shift in the dependent group from younger to older ages has resulted in an increased demand for government services to support older persons. While the American family has placed a high value on the rearing of young children, and most people would feel deprived if not allowed to rear their children, they have not held the same attitude toward their older family members. Americans appear to be anxious to shift the responsibility for older family members off themselves and onto the government. The result is an ever increasing demand for government services for older Americans.

The past 40 to 50 years have seen sociologists and other social scientists advocate a number of different perspectives with which to view the social realities of aging. The disengagement and activity perspectives were the earliest developed and appeared to be as much philosophies of life as they were theories. Subsequently continuity, symbolic interaction, and exchange theories were utilized to examine the problems and opportunities of later life.

The continuity theory seemed to bridge the gap between disengagement and activity theory by asserting that disengagement was more selective than inevitable; older persons carefully choose which roles they will maintain and which they will give up as they attempt to lead a preferred style of life. Moreover, they will choose how active or inactive they would prefer to be in the later part of the life cycle.

Symbolic interaction and exchange theories provided considerably different perspectives for viewing the social realities of aging. The symbolic interactionist basically argues that, in order to understand the lives of older Americans, you must understand the norms, values, and attitudes of society toward aging. The symbolic interactionist would like to know what roles older Americans assume and how important they are considered to be by others in the social system. The social reconstruction model which was derived from a symbolic interaction perspective indicates a number of inputs that could be made by others in the social system in order to assist older persons in maintaining their independence.

The exchange perspective looks carefully at the power exercised by the individual. Exchange theorists view older persons as involved in a number of exchanges of power with others in the social system; each exchange results in a loss of power for the elderly participant. Ultimately the older person has no choice but to surrender any power exercised in adult life in exchange for a retirement income.

Which of the theoretical perspectives offered to explain the social realities of aging will prove most valid is still undecided. These diverse perspectives certainly offer researchers a number of disparate approaches to take in examining the aging process.

References

1. Allen C, Brotman H: *Chartbook on Aging in America.* Washington, DC, Administration on Aging, 1981.
2. Bengston VL: *The Social Psychology of Aging.* Indianapolis, Bobbs-Merrill, 1973.
3. Blau PM: *Exchange and Power in Social Life.* New York, John Wiley, 1964.
4. Cooley CH: *The Nature of Human Nature.* New York, Charles Scribners' & Sons, 1902.
5. Cousert D: Symbolic Interactionist Approach to Attitudes of Older People toward Psychiatrist versus Medical Doctors. Unpublished paper, Indiana State University, 1977.
6. Cowgill D: *Aging around the World.* Belmont, CA, Wadsworth, 1986.
7. Cumming E, Henry WH: *Growing Old.* New York, Basic Books, 1961.
8. Dowd JJ: Aging as exchange: a preface to theory. *J. Gerontol* 30:584−94, 1975.
9. Foner A, Riley M: *Aging and Society: An Inventory of Research Findings,* Vol. 1. New York, Russell Sage, 1968.
10. Harris L. & Associates: *The Myth and Reality of Aging in America.* Washington, D.C., National Council on the Aging, 1975.
11. Havighurst RJ: Successful aging. In Williams RH, Tibbit, C Donahue W (eds): *Process of Aging.* New York Lieber-Atherton, 1963, p 229.
12. Jeffers FC, Nichols CR: The effects of aging on activities and attitudes to physical well-being in older people. In Palmore E (ed): *Normal Aging.* Durham, NC, Duke University Press, 1970, pp 301−310.
13. Kalish RA: Of social values and the dying: a defense of disengagment. *Fam Coord* 21:81−94, 1972.
14. Kuypers JA, Bengtson VL: Social breakdown and competence: a model of normal aging. *Hum Dev* 16 (2): 37−49, 1973.
15. Lemon BW, Bengtson VL, Peterson JA: Activity types and life satisfaction in a retirement community. *J Gerontol* 27:511−23, 1972.
16. Maddox G: Disengagement theory: a critical evaluation. *Gerontologist* 4:80−82, 1964.
17. Mead GH: *Mind, Self and Society.* Chicago, University of Chicago Press, 1934.
18. Parsons T: *The Social System.* New York, Free Press, 1951.
19. Peterson W: Lecture given at the Critical Problems of Aging workshop, Indiana State University, June 1976.
20. Sainsbury P: Suicide and depressions: recent development in affective disorders. In Cooper A, Walk A (eds): *British Journal of Psychiatry Special Publication,* No. 2, 1968.
21. Schick FL: *Statistical Handbook on Aging Americans.* Phoenix, AZ, Oryx Press, 1986.
22. Stryker S: Symbolic interaction as an approach to family research. *Marriage Fam Liv* 21:111−119, 1959.
23. Thomas WI: *Primitive Behavior: An Introduction to the Social Sciences.* New York, McGraw-Hill, 1937.
24. U.S. Bureau of the Census: Distribution of the Older Population by Age Group.
25. U.S. Bureau of the Census: Number of Persons Age 65 and Older and Under 18, per 100 Persons aged 18−64, 1930−1980 and Projections to 2050.
26. U.S. Bureau of the Census: Rates of Increase 65 and Older Population and Older vs. Total U.S. Population 1900−1975.
27. U.S. Bureau of the Census, Social Security Administration: U.S. Population Age 65 and Older 1900-2030.
28. Zusman J: Some explanations of the changing appearance of psychologic patients: antecedents of the social breakdown syndrome concept. *The Mullbank Memorial Fund Quarterly* 64 (1):2, 1966.

4 Physiology of Aging

RICHARD A. KENNEY

Editor's Note

The most tangible aspects of the normal aging process are those physical changes that frequently begin in middle adulthood and continue until death. Certainly, the physiology of aging (in the absence of any specific disease processes) has been extensively researched. In Chapter 4, author Kenney has synopsized the available literature into a compact but thorough manual of physiological aging. The reader should return to this chapter frequently as a reference source in understanding the physical aspects of aging and the potential effects of physiological changes upon communication behaviors and interventions. In particular, speech-language pathologists and audiologists will be interested in the sections on respiration, the cardiovascular system, the nervous system, the special senses, and the mouth. Kenney has carefully selected key references for those interested in further reading on a specific topic. Special note should also be made of the discussion of homeostasis early in the chapter. It is suggested that the process of aging can be viewed as a period of failing physiological homeostasis. Subsequent chapters highlight the potential disturbances in emotional and familial homeostasis created by communication breakdown. Thus, it is clear that our intervention programs must become responsive to the older adult's need for establishing and maintaining some form of intra- and interpersonal equilibrium, albeit an altered one.

Aging is a part of a continuum of changing function which begins at conception and is terminated by death. All too often, our interest is concentrated on just one part of this continuum—the adult years—so that differences in the function of the body in the years on either side of this central range come to be regarded as deviations from the normal rather than manifestations of a shifting state of normality. When we speak of a "physiology of aging," we are acknowledging that bodily function changes with the passage of years without there being any disease process involved. On the other hand, many disease processes profoundly affecting function show an increasing incidence with increasing age. Consequently, when one is confronted with a state of altered function, it is difficult to separate out the two components: one the effect of aging per se (sometimes termed the "eugeric" process) and the other the effect of disease (or "pathogeric") process (26).

When we examine the continuum of changing function over the whole life span, it becomes apparent that, while some alterations have clear milestones (such as the ability to handle solid food, eruption of teeth, and menarche), other changes are much more subtle and extremely variable in their time of occurrence. The changes of aging fall into this latter group and, in contrast with the changes of function which are part of development and maturation, are typically decremental in nature, linear with time rather than "step functions."

Physiological changes of aging can be classified in several ways. A typical scheme is as follows:

1. Functions which are totally lost; for example, reproductive capability or the ability to hear sounds above a critical frequency;
2. Functions which are impaired by the loss of functional units with surviving units showing essentially normal activity; for example, the kidney and, to a large extent, skeletal muscle;
3. Functions which become less efficient, an example being the slowing of speed of conduction in nerves;
4. Functions which are altered in a secondary fashion such as the elevated circulating levels of the gonadotrophic hormones when primary depression of the gonadal secretions there occurs;
5. The exceptional case of functional increases such as the tonic contraction of the vascular smooth muscle or the rate of secretion of the antidiuretic hormone in response to a change in the osmotic pressure of the body fluids.

Man possesses a wonderful set of mechanisms which serve to maintain within the body optimum conditions for the working of the constituent cells and tissues. The constancy of this internal environment, maintained by the process of homeostasis, makes possible life in a broad spectrum of external environments. Homeostasis is, in fact, our defense against the challenges of daily life on our planet—extremes of temperature, broad ranges of physical activity, and the like. At the two extremes of our time scale, this homeostatic defense is somewhat less perfect than in the young adult; both the very young and the very old need some additional protection from environmental challenges. In other words, the process of aging can be considered as a period of failing homeostasis.

Primitive man had very little chance of aging. Without the protections of a social organization and of technology, deterioration of physiological function made him easy prey to a hostile environment. Failing vision, failing hearing, loss of teeth, and loss of muscular strength all worked together to make a long survival unlikely.

In contrast, man's current life span makes him a special case in several ways. In general, the greater the body weight of a species among the mammals, the greater the life span; man's life span is greater than would be predicted on this basis. Life span shows a similar relationship with the weight of the brain and here man fits more nearly perfectly (32). Before assuming that our relatively oversized brain has in some ways provided for our longevity, however, it needs to be mentioned that the same relationship can be found with the weight of the adrenal gland. Another human peculiarity is that life span in the female is approaching twice the reproductive life span.

The concept of aging as a progressive failure of homeostasis implies nothing more than that in the total absence of disease and accidental death, man would die of "natural causes" (12, 13). The pace of decrement of function differs from individual to individual so that "biological age" bears a variable relation to chronological age. This raises the question of man's maximum potential life span (MPLS). Some believe that this MPLS has remained fixed for millenia at about 100 years; others believe that the MPLS is, in fact, far greater than any life span yet achieved (8). Taking the former position, medical progress of this century can be seen as enabling increasing numbers of people to more nearly achieve their potential for survival.

The powerful incentive of a desire to slow aging, and thereby defer death, has focused major attention on the fundamental cause of aging. While superficially we may say that aging and death are the product of deterioration and ultimately failure of homeostasis, we need to examine the process at the cellular level, since man's overall function is a product of the function of cells.

CELLULAR AGING (19, 33)

The cells of the body have a broad range of life spans: the cells lining the intestinal tract have a life of only 4 to 5 days before being replaced; the red blood cells live for about 120 days; and the cells of muscle and the nerve cells survive for our whole life span. Cells like the intestinal cells or the red blood cells are constantly being replaced by new cells formed by a population of primitive cells which continue to divide and mature. Muscle cells and neurons are fixed cells which are not replaced. Even in cells which run their course in a few days, signs of aging can be found either in their structure or their function. One common sign of cellular aging is the accumulation within the cell of a pigmented material, lipofuscin, which sometimes comes to occupy the greater part of the cell interior. This observation gave rise to the so-called "clinker" theory of aging; so much of this material accumulated in the furnace as to obstruct its normal function. Lipofuscin appears to be debris derived from membranes and other constituents of the cells which have been damaged in some way.

One way in which cells may be damaged is by oxidation of the lipid components by so-called free radicals. These are chemical entities which bear an extra electrical charge and which take part in many chains of metabolic processes within the cell. In this role, radicals are bound or confined to elements of subcellular structure. When free or unbound, they work adversely upon the cell. The resultant action of superoxidation is the basis of the free radical theory of aging of cells. This is an attractive theory since superoxidation can be prevented by the so-called antioxidants, of which vitamins C and E are well known examples. Another common and very powerful antioxidant is BHT, which is used to retard the development of rancidity in confectionery products. Vitamins C and E together with BHT enjoy large sales as agents to retard aging although evidence that they are effective in this role is, at best, scanty.

Another theory of aging is the so-called error theory. This places the phenomenon in the cell's informational system, the DNA and RNA molecules which govern and direct the synthesis of proteins within the cell. The theory proposes that errors occur either at the stage of transcription or translation of the genetic information. Errors lead to the synthesis of materials no longer capable of supporting the metabolism. These errors may arise because of damage (for example, by radiation or other environmental factors) coupled with an inadequate ability of the cell to repair the damage that occurs. The genetic material of the cells has a high degree of redundancy so that only about 1% or less is necessary for control of synthesis. As damage occurs, this redundancy is used up. The error theory of aging thus has two subtheories, one of repair failure and one of exhaustion of redundancy.

Another theory concerns the immune system which normally operates to defend the body against foreign materials which gain entry. Essential to this function is the ability of the immune system to recognize foreign material as distinct from the body's own structural materials. The immune theory postulates that as the system ages, this ability to distinguish "self" from "not-self" becomes impaired and the body mounts an immune response to its own tissues, damaging their function. This theory, like the free radical theory, is attractive because it is potentially accessible to manipulation via hormones which regulate the immune system and which are able to be isolated from the thymus gland. Through hormonal regulation, some believe aging might be delayed.

The theory which is perhaps best supported by direct experiment suggests that cells are in fact "programmed" to age and die (18). If some of the cells which provide the supporting tissues of the body, the fibroblasts, are removed and grown in artifical solutions, they will grow and divide and will double in number about 50 times if the source of the original cells was a young person and about 20 times if taken from an elderly person. Moreover, if cells are taken from a child suffering from "progeria" or any other disease which simulates aging (30), they divide only a few times. If a culture of cells from a young person is allowed to divide, say 20 times, and then is frozen in liquid nitrogen, the cells can be preserved for many years. If at the end of that time the deep-frozen cells are thawed, they again begin to grow and divide and do so the number times (e.g., 30 times) which remained uncompleted at the time they were frozen. Thus, the cells have a memory as well as a program. Fascinating as these experiments are, there can be no certainty that this programmed aging is important for cells in their normal situation in the body.

If an animal, maintained under controlled experimental conditions, is fed a diet which is less than adequate to support the normal rate of growth, the life span of the animal is increased, as is the time to reach maturity. While there is abundant evidence that the prevalent form of malnutrition found in our society, namely, excessive calorie intake, tends to shorten life, there is at present no evidence that relative undernutrition will change man's potential life span, although it may be a factor in letting him more nearly approach his potential.

BODY CONFORMATION AND COMPOSITION (31)

Significant changes occur in both the conformation and composition of the body as it ages. There is a tendency for loss of stature without there being any change in the length of the arms, so that one can obtain an appreciation of an individual's stature in youth from a measurement of arm span. This question of aging loss of standing height is an illustration of one of the difficulties in describing the normal aging changes. If we were to measure today the standing height of some hundreds of men with ages ranging from 20 to 80 years, we would certainly see an impressive difference in the height of those 20 and those of 80. Much of this difference, however, would have nothing to do with aging. It would simply be a reflection of the fact that 20 year olds in the 1980s are taller that 20 year olds of 60, 40, or 20 years ago. In other words, a change in height is a secular change. There is, however, a true but small aging loss in height which is accounted for by collapse of the arches of the foot, narrowing of the joint spaces of the legs, and an increasing curvature of the spine. The diameter of the chest tends to increase due to a loss of the elastic collapsing force of the lungs which normally prevents the chest wall from expanding. The nose and the ears continue to grow in length throughout life; the eyes become sunken into their sockets as fatty tissue from the orbit is lost. The circumference of the head enlarges as bone is laid down on the skull, although this change is often obscured by the loss of hair from the scalp. If one needs a mnemonic of these conformational changes, a good caricature is provided by the senior of Snow White's dwarfs.

The gross composition of the body also changes. We can divide the body weight into three basic elements: water, fat, and nonfat solids. A healthy average young man has about 60% of body weight as water, 18% as fat, and the remaining 22% as nonfat solids which are largely protein but include a substantial contribution from the mineral of bone. The equivalent figures for a healthy young female would show 30% of the body weight as fat and correspondingly lesser fractions as water and non-fat solids. With aging, there occurs in both sexes a loss of lean body mass and an increase in adipose tissue. Usually, this begins by 40 years of age and is progressive until about 70 in the male and somewhat later in the female. The total body weight tends to remain surprisingly constant until these latter ages. The extra adiposity which come with aging is largely situated within the body, in and around organs rather than in subcutaneous sites which, in fact, tend to lose fat. This is shown by the fall in skin fold thickness (the "you can't pinch an inch" test). The loss of lean tissue and the loss of the water component of body weight is of particular significance in establishing appropriate doses of drugs for older people, since many drugs distribute only in the water compartment. If drug dosage were to be based on body weight alone, there would be a chance of too high a concentration being reached.

AGING OF TISSUES (17)

Another basis on which to examine aging changes is in terms of major tissues: the supporting tissues which include bone, cartilage, tendons, ligaments, and the more diffuse connective tissue which serves to locate and support other tissues; the muscle, both that which serves posture and movement and the special muscle of the heart; and the epithelial tissues which cover the body and line the body spaces. All of these elements show significant change.

The supporting tissues of the body share a common origin in a cell called the fibroblast which can differentiate to fulfill several functions, all of which involve secretion of material by the cell. In the simplest of tissues this secretion is in the form of "ground substance" which is a gel around the cells. The next stage of elaboration is the secretion of fibers by the fibroblast, either very fine fibers (reticular fibers) which form a meshwork with the gel or more specialized fibers, one collagen which is used to provide rigidity and strength and the other elastin, which gives the property of elasticity. The ligaments which bind bones together are largely a mixture of these two types of fiber; the tendons which connect muscle to the bones of the skeleton are bundles of collagen fibers. Elastic tissue is found in the blood vessels, the heart, and the lungs as well as beneath the skin where it is responsible for holding the skin bunched and taut against the underlying tissue.

Fibroblasts can become converted to the formation of cartilage, which forms either unions or bearing surfaces between bones or sometimes provides the actual form to a body part such as the ears or part of the nose. This cartilage may be either clear and rubbery, or it may contain elastic or collagen fibers when strength and resistance are required. The fibroblast may also become converted to a bone cell which plays the special role of causing bone mineral to be deposited on a framework of fibrous connective tissue or cartilage.

The aging changes which occur in all of these varieties of supporting tissue have profound functional results. The gel of ground substance around the cells becomes less hydrated, and this can interfere with the diffusion of material from the blood into the tissue cells. Collagen fibers as they age tend to become bound more tightly together and become more rigid. When this occurs in the fibers surrounding the joints, the result is joint stiffness and extra effort in moving the limbs. Elastic fibers, on the other hand, tend to become frayed and to disintegrate, resulting in a loss of elasticity. The elastic tissue in the walls of arteries becomes replaced by collagen, so that the blood vessels "harden" and become more rigid. Loss of elastic tissue from the walls of veins leads to a weakening of these vessels so that varicosities develop. Changes in the connective tissue of the organs of phonation are revealed by a change in the timbre of the voice.

Cartilage as it ages becomes less pliable and is often invaded by fibers. In the joints, this results in the cartilaginous bearing surfaces becoming more friable and thus eroding with movement of the joint. The stiffening of the pads of cartilage which unite the ribs with the sternum makes movement of the chest wall in breathing more difficult. The pads of fibrous cartilage which form the discs between the vertebrae tend to shrink, causing some shortening of the spine. In the cervical portions of the spine, this shortening can cause a kinking of the vertebral arteries which supply blood to the brain and is thus an underlying cause of one of the varieties of transient ischemic attack, brief lapses of consciousness, to which old people are susceptible. When fibrous tissue or cartilage becomes sufficiently dense with aging, there is a tendency for calcium salts to be deposited on the matrix, and this process may go to the point where true bone is formed even within organs.

As true bone ages, it loses mineral, creating the condition of osteoporosis. This loss occurs in both sexes, usually with an onset around 40 years of age, but in the female proceeds at an accelerating rate after menopause. In the long bones, remodeling of the bones in response to changing stress is a lifelong process which involves bone being removed from some areas while mineral is laid down in other sites. As the long bones age, mineral continues to be laid down on the outside while the inner surface is being eroded. The result in that the diameter of the bone increases, and the wall becomes thinner. In the female, this weakening of the bone proceeds to such an extent that vertebrae are in danger of collapse and the spine becomes excessively curved (the "dowager's hump"). One woman in five at 80 years of age suffers a hip fracture. The maintenance of adequate density of bone mineral by a combination of dietary supplementation of calcium, the beneficial effects of the bone stress resulting from exercise, and possibly estrogen replacement could potentially save society the several billions of dollars annually which are the cost of hospitalization and subsequent institutionalization of old persons suffering disabling fractures. Decalcification of the ribs can so weaken them that they can no longer support the tension of the respiratory muscles. The chest becomes "pinched," with disastrous consequences for breathing.

A major part of the loss of lean tissue mass which is characteristic of aging is attributable to loss of muscle. Skeletal muscle consists of fibers which are organized into functional units termed motor units. Each motor unit receives its nerve supply from a single nerve cell. These motor units vary greatly in the number of muscle fibers which they contain. Massive muscles whose function is largely the maintenance of posture against the force of gravity have units each containing thousands of fibers; small muscles responsible for very fine movements have motor units of only 4 or 5 fibers. The typical aging process in muscles is a progressive loss of muscle fibers and loss of motor nerve fibers. The loss of the former occurs at a greater rate than the latter so that the individual motor units become smaller in size. The result can be a perception of increasing effort required for a muscular task since our perception of effort is measured in terms of the number of motor units which need to be recruited to provide the necessary power. A major cause of loss of muscle mass is disuse. Nowhere more than in muscle is there truth in the "use it or lose it" concept (3). Changes in muscle power relate closely to the loss of muscle mass. In the aging muscle fibers, there is accumulation of aging pigment, and there are signs that synthesis of protein continues to occur. Any new protein synthesized, however, fails to become organized for contraction and so makes no contribution to muscle strength. As fibers are lost within a muscle, part of the mass is replaced by fibrous connective tissue and fat. At the functional level, the speed with which the muscle contracts

is reduced as is also the speed of relaxation (34).

The cells covering the body surface are referred to as epithelia. Because they are exposed to the external environment, they are subjected to wear and tear and are replaced rather frequently. It is important to recall that in addition to the skin, the linings of the alimentary tract, the airways and the lungs, the bladder and the kidneys, and the vagina are all in contact with the external environment. The epithelial coverings are of several types; some are moist and delicately thin, while others are thick and have relatively impervious coverings. The function of the skin is protective and forms a barrier preventing loss of water vapor from the body and preventing entry of materials from the environment. The skin also serves as a major avenue by which heat can be exchanged with the environment. Associated with the skin are the so-called adnexa (hairs, glands, and nails); in addition, the skin contains nerve endings which serve as receptors of information from the environment.

As the skin ages (6, 16), the rate of renewal of the cells falls and the skin thins out, becoming in the very old almost transparent. It ceases to be an effective barrier against, for example, infection. Hair-producing follicles are lost, and in a few of the very old, the skin may become totally hairless. The glands of the skin are of three basic varieties: those producing an oily secretion which serves to reduce the water permeability of the skin; those situated in the axillae and the groin, which have a rather viscid odiferous secretion; and the sweat glands, whose role it is to provide, when necessary, large quantities of watery secretion which can be evaporated to cool the body. In the old person, all three types of glands are reduced in number; the skin tends to become drier as the oily or sebaceous secretion is lost; and, with the loss of sweat glands, the skin becomes less efficient in the regulation of the body temperature. Nails tend to thicken and become pigmented. Longitudinal ridges develop along the nail, and the typical half-moon at the base of the nail is reduced in size. Nervous receptors in the skin are lost, and this results in some impairment of the sensations which arise through the skin—sensations of heat and cold, touch, pressure, and pain (6). However, the fact that the skin is also becoming thinner tends to counter the loss of some receptors, and the older person may in fact have an increased sensitivity to pain.

The epithelial surfaces which form the inner surface of the body show mainly a reduction in the rate at which new cells are formed. Cells covering the surface of the alimentary tract, instead of being replaced every 4 days, may stay in place for 5 days. The moist, multilayered epithelia such as those lining the vagina or the mouth become thinned out. The cells covering the surface of the airways tend to lose their hair-like processes (cilia) and so are less well equipped to prevent inhaled particles from finding their way deep into the lungs. This lining epithelium contains cells which produce mucus which also serves to trap particulate matter. In the airways of the old, this secretion is reduced, further impairing the protective function.

AGING OF THE BLOOD (22)

For a long time, it was believed that a mild degree of anemia was a natural consequence of aging. However, more careful study has shown this not to be the case. Older people who are living a normal life within the community have a red cell concentration and a hemoglobin concentration which is within normal limits. The lower values are to be found in institutionalized individuals and are probably a reflection of less adequate nutrition and of a less active life-style.

The red blood cell has a life span of about 120 days; in other words, the red cell-generating tissue, the bone marrow, is called upon to generate each day nearly 1% of the body's complement of these special cells (approximately 25×10^{12} cells) and to synthesize about 7 g per day of the oxygen-carrying protein hemoglobin. Even in the oldest individual, the hemoglobin has exactly the same composition as in the youngest, evidence that this synthetic process is conducted without error for decades.

One impairment shown by the aged is in the response to a loss of blood. In a young person, the loss is rapidly made good by increasing the rate of formation of new cells. In the old person, restoration is no less complete but takes longer to accomplish. Fundamental to the maintenance of adequate levels of hemoglobin are the nutritional supplies of protein, iron, vitamin B_{12}, the secretion of an intrinsic factor in the gastric juice, and good absorption of these elements from the alimentary tract. All of these items may be threatened in one way or another in the older individual. Nonetheless, overall function is maintained at a perfectly adequate level.

The concentration of protein in the plasma fraction of the blood tends to fall slightly, and this can reduce the extent to which some substances, especially drugs, are bound to protein during their carriage in the blood. This can increase the free concentration of substances to which the tissues are exposed. The total blood volume falls with age at about the same rate as the lean body mass diminishes so that harmony is maintained between the oxygen-supplying tissue, blood, and the oxygen-using tissues.

THE AGING LUNG (4, 27)

The lung is designed to provide an interface between the atmosphere, with which the body exchanges gases, and the blood, which serves a role of mass transit for these gases to and from the active cells where oxygen is used and carbon dioxide produced. This interface is the "alveolar membrane," which consists of a very thin layer of epithelial cells, a layer of endothelial cells which form the wall of the capillary blood vessels, and a little fine connective tissue. Blood perfuses these fine blood vessels from the right side of the heart and returns to the left side of the heart for distribution to the body. Although the volume of blood perfusing this system is large (5 liters/minute at rest and as much as 25 liters/minute in heavy exercise), the pressure of the blood is low because the resistance to blood flow on this circuit is low. Oxygen is constantly being used and carbon dioxide produced, and so the air which is presented to the blood at the alveolar membrane must constantly be renewed by the rhythmical act of ventilation.

The lungs consist of a system of branching conduits or airways which terminate in collections of alveoli, partly spherical sacs formed by the alveolar membrane. In spite of their fine structure, the lungs are passive structures which are ventilated by being stretched by the changes in volume of the thorax occurring as a result of the muscular movements of breathing. The lungs are elastic and recoil when the stretching forces are removed. Inspiration, the entry of air to the lungs, is an active process while the exit of air is generally passive. The movements of the thorax are transmitted to the lungs by a layer of fluid which is constantly present between them and the layer of tissue which lines the entire cavity of the thorax.

There are two components to the changing volumes in the thorax. One occurs by movements of the ribs, the costal component, and the other by movement of the diaphragm. The ribs are joined by flexible pads of cartilage to the sternum in front and to the vertebrae in the back. Between the ribs run bands of muscle arranged in two discrete systems. One set of muscles—the external intercostals—are so arranged that when they contract, they pull the ribs upward. When the second set—the internal intercostals—shorten, they serve to depress the ribs. With elevation of the ribs, the diameter of the thorax increases; with depression, the volume is reduced. The diaphragm, which forms the partition between the thorax and the abdomen, is a flat sheet of muscle which when relaxed is convex upward. When the muscle contracts, the diaphragm loses its convexity and by lengthening the thorax, increases its volume. Additional muscles are brought into play when very large volumes of air are being exchanged. These include muscles of the shoulder which increase the elevation of the ribs and the abdominal muscles which augment the upward movement of the diaphragm. Movement of these component respiratory muscles is controlled and coordinated by a complex nervous center in the brain stem. This center receives input from many areas, including from the cerebral cortex, to integrate air movement with speech; from temperature-regulating areas of the brain; from the joints, so that the breathing movements may be coordinated with movements of the limbs; from the skin; as well as from specialized "chemoreceptors" which monitor the chemistry of the blood. These receptors which are impressively sensitive in youth become blunted with age, so that the concentrations of gases in the blood is not so precisely controlled.

The ventilatory function of the lungs is commonly described in terms of the volume of air within the lungs or the volume of air being moved in and out of the lungs. When a maximal forced expiratory effort is made, a volume of air known as the residual volume remains in the lungs. If a maximal inspiratory effort is then made, the volume of air in the lungs increases; the increase in volume is the vital capacity. The sum of residual volume and vital capacity is the total lung volume. When at rest we neither expire nor inspire to the maximal extent, so that we are using just a part of the vital capacity; the volume of air moved is called the tidal volume. Under these conditions we have an inspiratory and expiratory reserve of volume. The volume of air which remains in the lung at the end of a normal expiration is the functional residual capacity. We can not only vary the volume of air that is moved with each breath but also must alter the speed with which the air is exchanged. Several tests of lung function are directed toward measurement of the volumes of air which can be moved in a certain time interval or the maximal rate of flow which can be achieved.

All of the tissues of the respiratory system show significant changes with aging, and in the aggregate these changes make for major depressions of function (21). A healthy old person at rest has adequate and comfortable breathing,

but reserve is lost so that large volumes or high rates of breathing are not attainable. It is perhaps surprising that respiratory function is maintained as well as it is when one reflects that each day of our lives on the order of 10,000 liters of air, all too often rich in particles and pollutants, enters and leaves our lungs.

As the thorax ages, its volume and shape undergo change. The loss of mineral from the bones of the spine leads to curvatures which tend to reduce the volume of the thorax as well as impede its movements. Further, in the advanced stages of demineralization of the bony cage of the thorax the ribs may be pinched inward, still further reducing volume. The cartilage pads which normally, by their flexibility, permit movement of the ribs relative to the sternum and vertebrae become fibrous and ultimately calcified so that movement of the rib cage becomes difficult. The thorax is said to become less compliant. Changes in the volume of the thorax become increasingly dependent upon movement of the diaphragm. Even here a problem may arise with an increase in the quantity of intra-abdominal fat obstructing this movement. Most old people are more comfortable when they are somewhat reclining so that free movement of the diaphragm is encouraged.

As the smaller airways age, they become weakened so that when a forcible expiration is made they tend to collapse and trap air within some parts of the lung. The airways come to occupy an increasing fraction of the lung volume at the expense of the alveolar air sacs. These tend to become more flattened, leading to a fall in the total area of alveolar membrane available for gas exchange. In the young adult this area is about 80 sq meters; at the age of 75 it is about 60 sq meters.

The lungs tend to lose their elastic recoil with the passage of years, with the result that the chest steadily expands as the residual air volume increases. This loss of elasticity of the lung comes about through changes in the organization of the lung's collagen and elastin fibers. In contrast with the thorax (which becomes less compliant), the lungs become more compliant (i.e., more easily stretchable). The change in the thorax outweighs the lung change so that overall, the compliance is reduced and the work of breathing increases. This extra effort of breathing gives the sensation of breathlessness (dyspnea). The total lung volume falls only slightly in aging individuals who are able to avoid the crouched posture brought about by increasing spinal curvature. In the presence of this curvature, and especially if it is accompanied by weakening of the ribs, the loss of lung volume can be major. The most consistent alterations seen in aging are the increase in residual volume and a fall in vital capacity which undergoes a reduction of up to 1% each year after 40. As already noted the reserve of ventilatory function is substantially reduced so that rapid movements of large volumes of air, whether in exercise, coughing, or loud speech, cannot be accomplished. Elaborate and often computerized tests of ventilatory function are available, but a simple test is to have the subject take a deep breath and then attempt to blow out a kitchen match held 8 inches from the lips while keeping the mouth wide open. This test can also be used as a training procedure to motivate improvement of ventilation.

Depression of ventilatory function has many causative factors, and these can be divided into two groups: (a) factors which restrict ventilation (spinal curvature, collapse of the rib cage, weakening of the respiratory muscle, or obstruction of diaphragmatic movement) or (b) factors which obstruct ventilation (collapse of small airways, reduction in the area of the larger airways as a result of increased tension of the muscle in their walls or by the excessive secretion and accumulation of mucus). Removal of these secretions by coughing is impaired by both the restriction of ventilation and by the loss and reduced activity of the ciliary processes of the epithelial cells which otherwise provide a "mucus escalator" to keep the airways clear.

For ventilation of the lungs to serve its fundamental purpose of supplying oxygen to the body, it must be appropriately matched by blood flow and perfusion of lungs. This matching of ventilation and perfusion shows impairment with age and is especially marked in inactive individuals. The consequence is that the blood is less well oxygenated, and so activity becomes further depressed. Exercising the breathing apparatus, whether by whole body activity or by specific "respiratory gymnastics" is thus beneficial both in terms of improving air flow and in increasing the oxygen supply to the tissues (34).

Superimposed upon these physiological changes may be a number of pathological changes. The reduction in alveolar membrane area may be worsened by the obliteration of part of the surface by particulate matter (dusts, for example, from the polluted atmosphere of a coal mine or a stone quarry). Irritation of the alveolar surface by particles or noxious gases leads to a thickening of the alveolar membrane and changes in its structure so that diffusion of gases between air and blood is impaired. Further, this persistent irritation ultimately leads to a breakdown of alveoli and a weakening of the walls of the small airways—the condition of emphysema—an occupational disease of the smoker as well as those who work in a polluted atmosphere.

THE AGING CARDIOVASCULAR SYSTEM (15, 25, 28)

The basic design of the cardiovascular system is two circulations through which blood flow is provided by a pump. Anatomically, the two pumps—one servicing the circulation to the lungs and the other the circulation to all the other bodily tissues and organs—are combined into one organ, the heart. The pumps, which are usually referred to as the right and left hearts, respectively, each consist of two muscular chambers, an atrium and a ventricle. The whole continuous internal surface of the heart and the two circulations is lined with a variety of covering cells called endothelia.

The blood vessels of the two circulations each arise from a single large artery with thick walls containing muscle and connective tissue elements. This artery divides sequentially into major branch arteries, small arteries, arterioles, and capillary vessels. As the vessels divide, the wall becomes thinner and simplified until, when the capillary is reached, it consists of merely the thin layer of endothelium and a few wisps of connective tissue, which serves to locate these fine vessels in the tissue which they serve. The capillary vessels are about 1 mm in length and of a diameter of about 5×10^{-3} mm, just large enough to permit the passage of red blood cells in a single file. These vessels are the only site at which materials can gain entry to or leave the blood; they are, therefore, referred to as exchange vessels.

Capillary vessels converge into the system of veins which is a mirror image of the system of arteries. The smallest vessels, the venules, unite to form small veins which continue this process until the heart is reached. The venous drainage from the pulmonary circulation empties into the left atrium via three large veins. Venous blood from the systemic circulation enters the right atrium via the two terminal veins, the superior vena cava from the upper parts of the body and the inferior vena cava from the lower. The walls of veins are uniformly thinner than their corresponding arteries but also contain muscle and connective tissue. The muscle of the blood vessels is referred to as smooth muscle, and its contraction and relaxation is controlled by a special system of nerves as well as by chemical and physical factors acting directly upon it.

The atria and ventricles are muscular pumps. The atria receive the blood as it returns from the two circulations and provide a small pressure to drive it into the ventricle, from which it is then driven into the arterial circulations at a much higher pressure. As would be expected from this difference in function, the atria have a relatively thin muscular wall while that of the ventricles is massive. The muscle of the heart is of a variety intermediate between that of the skeleton and that of the blood vessels, with both of which it shares some characteristics. The muscular parts of the heart also contain fibrous connective tissue which arises from a rather dense plate of tissue separating the atria and the ventricles and in which are situated the valves which ensure the one-way flow of blood from the atria to ventricle to artery. These valves are simple passive flap-like structures of fibrous connective tissue covered with a fine endothelium.

The heart contains an electrical system by which excitation is delivered to the muscle to bring about rhythmical contraction. This system consists of cells which have some of the characteristics of the heart muscle and also of nerves. The cells are bunched into two "nodes"; one, the sinoatrial node (SAN) at the point where the veins enter the right atrium, and the second, the atrioventricular node (AVN) close to the junction of the right atrium and ventricle. From this node arises a bundle of fibers which conducts and delivers electrical impulses to the muscle of the ventricle. This electrical excitation originates in the SA node where the cells act as pacemakers by spontaneously generating electrical impulses which travel over the atrial muscle to reach the AVN, from which they are then delivered to the ventricular muscle. It is this spread of electrical activity through the heart that is examined by the physician as the electrocardiogram. The heart receives a nerve supply from the autonomic nervous system. This nerve supply controls both the frequency with which the heart muscle contracts (the heart rate) and the force and extent of the contraction which, in turn, regulates the volume of blood which will be ejected from the heart at each beat (the stroke volume). The product of heart rate and stroke volume is the cardiac output.

A young adult sitting quietly at rest has a heart rate of about 70 beats per minute and with each beat, about 70 ml of blood are ejected from each ventricle. Thus the right heart ejects 5 liters of blood each minute into the pulmonary circulation while the left heart drives a precisely equal volume through the systemic circulation. Both of these circulations offer resistance to flow of blood so that pressure is developed in the arteries. The pressure rises with each beat of the heart (the systolic pressure) and falls in the interval between beats (the diastolic pressure). The resistance of the systemic circuit is much greater than that of the pulmonary circulation so that pressures in the main artery of the systemic system, the aorta, are about 120 mm Hg at systole and 80 mm Hg at the end of diastole. In the pulmonary circulation, the values in health are 25 and 8 mm Hg, respectively. These pressures are commonly written as 120/80 or 25/8.

The 5 liters of blood driven into the systemic circulation each minute are distributed to the various organs in amounts governed by the resistance offered by the blood vessels of the organ. This resistance is a function of the state of opening of the arterioles as well as the total size of the vascular bed. In round numbers, the brain receives 750 ml of the 5 liters of available output; the heart itself receives 250 ml; the kidneys receive 1200 ml; and the alimentary tract and liver receive about 1500 ml. This leaves 1300 ml to service the needs of muscle, skin, and bone. When the level of physical activity increases to satisfy the demands for extra metabolism by the tissues, a well-trained young person can increase the cardiac output fourfold; we would describe such an individual as having a "cardiac reserve" of 15 liters of output per minute. This increase in output is provided by a combination of an increased rate of the heart coupled with an increase in the volume of blood ejected at each beat. The majority of the extra cardiac output in these circumstances is delivered to the active muscles where the resistance to blood flow is lowered, while at the same time, blood flow to the kidneys and alimentary tract is reduced by an increase in the vascular resistance.

As the heart ages, its weight remains almost constant, in sharp contrast with that of many other organs. The most striking change is in the accumulation of aging pigment within the muscle cells, but it is unknown to what extent this affects function. The muscle shows a slowing of the contraction process and also a slowing of relaxation. The connective tissue elements, the collagen and elastin, show typical aging change, and as a consequence, the heart becomes less compliant with a reduction in the volume of blood which can be accommodated by the chambers. There is also a loss of cells in the SAN and a smaller reduction of AVN cell numbers. As these specialized cells are lost, they are replaced by fibrous tissue. The speed with which excitation spreads through the conducting system is slowed but not to an extent which takes it outside the normal limits. The major change which occurs in the electrical system is a reduction in the maximum rate at which impulses can be generated. This is manifest in a fall in the limiting heart rate which is highly predictable from the age by the expression:

Limiting heart rate

$$= (220 - \text{age in years}) \text{ beats/minute}$$

Healthy aging of the arteries affects mainly the connective tissue components. The smooth muscle cells of the blood vessel walls show a slight change in the chemical composition of their interior which may account for an alteration in their resting state of contraction. A more subtle change occurs in the cell membranes that alters the responsiveness of the muscle to nervous control. The elastic fibers which in large arteries form two tabular sheets within the vessel walls fray and break. At the same time there is an increase in the amount of collagen which also becomes more rigidly bound into bundles. The net result is that the arteries lose their elasticity and become more rigid. A consequence of this is that the systolic pressure rises while the diastolic pressure falls. A further consequence is an increase in the velocity with which the arterial pulse is carried to the periphery. The accumulation of linked collagen can proceed to the point where it acts as a base for calcium deposition. Elastic fibers are also lost in the veins but there is little or no new accumulation of collagen so that the vessels weaken. The valves of the veins, which normally relieve the pressure exerted by gravity on the vein walls in dependent parts, tend to become incompetent so that the vessels develop varicosities. Within the microvasculature, there is very little age-related change save for an increase in the level of tone (resting state of contraction) of the arterioles. In some areas, the fine substrate (basement membrane) of the capillary endothelium shows an increase in thickness which may impair the exchange of materials between the blood and the fluid which bathes the cells.

Resting cardiac output falls at a rate of close to 1% each year with an onset at around 40 years of age. This rate of decline is less in individuals who maintain an active life-style and is, at least to some extent, another manifestation of hypokinetic disease. The cardiac reserve diminishes at a rate somewhat greater than the fall in resting cardiac output. This comes about by the reduction in the limiting heart rate combined with the inability of the ventricles to relax and allow good filling and an inability to augment the force with which the ventricles contract. Both the pacemaker tissues and the muscle

of the heart become less responsive to nervous control so that some of the automatic responses of the cardiovascular system to stresses such as change of posture become blunted. Spells of giddiness upon arising from bed, for example, are quite common in the old because the adjustment to gravity which is necessary to maintain a good blood flow to the brain does not occur sufficiently promptly.

The fall in resting cardiac output results in reduced perfusion of tissues and organs; the extent of this reduction is very variable. Blood flow to the kidney fails by 40% from the ages of 35 to 80; blood flow to the brain fails by about 10% over the same interval. Other organs show intermediate values. In many cases, the reduction in blood flow is in proportion to the reduction of active mass of tissue. Some argue that the reduction in perfusion is the cause of the reduction in active tissue mass; others regard it as a consequence.

THE AGING NERVOUS SYSTEM

In gross terms, the nervous system consists of a central portion (the brain, a brain stem, and the spinal cord) and a peripheral portion (consisting mainly of the very long processes, or nerve fibers, which arise from cells situated in the central part). These nerve fibers have the function of conveying information from the periphery to the center or conveying information from the center to the peripheral structures. The information traveling inward arises from specialized receptors situated in the skin, from receptors in the muscles and joints and from the special sense organs of vision, hearing, taste, and olfaction. We speak of this system in general terms as the sensory component of the nervous system. The outward traveling information provides for control of muscles and glands; this is the motor component.

The cells of the nervous system are of two basic types: neuron and supporting cells called glia (a term which derives from the Greek for "nerve glue"). The neurons are characterized by maintaining an electrical charge across the cell membrane and by synthesizing in the body of the cell specific chemical substances, neurotransmitters, which are used in communication between individual neurons and between neurons of the motor system and the structures which they control. Glial cells are extremely active cells with the responsibility of controlling the environment of the excitable neurons. They do this by taking up materials from the blood, sometimes processing the material, and then exchanging these materials with the fluid which surrounds the neurons.

Neurons are quite variable in their shape, but three major elements can be recognized: a cell body; the nerve fiber or axon, a single, often long, process; and at the side of the cell opposite the axon, a tree-like branching set of processes called dendrites. Neurons act as "valves" directing the flow of information through the nervous system. A cell receives information via the dendrites; an electrical change occurs in the membrane of the neuron which spreads across the body of the cell toward the point from which the axon arises. An electrical change then spreads rapidly down the axon (an axon potential) to its termination which lies close to the dendrites or the body of another neuron. The cells do not touch but form a narrow gap, on either side of which, the axon and the dendrite or cell body show a special structure of the cell membrane. These two special areas and the tiny gap between them form the synapse. The arrival of an axon potential at the axon termination gives rise to the liberation of a neurotransmitter which diffuses across the synaptic gap and excites the second neuron.

Within the central nervous system, the cell bodies lie together in the "grey matter" which forms the outer part of the brain while the fibers form bundles and bands of "white matter" which runs not only out of but also from area to area of the brain itself. In the spinal cord, the cellular grey lies inside while the fibers form the outer part. The white appearance of the nerve fibers is due to the fact that they are covered by a special type of glial cell which forms a fatty insulation around the axons, preventing the electrical message from short-circuiting and cross-talking between axons.

During development, cells are being formed and are constantly degenerating as the brain increases in size and is serially remodeled to provide the necessary circuits within the nervous system. At birth, the process of increasing cell number is virtually complete, but the brain continues to increase in size until an individual's 20s, largely by enlargement of cells and growth of the nerve fibers. From about 23 onward, the brain begins to lose weight, albeit very slowly. This loss of weight involves the loss of neurons and their processes, and the brain undergoes some change in shape. The extensive convolutions of the outer cortex become a little flatter, and the fluid-filled spaces in the interior of the brain become a little larger.

Loss of cells does not occur uniformly throughout the brain. In some parts of the brain, it is marked; in other areas there is virtually no reduction in cell density. The reduction in neuron numbers, and the associated loss of fibers in the peripheral nerves, shows acceleration beginning in the 6th decade of life. As cells are lost, new connections between surviving cells are established, remodeling the circuitry so that, in general, function is impaired less than might be expected from the loss of units. Blood flow to the brain falls at a rate in excess of the loss of brain substance so that the reserve of oxygen supply to support cellular activity is diminished. The aging brain is thus exposed to hazard when any further disturbance, for example a fall in blood pressure, is superimposed upon this already marginal situation.

At the cellular level, neurons show some changes which appear to fit the definition of physiological but which merge into states which are pathological. In common with most cells of the body, neurons accumulate lipofuscin. In the cell body, the fine fibrillar system changes its arrangement and grows in size. This process may go to the point where a large part of the cell interior is occupied by so-called neurofibrillary tangles, an appearance seen in Alzheimer's disease and in senile dementia of the Alzheimer's type. These tangles are believed to form the substrate upon which metals, notably aluminum, deposit. The dendrites lose complexity, and proteinaceous material may deposit around them. In the extreme, the dendrites become confluent to form a variety of the senile plaques found in the brains of individuals both functionally normal and those exhibiting signs of dementia.

The speed with which action potentials travel the nerve fibers falls by about 30% between the 20s and 80. This affects both sensory and motor systems so that informational exchange between the center and the periphery is not only embarrassed by the loss of "channels" (i.e, nerve fibers) but also by the increased time required for messages to pass. In the peripheral nerves there is a tendency for the insulating layer which surrounds the axons to become reduced in amount. In the extreme case, this produces the pathology of the demyelinating diseases of which multiple sclerosis is an example. Loss of the myelin insulation slows conduction in the nerve fiber as well as producing some loss of "discreteness" of the informational flow.

Nerve cells have a vigorous synthetic function in addition to maintaining their property of excitability. The products of this synthesis include protein, the specific neurotransmitter substances, enzymes involved in the metabolism of neurotransmitters, and substances which modulate structural changes in the nerve cell of origin as well as in adjacent glia cells and other neurones which they contact at the synapses. The substances are synthesized within the nerve cell body and then travel along the axons for considerable distances, in excess of 1 m in some cases. The process involved in this movement of material is active, utilizing energy and is termed axonal transport (AxT) (11). Different substances are transported at very different rates. Some only travel 1–2 mm per day, others 400 mm per day while a few move rapidly at a rate around 2 m per day. AxT has the responsibility for maintaining the supply of neurotransmitters at the axon termination as well as providing structural material at the synaptic membrane. In addition AxT has what is termed a neurotropic role in regulating activity and probably functions transsynaptically in the target cells of the nerve. AxT can also occur in the reverse direction from axon termination towards the cell body. By this means, the synaptic connection may be able to influence events in both the presynaptic and postsynaptic (target) nerve cells.

In the experimental animal, studies have shown major changes in AxT with aging, with the rate of transport falling by a factor of as much as 10. Impairment of AxT has been shown to be a fundamental change in diseases characterized by peripheral degeneration of nerve fibers as well as in the loss of nerve cells in the cerebellum which are the target of some nerve pathways. It is tempting to speculate that some of the typical aging loss of synapses and neurons has its origins in impaired AxT. Evidence is accumulating that the process of AxT can be modified with drugs. If true, this would make many of the impairments of the aging nervous system treatable.

The general pattern of aging change in the neurotransmitter systems is a reduction in the amount present within the nervous system—the result either of a reduction in the rate at which the chemical is synthesized or an increase in the rate at which it is destroyed or inactivated. Acetylcholine is a transmitter substance which, although not widely distributed within the central nervous system, is involved in several very important neuronal circuits including those for memory (10). Experiments directly manipulating the concentration of acetylcholine to which the brain is exposed have shown definite improvement in individuals suffering from loss of short-term memory. Another naturally occurring brain chemical, vasopressin (a hormone secreted by neurons of the hypothalamus), has also shown promise of ameliorating memory.

Another neurotransmitter substance, norepinephrine, falls in concentration in the brain as a result of an increase in the activity of the enzyme monoamine oxidase which inactivates it. This is in contrast with acetylcholine, in which case, the defect is too little production. Norepinephrine is involved in neural pathways which regulate the activity of the pituitary gland, and its depressed activity has been involved in onset of the menopause as well as a number of psychiatric conditions. Drugs which inhibit the action of monoamine oxidase have been proposed as potential "elixirs of youth" based on the concept that the norepinephrine depression is a fundamental step in aging. A common drug which has this action is the local anesthetic procaine; this is rather widely used in various formulations in Europe for its supposed antiaging properties. There is virtually no evidence, however, that it succeeds in that role.

A classical example of the reduced activity of a neurotransmitter being associated with a disease of aging (as distinct from physiological aging) is dopamine, a substance related to norepinephrine, the loss of which gives rise to the movement disorder parkinsonism. Fortunately, it is possible to combat this condition by administration of a chemical precursor of dopamine which can reach the cells of the brain in which the transmitter is normally synthesized.

Changes in posture and gait are common functional signs of aging of the nervous system. Both depend upon a constant flow of information about the position of the body in space and the relation of the limbs and trunk one to the other. This information is integrated in a posterior brain structure, the cerebellum, which then influences the outflow of information to the muscles. In the old, there are fewer positional receptors; nerve fibers have been lost from the pathways; cells have been lost from the integrating circuits of the cerebellum; and finally there is slower outflow of messages to the muscle. Other parts of the brain show equivalent changes and, furthermore, the changes which occur in the joints themselves tend to make movements coarse and often difficult. For these and other reasons, old people show excessive body sway when standing quite still. In many, standing erect with the eyes closed (so that auxiliary information about body position is removed) is impossible. Tremor is likely to be present both at rest and when movement is undertaken. This can take the form of decomposition of speech as well as obvious effects on the limbs. Gait becomes slow and shuffling without the heel-and-toe action characteristic of the young.

Changes in sensations arising from the skin have already been discussed under that topic and, of those sensations, that of vibration is the most affected. At 70 years of age, this modality of sensation can be totally absent.

Reaction time (that is, the time which elapses between a signal being given and a required motor response being undertaken) is prolonged with aging. As might be anticipated, the time required for the inflow of information and for the outflow of response to occur both increase, but a major part of the increased reaction time can be located centrally in the circuits of the brain which lie between perception of the signal and activation of the intention to respond.

THE AGING OF THE SPECIAL SENSES (23)

The systems which provide the senses of vision, hearing, taste, and smell begin their aging process early in childhood. All of them are at their most acute in the first decade and then show a slow progressive decrement. The aging of hearing is dealt with fully elsewhere in this book. Suffice it to say that, in the auditory system, we see a fine example of the accumulation of a series of small decrements of function attributable to the general processes of aging in tissues already described (stiffening of fibrous structures, loss of perfusion, rigidity of bony joints, loss of receptors and nerve cells, slowing of nervous conduction, etc.).

The aging of vision which begins in early childhood first comes to attention when the near point of clear vision (the nearest point to the eye at which type can be read) retreats to arm's length. For the vast majority of individuals, this has occurred by the age of 50, and glasses become necessary for reading. This condition of presbyopia is brought about by the lens of the eye becoming more rigid and unable to change its curvature and power to shift focus from distant to near objects. This loss of accommodation is merely the most apparent of the aging visual changes.

The pupil of the eye regulates the amount of light which reaches the photoreceptors of the retina and, in youth, adjusts promptly for changes in illumination. In the older person, the pupil becomes smaller and fixed in size with the consequence that older people require brighter illumination if they are to see clearly (three to four times brighter, in fact, than young people), and the eyes do not adjust when moving from a light to dark area, an important consideration in the design of indoor environments for old people.

The fluid which fills the anterior portion of the eye tends to become pigmented with a flourescent yellow material so that it becomes difficult to distinguish the colors blue and green. The eyes tend to sink a little more deeply into their sockets so that the field of vision becomes obstructed by the brows and temples. The aging lens also develops pinpoint opacities which act like dust on a windshield and produce dazzle from sources of bright light. The lens has no blood supply and has to rely on diffusion for its nutrition. As the aging lens thickens and cells become further removed from fluids which bathe the lens, metabolism of the lens is impaired, and the major opacity of cataract occurs. Some have suggested that if man's life span were to be extended to 120 or 130 all would eventually become blind by cataract. Another common condition of the eye, by no means limited to the aging, is glaucoma, an increase in pressure in the eyes caused by inadequate drainage of intraocular fluid. This elevated pressure can impair the circulation to the retina and destroy the rod and cone receptors. Glaucoma has an increased tendency to occur in the old since it is also a side effect of some common medications.

The chemical senses of taste and smell undergo significant impairment with aging. The special receptors for taste which are gathered in taste buds on the tongue and pharynx are reduced to about one-third of their number in youth. The receptors for salt taste are especially affected, and this commonly leads to oversalting of food. Not only is the pleasure of taste lost but also the protective function. Poisoning by harmful materials, a majority of which have an offensive taste, is an age-related hazard. The sense of smell is equally diminished by loss of the receptors and neurons, and some very old people become totally anosmic, unable either to enjoy the odors of flowers or cooking or to perceive the danger of a gas leak. The impairment of the channels of special sense all serve to increase the sense of isolation so commonly experienced by the old.

THE AGING OF THE MOUTH (36)

Aging of the structures of the mouth has impact upon nutrition, upon articulation and, not trivially, upon the senses both pleasurable and protective. The mouth is lined with a variety of epithelium called stratified squamous epithelium, which is kept moist by the secretion of saliva into the mouth from three sets of specialized glands and by other minor mucus secreting glands. The muscular tongue has its own specialized epithelium on the upper and lateral surfaces in which are found the sensory receptors for taste. The teeth are suspended in the alveolar bone of the jaws by sling-like bands of connective tissue and project from the gums, which form a cuff around the midportion of the teeth. The whole cavity of the mouth is abundantly supplied with nerve endings which provide sensations of temperature, touch, pressure, and pain. Sensation is especially acute in the lips; the muscles around the mouth have good proprioceptive (positional) sensation. The exquisitely fine motor control of the muscles involved in speech will be discussed elsewhere; suffice it to say that this part of the motor system is exceptionally well preserved in healthy aging.

Salivary secretion is reduced with aging so that lubrication for chewing, swallowing, or speech becomes rather inadequate and needs to be reinforced by frequent sips of water. A powerful stimulus to the secretion of saliva is the smell or taste of food; both of these senses show major impairment with aging. Acuity of taste at 70 years of age is only about 25% of what it was in youth, and olfaction shows a very similar decrement. Absence of this important avenue of stimulation coupled with the reduced secretory activity of the glands themselves makes dry mouth a significant problem for the old.

Teeth are remarkable structures; their material is so resistant to wear and tear that it is estimated that they could last us at least two lifetimes. The central bony part of the teeth which lies beneath the enamel continues to grow throughout the life of the tooth. This central growth ultimately obliterates the pulp cavity which normally contains nutrient blood vessels and nerves. In the old, surviving teeth are denervated and bloodless. However, loss of teeth to caries or periodontal disease is so common that until very recently, about half of the population over the age of 65 had no natural teeth in one or the other jaw, and about 20% had no natural teeth at all. The recent change for the better in this picture can be attributed to improved dental hygiene and in many places the fluoridation of the water supply.

In addition to these factors critical to retention of the teeth is pressure applying tension to the connective tissue attachments. Foods which call for energetic mastication provide such pressure. Another source of pressure is the matching tooth of the opposite jaw with which occlusion occurs. Loss of a tooth thus makes the retention of the occlusal partner less likely. Once the loss of teeth is started, it becomes progressive unless the missing tooth or teeth is replaced by a prosthesis. Although masticatory function can be replaced by dentures, this is accomplished at the expense of sensation from the mouth and of the quality of speech. Furthermore, progressive aging changes in the jaws and gums make necessary rather frequent adjustment of the fitting of dentures. If this is not done, the discomfort and inadequacy of ill-fitting devices leads to their abandonment and the adoption of a bland, nutritionally poor diet and resigned acceptance of poor speech.

THE AGING ALIMENTARY TRACT (14)

The alimentary tract is essentially a muscular tube lined with epithelium which provides an extensive surface by which the body interfaces with the environment. It displays three major functions: (a) it has motility by which ingested food is moved along the tract; (b) it secretes fluids containing specific enzymes by which the food is digested and broken down into small molecules prior to (c) absorption. There is voluntary control of the tract at either end; the initiation of swallowing and of defecation are consciously controlled. Between the upper esophagus and the rectum, the gut is autonomous with both motility and secretion being controlled by a system of nerve plexi within the walls of the gut and by a series of hormones secreted by cells of the gut lining.

Associated with the gut are secretory glands which either lie in the walls of the gut (e.g., the glands of the stomach which secrete the gastric juice and acid) or which lie outside the gut but communicate with it by means of a duct (e.g., the pancreas).

The liver has a special relation to the gut in that it secretes bile into the lumen and receives the venous blood which has perfused the gut by means of a major blood vessel, the portal vein. This provides a direct pathway by which substances absorbed in the gut can be delivered to the liver where synthesis and conversion of material take place.

The lining of the gut consists of epithelial cells. These are constantly undergoing some abrasion as food materials move over them. The life of these cells is limited to about 4 or 5 days, after which time they are shed from the surface and are replaced by new cells providing a population of constantly dividing stem cells. In the aged alimentary tract, the replacement rate of these cells is slowed, and the surface becomes thinned and reduced in area.

The process of alimentation begins with the act of swallowing. Food that has been chewed and mixed with saliva is driven by the action of the tongue and the muscles of the mouth into the upper part of the esophagus. This action initiates a wave of propulsive contraction which sweeps the food down toward the stomach. At the junction of the esophagus and stomach a sphincter of muscle relaxes to allow the entry of the swallowed food. Another wave of contraction travels down to clear any residual material from the esophagus.

This action is disrupted in a characteristic way in the old person. First, the act of swallowing does not always initiate the propulsive wave. Several swallowing actions may be necessary. The arrival of this wave at the sphincter may not lead to its relaxation; consequently, food may be held in the lower part of the esophagus, giving rise to a sense of pressure or fullness. Furthermore, the lower part of the esophagus in the old person frequently shows rings of contraction, further delaying the normal passage of food and increasing discomfort. These aging changes in the esophagus are so regular and common that one speaks of the condition of ''presbyesophagus.''

Food is normally held for some time in the stomach before being transported to the small intestine. In the old person, this delay is increased. The glands of the stomach secrete acid and digestive juice in response to a number of stimuli. These include the thought, sight, smell, and taste of food, the latter two of which are diminished in the old. Secretion of the glands is diminished by age, especially in the male, which may influence not only the early stages of digestion but also the absorption of some classes of drugs.

Movement of material and secretion in the small intestine is little changed by age, although the pancreatic secretion of the enzyme concerned in fat digestion may be somewhat less than in the young. However, there is such a safety factor involved here that this usually does not lead to fat intolerance.

The major aging problem in the large bowel arises from the thinning of the muscular walls and loss of the internal nerve supply. The consequence is the formation of blind sacs bulging into the muscle layers referred to as diverticuli and a loss of propulsive power to move material. Constipation is the result. This all too often leads to overenthusiastic use of laxatives which may worsen rather than aid the condition.

Blood flow through the gut falls to an extent equal to the fall in the cardiac output. This does not directly impair absorption, although it may prolong the time required for this process. The rates of absorption from the gut tend to fall with age but not to such an extent that nutrients are lost from the gut. In a minority, the impairment of fat digestion may lead not only to poor absorption of essential fatty acids but also of the fat-soluble vitamins. Calcium absorption may become only marginally adequate, especially where vitamin D_3 levels are less than optimal.

The liver shows a significant weight loss as it ages, and its blood flow, which is largely provided over the portal vein, falls. In most respects, function is well maintained. The rate of plasma protein formation is little changed, and the formation and secretion of bile is adequate. The liver has an important role in the detoxification of drugs and other substances foreign to the body. This function is subserved by a special class of enzymes which are induced in the presence of the foreign substance. These enzymes become significantly less inducible as the liver ages. This special impairment of liver function will be discussed elsewhere in this text.

THE AGING KIDNEY (5)

The kidney exercises the major role of maintaining the internal environment of the body by eliminating many of the products of metabolism and regulating the body's content of water and salts. The kidneys are simple in structure, consisting of about 2,000,000 (1,000,000 in each kidney) essentially similar units, the nephrons. Each nephron consists of a highly coiled tubule, closed at one end and, at the other, opening into the urinary space at the pelvis of the kidney. The tubule is lined with epithelial cells which, at the closed end, are specialized into a sheet of cells which interdigitate one with another, leaving ''slit pores'' in the membrane. This blind end of the tubule is invaginated by a tuft of capillary blood vessels arising from fine arterial blood vessels called the afferent arterioles. The capillary blood vessels, which form the glomerular tuft, unite to form a second arterial vessel, the efferent arteriole, which then divides into a second set of capillary blood vessels surrounding the tubule.

The function of the glomerular capillaries is to filter water and small molecules from the blood. This filtrate passes across the walls of the capillaries and the epithelial cells of the invaginated tubule into a space called Bowman's capsule. The membrane of the glomerulus (the capillary wall and the epithelial cells), impermeable to blood cells and the plasma proteins, is freely permeable to water and small molecules. The fluid entering Bowman's capsule is known as an ultrafiltrate of plasma. As the fluid flows down the tubule, it is modified by the epithelial cells lining the tubule which reabsorb some constituents from the tubular fluid and secrete substances from the blood into the fluid.

The two kidneys, which in youth weighed less than 400 g, receive perfused blood at a rate of 25% of the total cardiac output. From this enormous blood flow, glomerular filtrate is formed at a rate of 120 ml per minute. The tubules thus receive, each minute, 120 ml of water plus the salts, glucose, amino acids, urea, and other metabolic end products contained in the plasma. From this, they form about 1 ml of urine by reabsorbing 119 ml of the filtered water and other substances which the body needs to conserve while allowing waste products to escape. Glucose and amino acids are totally reabsorbed; about 99% of the sodium chloride is absorbed. Urea, the major route for elimination of excess nitrogen from the body, is reabsorbed less than 50%. Another end product of metabolism, creatinine, is not reabsorbed at all. The tubules secrete acid derived from the metabolism of the diet very efficiently. In fact, when challenged by a large acid load, a urine is formed which is 1000 times as concentrated with respect to acid as the plasma. One may summarize this function as one of conservation of materials essential to the body and elimination of materials present in excess of need. On a hot day, when the body is losing substantial volumes of water as sweat, the responsibility of the kidney is to keep water loss in the urine at a minimum. Consequently, a very small volume of concentrated urine is excreted. On the other hand, a large volume of beer increases the volume of body water. The kidney responds by reabsorbing less and forming a large volume of very watery urine. This same principle of regulated conservation or elimination applies to all the constituents of the body fluids.

The kidney is at its maximum size in the early 30s and then shows a slow progressive decline in weight and size. The loss takes the form of elimination of nephron units. The surviving units age with relatively little change in their function. By the age of 80, the number of nephrons has been halved. Along with this loss of renal mass goes a proportionate reduction in blood flow and formation of glomerular filtrate. Because the loss of tissue is of entire functional units, a balance is still maintained between the rate at which materials are filtered and the rate at which they can be reabsorbed by the tubules.

In a young person, if a part of the kidney mass is removed, the remaining tissue will hypertrophy so that after a time, function will be restored towards its original value. This property of hypertrophy makes the donation of a kidney an effective procedure. After a while, both the donor and the donee will each have something approaching the functional capacity of a pair of kidneys. This capacity for hypertrophy is lost as the kidney ages. For this reason, a kidney donation is not appropriate for individuals over 50 years of age.

The loss of functional units from the aging kidney reduces the efficiency of the regulation which it normally exercises. This occurs not so much in terms of absolute control, but rather in terms of how rapidly the composition of the body fluids can be restored to normal. If an old person is given a large load of water, it is eliminated more slowly than by a young person. Ultimately, correction of the body fluid volume will be achieved. Similarly, an old person can eliminate a load of acid end products only over an extended period of time. The aged kidney cannot conserve materials as well as can the young. The urine cannot be made as concentrated so that elimination of salts which are in excess or waste products becomes expensive in terms of the water in which they must be excreted.

The kidney has responsibilities beyond excretion. It is the locus for the formation of a hormone, erythropoietin, which regulates the formation of red blood cells. It is also the site at which a precursor of vitamin D_3 is activated. Loss of renal mass reduces these functions but not sufficiently to embarrass the body's economy.

The lower urinary tract shows aging changes which are mainly due to an impairment of muscular control through loss of nervous input. In addition, muscle tissue is lost with aging. Urinary incontinence, caused by the loss of sphincter control, is a source of inconvenience and embarrassment to older persons. It may also persuade the person to avoid drinking adequate fluid. Such voluntary dehydration leads to many widespread impairments of other systems of the body. In the male, overgrowth of the prostate gland (a eugeric change) can produce urinary retention, mechanically damaging the kidneys as well as increasing the likelihood of infections of the urinary tract.

THE AGING OF THE REGULATORY SYSTEMS (24)

This examination of the physiology of aging took origin from the concept of homeostasis, the maintenance within the body of a finely regulated internal environment in which the cells could operate at an optimum level. This internal environment serves to buffer the body from the external world with which, nevertheless, the body must constantly exchange materials. The regulated elements of the internal environment include the temperature, the level of acidity, the concentration of salts, the concentration of metabolic substrates and products, and the volume of the body fluids. Constancy of these elements is achieved by regulating the exchange with the external environment. The organs of exchange are the lungs, the alimentary tract, the skin, and the kidneys.

Part of this regulation of exchange is dependent upon conscious behavior. For example, although we have unconscious, automatic mechanisms which defend the volume of water within the body, these have to be assisted by voluntary behavior (e.g., by drinking in response to thirst). These supporting behaviors are very sensitive to aging; an old person with a mobility problem may not be physically capable of getting to the refrigerator for water or food. As a result, even the most delicate automatic regulation becomes ineffective. Each year thousands of old people die because of breakdown in homeostasis. Accidental hypothermia, the often fatal lowering of the body temperature, kills thousands each winter—not because of failure of the internal regulating mechanism but rather because of the individual's inability to respond to the need to turn up the thermostat or put on extra clothing. In a summer heat wave, people die as a result of dehydration all too often resulting from an inability to obtain access to adequate fluid. It is in this area of behavioral impairment that environmental protection becomes necessary for the old (1, 29).

The automatic regulation of the cellular environment is effected by two systems: (a) a special division of the nervous system, the autonomic nervous system which operates upon the involuntary muscles (i.e., muscles other than those used for movement of the body) and upon glands; and (b) the endocrine system, which regulates the activity of muscle and of cells which transport material into or out of the body. This is accomplished by means of hormones secreted into and transported in the blood. Common to both of these systems is the need for the regulated cell to be able to recognize the message which reaches it from the nerve ending or from the blood. To this end, the cells have membrane patches of receptors which are specific for the message which they will accept. When a receptor is engaged by either the specific neurotransmitter or hormone, a cascade of actions comes into play, and the cell reacts by contraction or relaxation (if it is a muscle cell) or by moving some material into or across the cell.

The autonomic nervous system shows most of the aging changes seen in the main (somatic) nervous system (7). There is a loss of nerve cells; cells accumulate pigment; and conduction through the system slows. Generally, however, these changes are not so marked as in the somatic nervous system. A major alteration occurs in the mechanisms which couple the receptors of the cell membrane with an action in the cell. Membrane receptors may also become very reduced in number or sometimes even change their specificity. The effect of this alter-

ation in the linkage between nerve and cell is to reduce the range of control of function which can be exercised.

The endocrine system consists of a number of glands scattered throughout the body. The majority of these glands are orchestrated in their function from the pituitary gland; others are autonomous and secrete their hormones in response to chemical changes within the blood. The pituitary gland exercises its control by way of "trophic" hormones which stimulate other endocrine organs. The pituitary gland is, in turn, regulated by means of releasing hormones produced by the hypothalamus, a part of the brain with mixed nervous and endocrine functions. The hypothalamus, the pituitary gland, and the other endocrine organs are subject to what is called feedback control, whereby the rate of secretion of a hormone is governed by the level of that hormone in the blood.

The hormones can be grouped by the function which they serve. Cellular metabolism of the substrates for energy, carbohydrates, and fatty acids is under the control of a variety of hormones, including two hormones secreted by the endocrine tissue of the pancreas—insulin and glucagon; growth hormone secreted by the pituitary; the thyroid hormone; epinephrine secreted by the medulla of the adrenal gland (epinephrine also functions as a neurotransmitter in the autonomic and central nervous system); and the glucocorticoids secreted by the cortex of the adrenal gland. Insulin and glucagon are autonomous secretions responding to the level of glucose in the blood. The aging effect upon them is essentially a loss of sensitivity, so that when the concentration of glucose in the blood is changed, it remains altered for longer than it does in a young person. This is called "glucose intolerance," and while it is a genuine physiological change, it merges almost imperceptibly into the disease diabetes mellitus. Growth hormone is secreted when exercise is undertaken and also is liberated in "bursts" during the deepest phases of sleep. In the old person, the exercise response is blunted and secretion during the night is reduced associated with the reduction in deep sleep which old persons show. Although anatomic changes can be seen in the thyroid gland, there is very little functional change with aging. This is interesting since at one time, many aging changes were seen as imitating thyroid deficiency. The epinephrine and glucocorticoid systems are relatively unaffected, and an adequate response to stress remains intact in the old. Glucocorticoid secretion is controlled from the pituitary by ACTH, and the feedback system of regulation remains unaffected.

ACTH also has a role in the second set of

hormones secreted by the adrenal cortex, the mineralocorticoids, of which the prime example is aldosterone. The major control, however, comes from a system originating in the kidney. This renin-aldosterone system is responsible for maintaing the salt content of the body. With age, this is very much blunted so that the old person has difficulty both in retaining salt and, when necessary, eliminating a salt load. This impairment is also due, in part, to the physiological loss of renal function which the old exhibit.

Embedded within the thyroid gland are four small endocrine masses, the parathyroid glands. These secrete two hormones, PTH (parathyroid hormone) and calcitonin. These hormones regulate the body's exchanges of calcium. The function of PTH is to promote the liberation of calcium from the bones into the blood; calcitonin promotes the deposition of bone mineral. In both males and females, the level of PTH rises with age from early middle age onward. The rise is severalfold greater in women than in men and coincides with the onset of menopause. Estrogen suppresses the secretion of PTH, and when its level fails at menopause, PTH secretion becomes unrestrained. Loss of bone mineral occurs in both sexes but as might be predicted, is far greater in women than in men. Mention has already been made of the great cost of the resulting osteoporosis.

Certain groups of neurons within the hypothalamus secrete hormones, vasopressin and oxytocin, which are stored before release in the posterior part of the pituitary gland. Oxytocin has well-defined functions in the females as an essential part of the mechanism of parturition and lactation. There is no certainty as to its possible role in the male; in neither sex is there a significant relationship between age and the circulating level. The same is true for vasopressin, otherwise known as the antidiuretic hormone, whose role is to control water loss through the kidney. Although circulating levels of the hormone remain relatively unchanged by age, there is an increased sensitivity of the secretion mechanisms so that a standard challenge by elevation of the solute concentration of the blood produces a greater secretion in the old than in the young. The target of vasopressin, the kidney, shows an almost compensatory reduction in the density of the cellular receptors for the hormone.

The most dramatic of the changes of the aging endocrine system is the fall in secretion by the ovary of the female sex hormones, estrogen and progesterone, which marks the end of reproductive cycles. The fall in ovarian production of these hormones interrupts the feedback control which they normally exercise on the pituitary gland, so that there is a great increase in secretion of the gonadotrophic hormones. The level of the male sex hormone, testosterone, remains within normal limits even in advanced old age; the gonadotrophic hormones do, however, show a small rise.

It is perhaps surprising that taken overall the regulatory system, which has such widespread influence on function, does not show more change with aging (9). In terms of percentage change of function, it is one of the least affected, running second only to the digestive and absorptive function of the alimentary tract.

NUTRITION IN AGING

All too little is presently understood about the nutritional requirements of the aging population. However, older individuals are inclined or are persuaded to purchase a disproportionate quantity of vitamins, minerals, and other dietary supplements.

The fall in lean body mass which is regarded as a typical physiological change in the elderly has given rise to the advice that caloric intake should be progressively reduced from early middle age onward. This advice is also appropriate in light of the typical reduction of physical activity which takes place at this time. However, it may be argued that dietary revision so as to maintain lean body mass might be effective in slowing down the aging process. In any event, matching caloric intake to energy consumption must be based upon individual evaluation of energy requirements.

If the reduction in caloric intake were to be achieved by simple reduction of the amount of food taken per day, malnutrition could easily result. The dietary content of some of the trace minerals, for example, is already marginal in the ample diet of young people and can easily reach the level of deficiency if the diet is cut down. Protein requirements remain unchanged in the aging in spite of loss of lean tissue mass due, perhaps, to a lowered efficiency of utilization by the body. Fats may be less well tolerated by old people and in any event, the intake can well be reduced so that not more than 25% of the calories come from this source. Reduction to lower levels offers the possibility of inadequate intake of fat-soluble vitamins and essential fatty acids which the body cannot synthesize. In terms of the gross composition of the diet, the advice should be an improvement in the quality of the diet by elimination of foods which provide empty calories, especially refined sugars and alcohol.

It is reasonable to consider supplementation of the diet in some of its elements. Calcium is a case in point; the recommended adult daily allowance of 800 mg is probably less than is necessary to combat the loss of mineral from bone in both sexes and especially in women. A target intake of 1500 mg per day would appear to be realistic. Unless the diet is very rich in dairy foods it may require a supplement in the form of a calcium salt, either the carbonate or the gluconate. For the extra intake of calcium to be effective, there must be adequate availability of vitamin D, which is another element which may be deficient in an old person. A precursor of vitamin D is formed in the skin under the action of sunlight. The aging skin has a sharply reduced synthetic capacity; the rate of formation of the vitamin in the 80 year old is half of that in the young adult. Moreover, some old people have a much lower exposure to sunlight. To be effective, vitamin D has to undergo activation by conversion in the kidney. This stage of the process is impaired as part of the overall reduction in renal mass and function. Reinforcement of the diet with respect to both calcium and vitamin D is protective against the two common bone diseases of the aging—osteoporosis and osteomalacia.

Mention has already been made of the trace elements, and some case could be made for attention to zinc intake. There is a possibility, whether remote or substantial is not established, that relative zinc deficiency is involved in loss of taste and olfactory sensitivity. An adequate intake of fiber may also become a problem in the old since natural sources of vegetable fiber call for hard chewing and, unless properly masticated, create difficulty in swallowing. It may sometimes be necessary to puree vegetables in order to maintain intake of this important dietary element.

Many medications which are in common use by the elderly interact with nutrition. Some may have a global effect by depressing appetite while others, such as diuretics, may rob the body of potassium.

The diminution of renal function and the blunting of some endocrine regulatory mechanisms impairs the body's ability to handle salt. Unfortunately, the reduction in the sense of taste leads many old people to salt their food so that intake is increased over and above the grossly high level common in our diet. Gratification of taste can readily be achieved by other spices.

Iron and vitamin B_{12} are well absorbed in the elderly and will not present a problem in the presence of a mixed diet. Self-selection of a bland, soft, mainly carbohydrate diet because of problems in the mouth or esophagus may lead to deficiency of these elements and a call for supplementation if hemopoietic function is to be maintained.

A SCALE OF BIOLOGICAL AGE (2, 20)

The point was made earlier that the physiological changes brought about by aging vary widely in their time of onset and proceed at different rates in different individuals. The aim in attempting to develop a scale of biological age is to obtain a measure of how quickly a person is moving through the continuum towards the maximal potential life span. Such a scale would have a number of uses. Society tends to base its expectations and to distribute benefits on a basis of chronological age rather than upon capability or need. It is interesting that primitive societies operate without chronological age and deal only in functional terms such as "old enough to herd goats," "old enough to carry a sibling," or "too old to hunt," "too old to eat meat," etc. Until recently, it was a tenet that at age 65, productive labor was no longer the norm, and so individuals were persuaded that their activity should be reduced with the consequence that many functions accelerated in their decline for want of use. So real is this accelerated decline that it was seen as causing "hypokinetic disease ." Parenthetically it should be noted that hypokinetic disease can also overtake the TV-addicted teenager. Another use of a scale of biological age would be as a yardstick in the evaluation of interventions designed to delay aging, changes in lifestyle, diet, even perhaps, drugs. It is also valuable for any professional working with an aging clientele to be able to make some assessment of an individual's potential regardless of chronological age.

Such a scale would need to be based on truly physiological changes which show a linear relationship with age. The procedure would then be to establish the average decline of function in a large group of healthy individuals. This could be done for a number of characteristics and measurable functions. By comparing observations on an individual with the norms for healthy people, one could then express an "equivalent age" for the item. The problem is to decide what should or could be measured. One of the least reliable assessments of age is greying of the hair of the head which is profoundly influenced by racial and familial traits. The greying of the hair of the axilla is a little more reliable but is tedious to quantitate. Several attempts have been made to establish a list of consistent aging features, and a sample list is given below. This list is arranged in order, with those showing the strongest relation to age ahead of those showing less change.

1. The time taken for a standard "pinch" of skin on the back of the hand to flatten;
2. The auditory threshold for a sound of 4000 Hz;
3. The sense of vibration tested by a tuning fork on the ankle or the great toe;
4. The volume of air which can be exhaled in 1 second;
5. The systolic blood pressure;
6. The time required to react to a visual stimulus;
7. The visual acuity measured by a standard Snellen test chart;
8. Strength of the hand grip.

No really successful list of measurements has yet been developed but the search would seem to be well worthwhile.

THE FUTURE OF AGING

Man's ability to survive and age depends upon the maintenance of a rather constant internal environment in the face of challenges, both internal and external. It is to this end of homeostasis that the body's systems work by reacting and adapting to these challenges. By these reactions and adaptations man is freed to live over the whole surface of the globe, to be idle or to achieve tremendous exertion, while still preserving for his cells and tissue comfortable surroundings in which they can perform optimally. The physiological changes which occur with the passage of years reduce the efficiency of these systems, so that the "world" available for man's activity closes about him. To some extent we can substitute technology for physiology by reducing the external challenges to which man is exposed.

It is highly likely however, that the more we come to understand about the fundamental nature of the aging process, the better we will be able to identify those processes which can be delayed in their onset or slowed in their progress. Already, changes in life-style, adjustments to the diet, and recognition of the dangers of environmental pollution are making it necessary to reexamine, critically, those physiological changes presently regarded as inevitable. The author is certain that when this chapter is rewritten 40 years hence, it will present a different picture of the capabilities of the elderly and aged.

ACKNOWLEDGMENTS

I would like to acknowledge the skilled secretarial assistance of Ms. Linda Vaughan during the preparation of this manuscript.

References

1. Besdine, RW: Accidental hypothermia: The body's energy crisis. *Geriatrics* 34:15–59, 1979
2. Borkan GA, Norris AH: Assessment of biological age using a profile of physical parameters. *J. Gerontol* 35:177–184, 1980.
3. Bortz WH: Disuse and aging. *JAMA* 248:1203–1208, 1982.
4. Brandsetter RD, Kazemi H: Aging and the respiratory system. *Med Clin North Am* 67:419–431, 1983.
5. Brown WW, Spry L, Davis BB: Alterations in renal homeostasis with aging. In Davis BB, Wood WG (eds): *Homeostatic Function and Aging.* New York, Raven Press, 1985, p 23.
6. Cavna N: The effects of aging on the receptor organs of the human dermis. *Adv Biol Skin* 6:63–69, 1965.
7. Collins KJ, Exton-Smith AN, James MH, et al: Functional changes in autonomic nervous responses with aging. *Age Aging* 9:17–24, 1980.
8. Cutler RG: Evolution of longevity in primates. *J. Hum Evol* 5:169–202, 1976.
9. Dolecek R: Endocrine changes in the elderly. *Triangle* 24:17–33, 1985.
10. Drachman DA, Leavitt J: Human memory and the cholinergic system: A relationship to aging? *Arch Neurol* 30:113–121, 1974.
11. Dravid AR: Axonal transport. *Triangle* 18:117–121, 1979.
12. Fries IF: Aging, natural death and the comprehension of morbidity. *N Engl J Med*, 303:113–123, 1968.
13. Fries JF, Crapo LM: *Vitality and Aging.* San Francisco, W.H. Freeman, 1981.
14. Geokas MC, Coneas CN, Majumdar APN: The aging gastro-intestinal tract, liver, and pancreas. *Clin Geriatr Med* 1:177–205, 1985.
15. Gerstenblith G, Lakatta EG, Weisfeldt ML: Age changes in myocardial function and exercise response. *Prog Cardiovasc Dis* 19:1–21, 1976.
16. Gomez ED, Berman B: The aging skin. *Clin Geriatr Med* 1:285–305, 1985.
17. Hall DA: *The Aging of Connective Tissue.* New York, Academic Press, 1976.
18. Hayflick L: Aging under glass. *Exp Gerontol* 2:123–135, 1967.
19. Hayflick L: The cell biology of aging. *Clin Geriatr Med* 1:15–27, 1985.
20. Hollingsworth JW, Haahizume A, Jablon S: Correlations between tests of aging in Hiroshima subjects: an attempt to define physiologic age. *Yale J Biol Med* 38:11–26, 1965.
21. Horvath SM, Borgia JF: Cardiopulmonary gas transport and aging. *Am Rev Resp Dis* 129:568–571, 1984.
22. Hyams DE: The blood. In Brockhurst JC (ed):

Textbook of Geriatric Medicine and Gerontology. Edinburgh, Churchill Livingston, 1973, 528.

23. Kenney RA: *The Physiology of Aging*. Chicago, Year Book Medical Publishers, 1982, pp 72–76.
24. Kenney RA: Physiology of aging. *Clin Geriatr Med*, 1:37–59, 1985.
25. Klausner SC, Schwartz AB: The aging heart. *Clin Geriatr Med* 1:119–141, 1985.
26. Korenchevsky V: *Physiological and Pathological Aging*. New York, Hatner, 1961.
27. Krumpe PE, Knudson RJ, Parsons G, et al: The aging respiratory system. *Clin Geriatr Med* 1:143–175, 1985.
28. Lakatta EG: Alterations in the cardiovascular performance that occur in advanced age. *Fed Proc* 38:163–167, 1979.
29. Lybarger JA, Kilbourne EM: Hyperthermia and hypothermia in the elderly: An epidemiological review. In Davis BB, Wood WG (eds): *Homeostatic Function and Aging*. New York, Raven Press, 1985, p 149.
30. Reichel W, Garcia-Bunvel R, Dilallo J: Progeria and Weiner's syndrome as models for the study of normal human aging. *J. Am Geriatr Soc* 19:369–375, 1971.
31. Rossman I: Anatomic and body composition changes with aging. In Finch CE, Hayflick L (eds): *Handbook of the Biology of Aging*. New York, Van Nostrand-Reinhold, 1977, p 203.
32. Sacher GA: Relation of life span to brain weight and body weight in mammals. In Wolstenholme GEW, O'Connor M (eds): *Ciba Foundation Colloquia on Aging*, vol 5, *The Life Span of Animals*. London, Churchill-Livingstone, 1959, p 74.
33. Schofield JD, Davies I: Theories of aging. In Brockelhurst JC (ed): *Textbook of Geriatric Medicine and Gerontology*, ed 2. Edinburgh, Churchill-Livingstone, 1979, p 37.
34. Shepard RJ: *Physical Activity and Aging*. London, Croom Helm Ltd, 1978.
35. Vernadakis A: The aging brain. *Clin Geriatr Med* 1:61–94, 1985.
36. Zack L: The oral cavity. In Rossman (ed): *Clinical Geriatrics*. Philadelphia, Lippincott, 1979, p 618.

5 Cognition and Aging

DONALD H. KAUSLER

Editor's Note

Perhaps no area of gerontological research and theory is more controversial than the exploration of cognitive changes associated with aging. Certainly no body of research has yielded more contradictory results. In Chapter 5, Kausler summarizes many of the methodological issues in exploring cognitive processes in the aged and reviews two of the more common theories concerning the underlying mechanisms for observed cognitive decline. These theories of diminished processing resources or reduced speed of processing have important communicative implications, since the linguistic elements of communication are cognitively derived. The remainder of the chapter is devoted to an overview of current knowledge concerning the cognitive skills of the elderly in the following domains: (a) perception; (b) learning, transfer, and retention; (c) memory; and (d) problem solving and reasoning. Each of these topic areas relates specifically to the content of subsequent chapters in one of three ways. The cognitive behavior of interest may directly affect auditory processing or linguistic functioning in the older adult. The cognitive behavior or deficit may also influence task performance in assessment situations and learning skills and strategies in intervention. Finally, beliefs about the relative competence or incompetence of the elderly tend to relate more to perceptions of cognitive status than to any other characteristic. These perceptions have a profound influence on self-image and on social expectations. Thus they directly affect the quality and frequency of interpersonal interactions with older individuals.

Remembering where you parked your car in the shopping center's lot, learning the locations of stores in a new mall, understanding the implications of a new tax law, trying to attend to your spouse's conversation while driving through heavy traffic, solving the problem of serving a tasty dinner to guests who are on restricted diets, balancing your checkbook, and comprehending the instructions given to you by your physician—all familiar everyday cognitive activities. Cognitive processes direct our attention to specific events present in our environment, enable us to perceive and interpret those events, guide the acquisition of new information about our environment, determine the subsequent memorability of that new information, and find the means of solving problems created by novel environmental demands. Any impairment in cognitive functioning results in the diminished ability to adapt to our physical and social environments. To the extent that cognitive processes decline in proficiency from early to late adulthood, older adults are likely to adapt less effectively than younger adults. Given the basic role played by cognitive processes in communication, researchers and practitioners concerned with the communicative skills of older adults should be well aware of age-related changes in those processes. Cognitive geropsychologists have discovered a great deal about aging's effects on cognition, although

much remains to be discovered. The purpose of this chapter is to summarize what is presently known about cognition and aging (see 15, 61, and 103 for more detailed summaries).

In this summary, several important issues need to be considered. Foremost among them is the extent of adult age differences in the basic components of cognition, namely, perception, attention, learning, memory, and problem solving/reasoning. Conceivably, some cognitive processes are adversely affected by normal aging, while other processes are largely unaffected. For those that are affected by aging, there is the important related issue of the possible reversibility, at least in part, of the decrement in cognitive proficiency through effective intervention, such as training programs.

Another important issue concerns the causes for the adult age differences in cognitive proficiencies that do seem to exist. Causation, in turn, needs to be considered at three levels. The first is in terms of whether or not it is aging per se that is responsible for adult age differences in cognitive performances. The problem here is that adults of greatly different ages may differ in many respects besides their degree of biological aging, such as in years of formal education and in health status. These differences, rather than aging itself, could account for at least some of the cognitive deficits commonly found for elderly adults. At the second level, cognitive geropsychologists are confronted with the problem of determining whether or not there is some general causative factor for aging deficits. That is: Is there a decline with aging in some broad cognitive resource or process that affects many specific cognitive abilities? Finally, specific causative mechanisms for age changes in cognitive performances need to be identified. For example: Are aging decrements in memory proficiency attributable primarily to encoding or to retrieval processes—or to both, as implied by a decrement in general resources? Much of this review of each component of cognition will focus on attempts to identify specific age-sensitive and age-insensitive processes.

The approach of this chapter will be to examine first the issue of age differences versus true age changes. We will then turn to explanations of aging deficits in terms of a postulated general causative factor. The remainder of the chapter will be devoted to an overview of aging research in the specific content areas of cognition. No specific section will be concerned with the concept of intelligence. Intelligence is viewed by cognitive psychologists as being composed of a number of specific abilities. Many of these specific abilities, such as memory span, vocabulary, problem solving, and reasoning, will be touched upon in various sections of this review. General issues concerned with aging's effects on intelligence will be considered in the final section dealing with problem solving and reasoning.

ADULT AGE DIFFERENCES VERSUS ADULT AGE CHANGES

Cohort Effects

The presence of adult age differences on cognitive tasks is usually detected through the use of the traditional cross-sectional method in which adults of different ages are compared at the same time in their performance levels on a given task. Consider, for example, the use of the method with a paired-associate learning task. Groups of young and elderly adults, each representative of their underlying like-age populations, practice on a list of pairs of unrelated words (e.g., *table-pencil*) until the list is mastered. As indicated in Figure 5.1, an age difference in performance scores, favoring the young adults, is highly likely to be the outcome. Although the age difference is quite apparent, the reason for it is less so. One definite possibility is that the age difference is the result of a true age change in ability to learn paired words. Our assumption is that the present

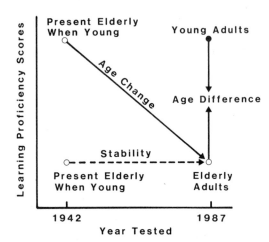

Figure 5.1. Contrast between an observed age difference and a true age change for performance on a learning task.

elderly adults would have scored much higher if they had been tested in 1942 when they too were young, rather than in 1987 when they were old. The resulting decline, depicted by the *solid arrow* in Figure 5.1, would constitute a true age change.

There is another possibility that must be considered, however. It is possible that the present elderly adults were really never much more proficient in learning ability than they are now. That is, their learning abilities may have been the same as young adults as they now are as elderly adults (represented by a *dashed arrow* in Fig. 5.1). For whatever reason, members of the earlier generation may simply have developed less proficiency for learning than did members of the later generation. If true, the resulting age difference apparent in 1987 would be the consequence of a cohort effect, rather than an aging effect. In other words, age as a causative variable is potentially confounded in cross-sectional comparisons by the very fact that the age groups being compared necessarily have their origins in widely separated cohorts or generations.

There are undoubtedly many variables and attributes that distinguish between members of widely separated generations. For example, child-rearing practices probably differed greatly when the members of the two generations were growing up. This difference could produce personality differences between present young and present elderly adults, and cohort effects for various personality traits have indeed been reported by a number of investigators (e.g., ref. 37). However, it seems unlikely that differences in child rearing practices would affect greatly cognitive processes. In fact, the only variable linked to cohort membership that is known to be related to performances on many cognitive tasks is that of education. Years of formal education have increased progressively from generation to generation in our society, meaning that there is a negative correlation between age and years of education for present members of our adult population. This fact of life was demonstrated recently in our laboratory when 128 adults, ranging in age from 20 to 79 years, received a paired-associate learning task (Kausler, Salthouse, and Saults, manuscript in preparation). The correlation between age and years of education was modest ($r = -0.24$), but statistically significant. The expected age differences in cognitive performance were confirmed by the presence of a significant correlation between age and paired-associate learning scores ($r = -0.30$). The problem in interpretation becomes apparent when it is realized that the correlation between years of education and paired-associate learning scores was also significant ($r = -0.26$). Is the age difference on our learning task the result of a true age decrement in learning proficiency or the result of a cohort effect reflecting the generational disparity in education?

The use of the cross-sectional method in cognitive aging research clearly calls for modification if it is to be effective in identifying age as the true causative factor for observed age differences in cognitive performances. Two modifications have been frequently employed. In the first, subjects of varying ages, selected to be representative of their underlying like-age populations, continue to be evaluated on the task in question. Statistical control over age differences in education is then applied by means of determining the correlation between age and performance scores after the effect of variation in educational level is partialled out. When this adjustment was made in our study, the correlation between age and learning scores remained statistically significant. The implication is that aging affects learning proficiency independently of the variation in education that accompanies variation in age.

The second modification calls for abandoning the use of subjects who are representative of their generations. Instead, age groups are selected in a manner that balances them on the critical nonage attribute of education. Thus, when college students serve as the members of the young group, as they commonly do, the older adults selected for comparison are equated with the students in years of education. When educationally balanced age groups are contrasted in paired-associate learning proficiency, a substantial age difference, still favoring the young adults, persists. The implication is again that

aging itself bears a causative relationship with the decrement in learning proficiency found for elderly adults.

Of course, it may be argued that there are other important attributes besides educational level that differ among different generations and remain undetected in their influence on age differences in cognitive performances. If true, age effects would continue to be confounded by cohort effects in cross-sectional comparisons despite the equality of education across the age groups. For those geropsychologists who accept this argument, the only solution is to find a better method than the cross-sectional one for comparing performances at different age levels. There are indeed other methods available. The traditional alternative is the longitudinal method whereby the same subjects are evaluated more than once on the same cognitive task, each time at a different age. Thus, for the earlier paired-associate example illustrated in Figure 5.1, longitudinal evaluation of age differences would require that the elderly adults tested in 1987 were also tested on a comparable task in 1942 when they were young adults. Since the same subjects are assessed at each age, each age group necessarily contains subjects from the same generation, therefore avoiding the potential confoundings of cohort effects.

Unfortunately, however, the longitudinal method has its own shortcomings. Most important, for it to be effective, a lengthy segment of the adult life span should enter into the separate assessments, meaning that many of the adults who were tested when they were young may not be available years later when they are to be retested. Those subjects who continue in the study may differ in initial performance level from those who drop out of the study. In addition, the time of measurement differs greatly between widely separated assessments. Consequently, the conditions present at one time of measurement may affect performance differently than the conditions present at a later time (e.g., an economic depression at Time 1, economic prosperity at Time 2). Uncontrolled variation in time of measurement could, in principle, be as potent a source of confounding age effects as uncontrolled generational variation (111). To these, and other methodological concerns (see ref. 61 for elaboration), add the problems of the high cost of longitudinal research and the demand placed on the patience of the investigator, and it is little wonder that, with the exception of research on adult age differences in intelligence (e.g., ref. 86), there has been little longitudinal research on cognitive aging. What has been done in such areas as learning (2), vigilance (97), and problem solving (1) has demonstrated age effects comparable to those found with the cross-sectional method.

The remaining alternatives consist of more recent additions to the methodological arsenal contributed by Schaie (111). Each involves a sequential analysis in which cross-sectional age comparisons, longitudinal age comparisons, and time lag cohort comparisons of like-age subjects are combined within the same study. Either cohort membership or time of measurement is treated as an independent variable, along with age as an accompanying independent variable, yielding a cross-sequential and a time-sequential design, respectively. Thus, rather than treating either cohort or time of measurement variations as nuisance variables to be controlled (or, more likely, ignored), the investigator varies one or the other systematically as an independent variable. Unfortunately, time of measurement remains uncontrolled in a cohort-sequential design, and cohort membership is uncontrolled in a time-sequential design.

Despite this shortcoming, the careful use of sequential methodology does hold promise for unraveling the separate effects of age, cohort membership, and time of measurement on adult age differences in cognitive performances. However, its application in gerontological research thus far has been limited largely to age differences in intelligence (e.g., 112) and age differences in personality (e.g., 37). Moreover, the extent to which sequential methods are needed in cognitive aging research on perception, attention, learning, memory, and problem solving/reasoning is debatable. For example, the magnitude of cohort effects, other than those associated with education, is probably slight for these components of cognition (see ref. 61 for further discussion). Consequently, the effective use of the cross-sectional method is probably adequate for evaluating the presence of true aging deficits on most cognitive tasks.

Competence versus Performance

A more serious challenge to the internal validity of cognitive aging studies (i.e., their ability to identify correctly age as the true causative factor for observed age differences) rests in the important distinction between competence for performance on a given cognitive task and the degree of utilization of that competence in actual task performance. Conceivably, young and elderly adults differ little in their competence, or true ability, to perform on a given task but, for whatever reason, elderly adults perform farther below their ability level than do

young adults. The implication is that the observed age difference for many cognitive tasks would virtually disappear if the reasons for elderly adults' performance deficits could be eliminated. The nature of the performance/competence distinction is illustrated in Figure 5.2 in reference to our earlier paired-associate learning example. Note that the age difference present under usual performance conditions (i.e., the conditions present for the results shown in Fig. 5.1) diminishes greatly as both age groups approach their true competence levels under more ideal performance conditions. If this were the case, the observed age difference apparent in Figure 5.1 would have its origin in a vastly different source than a cohort effect.

A number of performance variables have been postulated to be responsible for much of the magnitude of the adult age differences commonly found on cognitive tasks, and many of them have been investigated in the laboratory. Only a brief overview of this research can be given here (see ref. 61 for an extended review).

One potential performance variable enters the picture because of the familiar practice of comparing task performances of elderly adults with those of college students representing young adults. Perhaps being a student is in itself a cognitively stimulating activity that maintains performance levels close to true ability levels. If true, then we would expect elderly adults who are themselves presently college students to perform more proficiently than typical nonstudent elderly adults, with, perhaps, the former even approaching the performance levels of young college students. Alas, however, the evidence here is not very convincing.

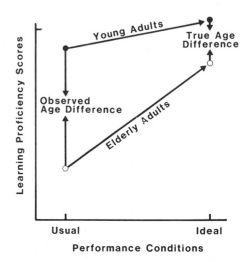

Figure 5.2. Hypothetical age differences in performance on a learning task under ideal performance conditions relative to usual conditions.

Parks et al (88) found no difference in paired-associate learning proficiency between student and nonstudent elderly adults, with the proficiency of each group falling well below that of young college students. A comparable outcome was reported by Hartley (48) for memory of discourse content.

Another popular performance hypothesis is that elderly adults are simply less motivated to perform well on most laboratory cognitive tasks than are young adults, resulting in a larger competence-performance discrepancy for the former than for the latter. Interestingly, others have postulated that elderly adults perform less well than young adults for the opposite reason, that is, because they are "overaroused" to the point where excessive arousal interferes with effective performance. The evidence supporting each of these motivational positions has not been very convincing. The fact is, adult age differences in many cognitive performances persist even under seemingly optimal motivating conditions (see ref. 61).

A third condition of the organism that may affect cognitive performance is health status. Elderly adults are considered, in general, to be in poorer health than young adults, and are therefore more likely to experience health-related deficits in performance. There is evidence indicating that elderly adults reporting poor health perform less proficiently on a serial learning task than elderly adults reporting excellent or good health (80), and that elderly adults with cardiovascular problems experience lowering of intelligence test scores (51). Cognitive aging researchers are well aware of the potential problems for interpreting age differences in performance when age groups differ in health status as well as in age. Their standard practice is to employ as subjects only elderly adults who rate their physical health status as being good or better. There is considerable evidence of substantial agreement between self-rated health status and health status as determined by a physician's examination (e.g., 69). Thus, there is good reason to believe that the age deficits reported in the cognitive aging literature are not the result of reduced performance proficiency attributable to poor health for the elderly participants.

Mental health status also needs to be considered, especially in light of the high instance of depression commonly reported in late adulthood (e.g., 46), and the popular belief that depression interferes with effective cognitive performances, especially those involving memory. The implication that the differential incidence of depression among the young and old segments of our population markedly affects adult age differences in cognitive performances has to be challenged seriously, however. In the first place, the incidence of depression in late adulthood seems to be inflated by the nature of the procedure used to assess its presence. As measured by clinical tests, depression is identified by the self-reporting of both psychological symptoms (e.g., the feeling of despair) and physical symptoms (e.g., loss of appetite and difficulty in sleeping). Many of the so-called physical symptoms are probably indicators of depression when experienced by young adults, but they are likely to be simply "signs" of normal aging when experienced by elderly adults. For example, sleep disturbances seem to be prevalent among normally aging elderly adults (e.g., 96,141). When these physical symptoms are eliminated from diagnostic tests of depression, the incidence of depression in late adulthood seems to be no greater than in early adulthood (13). Moreover, a number of studies (e.g., 93) have reported that elderly adults who score high on tests of depression do not differ on memory tasks from those who score low, even though the former do complain more frequently about having "memory problems." Depression as a causative variable for adult age differences in performances on cognitive tasks seems to have no more validity than does motivation or physical health status.

The final potential performance variable that may differ between young and elderly adults is especially intriguing. Ever since the early research of Thorndike (128), it has been argued that the cognitive skills of elderly adults become "rusty" through their disuse late in life. With sufficient practice, these latently available skills should begin to approach their true competence levels, presumably levels close to those of young adults. The validity of the disuse principle has been given a number of tests in recent years on such tasks as memory scanning (110), visual discrimination (110), and sorting cards on the basis of target letters they contain (91). In these studies, both young and elderly subjects are given many trials on the task in question, and scores are related to the degree of practice. The disuse principle predicts that as practice progresses, performances of elderly subjects should begin to "catch up" with those of young adults. This is not the case, however. Elderly subjects do indeed improve dramatically with practice, in agreement with the disuse principle—but so do young adults. The lesson is clear. Adults of all ages generally perform below their true ability levels, and with practice they begin to approach their optimal levels. The net effect is that the magnitude of adult age differences in performances remains essentially unaffected by degree of practice. Nevertheless, the striking increment with practice manifested by elderly adults does have important practical implications that will be discussed later in this chapter.

Other Methodological Issues

Our focus thus far has been entirely on subject characteristics that complicate the interpretation of the meaning of adult age differences in laboratory cognitive performances. There are many nonsubject issues as well. (Obviously, cognitive aging research is not for the fainthearted!) These issues have been discussed thoroughly elsewhere (62, 107), and two of the most important will be touched upon here.

The first concerns the difficulty level of the task serving to evaluate the magnitude of adult age differences in performance. If the task is excessively difficult, both young and elderly subjects will perform poorly on it. A floor effect will be present for all age groups, giving the false appearance of the absence of an age difference. If the task is very easy, both young and elderly subjects will perform extremely well on it, again giving the false impression of age equality. To test adequately for the presence of adult age differences in cognitive performances, tasks of intermediate difficulty clearly need to be employed.

The second issue concerns the generalizability of the age differences found in the laboratory to age differences found in the everyday world. At stake is the "ecological validity" of laboratory performances—that is: Are they valid indices of their everyday counterparts? Much of the concern expressed by critics of laboratory assessments (e.g., 85, 100) has centered on learning/memory and problem solving/reasoning tasks. Consider, for example, the laboratory-based paired-associate learning task described earlier. What does the aging deficit found with it tell us about everyday aging deficits in learning? Answers to this question can be given only after cognitive geropsychologists have developed effective means of evaluating everyday performances, thereby permitting the determination of the extent to which laboratory assessments relate to everyday performance levels. Thus far, everyday evaluations have been restricted to self-ratings of functioning in the real world. Laboratory performances have been found by some investigators (e.g., 138), but not by others (e.g., 137), to correlate significantly with self-ratings of everyday learning/memory proficiency. Unfortunately, many individuals at all ages are probably not the best judges of their own learning/memory proficiencies. Interestingly, Sunderland et al (125) found that ratings given by significant other people (e.g.,

spouses) correlated substantially higher with scores on a laboratory paired-associate learning task than did self-ratings.

THE SEARCH FOR A GENERAL EXPLANATION OF AGING DEFICITS

Assuming that there are widespread aging deficits in cognitive performances, it makes sense to believe that there is an age-related decline in some basic cognitive mechanism that affects the proficiency of many specific cognitive processes. Two such mechanisms have been proposed by cognitive geropsychologists. The first proposes an age-related decrement in overall processing resources, the second an age-related "slowing down" of cognitive processes. Each of these mechanisms will be examined in the present section, along with the evidence supporting (or failing to support) them.

Diminished Resources

There are several versions of the diminished resources principle. They all argue, however, that the resources available for engaging in most cognitive performances, whether they be viewed in terms of space for conducting cognitive operations or the mental energy needed for those operations, are less for elderly adults than for young adults. Cognitive tasks that must draw upon those resources will show aging deficits, while tasks that bypass those resources will show little, if any, aging deficits (49). The most popular versions of this principle place those resources in what is called a working memory. Working memory is a cognitive structure viewed as having a limited capacity both for the temporary storage of information (i.e., short-term memory) and for the manipulation, or processing, of that information while it is held in storage (e.g., encoding it for transmission to a long-term store). The concept of a limited capacity working memory has been successfully applied in basic cognitive research with young adult subjects. For example, it explains nicely differences in performing a secondary task (responding when a click is heard) as affected by the difficulty of material being read simultaneously for later memory testing (the primary task) (19). Shown in Figure 5.3 are several possible effects of aging on working memory. (a) Storage capacity decreases, with processing capacity unaffected; (b) Processing capacity (or energy supply) decreases, with storage capacity unaffected; and (c) both stor-

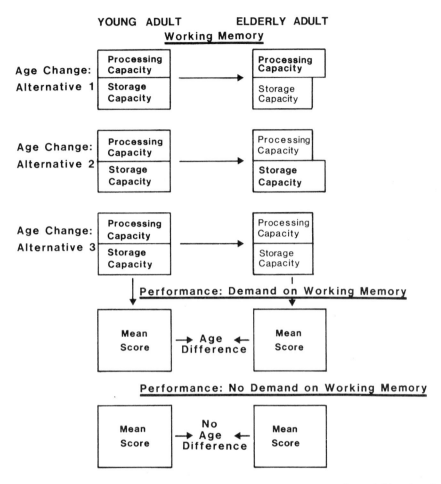

Figure 5.3. Alternative views of diminished capacity of working memory in late adulthood and expected effects on age differences in performance contingent on the involvement or noninvolvement of working memory.

age and processing capacity decrease. The net effect is the same for each—task performances that make demands on working memory are age sensitive; those that do not are age insensitive.

A major problem with the diminished resources principle has been the difficulty of obtaining direct support for its involvement in aging deficits. Ideally, one would like to operationalize the concept of working memory and measure its capacity independently of the particular cognitive task for which it is postulated to determine aging deficits. Elderly adults who score low on this measure would be expected to perform far less proficiently on the task at hand (e.g., a paired-associate learning task) than elderly adults who score much higher. Conventional measures of short-term memory, such as forward and backward digit span, prove to be ineffective as measures of working memory capacity, and therefore fail as predictors of per-

formance scores on cognitive tasks (29, 71). As a result, cognitive aging researchers have turned to the more demanding measure of reading span introduced by Daneman and Carpenter (29). Subjects read a series of sentences for which the last word in each sentence is to be recalled at the end. A subject's reading span is the longest number of sentences that can be read with perfect recall of their terminal words. This measure has been found to correlate significantly with young adults' comprehension and recall of sentences (29). Unfortunately, however, it has not been found to be very predictive of individual differences among elderly adults in their memory for sentences and story content (48, 71). Nor have other measures that, on the surface, seem closely related to working memory capacity proved to be any more effective in predicting elderly adults' scores on other kinds of cognitive tasks (e.g., 108). In addition, there are conceptual problems inherent in the concept of diminished resources with aging that add further to its questionable validity as a general mechanism for explaining aging deficits (105, 106).

Speed of Processing

The possibility that the overall rate of processing information in the central nervous system is slower for elderly adults than for young adults was proposed some years ago by Birren (14). Neural events were simply regarded as requiring increasing time to complete their cycles with increasing age, and their increasing cycle times were believed to affect adversely a wide range of cognitive activities. The "slowing down" mechanism has been championed in recent years by Salthouse (105, 106). A number of possible reasons for the slower rate of neural events with aging are considered by Salthouse, but the favorite seems to be that "neural events are slower in the older nervous system because of its need to integrate information samples for a longer time to compensate for increased levels of 'neural noise' (105, p. 415)." The same processes are engaged in by older as by younger individuals, but the cycle-time to complete each process is longer as age increases. As noted by Salthouse, "One implication of the cycle-time hypothesis is that no single information processing stage should be found to be 'critical,' or uniquely responsible, for the age-related slowing, but instead the slowing should be generalized and evident in nearly all stages of processing (105, p 415)." In general, as the number of processes involved in performing a cognitive task increases, the magnitude of the aging deficit in task performance should increase simply because each additional process adds to the overall slower rate of completing the processing of task information.

Just as the limited capacity principle needs operationalization and independent measurement of individual differences, so does the speed of processing principle. For Salthouse (106), measurement is by means of scores on such speed-oriented tests as the digit symbol test. Here subjects have to substitute numbers for the geometric figures they represent in a coding system. Their scores are the time it takes to complete a set number of substitutions. Elderly adults do indeed take considerably longer to complete this task than do young adults, presumably because of their slower processing rate. Slower processing rate, as indexed by time scores on the digit symbol test, does seem to account for aging deficits on a number of cognitive tasks,

but not on others, such as paired-associate learning (106). Thus, the slowing down principle, as a general explanation of cognitive deficits for older individuals, has its own limitations.

At this time, both the diminished capacity hypothesis and the "slowing down" hypothesis continue to attract many proponents, and with good reason—they both give adequate accounts of many aging deficits. From the perspective of the capacity hypothesis, aging deficits are expected only when performance requirements exceed the capacity of older adults, but not that of younger adults. From the perspective of the "slowing down" hypothesis, aging deficits are expected only when performances are affected by the rate at which their component processes are completed. In most cases, predictions regarding age differences derived from the two hypotheses are indistinguishable.

PERCEPTION

Perception refers to the meaning assigned to the sensory information we receive from our environment. Thus, the visual stimuli reaching our eyes as we stroll down the street are perceived as cars, trees, and people; the auditory stimuli as screeching brakes, the crying of a child, and speech; and the olfactory stimuli as the burning of leaves and a passer-by's potent after shave lotion. It should be obvious that perception per se changes little qualitatively with advancing age—a kiss is still a kiss; a sigh is still a sigh; and a tree is still a tree. What does change with aging is the rate at which sensory information is processed on its way to being recognized and identified. In cognitive psychology, the analysis of incoming sensory information and the subsequent identification of that information (i.e., perception) are known as pattern recognition. Adult age differences in both visual and auditory pattern recognition will be our major concern in this section. However, there is a preliminary topic to consider. Pattern recognition operates on information registered by the senses. To the extent that sensory sensitivity diminishes with aging, the pattern recognition processes of elderly adults will have less sensory input upon which to operate than will the processes of young adults.

Sensory Sensitivity

Sensory sensitivity refers to both the ability to detect the presence of low intensity stimuli (i.e., they are near threshold value) and the ability to detect variation in the intensity of stimuli that are well above threshold value. Tests of age differences in low intensity sensitivity are complicated by the possibility that elderly adults are more conservative than young adults in their sensory decision-making characteristics. That is, older adults may require greater intensity of a stimulus to be present before they will risk saying it is there, even though they may actually be able to detect low levels of intensity. Tests of age differences in low intensity sensitivity therefore require a methodology that permits separating sensitivity per se from decision-making characteristics. The methodology that accomplishes this objective is that of signal detection (45).

To apply signal detection methodology, subjects receive a number of trials, say, 200. On 100 of the randomly ordered trials a weak stimulus, such as a faint tone, is actually presented; on the other 100 trials, no stimulus occurs. Subjects respond "Yes" on those trials in which they believe they heard the tone, and "No" on those trials in which they believe the tone was absent. From a subject's pattern of hits (correctly responding "Yes" to a true stimulus and "No" to an absent stimulus), misses (incorrectly responding "No" to a true stimulus), and false alarms (incorrectly responding "Yes" to an absent stimulus), both an index of sensitivity (d') and an index of conservatism in decision-making (beta) may be determined for that subject. Studies with this method have revealed that elderly adults are both less sensitive to low intensity tones and more conservative in decision-making than are young adults (96, 99). Research on the other senses, such as smell, has also revealed the elderly adult's diminished sensitivity for low intensity stimuli.

Diminished sensitivity for low intensity stimuli has many practical implications for elderly people. For example, the slight odor of a gas leak from a stove may go undetected; a whispered conversation may not be heard; and the faint light on a roadblock in the distance may not be seen. However, most sensory stimuli in our daily lives are well above threshold value. Diminished sensitivity to low intensity stimuli is probably a good indicator of diminished sensitivity to suprathreshold stimuli as well. An age-related decline in suprathreshold sensitivity has, in fact, been found for odors (24, 81, 101), and is likely to be found for the other senses as well. The procedure calls for presenting an odorous substance varying in degree of concentration and asking subjects to rate the intensity of their subjective experience of smell at each level of physical intensity. Elderly subjects reveal a much flatter function than do young adults, indicating that a given increase in physical intensity produces far less of a gain in experienced intensity for elderly than for young adults. That is, elderly adults appear to be less sensitive to sensory increments than are young adults. It is declining sensitivity with age that accounts for the frequent statement by elderly adults that "everything tastes alike." Although this is likely to be a gross exaggeration for most elderly people, it is true that elderly people have greater difficulty identifying foods by taste than do young adults (82, 115) and identifying familiar substances, such as ammonia and bleach, by smell (114).

Our focus on pattern recognition should not prevent us from realizing that structural changes with aging in the sensory receptors themselves result in impairments in perceptual phenomena other than those of pattern recognition. For example, depth perception appears to decline progressively in proficiency from age 40 or so on (9), most likely the consequence of such factors as an age-related decrease in illumination reaching the retina. More frequent "fender benders" while attempting angular parking of a car as people get older should not be surprising. Similarly, the "yellowing" of the lens with aging presumably accounts for the age-related decline in color perception reported by some investigators (e.g., 43). However, recent evidence (123) indicates that the color weakness of older individuals may be manifested only when finer contour discriminations are required. Fine contour discriminations are involved, for example, in distinguishing among the colors in a tie that contains a complex, mutable pattern of shapes and colors.

Diminished sensory sensitivity with aging carries with it special responsibilities for cognitive aging researchers. For cognitive tasks having rigorous visual or auditory demands on subjects, assurance of the absence of sensory impairments that would unduly handicap the performances of elderly subjects is sorely needed. Ample testimony to the dangers of the failure to give such assurance comes from evidence demonstrating negative correlations between degree of auditory sensitivity in elderly subjects and scores earned on both an intelligence test (44) and a memory task (127).

Visual Pattern Recognition

Most of the research on aging deficits in visual pattern recognition has concentrated on the peripheral versus central locus of those deficits. Anatomically, peripheral refers to sensory pathways and the lower brain centers with which they connect, central to the higher brain centers where the processing initiated in the lower centers is completed. Translated to cognitive terms, peripheral processes are presumed to analyze the features of patterns registered by the visual system, and central processes to match those features with information stored permanently in generic memory (see the later section on memory), leading to the identification of the pattern. Thus, for the visual pattern "*H*," feature analyzers segregate the pattern into component vertical lines and a single horizontal line that bisects both vertical lines. These features are then compared with the permanently stored information that identifies them as being those of the letter *H*. At this point, the pattern has been identified, that is, perceived. As illustrated in Figure 5.4, the transition from a sensory registration stage to a feature analytic stage and to a matching/identification stage requires real time. Accuracy in identifying such simple patterns as single letters of the alphabet is not at stake—young and old perceivers are not expected to differ. Of interest instead are questions pertaining to age differences in the rate of completing pattern identifications. Is there a "slowing down" with aging only in the peripheral stage (i.e., in feature analysis)? only in the central stage (i.e., in matching features with stored information and a subsequent identification)? or in both stages? Most important: What is the magnitude of slowing down, wherever it does occur?

Two methods have been employed to answer these questions. The first is called chronometric analysis (94). Pairs of letters, such as HH, Hh, HB, and Hd, are presented to subjects. Their job is to respond, as rapidly as possible, in some way to signify "Yes" if the letters have

the same name and "No" if they have different names. Note that the answer for both HH and Hh pairs is "Yes." However, in the case of HH only the peripheral process of feature analysis is needed in that this analysis reveals identical features, and therefore necessarily identical names, for the two letters. Feature analysis alone is insufficient for Hh-like pairs. It must be followed by the central process of matching both letters' unique features with the same name before a "Yes" decision can be made. The time to respond to HH-like pairs yields an estimate of peripheral processing time combined with the time to make the physical response signifying "Yes," and the time to respond to Hh-like pairs adds to this total time the time to conduct central processing (Fig. 5.4). By subtracting the first time from the second time, an estimate of central processing rate can be obtained. The use of this method in aging research (e.g., 73) indicates a slower rate of central processing by elderly than by young adults, with the differential being about 100 milliseconds. Peripheral processing rate also appears to be slower for elderly than for young adults, although the magnitude of the age differential is more difficult to determine in that it is inflated by the elderly adult's slower execution of the response (e.g., moving a lever in a specified direction) signifying "Yes."

The second method involves a backward masking procedure in which a letter, as a target stimulus, is exposed briefly (e.g., for 50 milliseconds), and is followed after a varying interval by a masking stimulus that disrupts the processing of the target. The subject's task is simply to identify the target stimulus—and the slower the processing of its information, the

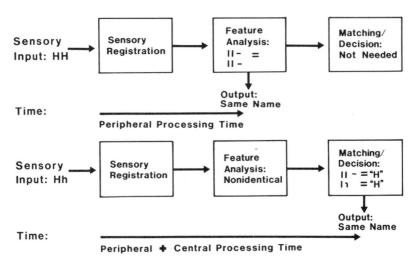

Figure 5.4.   Peripheral (feature analytic) and central (matching/decision) stages of pattern recognition.

longer the time interval before the occurrence of the masking stimulus that is needed to permit identification. By introducing several variations of this procedure, it is possible to estimate separately peripheral and central processing rates. These estimates also indicate slower processing rates for elderly adults, both peripherally and centrally, with the age difference for each being about 100 milliseconds (e.g., 35, 131). The finding of a slower rate for elderly adults in *both* stages is, of course, in agreement with Salthouse's position of a *general* slowing down with aging.

While the absolute difference in processing rates between young and elderly adults is not great, it should be noted that only simple patterns need to be identified with letters as stimuli. With more complex patterns, the multiple features requiring analysis and eventually synthesis in the form of identification are likely to result in a more pronounced age differential in the total time needed for identification. This could be the case, for example, when an object in the road ahead of a driver may be either a tumbleweed or an animal—with the consequence dependent on the driver's time to make the identification. However, expertise in the pattern recognition of complex stimuli is possible after years of experience with those stimuli. This is the case, for example, with expert typists (104) and chess masters, (25). Expert typists well into their 60's and early 70s type as rapidly as young expert typists, even though the elderly typist displays a far slower rate of performance on other tasks unrelated to typing. The apparent reason is that elderly experts have increased sensitivity to characters well in advance of the character they are currently typing, a sensitivity that is absent in the young expert and that compensates for the overall slower responding of the older expert. Similarly, older chess masters can briefly examine a chess board having the pieces arranged meaningfully and then reproduce their placements exactly, an achievement younger novices cannot accomplish. On the other hand, when the pieces are arranged randomly, the older master has greater difficulty in reproducing the placements than does the younger novice.

Auditory Pattern Recognition

There has been far less research on adult age differences in auditory pattern recognition than in visual. What evidence there is comes from a variation of chronometric analysis by Elias and Elias (39), in which subjects were given successive tones and asked if they were the same or different. Such judgments would seem to require only peripheral processing in that identify may be determined by featural commonality. Not surprisingly, peripheral processing was found to be slower for elderly than for young subjects, with the age difference in reaction time being about 169 milliseconds. Determining the extent of slowing down in central processing rate could perhaps be determined by presenting pairs of successive words. For some pairs, the members would be identical words (e.g., *pretty-pretty*); for other pairs they would be synonyms (e.g., *pretty-beautiful*); and for the remaining pairs they would be words unrelated in meaning (e.g., *pretty-stingy*). Subjects would be asked to respond "Same" if the successive words have a common meaning and "Different" if not. Central processing is required for synonym pairs, but not for the other kinds of pairs where decisions can be made solely on the basis of featural commonality.

Information obtained in such studies would be important in determining the effects of aging on speech comprehension as a form of auditory pattern recognition (see Chapters 8 and 9). In general, age differences in speech comprehension have been studied by presenting sentences that vary either in rate of presentation or in amount of distortion. These studies usually indicate little aging deficit in comprehension when sentences are spoken at a normal conversational rate, but a pronounced aging deficit under conditions of distortion (e.g., 11). Conceivably, the deficits that do occur in the presence of distortion are the consequence of the slower central processing rate of elderly adults, relative to young adults.

ATTENTION

In an earlier review of attention, the present writer commented that "some idea of the importance of attention in our everyday lives may be gleaned from the many statements we hear or read that refer to some aspect of attention: " 'Be alert!,' 'Watch for any sign of activity,' 'Get ready, get . . . .' 'He's listening, but he's not hearing,' 'Probable cause of the accident—inattention of the driver in vehicle A,' 'He can't walk and chew gum at the same time' (61, p 221)." As these examples suggest, attention is a complex phenomenon that takes three forms: vigilance, selective attention, and divided attention. Each form is of considerable relevance to potential impairments in the everyday functioning of elderly adults.

Vigilance

"Watch for any sign of activity!" The implication of this command is that there will be a steady stream of inactivity, and the observer's job is to detect any change in that pattern. This situation demonstrates the attentional demands of a vigilance task—monitoring a series of constant stimuli in order to detect the occasional occurrences of a deviant stimulus. These demands are encountered, for example, by a security guard who must monitor a video screen displaying the presumably deserted hallways of a building.

Age differences in the ability to maintain vigilance are studied by means of a clock-like device in which the single hand of the clock moves one space at a time over a lengthy interval, and then unexpectedly jumps two spaces. The subject's task is to detect each aberrant movement of the hand. An early study by Surwillo and Quilter (126) found a modest, but statistically significant, aging deficit for this task, even though the "young" subjects in their study were actually middle-aged. Interestingly, the investigators examined the age difference separately for each 15-minute segment of the total 60 minutes of clock monitoring and found the aging deficit to be restricted to only the final 15 minutes. Apparently, fatigue accounts for the modest aging deficit—and no aging deficit in simple vigilance is apparent in the absence of fatigue's accumulation over a lengthy performance session. Essentially the same outcome was reported in a longitudinal reassessment 18 years later of many of the original subjects in this study (97). This outcome should not be surprising. The simple monitoring of constant stimuli makes little demand upon cognitive resources and should therefore be largely unaffected by any age-related decrement in those resources. Nor should the slowing down of processing rate be expected to affect markedly the monitoring of a series of simple stimuli.

It is a different matter, however, when vigilance is complicated by adding a memory demand. This is the case when subjects must monitor a pattern of light stimuli in which each stimulus requires its own specific response to be made (e.g., pushing one button for stimulus 1, a different button for stimulus 2, and so on). Instead of responding to the just presented light, subjects must respond to the light presented one or two steps earlier. Thus, they must hold in memory information about previously seen lights while continuing to monitor the flow of changing stimuli. Under these conditions, elderly adults perform at a level considerably below that of young adults, with the degree of the aging deficit increasing as the memory demand increases (68). The aging deficit here may be readily explained in terms of either the diminished resources or the slowing down hypothesis.

Selective Attention

A student listening to a professor's lecture is presumably focusing attention on the scintillating flow of the professor's words while screening out such extraneous auditory stimuli as the whispering going on among nearby students. The ability to restrict attention to relevant stimuli (e.g., the professor's words) while ignoring irrelevant stimuli (e.g., the whispering) is known as selective attention. The importance of selective attention in our daily lives is apparent from the fact that we are often bombarded by many stimuli, and we must attend to only those relevant to our ongoing performances. Beginning with the pioneering research of Broadbent (20), psychologists have postulated that selective attention is accomplished by the presence of a filtering mechanism in the attentional/perceptual system. The filter permits relevant information to be processed fully (i.e., perceived), while rejecting, or at least attenuating, the processing of irrelevant stimuli. The fact that the filter attenuates rather than rejects irrelevant stimuli is made readily apparent when irrelevant information of high pertinence to the receiver is perceived. For example, the student's attention is highly likely to be diverted to the whispering if his or her name is embedded within the irrelevant information.

Our interest in selective attention rests in the considerable evidence indicating the diminished ability of elderly adults to "tune out" irrelevant sources of information. One form of evidence comes from the use of the Stroop task. Subjects are asked on some trials simply to name the color of a square displayed on each card in a series of cards and on other trials to name the color of the ink in which a word present on the card is printed. For the latter trials, naming the ink color is interfered with by having the accompanying word be the name of a different color. For example, the word *blue* may be printed in red ink, with subjects being required to say "red." The word name, as an irrelevant stimulus, must be ignored as much as possible while attending to the ink color as a relevant stimulus. Young and elderly subjects differ only slightly in the time taken to name colors on the cards in the absence of competing word stimuli. However, a pronounced aging deficit is found for the time to name relevant ink colors in the presence of irrelevant, competing word stimuli (26). An aging deficit is also found (e.g., 98) when subjects must sort a stack of cards on the basis of which of two target letters appear on each card. For example, if the letter Q is on a card, the card belongs in the left pile; if the letter V is on a card, it belongs in the right pile. The targeted letters therefore constitute relevant stimuli. If no other letters appear on the cards, the age difference in sorting time is a modest one. The age difference increases, however, when other letters (e.g., B and W), constituting irrelevant stimuli, are also present on the cards to be sorted. Moreover, the magnitude of the aging deficit increases progressively as the number of irrelevant letters present on each card increases.

The reason for the age difference in distractability by irrelevant stimuli is not fully understood. Conceivably, young adults simply terminate their analysis of irrelevant stimuli after peripheral processing identifies them as being nontargeted information. Further analysis of the identity of the irrelevant stimuli through central processing is not required to perform the task at hand, and serves merely to retard performance. By contrast, elderly adults may have difficulty "turning off" the processing of irrelevant stimuli until it has been completed to the point of identifying them. The net effect would be increased time for elderly adults to reach a "reject" decision for each irrelevant stimulus. Evidence for this position comes from a study by Farkas and Hoyer (41). In one condition of their study highly dissimilar irrelevant stimuli (i.e., dissimilar with respect to the targets) were included along with targeted relevant stimuli. When no irrelevant stimuli were present on the cards, an increase in sorting time was found for elderly subjects, but not for young subjects. The dissimilar stimuli were sufficiently distinctive to permit their rejections as targets after peripheral processing alone. Nevertheless, elderly adults appeared to engage in redundant central processing of their contents.

Age differences in distractability by irrelevant stimuli may also be explained in terms of either the overall slower processing rate of elderly adults or the diminished processing resources of elderly adults. In the former case, young and elderly individuals are presumed to engage in the same kind of processing, whether it be peripheral alone or peripheral plus central. It simply takes longer for elderly adults to complete the identification of irrelevant stimuli as irrelevant. In the latter case, the assumption is that the discrimination between relevant and irrelevant information requires cognitively

effortful, or controlled, processing (116). The diminished resources of elderly adults may then be presumed to increase the difficulty of making such discriminations. Interestingly, elderly adults appear to be as capable as young adults in decreasing dramatically their decision times when the same target and nontarget letters are repeated many times in a lengthy series of trials (77, 92) (a condition known as "consistent mapping," in contrast to a "varied mapping" condition where the targets and nontargets keep changing in content over the trials). Under these conditions, the discrimination between relevant and irrelevant stimuli is postulated to be guided by automatic processes that bypass the limited resources needed for controlled processing under varied mapping conditions(116).

Divided Attention

Driving your car while listening to the conversation of a passenger is a familiar example of divided attention. Note that there are two sources of relevant information that require attention—the visual information from the flow of traffic and the auditory information from the passenger's conversation. Dividing attention between the two should be easy when the traffic is light, but it should become increasingly difficult as the amount of traffic increases. Of interest to us are age differences in the ability to allocate attentional resources to the separate informational sources in accordance with the demands of the task at hand. When traffic is very heavy, nearly 100% of the driver's resources are likely to be devoted to it, and virtually 0% to the conversation. With moderate traffic, the attentional resources may be fairly equally divided between the two sources, and with the total absence of traffic, as in driving through some sections of Nevada, most of the allocation may be devoted to the conversation.

There are many complex methodological problems in determining the extent of age differences in the proficiency of allocating resorces under conditions of divided attention. Fortunately, many of these problems were resolved in two recent studies by Salthouse (109, 120). The results of these studies suggest that aging deficits in allocating resources to simultaneously present stimuli are negligible when the underlying tasks are simple to perform, but they become more substantial with more difficult tasks. In the former case, subjects simply had to detect the presence or absence of each of two different visual targets. In the latter case, subjects had to remember each of two visually presented series of items, one consisting of letters, the other of digits. Returning to our driver analogy, we might expect to find little effect of aging on dividing attention between traffic and conversational content when the latter is confined to simple topics like the weather. The effect could be magnified considerably, however, when the conversation is about difficult topics like cognitive psychology.

LEARNING, TRANSFER, AND RETENTION

The distinction between learning and memory in contemporary cognitive psychology is a dubious one. It may be argued that memory is simply a broader concept than is learning. Learning is one means of assuring memory of our interactions with the environment, but not the only means. We have memory for the rules of a new word game we have been playing recently, but we also have memory of birthday gifts received months and even years ago. In the former case, memory is the product of learning, defined in terms of intentionally practicing and rehearsing the information to-be-retained. In the latter case, memory seems to be present in the absence of any apparent intent to remember or to practice/rehearse the information in question. Similarly, we have memory of people's names and memory of how to operate a word processor, both the likely products of prior learning—but we also have memory of having turned off the gas on the stove before leaving the kitchen and memory for the content of a recently viewed television program, both the unlikely products of learning, but memories nonetheless.

The distinction is complicated further by the fact that learning is a concept long favored by traditional stimulus-response associationists, while memory is a concept favored by contemporary information-processing psychologists. To associationists, learning is viewed as the acquisition of connections, or associations, between stimulus and response events via practice and rehearsal. To information-processing psychologists, memory is the product of the operations we perform on incoming information, regardless of our intent to remember the content of that information or the extent to which practice and rehearsal determine its memorability.

In this section our concern will be with learning as a rehearsal-dependent form of memory in which tasks analyzable in terms of stimulus-response associations are practiced, and performed with increasing degrees of proficiency as practice continues. Among these tasks are those of classical (or Pavlovian) conditioning, motor skill acquisition, and verbal learning. Our focus will be on the learning of paired associates in which verbal elements (e.g., words or nonsense syllables) serve as both stimulus and response elements. Age differences in learning paired-associate lists are fairly well representative of age differences in learning other tasks that are also analyzable in terms of stimulus-response elements. The aging deficits found with paired-associate learning have also been found, for example, with classical conditioning (e.g., 18), motor skill learning (e.g., 102), and serial verbal learning (e.g., 38). We will also touch upon two other phenomena closely related to learning, namely, transfer and retention.

Paired-Associate Learning

Age differences in paired-associate learning have been examined in many studies employing different kinds of materials (e.g., pairs of unrelated words, pairs of related words, and pairs of nonsense syllables), different numbers of pairs within a list, different rates of presenting the materials, and so on. Regardless of the specific conditions, the result is much the same—aging deficits exist in the rate of learning paired associates. This may be seen in Figure 5.5 for several representative studies. Note that the number of trials to master the list varied considerably from study to study, depending on the learning conditions employed in each study, but the extent of the aging deficit remained fairly constant.

The implication is that the everyday learning of new stimulus-response associations proceeds more slowly for elderly than for young adults (but learning occurs regardless of age). There are frequent occasions when we do learn new paired associates. For example, we learn names to go with the faces of new acquaintances, names of athletic teams to go with the cities in which they are located when a new league is created, and so on. However, it is likely that laboratory assessments of age differences in paired-associate learning proficiency overestimate the magnitude of age differences in everyday paired-associate learning proficiency, at least in many instances. In the laboratory, subjects are required to learn as many as 10 to 12 new associations simultaneously, resulting in considerable interpair interference (8). The degree of such interference is likely to be greater for elderly adults than for young adults, resulting in an overall retarding of learning the individual associations by elderly adults (135). Massive interpair interference is unlikely to be encountered in learning, for

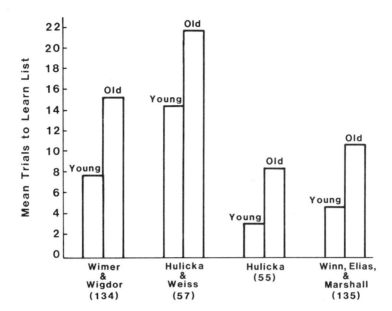

Figure 5.5. Result obtained in representative studies comparing young and elderly subjects in paired-associate learning proficiency.

example, new face-name associations in the everyday world. Here we are likely to have to struggle with the names of no more than one or two new acquaintances at any one time.

Even when interpair interference is minimized, however, it is likely that the rate of learning paired associates declines somewhat with advancing age. There are two probable reasons for this decline. The first is the slower rehearsal rate of older adults, relative to younger adults. Rehearsal in this case refers to the rote repetition of the elements of a paired associate, for example, repeating "table pencil" over and over in order to learn the *table-pencil* association. The opportunity to rehearse is limited to the time the paired elements are actually exposed to a subject. Exposure time is often no more than a few seconds. With fast pacing, the slower rate of rehearsal of elderly adults places them at a pronounced disadvantage. With slower pacing, the disadvantage decreases as more rehearsal time is available to compensate for their slower rate of rehearsal (e.g., 23). The second reason is the diminished use by elderly adults of such mnemonics as generating either an interacting image of paired elements (e.g., imagining a very large *pencil* on top of a very small *table*) or a verbal chain connecting the elements (e.g., the sentence, "The *table* has a large *pencil* on top of it."). These devices permit the "short circuiting" of learning the association by bypassing the necessity of rote rehearsal. For whatever reason, elderly adults appear to be less likely than young adults to engage spontaneously in mnemonic activity (56). However, when trained in the use of such mnemonics as imagery, elderly adults can improve dramatically in their rate of paired-associate learning (e.g., 129).

Transfer

If one learned the name "Johnson" for someone with a round, moonish face, it may make it difficult to associate the name "Bradley" with someone having the same type of face. The previously learned face-Johnson association interferes somewhat with learning the new face-Bradley association. That is, the rate of learning the new association is retarded by interference from the prior association. In terms of the classical interference theory of associationism, negative transfer is the result of learning successive associations in which identical, or similar, stimulus elements are paired with different response elements. In the laboratory, negative transfer is investigated by having subjects practice on successive lists in which List 1 contains such pairs as *table-pencil* and List 2 such pairs as *table-apple* (i.e., identical stimuli, different responses across the lists). A longstanding hypothesis in geropsychology is that elderly adults are more "interference prone" than young adults (60), and should therefore manifest a greater amount of negative transfer under these list conditions. Support for this hypothesis has not been very convincing, however. Negative transfer occurs for both young and elderly subjects, but the amount doesn't seem to differ greatly between age levels (42).

Of course, previous learning is often expected to facilitate new learning, rather than to hinder it. That is, positive transfer should occur under appropriate conditions. Suppose, for example, that the new name to be associated with the moonish face had been Kennedy instead of Bradley. Here the historical relatedness between the names of Johnson and Kennedy may facilitate new learning via activation of the chain "face→(Johnson)→Kennedy." Laboratory simulation of this condition requires such pairs as *table-pencil* in List 1 and *table-paper* in list 2. Note that identical stimuli and related responses enter into old (list 1) and new (list 2) learning. In this case, the mediating chain for new learning is "table→(pencil)→paper." That is, the association from list 1 prods the response element of list 2 via its relatedness to the response element of list 1. Positive transfer is usually found for young adults under this list condition. However, the little evidence available for elderly adults suggests that negative, rather than positive, transfer is the more likely outcome (42). The absence of positive transfer for elderly adults is in agreement with the evidence cited earlier indicating that elderly adults are unlikely to employ mnemonic mediators spontaneously in learning new associations. In the absence of the mediating "pencil→paper" sequence, the "table→pencil" and "table→paper" associations conform to an interference relationship (same stimulus, different responses), with negative transfer the expected outcome.

Retention and Forgetting

What learning giveth, forgetting taketh away—at least partially. Forgetting is as much a part of our daily lives as is the learning of new associations. How well can you recall the names of television programs from 10 years ago, the titles of songs popular 20 years ago, the names and locations of streets in your college community, a foreign language vocabulary learned in a high school course, and the names of your high school teachers and classmates? A number of studies have demonstrated a remarkable commonality in the forgetting of these materials over the course of the adult lifespan (3–5, 7, 117, 122). As may be seen in Figure 5.6, forgetting occurs rapidly for the first 3 to 6 years after material has been learned, and then levels off such that there is little additional forgetting over the rest of the life span. Years after initial learning, it is likely that from 20 to 40% will remain recallable from what Bahrick (4) has called a permastore. Presumably, what remains in permastore is that portion of the originally learned material that was highly overlearned at the time of acquisition. The implication, of course, is that the ability of elderly adults to recall what had been learned 50 years earlier differs little from the ability of

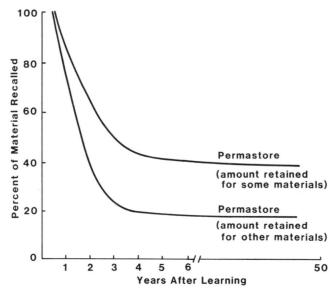

Figure 5.6. Forgetting over time of material learned in early adulthood, with variation in the amount attaining permastore status.

younger adults to recall what had been learned 5 to 10 years earlier.

Our reference thus far has been to the forgetting of material learned as young adults, and retained as we grow older. There remains the important question of the rate of forgetting for material learned by elderly adults per se, relative to the rate of forgetting for the same material learned by young adults. Forgetting, like negative transfer, is postulated by interference theory to be the product of learning competing associations involving identical (or similar) stimulus elements and different response elements. Interference, and the subsequent loss of associations (i.e., forgetting), may result from competing associations acquired either before (proactive interference) or after (retroactive interference) the associations to be retained. Laboratory simulation of these conditions requires subjects to practice successive lists containing such pairs as *table-pencil* in list 1 and *table-apple* in list 2. Difficulty in recalling "apple" to "table" after having learned the *table-pencil* association defines proactive interference, and difficulty in recalling "pencil" to "table" after learning the *table-apple* association defines retroactive interference. For example, prior to living in Collegetown, USA, the names and locations of streets in one's home town had been well learned, and, after leaving college, the names and locations of the streets in other communities must now be learned, thus accounting for proactive and retroactive sources of interference, respectively, for the forgetting of some names and locations of streets in one's college community. Given the heavy interference produced under laboratory list conditions, the forgetting of associations progresses rapidly, with much of the content of either list 1 or list 2 being lost after a week. However, the rate of forgetting appears to be no more accelerated for elderly adults than it is for young adults, provided the lists have been learned equally by the two age groups (55, 57, 134). Again, there is no evidence to indicate that elderly adults are more "interference prone" than are young adults. The secret of assuring retention of newly learned material by elderly adults that is equivalent to that of young adults is to assure thorough initial learning of that material.

MEMORY

The human memory system has four major components: generic (or semantic) memory, episodic memory, working memory, and metamemory. Generic memory and episodic memory involve separate long-term stores, each having essentially unlimited capacities. (Some contemporary cognitive psychologists, however, believe that it is unnecessary to postulate the existence of two long-term stores, and argue that a single long-term store may account for both generic and episodic memory phenomena; see ref. 79). The stores differ in terms of the kind of information, or knowledge, they contain (130). Permanent knowledge that is stored without reference to when and where it was acquired resides in the generic store; personally experienced knowledge that is stored in reference to when and where it was acquired resides in the episodic store.

An important component of the generic store is that of an internal lexicon or "mental dictionary." It is an organized network containing our knowledge of words in terms of the concepts they represent, their orthographic and phonemic features, their meanings, and their relatedness to other words. Other forms of permanent knowledge are also present in the generic store, such as knowledge of the rules of arithmetic and factual information. Note that it is highly unlikely that your knowledge of the word *psychology* is stored with reference to the context in which it was acquired (in grade school? high school?). Equally unlikely is the storage of information revealing when and where you learned that Jefferson City is the capital of Missouri.

By contrast, episodic memory is a context-based system. Memories are stored in reference to the spatial and temporal context in which personally experienced events occurred (e.g., memory for when and where you dropped your tray in a cafeteria). From a memory theory perspective, the association between two unrelated words in a paired-associate list is an episodic memory phenomenon. The words entering into the association certainly aren't being "learned"—they were in subjects' generic memories long before they entered the laboratory. What is being learned instead is the co-occurrence of these specific words (the content of the resulting memory) in an arbitrary list practiced while in the laboratory (contextual information in the resulting memory). Rehearsing the paired words is assumed to establish a memory trace composed of both content and contextual information that is transmitted to the long-term episodic store. Similarly, memory for having turned off the gas before leaving the kitchen is stored episodically. The trace again consists of content (the action of turning a dial on the stove) and context (when and where the action took place). In this case, however, transmission to the store seemingly occurs automatically, that is, without intent and without rehearsal, in contrast to the transmission of learned episodic events where the intent to remember assures the activation of rehearsal processes.

Working memory is the locus of the encoding, transmission, and retrieval processes involved in episodic memory. Encoding begins with matching the content of an episodic event with information stored in generic memory (i.e., pattern recognition). Some, but not necessarily all, of this information is copied to become part of an ensuing memory trace. What kind and how much information enter the memory trace is contingent on the nature of the encoding processes engaged in by the memorizer. For nonautomatic forms of memory, transmission of the trace to the long-term store requires rehearsal of the information while it resides in working memory. Retrieval processes are directed at gaining access to stored traces and outputting them in the form of recall or recognition. As discussed earlier, working memory is postulated to have a limited capacity for both processing information and for holding information briefly within its storage "bins," a capacity commonly assumed to decrease from early to late adulthood (Fig. 5.3).

Metamemory, like generic memory, is a store of general knowledge. However, in this case, the knowledge is of one's own memory system. Especially important for proficient episodic memory is knowledge about the rehearsal processes needed to assure the registration of memory traces in the episodic long-term store. That

is: What kind of rehearsal is required, and how much, in order to meet the demands of the task at hand? Failure to activate an appropriate memory strategy is likely to result in little, if any, long-term episodic memory.

The interactions among the components of the memory system are summarized in Figure 5.7. Represented there is the sequence of operations postulated to enter into both short-term and long-term memory for episodic events requiring rehearsal in order to be remembered. As observed earlier, some episodic events appear to be registered in long-term memory without intervening rehearsal. Our interest is in age differences for each component of the total memory system.

Generic Memory

Research on adult age differences in generic memory has centered on questions about the internal lexicon. One question concerns the possibility of a change with aging in the structure of the lexicon. If structural changes do occur, they should be reflected in age differences in the nature of both free and constrained associations to stimulus words. Free associations are obtained by providing subjects with such stimulus words as *table* and *bread* and asking them to give the first word that comes to mind for each stimulus. The responses given by elderly adults have been found to differ little from those of young adults in terms of such attributes as the most common response (e.g., "chair" to *table*)

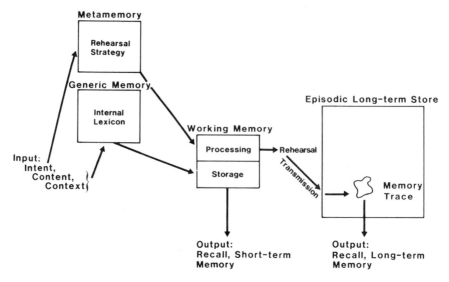

Figure 5.7. A model of the human memory system illustrating the processes and structures involved in the encoding and retrieval of episodic events.

and the proportion of total responses that are paradigmatic (i.e., come from the same grammatical class as the stimulus word) (22, 74). Constrained associations (word fluency tasks) are obtained by asking subjects to name several instances for each of a number of different taxonomic categories (e.g., "names of animals," and "names of professions"). The responses of elderly adults again differ little from those of young adults (53). There is no reason to believe that there are major structural changes with aging in the organization of the internal lexicon.

A second question is concerned with possible age differences in gaining access to information stored in the lexicon. For young adults, much of the accessing of lexical information occurs through an automatic process known as spreading activation. Activation of one word's representation in the lexicon spreads without intent to the representations of other words that are semantically related to the activated word and therefore stored in close proximity to the activated word. Spreading activation is readily demonstrated in the laboratory by means of the lexical decision task. A series of letter strings, some of which are words, the rest nonwords, are displayed one at a time and in a seemingly random order. For each exposed item, subjects respond as rapidly as possible to indicate if it is a word or a nonword. For young adults, the time to respond to a word, say, *nurse*, is significantly faster if it had been preceded by a related word, such as *doctor*, than if it had been preceded by an unrelated word, such as *pencil*. Activation of *doctor* spreads to *nurse* in advance of actually seeing *nurse*, thus accelerating *nurse's* processing when it does appear. The unrelatedness of *pencil* to *nurse* means that the latter receives no indirect activation prior to its appearance. There is considerable evidence indicating that spreading activation functions in late adulthood much the way it does in early adulthood (e.g., 54, 78). That is, the magnitude of the facilitation effect is about the same as that found for young adults. Thus, stability of generic memory seems to apply to its functioning as well as to its structure.

There is, however, one component of generic memory functioning that may be age sensitive. The nature of this component is revealed in a recent study by Bowles and Poon (17). They gave their subjects two different tasks. The first was essentially a vocabulary test in which young and elderly subjects gave definitions of words. In agreement with the results obtained by many other investigators (see refs. 61 and 103 for detailed summaries), elderly subjects scored, if anything, higher than young subjects. Vocabulary does seem to be an ability that remains stable over the adult life span, and may even increase somewhat from early to late adulthood. The second task was the reverse of a vocabulary test. That is, subjects were given the definitions of words, and they were asked to provide the words fulfilling those definitions. Here elderly subjects performed at a level significantly below that of young adults. Comprehending speech, of course, requires "traveling" in the lexicon from words to other words that define the words being comprehended, a progression that, as indexed by performances on vocabulary tests and lexical decision tasks, shows little effect of aging. By contrast, speech production requires "traveling" from concepts to the words conveying those concepts, a progression that may be adversely affected by aging. Given the importance of speech production in the everyday lives of elderly people, further research along the lines begun by Bowles and Poon is clearly needed. Chapter 9 provides a summary of the available literature in this area.

Episodic Memory: Short-Term

Short-term memory is defined by memory researchers as the retention of information (e.g., a telephone number) over a brief interval, usually no longer than 20 to 30 seconds. Retention beyond that interval is commonly accepted as being of information rehearsed sufficiently to have entered the episodic long-term store from which it is then recalled. Our interest rests in age differences in the storage capacity of working memory from which information may be directly recalled (i.e., the short-term store) and in the rate of loss of information from working memory. It should be noted in advance that not all memory theorists accept the idea that short-term memory is mediated by direct recall from a separate short-term store (e.g., 28). To these theorists, both short-term and long-term episodic memory are hypothesized to involve a single episodic store. From this perspective, the rapid rate of forgetting over a brief interval reflects the fragile nature of memory traces resulting from shallow encoding (to be discussed more fully later).

The traditional means of comparing age groups in their short-term storage capacities is to contrast their memory spans for such materials as a series of digits. Digit span is defined as the longest series of digits recalled without an error. Elderly adults have consistently been found to have a slightly shorter span (about 6.5 digits, on the average) than young adults (about 7 digits) (e.g., 16). The implication is that working memory's storage capacity declines modestly from early to late adulthood. However, many researchers believe that memory span reflects recall from the long-term store as well as from the short-term store, and that other measures of short-term storage capacity are needed to evaluate the true extent of an aging decrement in capacity. A favored alternative is to give subjects a number of free recall lists (e.g., 15 lists), each containing a number of unrelated words (e.g., 16 words). A single presentation of each list is followed by the recall of the words in whatever order they come to mind (thus, the term "free" recall). Of interest is the number of words recalled from the end of a list, averaged over all of the lists. These words are presumably still residing in the short-term store when recall begins, and the number recalled (e.g., three—the 14th, 15th, and 16th words in the list) depends on the capacity of the store. The estimated decline with aging in capacity found with this method (87) is somewhat greater (about 20%) than that found with the span method (about 10%). Since information needs to be held in storage in order to be rehearsed for transmission to the long-term store, the decrement in capacity may explain, at least in part, the pronounced aging deficits found for long-term episodic memory. The problem with accepting this position stems from the fact, as noted earlier, that measures of working memory capacity correlate poorly with long-term memory scores (e.g., 71).

Forgetting is assumed to occur for information held in the short-term store by its displacement by other new information arriving in the store. The rate of forgetting is determined through the use of a method introduced some years ago by Peterson and Peterson (90). It calls for giving subjects a number of short-term memory trials. On each trial an individual item is exposed, such as a triad of letters (e.g., PQJ), followed by a retention interval filled with a rehearsal preventing activity, such as counting backwards by threes from a designated number. At the end of the interval, the item to be remembered is recalled. The interval itself varies from trial to trial, sometimes being 0 seconds (i.e., immediate recall without intervening distraction), sometimes 3 seconds (filled with the distracting activity), sometimes 6 seconds, and so on. Forgetting occurs rapidly under these conditions, with recall being quite low after no more than 15 to 20 seconds of distracting activity. Some researchers who have used this method have found little difference between young and elderly subjects in their rates of forgetting (e.g., 118), while others have found a more rapid forgetting for elderly than for young subjects (e.g., 59). Consequently, the issue of an age difference in rate of forgetting remains unresolved.

Episodic Memory: Effortful Long-Term Memory

The free recall task has been the standard one used to evaluate the extent of aging deficits in effortful long-term memory and the reasons for those deficits. Again, effortful memory involves the limited processing resources of working memory. Items other than those near the end of a list are recalled from the long-term store following their encoding as traces and the transmission of these traces to the store. The extent of the aging deficit in effortful memory may be seen in the top panel of Figure 5.8 where the proportions of items recalled by both young and elderly subjects after one study trial are plotted for three representative studies. A number of explanations have been offered to explain this aging deficit, most of which place the responsibility on less proficient encoding of episodic events by elderly than by young adults. For example, some psychologists (e.g., 27) have hypothesized that elderly and young adults differ with respect to where they fall on a level of encoding dimension which varies from "shallow" to "deep." "Shallow" refers to encoding sensory information about an episodic event, such as the phonemic content of a word, and "deep" to the encoding of semantic information, such as a word's meaning. Memory traces based on semantic information are viewed as being more durable and less susceptible to decay over time than traces based on sensory information. Elderly adults are likely to engage in shallow encoding and young adults in deep encoding, thus accounting for aging deficits in effortful memory. Deep encoding is assumed to require greater processing resources than shallow encoding, and is therefore adversely affected by the elderly adult's diminished resources (Fig. 5.3).

Alternatively, encoding deficits may be the result of less elaborative rehearsal by elderly than by young adults (61). Elaborative rehearsal consists largely of generating imaginal representation of episodic events to supplement the semantic information embedded in memory traces. The result is to make traces more distinctive, and therefore more accessible for recall, than they would be if only sensory and semantic information had been encoded. Other possibilities include less encoding of contextual information by elderly than by young adults (21), and less organization of events in terms of their relatedness by elderly than by young adult (58). Each of these encoding explanations has received empirical support to some degree,

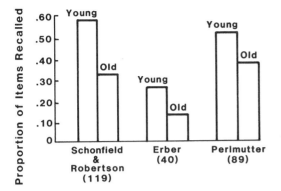

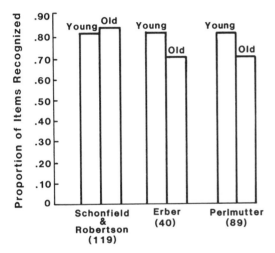

Figure 5.8. Results of representative studies comparing young and elderly subjects in the recall (*top panel*) and recognition (*bottom panel*) of the items in a free recall list.

and each may contribute to the aging deficits found for effortful memory.

Not to be overlooked is the possibility that much of the aging deficit in long-term memory stems from the diminished retrieval proficiency of elderly adults. Recall requires an effortful search of the long-term store, and may therefore be affected by a reduction in cognitive resources. Of interest is the fact that, as shown in the *bottom panel* of Figure 5.8, recognition deficits are usually less pronounced than recall deficits (e.g., 40, 89, 119). Recognition demands less effort than recall, and should therefore be less affected by diminished resources.

The processes governing memory for list items are viewed as being generalizable to other effortful memory tasks as well, such as memory for discourse. Thus, the reasons for aging deficits in free recall memory, once they have been fully identified, are expected to apply to more ecologically relevant forms of memory. The extent of this generalizability is debatable, but the fact remains that aging deficits have been reported for discourse by a number of recent investigators (e.g., 36, 121, 140). Less certain, however, is the level, or levels, of text structure at which the deficit occurs. Structural level refers to the propositional, or idea, content of the discourse to be remembered. Propositions range from top to bottom in a hierarchy in accordance with their importance to the discourse's content. Some investigators (21, 140) have found an aging deficit only for the recall of lower level propositions (i.e., memory for irrelevant details), while others (e.g., 36) have found deficits for the recall of higher order propositions (i.e., central themes basic to the discourse's content) as well as for lower order propositions. In addition, there is evidence to indicate that these deficits reflect memory problems per se rather than problems in comprehending discourse materials by elderly adults (139), although difficulty in comprehending complexly related sentences may add to the memory problems of elderly adults (72).

Episodic Memory: Automaticity

As noted earlier, some episodic events are believed by some memory researchers to be encoded automatically. Automaticity means that encoding occurs with little cognitive effort being exerted, and with little, if any, demand on working memory's limited processing resources. Some attributes of episodic events, such as their frequencies of occurrence and their temporal sequencings, are considered to be so essential for maintaining continuity with the everyday world that they are programmed innately for automaticity of encoding (49).

One of the criteria of automaticity is that intent to memorize the attribute in question should have no effect on that attribute's memorability, as compared with memorability under incidental memory conditions. To test the validity of this assumed equality for the frequency attribute, subjects are shown a series of words, some of which appear once, some twice, some three times, and so on, in a random order. Afterwards they are asked to judge the frequency of each event's (i.e., word's) occurrence in the series. Under intentional memory conditions, subjects know in advance that their memory for frequency information will be tested. Under incidental memory conditions, subjects have no forewarning of the future test, and they are given a disguised reason for attending to the events in the series. In general, considerable support has been obtained for the equality of intentional and incidental memory for both young and elderly adults (e.g., 67), although there have been some exceptions in which intentional memory has exceeded incidental memory (e.g., 84), at least for young adults.

It is the second criterion of automaticity that is of particular concern, namely, its insensitivity to adult age differences. That is, elderly adults are expected to be as proficient as young adults in memory for an automatically encoded attribute (49). The reason for the expected age equality is that automatic encoding should be unaffected by working memory's processing capacity (Fig. 5.3). Unfortunately, however, evidence is beginning to accumulate to indicate that the so-called automatic memory of non-content attributes is age sensitive, even though it is rehearsal-independent in the sense of intent to remember having no effect on its proficiency. Age differences have been found for both memory of frequency information (66) and memory for temporal information (65; Kausler, Salthouse, and Saults, in preparation). Temporal memory is tested by presenting a series of events (e.g., words) in a designated order and then asking subjects to reconstruct the order in which the events occurred. Correlations between true order and reconstructed order are substantially higher for young than for elderly subjects, contrary to the age equality expected on the basis of the assumed automaticity of encoding temporal information.

There are at least two other important types of memory that could be considered automatic, and therefore immune to aging deficits in proficiency. The first is memory for one's own performed activities. We all experience memory (or the frequent absence of memory) for having mailed a letter, having locked the door, having balanced the checkbook, and so on. Memory for such activities exists in the everyday world in the apparent absence of intent to remember and in the absence of deliberate rehearsal to promote memorability. Laboratory simulation of activity memory calls for giving subjects a series of tasks to perform, such as solving anagrams and tracing mazes, and then asking them to recall the just performed activities. In agreement with the automaticity principle, incidental memory for prior activities is as proficient as intentional memory for both young and elderly adults (see 63, 67, 70). However, substantial age differences favoring young adults have been found consistently. The aging deficit persists whether the activities are verbal or motor in nature (70) and regardless of how long the activities are performed (66). For whatever reason, activity memory, like memory for non-content attributes, appears to decrease in

proficiency from early to late adulthood.

The second is memory for conversations. In the everyday world, we have memory for our conversational exchanges with other people, imperfect though it may be. Here too there seems to be no intent to remember and no active rehearsal of conversational content. There has been surprisingly little research on this important form of memory. Kausler and Hakami (64), however, did find superior recall of conversational topics by young relative to elderly subjects, despite the equality in memory for the topics under incidental and intentional memory conditions, regardless of age.

Given the pervasiveness of aging deficits across both effortful and rehearsal-independent forms of episodic memory, it is little wonder that problems with memory are ranked high by elderly adults when they are asked to describe the problems they face in their everyday lives (76). However, there is one positive sign. A recent study by Cavanaugh (24) revealed little aging deficit in memory for the content of television programs!

Metamemory

Elderly adults may be less proficient than young adults in episodic memory performances not because of their diminished competence in encoding/retrieval processes, but rather because they monitor their own memory processes less effectively. For example, elderly adults may underestimate the difficulty of encoding task materials, and therefore devote less effort to encoding than is necessary to assure memorability. Some researchers have found elderly subjects to be more likely than young subjects to underestimate the difficulty of learning individual pairs in a paired-associate list (75), while others have found elderly subjects to terminate their rehearsal processes prematurely while studying a list for recall (83). Inappropriate evaluation of the amount of rehearsal needed to master a memory task could certainly contribute to the memory problems of elderly adults. However, it seems unlikely that it would account for any more than a minor proportion of the aging deficits found for many memory tasks.

PROBLEM SOLVING AND REASONING

Problem Solving

Familiar everyday problems to be solved are those of finding a way into a locked apartment when the key has been lost, finding a way of stretching the budget to make it to payday, and finding a room when all nearby hotels appear to be filled. In each case, there is no response provided for a subject to learn to associate with a specific stimulus. Instead, the problem solver has to discover an appropriate response that eliminates the problem presented by a stimulus situation (e.g., a locked door and no key). Our concern is with the extent of age differences in the discovery of solution responses and with the probable reasons for those differences.

Laboratory research on problem solving has concentrated on the use of variations of the 20 Questions game. In one laboratory version of the game, pictures of a number of familiar objects (e.g., a cup, a dinner plate, a hat, a sweater, and so on) are displayed simultaneously on a board. The subject's task (i.e., the problem situation) is to pick the one picture the experimenter has in mind by asking only questions that can be answered "Yes" or "No." Elderly adults average a considerably greater number of selections than young or middle-aged subjects before solving the problem (i.e., picking the correct picture) (31, 34). Other investigators (e.g., 47) have found comparable aging deficits when subjects are asked to find the single square in a matrix of many squares that the experimenter has in mind. The reason for the aging deficit on these tasks is quite clear. Elderly subjects ask far fewer constraining questions than do younger subjects. A constraining question is one that by its answer serves to eliminate a number of remaining pictures or squares from consideration (e.g., "Is it living?"; "Is it in the top half of the matrix?"). Instead, elderly subjects ask an inordinate number of questions that eliminate only one picture or square at a time (e.g., "Is it the hat?").

It seems unlikely that the failure to employ frequent constraining questions is the result of an elderly adult's diminished processing resources. Denney (30) has argued instead in favor of the disuse principle. That is, there is little demand for asking constraining questions in late adulthood, and the underlying skill becomes "rusty" (but still latently available) as a result. However, Denney (e.g., 34) has found that elderly subjects who have difficulty solving 20 Questions problems also have difficulty solving life-like problems, such as the locked room problem, when confronted by them in a paper and pencil form. Disuse seems an unlikely reason for difficulty in solving such everyday problems. A more feasible explanation is in terms of diminished resources. There is evidence (136) indicating that elderly adults have greater difficulty than young adults in solving fairly simple addition problems when another task (holding a 3-digit number in memory) must be performed simultaneously. The added task places an undue strain on the more limited resources available to elderly adults for solving the addition problem, but not on the more abundant resources available to young adults.

Reasoning

Age differences in inductive reasoning are assessed by paper and pencil tests in which subjects receive items containing a series of stimuli related in some way, and they are to select from several alternatives the stimulus that completes each item. For example, the item "15 32 66" may be given, followed by the alternatives "100 116 132 134." When assessed cross-sectionally, age differences on inductive reasoning tests are quite pronounced (e.g., 50, 113), with young adults scoring substantially higher than elderly adults. In terms of the currently popular distinction between fluid intelligence and crystallized intelligence, inductive reasoning is considered to be one of the major components of fluid intelligence (52). The optimal level of fluid intelligence is attained in early adulthood and is assumed to be determined by heredity. Consequently, inductive reasoning, as a component of fluid intelligence, is believed to be relatively unaffected by education and acculturation. By contrast, crystallized intelligence is largely the product of education and acculturation. Fluid intelligence, as measured by performances on tests of inductive reasoning, presumably declines progressively with neurological degeneration beyond early adulthood, while crystallized intelligence, as measured by tests of vocabulary and general information, increases moderately from early to late adulthood (e.g., see refs. 12, 61, and 103).

Training and Modification

Problem solving ability and inductive reasoning ability have been the favorite targets of training programs designed to facilitate the higher mental functioning of elderly adults. The implication is that much of the decline in fluid intelligence is the result of disuse of the underlying abilities during late adulthood, and that, with sufficient training and practice, elderly adults have the plasticity to restore their performance levels close to what they had been earlier in life (10). Denney and colleagues (31–33) have demonstrated that training on the appropriate strategy to apply in the 20 Questions game does indeed facilitate the performances of elderly adults on the game. Similarly, a number of investigators (e.g., 6, 132, 133) have found that intensive training and practice on inductive reasoning problems facilitates subsequent performance on similar problems. Moreover, training has been discovered to benefit not only those individuals whose longitudinal assessments of inductive reasoning ability revealed decline over the years, but also those individuals whose ability had remained relatively stable over the same time period (133).

On the other hand, training specifically on inductive reasoning problems seems to show little transfer in the form of improved performances on other components of fluid intelligence—and even the facilitation of inductive reasoning performance seems to dissipate within a few months after completing the training program. In addition, it seems unlikely that training would affect markedly the extent of age differences found for either problem solving or inductive reasoning. As noted earlier in this chapter, young adults, if given equivalent training, would probably show comparable facilitation in their performance levels. Nevertheless, it is encouraging to know that elderly adults do possess a degree of resilience for their higher mental processes, and appropriate training programs can facilitate their mental performances. Hopefully, improved means of training will be discovered in the near future that: (a) transfer to fluid intellectual abilities other than the specifically trained ability; (b) transfer to everyday problem solving and reasoning; and (c) retain the facilitative effects of training long after the training program itself has been completed. The belief in the eventual fulfillment of these objectives enables us to end this chapter on a somewhat optimistic note.

SUMMARY

Adult age differences in cognitive abilities are of importance in understanding the effects of aging on communication. However, age differences in performances on cognitive tasks, as revealed by cross-sectional age comparisons, do not necessarily mean that age changes have occurred in the processes underlying those performances. Such differences may result from uncontrolled variation in cohort, or generational, membership. Various methods have been employed in cognitive aging research to control for potential cohort effects. These methods include the use of age groups balanced on such critical attributes as educational level, the use of longitudinal assessments of the same individuals at different ages, and the use of sequential analyses in which age variation is combined with variation in either cohort membership or

time of measurement. Age differences may also reflect age variation on performance variables rather than age variation in true competence. However, considerable research has revealed aging deficits even when such critical performance variables as motivation and health status are equated across age groups.

A common approach to explaining aging deficits in cognitive performances is in terms of a broad mechanism that is presumed to be adversely affected by aging. The two mechanisms postulated by contemporary geropsychologists are those of diminished cognitive resources with increasing age and decreasing speed of processing information with increasing age. Both mechanisms account adequately for many aging deficits in cognitive performances. However, neither mechanism has thus far received convincing direct support.

Age differences are apparent in sensory functioning for both threshold and suprathreshold levels of performance. For low intensity stimuli, elderly adults are both less sensitive in detecting their presence and more cautious in reporting their presence than are younger adults. For suprathreshold stimuli, elderly adults experience less change in intensity as the physical intensity changes than do younger adults. The most prominent perceptual change with aging is in the rate of identifying, or recognizing, stimulus patterns. The slower rate of processing is apparent both peripherally and centrally. There is little change with aging in vigilance unless a memory demand is required to monitor a series of stimuli. Selective attention appears to be adversely affected by aging in the sense that elderly adults have greater difficulty than young adults in ignoring the presence of irrelevant sources of stimuli. Dividing attention between two simultaneous sources of stimulation appears to diminish in proficiency with aging only when the tasks to be performed are complex ones.

Learning progresses more slowly for elderly adults than for younger adults. However, the rate of forgetting what has been learned appears to be independent of age level. Memory involves a complex system than includes generic and episodic components. Generic memory, as manifested in the structure and operations of an internal lexicon, is largely age insensitive. Episodic memory consists of short-term and long-term as well as effortful and automatic subcomponents. Short-term memory is only modestly affected by aging. More pronounced aging deficits are commonly found for effortful long-term episodic memory. Although automatic long-term episodic memory is commonly hypothesized to be immune to age changes in proficiency, a number of its forms have been found recently to be age sensitive. Problem solving and reasoning are higher mental processes associated with the concept of fluid intelligence. Aging deficits on tasks involving these processes have been found to be at least partially reversed by effective training procedures.

References

1. Arenberg D: A longitudinal study of problem solving in adults. *J Gerontol* 29:650–658, 1974.
2. Arenberg D, Robertson-Tchabo EA: Learning and aging. In Birren JE, Schaie KW (eds): *Handbook of the Psychology of Aging*. New York, Van Nostrand Reinhold, 1977, p 421.
3. Bahrick HP: Maintenance of knowledge: Questions about memory we forgot to ask. *J Exp Psychol (Gen)* 108:296–308, 1979.
4. Bahrick HP: Semantic memory content in permastore: Fifty years of memory for Spanish learned in school. *J Exp Psychol (Gen)* 113:1–29, 1984.
5. Bahrick HP, Bahrick PO, Wittlinger RP: Fifty years of memory for names and faces: A cross-sectional approach. *J Exp Psychol (Gen)* 104:54–75, 1975.
6. Baltes PB, Dittman-Kohli F, Kliegl R: Reserve capacity of the elderly in aging-sensitive tests of fluid intelligence: Replication and extension. *Psychol Aging* 1:172–177, 1986.
7. Bartlett JC, Snelus P: Lifespan memory for popular songs. *Am J Psychol* 93:551–560, 1980.
8. Battig WF: Paired-associate learning. In Dixon TR, Horton DL (eds): *Verbal Behavior and General Behavior Theory*. Englewood Cliffs NJ, Prentice-Hall, 1967, p 149.
9. Bell B, Wolf E, Bernholz CD: Depth perception as a function of age. *Aging Hum Dev* 3:77–88, 1972.
10. Bellucci G, Hoyer WJ: Feedback effects on the performance and self-reinforcing behavior of elderly and young adult women. *J Gerontol* 30:456–460, 1975.
11. Bergman M, Blumfield VG, Cascado D, et al: Age related decrement in hearing for speech. *J Gerontol* 31:533–538, 1976.
12. Berkowitz B: The Weschsler-Bellevue performance of white males past 50. *J Gerontol* 8:76–80, 1953.
13. Berry JM, Storandt M, Coyne A: Age and sex differences in somatic complaints associated with depression. *J Gerontol* 39:465–467, 1984.
14. Birren JE: Age changes in speed of responses and perception and their significance for complex behavior. In: *Old Age in the Modern World*. Edinburgh, Livingstone, 1955, p 235.
15. Birren JE, Schaie KW (eds): *Handbook of the Psychology of Aging*, ed 2. New York, Van Nostrand Reinhold, 1985.
16. Botwinick J, Storandt M: *Memory, Related Functions and Age*. Springfield, IL, Charles C Thomas, 1974.
17. Bowles NL, Poon LW: Aging and retrieval of words in semantic memory. *J Gerontol* 40:71–77, 1985.
18. Braun HW, Geiselhart R: Age differences in the acquisition and extinction of the conditioned eyelid response. *J Exp Psychol* (Gen) 57:386–388, 1959.
19. Britton BK, Westbrook RD, Holdredge TS: Reading and cognitive capacity usage: Effects of test difficulty. *J Exp Psychol: Hum Learn Mem* 4:582–591, 1978.
20. Broadbent DE: *Perception and Communication*. London, Pergamon, 1958.
21. Burke DM, Light LL: Memory and aging: The role of retrieval processes. *Psychol Bull* 90:513–546, 1981.
22. Burke DM, Peters L: Word associations in old age: Evidence for consistency in semantic encoding during adulthood. *Psychol Aging* 1:283–292, 1986.
23. Canestrari RE Jr: Paced and self-paced learning in young and elderly adults. *J Gerontol* 18:165–168, 1963.
24. Cavanaugh JC: Comprehension and retention of television programs by 20- and 60-year olds. *J Gerontol* 38:190–196, 1983.
25. Charness N: Visual short-term memory and aging. *J Gerontol* 36:615–619, 1981.
26. Comalli PE Jr, Wapner S, Werner H: Interference effects of Stroop color-word test in childhood, adulthood, and aging. *J Genet Psychol* 100:47–53, 1962.
27. Craik FIM: Age differences in human memory. In Birren JE, Schaie KW (eds): *Handbook of the Psychology of Aging*, ed 1. New York, Van Nostrand Reinhold, 1977, p 384.
28. Craik FIM, Lockhart RS: Levels of processing: a framework for memory research. *J Verb Learn Verb Behav* 11:671–684, 1972.
29. Daneman M, Carpenter PA: Individual differences in working memory and reading. *J Verb Learn Verb Behav* 19:450–466, 1980.
30. Denney NW: Cognitive change. In Wolman BB, Stricker G (eds): *Handbook of Developmental Psychology*. Englewood Cliffs, NJ, Prentice-Hall, 1982, p 807.
31. Denney NW, Denney DR: Modeling effects on the questioning strategies of the elderly. *Dev Psychol* 10:458, 1974.
32. Denney NW, Denney DR: The relationship between age and questioning strategies among adults. *J Gerontol* 37:190–196, 1982.
33. Denney NW, Jones FW, Krigel SH: Modifying the questioning strategies of young children and elderly adults with strategy modeling techniques. *Hum Dev* 22:23–36, 1979.
34. Denney NW, Pearce KA, Palmer AM: A developmental study of adults' performance on traditional and practical problem-solving tasks. *Exp Aging Res* 8:115–118, 1982.
35. DiLollo V, Arnett JL, Kruk RV: Age-related changes in rate of visual information processing. *J Exp Psychol (Hum Percept Perform)* 8:225–237, 1982.
36. Dixon RA, Simon EW, Nowak CA, Hultsch DF: Text recall in adulthood as a function of information, input modality, and delay interval. *J Gerontol* 37:358–364, 1982.
37. Douglas K, Arenberg D: Age changes, cohort differences, and cultural change on the Guil-

ford-Zimmerman Temperament Survey. *J Gerontol* 33:737–747, 1978.

38. Eisdorfer C, Service C: Verbal rote learning and superior intelligence in the aged. *J Gerontol* 22:158–161, 1967.

39. Elias MF, Elias PK: Matching of successive auditory stimuli as a function of age and ear of presentation. *J Gerontol* 31:164–169, 1976.

40. Erber JT: Age differences in recognition memory. *J Gerontol* 29:177–181, 1974.

41. Farkas MS, Hoyer WJ: Processing consequences of perceptual grouping in selective attention. *J Gerontol* 35:207–216, 1980.

42. Freund JS, Witte KL: Paired-associate transfer: age of subjects, anticipation interval, association value, and paradigm. *Amer J Psychol* 89:695–705, 1976.

43. Gilbert JG: Age changes in color matching. *J Gerontol* 12:210–215, 1957.

44. Granick S, Kleban MH, Weiss AD: Relationships between hearing loss and cognition in normally hearing aged persons. *J Gerontol* 31:434–440, 1976.

45. Green DM, Swets JA: *Signal Detection Theory and Psychophysics*. New York, Wiley, 1966.

46. Gurland BJ: The comparative frequency of depression in various adult age groups. *J Gerontol* 31:283–293, 1976.

47. Hartley AA, Anderson JW: Task complexity and problem-solving performance in younger and older adults. *J Gerontol* 38:72–77, 1983.

48. Hartley JT: Reader and text variables as determinants of discourse memory in adulthood. *Psychol Aging* 1:150–158, 1986.

49. Hasher L, Zacks RT: Automatic and effortful processing in memory. *J Exp Psychol (Gen)* 108:356–388, 1979.

50. Heron A, Chown SM: *Age and Function*. London, Churchill, 1967.

51. Hertzog CK, Schaie KW, Gribbin K: Cardiovascular disease and changes in intellectual functioning from middle to old age. *J Gerontol* 33:872–883, 1978.

52. Horn JL, Cattell RB: Age differences in fluid and crystallized intelligence. *Acta Psychol* 26:107–129, 1967.

53. Howard DV: Category norms: a comparison of the Battig and Montague (1969) norms with the responses of adults between the ages of 20 and 80. *J Gerontol* 35:225–231, 1980.

54. Howard DV, Lasaga MI, McAndrews MP: Semantic activation during memory encoding across the adult life span. *J Gerontol* 35:884–890, 1980.

55. Hulicka IM: Age differences in retention as a function of interference. *J Gerontol* 22:180–184, 1967.

56. Hulicka IM, Grossman JL: Age-group comparisons for the use of mediators in paired-associate learning. *J Gerontol* 22:46–51, 1967.

57. Hulicka IM, Weiss RL: Age differences in retention as a function of learning. *J Consult Psychol* 29:125–129, 1965.

58. Hultsch DF: Adult age differences in the organization of free recall. *Dev Psychol* 1:673–678, 1969.

59. Inman VW, Parkinson SR: Differences in Brown-

Peterson recall as a function of age and retention interval. *J Gerontol* 38:58–64, 1983.

60. Kausler DH: Retention-forgetting as a nomological network for developmental research. In Goulet LR, Baltes PB (eds): *Life-Span Developmental Psychology: Research and Theory*. New York, Academic Press, 1970, p 305.

61. Kausler DH: *Experimental Psychology and Human Aging*. New York, Wiley, 1982.

62. Kausler DH: Comments on aging memory and its everyday operations. In Poon LW, Rubin DC, Wilson BA (eds): *Everyday Cognition in Adulthood and Aging*. New York, Cambridge, in press, 1987.

63. Kausler DH, Hakami MK: Memory for activities: adult age differences and intentionality. *Dev Psychol* 19:889–894, 1983.

64. Kausler DH, Hakami MK: Memory for topics of conversation: adult age differences and intentionality *Exp Aging Res* 9:153–157, 1983.

65. Kausler DH, Lichty W, Davis RT: Temporal memory for performed activities: intentionality and adult age differences. *Dev Psychol* 21:1132–1138, 1985.

66. Kausler DH, Lichty W, Hakami MK: Frequency judgments for distracting items in a short-term memory task: instructional variation and adult age differences. *J Verb Learn Verb Behav* 23:660–668, 1984.

67. Kausler DH, Lichty W, Hakami MK, et al: Activity duration and adult age differences in memory for activity performances. *Psychol Aging* 1:80–81, 1986.

68. Kirchner WK: Age differences in short-term retention of rapidly changing information. *J Exp Psychol* 55:352–358, 1958.

69. LaRue A, Bank L, Jarvik L, Hetland M: Health in old age: how do physicians ratings and self-ratings compare? *J Gerontol* 34:687–691, 1979.

70. Lichty W, Kausler DH, Martinez DR: Adult age differences in memory for motor versus cognitive activities. *Exp Aging Res*, in press, 1987.

71. Light LL, Anderson PA: Working memory capacity, age, and memory for discourse. *J Gerontol* 40:737–747, 1985.

72. Light LL, Capps JL: Comprehension of pronouns in young and older adults. *Dev Psychol* 22:580–585, 1986.

73. Lindholm JM, Parkinson SP: An interpretation of age-related differences in letter matching performance. *Percept Psychophys* 33:283–294, 1983.

74. Lovelace EA, Cooley S: Free associations of older adults to single words and conceptually related word triads. *J Gerontol* 37:432–437, 1982.

75. Lovelace EA, Marsh GR: Prediction and evaluation of memory performance by young and old adults. *J Gerontol* 40:192–197, 1985.

76. Lowenthal MF, Berkman PL, Beuhler JA, et al: *Aging and Mental Disorder in San Francisco*. San Francisco, Jossey-Bass, 1967.

77. Madden DJ: Aging and distraction by highly familiar stimuli during visual search. *Dev Psychol* 19:499–507, 1983.

78. Madden DJ: Adult age differences in visual word recognition: semantic encoding and episodic retention. *Exp Aging Res* 12:71–78, 1986.

79. McCoon G, Ratcliff R: A critical evaluation of the semantic-episodic distinction. *J Exp Psychol (Learn, Mem, Cogn)* 12:295–306, 1986.

80. Milligan WL, Powell DA, Harley C, et al: A comparison of physical health and psychosocial variables as predictors of reaction time and serial learning. *J Gerontol* 39:704–710, 1984.

81. Murphy C: Age-related effects on the threshold, psychophysical function, and pleasantness of menthol. *J Gerontol* 38:217–222, 1983.

82. Murphy C: Cognitive and chemosensory influences on age-related changes in the ability to identify blended foods. *J Gerontol* 40:47–52, 1985.

83. Murphy MD, Sanders RE, Gabriesheski AS, Schmitt FA: Metamemory in the aged. *J Gerontol* 36:185–192, 1981.

84. Naveh-Benjamin M, Jonides J: On the automaticity of frequency coding: effects of competing task load, encoding strategy, and intention. *J. Exp Psychol (Learn, Mem, Cogn)* 12:378–386, 1986.

85. Neisser, U. *Memory Observed: Remembering in Natural Contexts.* San Francisco, WH Freeman, 1982.

86. Owens WA Jr: Age and mental ability: a second follow-up, *J Educ Psychol* 57: 311–325, 1966.

87. Parkinson SR, Lindholm JM, Inman VW: An analysis of age differences in immediate recall. *J Gerontol* 37: 425–431, 1982.

88. Parks CW Jr, Mitchell DB, Perlmutter M: Age and student status effects on adult performance. *Psychol Aging* 1:248–254, 1986.

89. Perlmutter M: Age differences in adults' free recall, cued recall, and recognition. *J Gerontol* 34:533–539, 1979.

90. Peterson LR, Peterson MJ: Short-term retention of individual verbal items. *J Exp Psychol* 58: 193–198, 1959.

91. Plude DJ, Hoyer WJ: Adult age differences in visual search as a function of stimulus mapping and processing load. *J Gerontol* 36: 598–604, 1981.

92. Plude DJ, Kaye DB, Hoyer WJ, et al: Aging and visual processing under consistent and varied mapping. *Dev Psychol* 19: 508–512, 1983.

93. Popkin SJ, Gallagher D, Thompson LW, et al: Memory complaints and performance in normal and depressed older adults. *Exp Aging Res* 8: 141–145, 1982.

94. Posner MI, Mitchell RF: Chronometric analysis of classification. *Psychol Rev* 74: 392–409, 1967.

95. Potash MI, Jones B: Aging and decision criteria for the detection of tones in noise. *J Gerontol* 32: 436–440, 1977.

96. Prinz PN: Sleep patterns in the healthy aged: relationship with intellectual function. *J Gerontol* 32: 179–186, 1977.

97. Quilter RE, Giambra LM, Benson PE: Longitudinal age changes in vigilance over an eighteen year interval. *J Gerontol* 38:51–54, 1983.

98. Rabbitt PMA: An age-decrement in the ability to ignore irrelevant information. *J Gerontol* 20:233–238, 1965.

99. Rees JN, Botwinick J: Detection and decision factors in auditory behavior of the elderly. *J Gerontol* 26:133–136, 1971.

100. Riegel KF: History of psychological gerontology. In Birren JE, Schaie KW (eds): *Handbook of the Psychology of Aging*, ed 1. New York, Van Nostrand Reinhold, 1977.

101. Rovee CK, Cohen RY, Shlapack W: Lifespan stability in olfactory sensitivity. *Dev Psychol* 11:311–318, 1975.

102. Ruch FL: Adult learning. *Psychol Bull* 30:387–414, 1933.

103. Salthouse TA: *Adult Cognition.* New York, Springer, 1982.

104. Salthouse TA: Effects of age and skill in typing. *J Exp Psychol (Gen)* 113:345–371, 1984.

105. Salthouse TA: Speed of behavior and its implications for cognition. In Birren JE, Schaie KW (eds): *Handbook of the Psychology of Aging*, ed 2. New York, Van Nostrand Reinhold, 1985, p 176.

106. Salthouse TA: *A Theory of Cognitive Aging.* Amsterdam, North-Holland, 1985.

107. Salthouse TA, Kausler DH: Memory methodology in maturity. In Brainerd CJ, Pressley M (eds): *Basic Processes in Memory Development.* New York, Springer, 1986, p 279.

108. Salthouse TA, Prill KA: Inferences about age impairments in inferential reasoning. *Psychol Aging*, in press, 1987.

109. Salthouse TA, Rogan JD, Prill KA: Division of attention: age differences on a visually presented memory task. *Mem Cogn* 12:613–620, 1984.

110. Salthouse TA, Somberg BL: Skilled performance: effects of adult age and experience on elementary processes. *J Exp Psychol (Gen)* 111:176–207, 1982.

111. Schaie KW: A general model for the study of developmental problems. *Psychol Bull* 64:92–107, 1965.

112. Schaie, KW, Hertzog C: Fourteen-year cohort-sequential analyses of adult intellectual development. *Dev Psychol* 19:531–543, 1983.

113. Schaie KW, Rosenthal F, Perlman RM: Differential mental deterioration of factorially "pure" functions in later maturity. *J Gerontol* 8:191–196, 1953.

114. Schemper T, Voss S, Cain WS: Odor identification in young and elderly persons: sensory and cognitive limitations. *J Gerontol* 36:446–452, 1981.

115. Schiffman S: Food recognition by the elderly. *J Gerontol* 32: 586–592, 1977.

116. Schneider W, Shiffrin RM: Controlled and automatic human information processing. I. Detection, search, and attention. *Psychol Rev* 84:1–66, 1977.

117. Schonfield D: In search of early memories. Paper, International Congress of Aging. Washington, DC, July 1969.

118. Schonfield D: Age and remembering. *Proceedings of Seminars.* Durham, NC, Duke University, 1969.

119. Schonfield D, Robertson BA: Memory storage and aging. *Can J Psychol* 20:228–236, 1966.

120. Somberg BL, Salthouse TA: Divided attention abilities in young and old adults. *J Exp Psychol (Hum Percept Perf)* 8:651–663, 1982.

121. Spilich G: Life-span components of text proc-

essing: structural and procedural differences. *J Verb Learn Verb Behav* 22:231–244, 1983.

122. Squire LR, Slater PC: Forgetting in very long-term memory as assessed by an improved questionnaire technique. *J Exp Psychol (Hum Learn Mem)* 104:50–54, 1975.

123. Stanford T, Pollack RH: Configuration in color vision tests: the interaction between aging and the complexity of figure-ground segregation. *J Gerontol* 39:568–571, 1984.

124. Stevens JC, Cain WS: Old age deficits in the sense of smell as gauged by thresholds, magnitude matching, and odor identification. *Psychol Aging* 2:36–42, 1987.

125. Sunderland A, Harris JE, Baddeley AD: Do laboratory tasks predict everyday memory? *J Verb Learn Verb Behav* 22:341–357, 1983.

126. Surwillo WW, Quiller RE: Vigilance, age, and response time. *Am J Psychol* 77:614–620, 1964.

127. Thomas PD, Hunt WC, Garry PJ, et al: Hearing acuity in healthy elderly population: effects on emotional, cognitive, and social status. *J Gerontol* 38:321–325, 1983.

128. Thorndike EL, Bergman EO, Tilton JW, Woodyard E. *Adult Learning*. New York, Macmillan, 1928.

129. Treat NJ, Reese HW: Age, imagery, and pacing in paired-associate learning. *Dev Psychol* 12:119–124, 1976.

130. Tulving E: Episodic and semantic memory. In Tulving E, Donaldson W (eds): *Organization of Memory*. New York, Academic Press, 1972, p 41.

131. Walsh DA, Till RE, Williams MV: Age differences in peripheral perceptual processing: a monoptic backward masking investigation. *J Exp Psychol (Hum Percept Perf)* 4:232–243, 1978.

132. Willis SL, Blieszner R, Baltes PB: Intellectual training research in aging: modification of performance on the fluid ability of figural relations. *J Educ Psychol* 73:41–50, 1981.

133. Willis SL, Schaie KW: Training the elderly on the ability factors of spatial orientation and inductive reasoning. *Psychol Aging*, in press, 1987.

134. Wimer RE, Wigdor BT: Age differences in retention of learning. *J Gerontol* 13:291–295, 1958.

135. Winn FJ Jr, Elias JW, Marshall PH: Meaningfulness and interference as factors in paired-associate learning. *Educ Gerontol* 1:297–306, 1976.

136. Wright RE: Aging, divided attention, and processing capacity. *J Gerontol* 36:605–614, 1981.

137. Zarit SH, Cole KD, Guider RL: Memory training strategies and subjective complaints of memory in the aged. *Gerontologist* 21: 158–164, 1981.

138. Zelinski EM, Gilewski MJ, Thompson LW: Do laboratory memory tests relate to everyday remembering and forgetting? In Poon LW, Fozard JL, Cermak L, Arenberg D, Thompson LW (eds): *New Directions in Aging*. Hillsdale, NJ, Erlbaum, 1980, p 519.

139. Zelinski EM, Light LL: Reading comprehension and the older adult. In Lovelace T (ed): *Reading and Older Adults*. New York, International Reading Association, in press, 1987.

140. Zelinski EM, Light LL, Gilewski MJ: Adult age differences in memory for prose: the question of sensitivity to passage structure. *Dev Psychol* 20:1181–1192, 1984.

141. Zeppelin H, McDonald CS, Zammit GK: Effects of age on auditory awakening threshold. *J Gerontol* 39:294–300, 1984.

6 Common Psychiatric Problems in the Elderly

JAMES T. MOORE

Editor's Note

In Chapter 6, Moore emphasizes strongly the fact that signs of emotional or psychiatric disturbance in an older person may be recognized first by other health professionals providing medical or therapeutic services to that individual. Thus this chapter is designed to make professionals aware of the most common psychiatric illnesses in late life, with particular emphasis upon dementia, depression, and paranoia. The DSM-III is used as the basis of classification in order to enhance interdisciplinary communication. After describing briefly the nature of the psychiatric examination, Moore provides a core of diagnostic, descriptive, and management data concerning organic mental disorders, adjustment disorders, affective disorders (mania, depression, and dysthymia), and paranoia. Anecdotal examples are used to illustrate elements of a number of these disorders as they involve older persons. When appropriate, the reader's attention is drawn to potential sources of diagnostic confusion, particularly as related to dementia.

INTRODUCTION

While the prevalence of most psychiatric illnesses may not increase with age, there is a dramatic increase in physical illness. By the age of 70, most persons have at least one significant physical health problem. Because of this, any health professional working with elderly persons is likely to see patients with psychiatric illness—usually coexisting with physical/medical conditions.

Most elderly patients with psychiatric illness are not seen by a psychiatrist; they either receive their health treatment from a primary physician or receive no treatment at all. Frequently, it is the health professional who spends the most time with such patients (e.g., nurses, physical therapists, occupational therapists or speech-language pathologists) who first recognizes psychiatric disturbance.

The most common psychiatric illnesses in late life are dementia, depression, and paranoia. Depression and dementia are increased in patients who have had a stroke; these same patients are commonly found in the caseloads of speech-language pathologists. It is estimated that 10% of persons over age 65 have symptoms of dementia, while 20% of those over 80 are so affected. Depending on the definition of depression, 2 to 4% of the elderly have symptoms of depressive illness, while many more suffer from other psychiatric illnesses, such as adjustment disorders (especially to loss) and paranoia.

In this chapter we will review the most common psychiatric problems likely to be seen by speech-language pathologists or audiologists. The review begins with consideration of the mental status examination. Some of the most common psychiatric conditions, such as dementia, depression, and paranoia, will be discussed in the second portion of the chapter.

APPROACHES TO PSYCHIATRIC EVALUATION

An individual's psychosocial functioning is the result of several factors. Some of these (e.g., personality type and presence or absence of serious psychiatric illness such as schizophrenia) are direct and obvious. Psychosocial stressors such as bereavement are also clearly important. Other important factors affecting mental health include physical illnesses. Whenever a psychiatric evaluation is conducted, it is essential to know the level of functioning of the individual before the onset of the psychiatric condition. Thus, a thorough psychiatric evaluation not only establishes a "psychiatric diagnosis" but also evaluates previous level of function, the presence or absence of stressful life experiences, and overall physical health, as well as describing the individual's personality or characteristic way of dealing with life experiences.

The most widely used, standardized classification system of psychiatric disorders in the

United States is the third edition of the Diagnostic and Statistical Manual of Mental Disorders (DSM-III), published by the American Psychiatric Association (1). The DSM-III evaluates the level of function in five areas, or axes.

1. Axis I is what is usually thought of as the "psychiatric illness." Examples of Axis I diagnoses include major depressive episode, paranoia, primary degenerative dementia, or Alzheimer's disease.

2. Axis II describes personality disorders. Personality disorders reflect inflexible and maladaptive personality traits. These disorders are generally recognizable early in life and, if anything, tend to become less severe with aging. However, some personality traits (such as an extreme need for independence) may be relatively adaptive earlier in life but begin to produce symptoms as a person becomes older and begins to need help for the first time in his or her life. Personality disorders in DSM-III include schizoid, avoidant, antisocial, passive aggressive, and borderline personality disorders.

3. Axis III describes physical disorders and conditions. It is important to recognize that physical illnesses can have profound effects on emotional well-being. Most elderly patients have at least one chronic medical condition. As we will see, loss of physical health is one of the most difficult losses for older people.

4. Axis IV describes the severity of psychosocial stressors associated with a psychiatric illness. A seven-point scale is used to rate severity of such stresses. This scale goes from no stress to catastrophic stress. An illness such as depression which occurs "out of the blue" usually requires a different approach than one that is associated with a loss such as bereavement.

5. Axis V describes the highest level of adaptive function in the previous year. As with Axis IV, adaptive function is rated on a seven-point scale ranging from superior to grossly impaired. Whenever we see a person with a psychiatric illness, it is important to determine at what level the person functioned prior to an illness. It is unusual for a person to function better after an illness than he or she could before.

MENTAL STATUS EXAMINATION

Before discussing clinical syndromes, it is important to understand the nature of a psychiatric examination. As with other fields of medicine, psychiatric diagnosis rests on history, physical examination, and ancillary studies such as laboratory tests. The mental status examination is part of the physical examination. The mental status examination character-

istically includes five major areas: (a) general appearance; (b) mood and affect; (c) speech; (d) thought processes; and (e) sensorium.

General Appearance

Many psychiatric illnesses produce characteristic patterns of physical appearance. Demented patients may be unkempt: depressed persons may sit slumped with poor eye contact and little attention to their environment. The general appearance section of the exam typically begins by describing the patient in terms of age and physical location (e.g., sitting in a chair, in bed, wheelchair-bound, etc.). Appearance relative to the patient's chronologic age, posture, and general social awareness is noted. Personal cleanliness and grooming are described, including notation as to the type and state of clothing. Level of psychomotor activity is an important observation. Depressed patients frequently have reduced psychomotor activity or show agitation through behaviors such as pacing and hand wringing.

Mood and Affect

Mood generally refers to how the patient feels, while affect describes the way the person appears. It can sometimes be difficult to determine whether abnormalities in mood and affect are due to an organic or an affective illness. For example, demented patients may cry easily during an interview, but this may reflect emotional lability related to their organic illness rather than an affective disorder. If a patient feels sad, it is important to describe the depth of the feeling. Patients with normal bereavement, for example, do not typically feel hopeless while depressed persons frequently do. Elderly persons with a depressive illness often deny a depressed mood but appear depressed, and are apathetic and withdrawn.

Mood is characterized in terms of its appropriateness to the situation, and is often described in the patient's own words. The stability or fluctuation of mood is important, since organic brain syndromes produce labile changes of mood and affect. While depression or elation are perhaps the most common symptoms of mood disorder, suspiciousness, hostility, and irritability are other important and relatively commonly observed affects.

Speech

In a psychiatric examination, some assessment of speech and language is important. Manic patients frequently show "flight of ideas" as they speak exceedingly rapidly. They quickly jump from subject to subject without being able to complete a thought. Speech is characteristically described as "forced" in a manic episode. In contrast, depressed patients frequently speak very slowly in association with psychomotor retardation. Aphasia is a common problem in dementias.

Thought

Assessment of thought includes an evaluation of delusions (i.e., falsely held beliefs that are not part of a cultural heritage), preoccupations, and general level of thought. While delusions are usually considered a symptom of schizophrenia, depression frequently produces delusional behavior in older people. These delusions are typically somatic or nihilistic. It is not uncommon for a depressed elderly person to be convinced that his or her misery is caused by a terminal illness that physicians cannot identify. Other depressed patients may be convinced that they are going to lose their home because of failing to pay a light bill.

Paranoid delusions can also develop for the first time in late life. An interesting difference between delusions of younger and older patients is that younger persons characteristically are suspicious of an object at a distance. That is, young schizophrenics most typically have paranoid delusions about the FBI, the CIA, or some other distant and faceless entity. In contrast, older persons are usually suspicious of someone in their immediate environment— especially persons on whom they are dependent, such as family members or other caregivers.

Sensorium

An assessment of the level of consciousness is routinely included in the mental status exam. The essential distinction between delirium and dementia is that delirium occurs in a "clouded" level of consciousness while dementia occurs in a clear level. A clouded state of consciousness refers to a reduction in the level of awareness of the environment. Memory is typically evaluated as part of the psychiatric examination. Short-term memory is often assessed by asking the person to remember three objects for a period of 3 to 5 minutes. This ability is typically impaired in dementia but can be affected in other illnesses such as depression. Calculations are frequently performed, with "serial 7s" being among the most common. Persons

are asked to start with 100 and subtract 7 from each final answer. Constructions assess an individual's ability to draw or to construct two- or three-dimensional figures. This ability is frequently impaired in dementias.

ORGANIC MENTAL DISORDERS

In DSM-III terminology, "organic brain syndrome" refers to a constellation of signs and symptoms without reference to etiology, while the term "organic mental disorder" designates a specific illness such as primary degenerative dementia. Symptoms of organic brain syndrome typically include memory impairment (especially short-term), emotional lability, disorientation, and impaired judgment. Anything which diffusely impairs the brain's function produces an organic syndrome. Thus, in the older patient, illness in virtually any organ system can produce an organic mental disorder.

A broad distinction can be made between delirium and dementia. As noted above, the essential feature of delirium is a clouded state of consciousness. Delirious patients cannot sustain attention and frequently have sensory misperceptions or even visual hallucinations. They are often agitated, picking at bedcovers or clothes, attempting to get out of bed, and lashing out at people.

Acute confusional episodes associated with delirium are very common among medically ill elderly patients, as a result of both the illness itself and accompanying medications. Medications with anticholinergic properties such as antidepressants are a relatively frequent cause of delirium. One 85-year-old man became delirious while taking an antidepressant and cut open a mattress with a knife because he was convinced money was hidden in the mattress. "Sundowning" is also a frequent problem in elderly patients—particularly with a change in environment. Persons who are admitted to nursing homes or hospitals frequently become confused and agitated at night. It is not completely clear whether the confusion is the result of being in a foreign environment, reduced sensory input at night, fatigue, or other factors.

Dementia

Dementia is one of the most common and feared illnesses associated with aging. Increasing age is the single greatest risk factor for dementia. Approximately 10% of individuals over age 65 have mild or moderate dementia while more than 20% of persons aged 85 and over have this illness. It is important to remember, however, that these statistics also suggest that 80% of patients over age 85 do not suffer from intellectual decline. The diagnostic criteria used to define dementia are shown in Table 6.1.

While primary degenerative dementia or Alzheimer's disease is responsible for most cases of dementia in the elderly, several other illnesses could produce dementia. After Alzheimer's disease, multi-infarct dementia is probably the most common cause of dementia. Both of these illnesses are presently irreversible and without a dramatically effective treatment. Because, like delirium, diseases in virtually any organ system can produce dementia and because many of these illnesses can be reversible, a careful diagnostic evaluation is important in any elderly person who develops dementia.

Evaluation of the Patient with Dementia

Evaluation of the patient with dementia attempts to establish a diagnosis. As with any other illness, diagnosis depends on history, physical examination, and use of ancillary studies such as laboratory and imaging techniques.

History. The nature of dementia demands that the history be obtained from a friend or relative as well as from the patient. There are several important questions included in the history. Was the onset of symptoms insidious or dramatic? An acute onset with "stepwise" deterioration is characteristic of multiinfarct dementia whereas an insidious onset is characteristic of Alzheimer's disease. It is important to determine what medications the patient is taking. Adverse reaction to medication is probably the most common cause of a reversible dementia. It is also important to know whether illnesses or life stress were associated with the intellectual impairment. Depression associated with bereavement or other losses can produce memory dysfunction.

Physical Examination. A thorough physical examination is important in evaluating a patient with dementia. Pneumonia, metabolic disturbances such as thyroid disease, and myocardial infarction can produce a dementia or exacerbate an existing dementia.

The Mental Status Examination is extremely important in evaluating the patient with dementia. Many clinicians think that they can evaluate a patient's intellectual capacity while performing a routine history. It is important to know that a standard medical interview assesses social skills rather than intellectual ability. A formal assessment of intellectual function should be conducted with all elderly persons. The Mini-Mental State Inventory developed by Folstein (Table 6.2) is one of the most widely used clinical instruments (9). It assesses several areas of intellectual function, including calculations, orientation, short-term memory, constructions, and aphasia.

Laboratory Evaluation. Ancillary studies are usually part of the evaluation of a patient with dementia, especially if the onset has been relatively recent. Most authorities recommend a standard metabolic workup, including thyroid hormone, B_{12}, and folate, among others.

The Role of Depression in Dementia. Depression frequently induces an apathetic, withdrawn state in elderly persons. This, plus the impairment of concentration associated with depression, can produce intellectual impairment. Depression is often considered as one of the reversible causes of dementia. The terms "pseudodementia" or, more properly, the dementia syndrome of depression, have been used to describe this condition (10, 23).

When there is the suspicion that intellectual decline is the result of depression, the single most useful question to ask is who is bothered by the impairment. If the patient is complaining of memory impairment, depression is quite likely; if family or friends are reporting the symptom, dementia is more likely. As with many either/or questions, it now appears that the problem is more often one of coexistence than of distinguishing depression from dementia. Follow-up studies of depressed persons with memory impairment show that the majority will develop dementia within the next 1 to 2 years (19). This phenomenon will be discussed more fully below when we describe Alzheimer's disease.

Table 6-1
Diagnostic Criteria for Dementia, According to DSM-III[a]

1. Loss of intellectual abilities sufficient to impair social or occupational function
2. Memory impairment
3. At least one of the following:
   (a) Impaired abstract thinking
   (b) Impaired judgment
   (c) Other impairments such as aphasia, apraxia, agnosia, or constructional difficulty
4. State of consciousness not clouded

[a]Modified from American Psychiatric Association: *Diagnostic and Statistical Manual of Mental Disorders*, ed 3. Washington, DC, American Psychiatric Association, 1980.

Table 6.2
Mini-Mental State Inventory[a]

Maximum	Score	Behavior
		Orientation
5	( )	What is the (year) (season) (date) (month)?
5	( )	Where are we: (state) (county) (town) (hospital) (floor).
		Registration
3	( )	Name 3 objects: 1 second to say each. Then ask the patient all 3 after you have said them. Give 1 point for each correct answer. Then repeat them until he learns all 3. Count trials and record.
		Trials
		Attention and Calculation
5	( )	Serial 7's. 1 point for each correct. Stop after 5 answers. Alternatively spell "world" backwards.
		Recall
3	( )	Ask for the 3 objects repeated above. Give 1 point for each correct.
		Language
9	( )	Name a pencil, and watch (2 points)
		Repeat the following "No ifs, ands or buts." (1 point)
		Follow a 3-stage command:
		"Take a paper in your right hand, fold it in half, and put it on the floor." (3 points)
		Read and obey the following:
		CLOSE YOUR EYES (1 point)
		Write a sentence (1 point)
		Copy Design (1 point)
		Total Score
_____		ASSESS level of consciousness along a continuum _____
		Alert Drowsy Stupor Coma

[a](Adapted with permission from Folstein MF, Folstein SE, McHugh PR: "Mini-Mental State": a practical method for grading the cognitive state of patients for the clinician. *Psychiatry Res* 12:189–198, 1975.)

Alzheimer's Disease

Because it is the most common cause of dementia, the natural history and management of primary degenerative dementia or dementia of Alzheimer's type will be considered in some detail. Many of the management principles of Alzheimer's disease apply equally to other forms of dementia. A number of clinical rating scales have been developed to describe the natural history of Alzheimer's disease. One of the more widely used is the seven-point Global Deterioration Scale (GDS) shown in Table 6.3 (20). For purposes of simplicity, the illness can be thought of as having three relatively distinct stages. Each stage has its own problems and issues for the clinician and the caregiver.

Stage I

Alzheimer's disease begins insidiously and therefore cannot be recognized with certainty in its earliest stages. The diagnosis of Alzheimer's disease rests on documenting deteri-

oration over time and excluding other causes. In its earliest stage, Alzheimer's disease characteristically produces personality changes, marital distress, depression, and other symptoms more dramatically than it impairs memory.

Unfortunately, the natural reaction of family, friends, and colleagues in this early stage is to try to help the individual in ways that are actually harmful. For example, a person who begins having problems at work is frequently assigned a different and presumably easier task. Unfortunately, learning a new task is extremely difficult for a patient with Alzheimer's disease early in the course. Similarly if an individual is depressed, counseling or efforts to involve the person in new activities may do more harm than good if their nature is to make intellectual demands beyond the patient's ability.

This is a difficult stage for patient, caregiver, and clinician because the diagnosis can only be considered and not made at this time. It can also be extremely difficult to evaluate if the individual has two problems, such as aphasia from a stroke as well as Alzheimer's disease. The first stage of Alzheimer's disease typically lasts 1 to 3 years.

Table 6.3
Global Deterioration Scale*[a]*

Stage	Characteristics
Stage 1 No cognitive decline	No evidence of memory impairment
Stage 2 Very mild cognitive decline	Person complains of misplacing items, etc.
Stage 3 Mild cognitive decline	Earliest clear-cut deficits; decreased performance in demanding social, occupational settings
Stage 4 Moderate cognitive decline	Can no longer perform complex tasks. Can usually travel to familiar locations.
Stage 5 Moderate-to-severe cognitive decline	Can no longer survive without some assistance.
State 6 Severe cognitive decline	May occasionally forget the name of spouse.
Stage 7 Very severe cognitive decline	Loss of verbal abilities, often incontinent.

[a](Adapted from Reisberg B, Ferris S, De Leon MJ, Crook T: The global deterioration scale for assessment of primary degenerative dementia. Am J Psychiatry 139:1136–1139, 1982.)

Stage II

The second stage of Alzheimer's disease typically lasts several years. The beginning of the second stage might be thought of as the time at which a clinical diagnosis can be made with reasonable certainty. That is, patients have deteriorated sufficiently that deficits are apparent and have developed in a slowly progressive manner. In addition to memory impairment, additional symptoms such as aphasia, agnosia, apraxia, wandering, and emotional lability appear. While depression frequently coexists in the early phases of dementia, as patients deteriorate they typically lose symptoms of depression. Combativeness and agitation, however, may emerge as problems during the course of the illness. Of all the problems associated with dementia, the nighttime wandering and violence are the two that are least well tolerated by caregivers. These two behavioral manifestations are among the most common causes of institutional placement.

The concept of "catastrophic reaction" is helpful in understanding emotional outbursts of Alzheimer's patients. Catastrophic reaction refers to the emotional outburst associated with the sense of being overwhelmed. As the disease progresses, it takes less to overwhelm a patient, and catastrophic reactions become common. Going to a physician's office and bathing are two relatively common precipitants of catastrophic reactions. It is helpful for caregivers to understand that these reactions are symptoms of the illness and cannot be voluntarily controlled by the patient.

Throughout the long second stage of the disease, most patients are at home. Caring for an Alzheimer's patient places a tremendous burden on the caregiver. In most cases, there is a single caregiver responsible for the patient. The main issues the caregiver and clinician deal with during this stage of the illness revolve around balancing concerns for protecting the patient versus the risk of independent activities. Driving a car, using a stove, and going for walks are examples of behaviors that at some point in the illness become dangerous.

Stage III

The third stage of Alzheimer's disease can be considered an institutional phase. This does not mean that patients inevitably are institutionalized, as many patients continue to be cared for at home. It does mean that if a patient is at home, it is because the home has essentially been converted to an institutional environment with 24-hour-per-day care and supervision. In this stage of the illness patients frequently fail to recognize their spouse, children, or friends. An important role of the clinician in this stage is to help caregivers anticipate issues they will have to face and help resolve them. One of the main decisions is how to provide the 24-hour-per-day care required.

Two excellent resources for the clinician and caregiver are the books *The 36-Hour Day* (17) and *Alzheimers Disease: A Manual for Nursing Home Staff* (12). Readers are referred to these books for more thorough description of symptoms associated with Alzheimer's disease as well as coping strategies.

ADJUSTMENT DISORDERS

An adjustment disorder is defined as a maladaptive reaction to an identifiable psychosocial stressor. The maladaptive reaction must occur within 3 months of the stressor. Emotional symptoms to a stress such as bereavement are, of course, to be expected. It is not the presence of symptoms per se but the maladaptive nature of the response that warrants the diagnosis of an adjustment disorder. An adjustment disorder must not be just an exacerbation of an independent psychiatric disorder. It is the maladaptive response which distinguishes adjustment disorder from other entities which might include many emotional symptoms such as normal bereavement.

By far the most frequently observed adjustment disorders of late life are those with depressed mood, anxious mood, or mixed emotional features. The most common precipitant is loss, and bereavement and loss of physical health are the most common losses leading to adjustment disorders.

AFFECTIVE DISORDERS

The main categories of affective illness in the DSM-III are manic episodes, major depressive episodes, and dysthymic disorders. The primary distinction between a major depressive episode and dysthymia is the severity and number of symptoms.

Mania

Characteristics

The distinction between bipolar disorder and major depression is based on whether there has been a manic episode. If there has ever been a manic episode, the illness is considered bipolar; if there have been only major depressive episodes, the illness is considered major depression. The diagnostic criteria for a manic episode are shown in Table 6.4. The essential feature of a manic episode is the disturbance of mood which may be predominantly elevated, expansive, or irritable. Patients may be silly

Table 6.4
Criteria for Diagnosis of Manic Episode, According to DSM-III

1. A distinct period when mood is predominately elevated, expansive, or irritable. The elevated or irritable mood must be prominent and persistent, though a depressed mood may alternate or intermingle.
2. At least three of the following symptoms (four if mood is only irritable) persist at least a week, or hospitalization is required:
   (a) increase in activity or restlessness;
   (b) talkative, pressure to keep talking;
   (c) flight of ideas, racing thoughts;
   (d) grandiose self-image;
   (e) decreased need for sleep;
   (f) distractibility;
   (g) overactive in ways that are likely to produce painful consequences such as buying sprees, foolish investments, reckless driving, etc.

[a]Modified from American Psychiatric Association: *Diagnostic and Statistical Manual of Mental Disorders*, ed 3. Washington, DC, American Psychiatric Association, 1980.

and irritable, especially when thwarted. In addition to the disturbance of mood, several associated symptoms can occur, and at least three must be present to warrant the diagnosis of manic episode. Patients are frequently restless and extremely active. As with the other symptoms of mania, these symptoms must be present to a pathologic degree. If a person is more active than usual and remains productive, this is not considered a characteristic of mania. In a manic episode patients may report increased energy and activity, but the increase in activity does not lead to productivity. For example, an individual might start multiple projects and not finish any and in fact might only create problems by partially completing activities.

Manic patients are extremely talkative, and there is usually a pressure to keep talking. They are extremely difficult to interview because of their need to control the interview. In addition to the pressure to keep talking or forced speech, these patients demonstrate flight of ideas, jumping from topic to topic in a disconnected way. They may describe their thoughts as racing through their head. Persons during a manic episode frequently have a grandiose self-image along with unwarranted optimism. They may perceive themselves as incapable of failing. Patients in a manic episode are highly distractible. As noted earlier, they may start several projects but not sustain attention to actually complete something successfully. Manic patients are typically overactive in ways that will cause harm to themselves or others. An elderly person may make foolish business investments, give money away, etc.

While bipolar illness usually begins during the 4th decade of life, the first manic episode can occur in late life. A hypomanic state is also recognized, and many highly successful productive people probably function in such a state.

Patients in a manic episode typically do not seek psychiatric care. In fact, almost invariably they avoid it, and it is not at all uncommon for patients in a manic episode to require involuntary commitment in order to be treated. It is understandable that an illness that produces feelings such as intense optimism, increased energy, or grandiosity and that affects judgment would not be likely to lead the patient to seek treatment.

Treatment

Treatment of manic episodes usually includes lithium carbonate and/or antipsychotic drugs. Hospitalization is frequently required, both because patients may be dangerous to themselves through impaired judgment and other symptoms and/or because patients refuse to take their medication otherwise.

During an acute phase, antipsychotic medications are frequently used to control the symptoms. Lithium carbonate not only controls symptoms during the acute episode but also is prophylactic for this recurrent illness. The side effects of lithium are important and potentially dangerous. Lithium is similar to digitalis in that there is a small difference between a therapeutic and a toxic blood level. For this reason, patients taking lithium need to have their blood level checked regularly. Symptoms of toxicosity are related to blood level. The initial symptoms of toxicosity are tremor and gastrointestinal disturbances such as nausea, vomiting, and diarrhea. At higher levels, central nervous system symptoms develop, such as seizures and ultimately respiratory arrest. Unlike other psychoactive medications, lithium is not metabolized but is excreted through the kidney. Thus, any medication or other physiologic change that affects kidney function can significantly change the blood level of lithium. Patients taking lithium need to be very careful of dehydration, diuretics, or other factors that could dramatically increase the blood level of this drug. (Important side effects of the antipsychotic drugs are discussed further in Chapter 7.)

When working with a bipolar patient, it is important to identify characteristic symptoms that develop early in the course of a manic episode. Identification of such symptoms is usually done by interviewing a spouse or someone else who knows the individual well. The first warning sign for one patient is an increase in the long-distance phone bill. Another patient can be followed by watching her credit card charges, while a third can be followed by monitoring alcohol intake.

The prognosis for manic episodes is good if the patient can be treated. Because of the potential harm they can cause themselves and others, it is important to treat patients with manic episodes as quickly as possible. It is possible for clinicians to miss manic episodes. One elderly patient with a predominantly irritable mood expressed her increased energy primarily through complaining of multiple somatic complaints. During a 6-week period she saw eight different physicians, had three emergency room visits and several diagnostic procedures, and was not recognized to be manic by any of the physicians who evaluated her. It was only with additional history obtained from her husband that the diagnosis was apparent. She was sleepless, going on buying sprees (17 trash bags of items bought at yard sales were stored in a hallway of her home because the rooms were already filled with overflow from previous purchases). While it is obvious after the diagnosis is made, it is important to remember that manic patients do not come in complaining of being manic. The clinician must be able to recognize the forced speech, distractibility, and other characteristic features of this illness.

Depressive Disorders

The term depression has been used to describe several different entities from a passing mood to a relatively well-defined clinical entity. In DSM-III terminology, there are three main groups of depressive disorders. The term major depressive episode refers to a severe and pronounced disorder which appears to have a significant biological component. Criteria for the diagnosis of major depressive episode are shown in Table 6.5. It should be noted that the primary feature of a major depressive episode is either a depressed mood or loss of interest in usual activities. One of the important features of late life depression is that individuals frequently deny a depressed mood but manifest their depression primarily by withdrawing from usual activities. In addition to the depressed mood or loss of interest in usual activities, patients evidence at least four associated symp-

Table 6.5
Criteria for Major Depressive Episode,
According to DSM-III[a]

1. Dysphoric mode or loss of interest in all or almost all usual activities and pastimes.
2. At least four of the following are present consistently for 2 weeks:
   (a) change in appetite or weight change when not trying to gain or lose weight;
   (b) insomnia or hypersomnia;
   (c) psychomotor agitation or retardation;
   (d) loss of interest or pleasure in usual activities or decrease in libido;
   (e) loss of energy, fatigue;
   (f) feelings of worthlessness, guilt, and/or slowed thinking;
   (g) decreased concentration, indecision;
   (h) suicidal thoughts or recurrent thoughts of death.

Can be further described as psychotic (i.e., presence of delusions or hallucinations) and melancholic (loss of pleasure, inability to enjoy pleasurable events, and three other associated symptoms such as early morning waking, depression worse in A.M., etc.)

[a]Modified from American Psychiatric Association: *Diagnostic and Statistical Manual of Mental Disorders*, ed 3. Washington, DC, American Psychiatric Association, 1980.

toms, such as change in appetite, sleep patterns, loss of energy, etc.

The two other DSM categories wherein depressive illness can be described are adjustment disorder with depressed mood and dysthymia. An adjustment disorder with depressed mood is diagnosed when depressive symptoms are associated with a specific event but are excessive and interfere with the individual's function. Perhaps the most common cause of an adjustment disorder with depressed mood in late life is loss. Longitudinal studies suggest that, of all the losses associated with late life, loss of one's own health is the most difficult to deal with. Dysthymia is a chronic low level of depressive symptoms. From looking at Table 6.6, it is clear that many of the symptoms of dysthymia are the same as those of a major depressive episode. The characteristic feature of dysthymia is that it is persistent. That is, symptoms must be present all or nearly all of the time for 2 years but are either less intense than those in a major depression or last for less than 2 weeks at a time, as with the case of major depression. Clinically, when talking to patients, it is useful to make the distinction between

depression (i.e., major depressive episode) and unhappiness (dysthymia).

Prevalence and Incidence of Depressive Illness

Estimates of the prevalence of depressive illness vary widely, depending on the population surveyed and definition of depressive illness. Generally speaking, patients seen in either medical or psychiatric settings have substantially higher rates of depressive symptoms than individuals in the general community. In recent epidemiologic surveys, approximately 1% of elderly persons in the community have signs and symptoms of major depression at any particular time. Approximately 2 to 4% have dysthymia (4). One thing that community sur-

Table 6.6
Criteria for Dysthymic Disorder, According to DSM-III[a]

1. For most or all of a 2-year period the person has been troubled by symptoms characteristic of depressive syndrome but the symptoms were of insufficient severity or duration to warrant diagnosis of major depressive episode.
2. Symptoms may be relatively persistent or separated by periods of relatively normal mood.
3. During the symptomatic time there is either significant depressed mood or marked loss of interest or pleasure in activities.
4. During the depressive periods at least three of the following are present:
   (a) Insomnia or hypersomnia;
   (b) Decreased energy or tiredness;
   (c) Feelings of inadequacy, decreased self-esteem;
   (d) Decreased effectiveness, productivity;
   (e) Decreased concentration;
   (f) Social withdrawal;
   (g) Loss of interest in pleasurable activities;
   (h) Irritability;
   (i) Inability to respond with pleasure to praise or rewards;
   (j) Pessimistic, brooding about the past;
   (k) Tearfulness;
   (l) Recurrent thoughts of death and suicide.
5. No psychotic features.

[a]Modified from American Psychiatric Association: *Diagnostic and Statistical Manual of Mental Disorders*, ed 3. Washington, DC, American Psychiatric Association, 1980.

veys consistently demonstrate is that individuals in a community warranting a diagnosis of major depression are untreated.

Recognition of Depression

As noted above, it is extremely important to identify withdrawal and loss of interest as a cardinal feature of major depression. It is not at all uncommon for the nursing staff, physical therapist, speech-language pathologist, or others working in a rehabilitation setting to be the first to recognize depression because the patient stops trying and/or loses interest in the rehabilitation program.

Some concerns have been expressed about using the DSM-III criteria for major depressive episodes in older people, because many of the symptoms (such as weight loss and sleep disturbance) could be associated with other age-related illnesses. However, there is good evidence that the criteria for major depression are equally helpful in diagnosing older people if one remembers that loss of interest or pleasure in usual activities can be the cardinal symptom (21).

Depressive illness can produce difficulties with concentration and attention that show up as a memory impairment. This can be pronounced enough to raise the question of dementia. Indeed, the term "pseudodementia" or, more correctly, the dementia syndrome of depression has been well described. While earlier much attention was given to making a distinction between depression and dementia in an either/or approach, more recent studies have shown that a substantial number of patients with "pseudodementia" will develop clear-cut dementia within the following year (5). In other words, it is perhaps more common for dementia and depression to coexist than it is for depression to mimic dementia. This is particularly the case during the first phase of Alzheimer's disease as described above.

Because depressive illness can be associated with biological and social factors, it is useful to have methods of measuring potential contributions in each of these areas. In terms of biological markers of depression, the dexamethasone suppression test (DST) and sleep polysomnography are the most widely used. In the DST, the person takes 1 mg of dexamethasone (a potent synthetic steroid) at 11:00 PM. In a normal individual, the presence of the exogenous steroid produces feedback though the hypothalamic-pituitary axis so that production of cortisol from the adrenal glands is diminished. Thus a normal individual will have a cortisol level less than 5 μg/dl when measured at 4:00 and 11:00 PM the following day.

Approximately 50% of persons with major depressive episodes with melancholia have a positive DST (i.e., they have levels greater than 5)(7).

Sleep polysomnography has also been used as a biological marker of major depressive episode. In major depression, characteristic changes include earlier onset of rapid eye movement (REM) sleep (i.e., decreased REM latency) and increased density of REM sleep (15, 16). These and other biological markers of major depression have been useful in confirming the presence of a biological component and are presently being studied to determine their role in monitoring response to treatment.

Treatment

Biological, psychological, and social interventions all have roles in treating depressive illnesses. The two main categories of biological treatment are antidepressant medications and electroseizure therapy (EST or ECT). EST treatments are the most effective treatment for major depressive illness and especially for the subgroup with melancholic features (3, 8, 22). Several studies have shown a response rate as high as 80% even with patients who have failed to respond to other treatments. There is some evidence that subgroups of dysthymic patients may also respond to biological treatment, but most of this research has been done on persons younger than 65 years of age.

Electroseizure therapy (EST) is a much maligned, poorly understood treatment. Not only is it considered the most effective treatment for severe depressive illness but, surprisingly, it is also generally considered to be safer than medications. There have been three major modification of EST since its discovery as a treatment in the 1930s. These are the use of anesthesia, muscle relaxants, and oxygenation. Physiologically, the two important modifications are muscle relaxation and oxygenation. Prior to the use of succinyl choline as a muscle relaxant, fractures (particularly vertebral body compression fractures) were the most common complication of the EST. Succinylcholine has virtually eliminated this problem. Oxygenation is extremely important because individuals do not breathe during a seizure and certainly not if they have been paralyzed with succinylcholine. Prior to induction of the seizure, patients are oxygenated so that blood oxygen levels are high throughout the procedure. The use of anesthesia allows the patient to be unaware of events during the treatment.

EST is most often used for patients who cannot tolerate antidepressant medications, those who fail to respond to adequate trials of antidepressants, and those who are so severely depressed that their illness is life-threatening (either through overt suicidal behavior or in other ways, such as starvation). The major side effect of EST is a short-term memory impairment which typically increases through the course of a series of treatments. Patients usually have 7 to 12 treatments during a treatment episode. The degree of EST-related confusion can be significant, making it difficult to perform such interventions as psychotherapy or other activities that require good memory. Occasionally patients will have conversations and appear to be completely alert and oriented, but will then have no memory of the content of the conversation the following day. Fortunately, this problem is short-term; within 2 to 4 weeks following treatment the individual's intellectual functions should have returned to baseline.

Antidepressant medications are the most widely used biological intervention in treating depressive illnesses. There are two main classes of drugs; tricyclics and monoamine oxidase inhibiters (MAOIs) are the presently available medications. There are a number of new chemicals including "tetracyclics." The search for new antidepressant medicines continues in an effort to find medications that are either quicker acting, have fewer side effects, or are more efficacious. All of these factors are important because presently available antidepressants typically require 2 to 4 weeks at therapeutic level to have maximum effect. Although approximately two-thirds of patients with major depressive episodes can be expected to respond to these medicines, a substantial portion remain symptomatic.

Adverse side effects also limit the usefulness of these agents in a number of people. Perhaps the most common side effects associated with tricyclic antidepressants are anticholinergic side effects, orthostatic hypotension, and cardiovascular effects. Many of these drugs cause significant orthostatic hypotension in the elderly. This is of great concern with frail older people who are at risk for falls resulting in a fractured hip, subdural hematoma, or other serious complications. Similarly, because these drugs tend to slow interventricular conduction, they have to be used cautiously in patients with heart block. Anticholinergic side effects produce symptoms such as constipation and urinary retention and can precipitate narrow angle glaucoma. The anticholinergic side effects of tricyclic antidepressants can also produce delirium.

Psychological and social interventions are also an important part of treating depressive illnesses in older people, particularly in dys-

thymia and adjustment disorders with depressed mood. Losses and a sense of decreased mastery of the environment are common problems in both depressive disorders and paranoid disorders in late life. It is extremely important to help individuals feel maximally "in charge" of their lives, which involves minimizing the effect of significant losses—social, economic, physical.

Dysthymic persons, especially if they loudly voice their complaints, can be extremely difficult to work with. Interestingly, there is a far less developed literature about dysthymia than there is about major depressive illness. Yet in community samples and clinical settings, dysthymia is roughly twice as common as major depression. In one of the few good studies, Gillis and Zabow compared dysthymic patients with those who probably met DSM-III criteria for major depression (11). Interestingly, depressed persons were similar to normals in socioeconomic level, income, education, and degree of social interaction with family. Dysthymics, on the other hand, were significantly different from normals or depressed persons in having less income, less education, and dramatically less interaction with their families. The authors speculate whether decreased interaction is a cause or a result of their dysthymia. In their study, dysthymics tended to be unpleasant, demanding, and complaining individuals.

As mentioned earlier, it appears that there are subsets of dysthymic patients who respond to biological intervention (2). It is also important to know that a significant number of persons have both a major depressive illness and dysthymia. Thus, they may partially respond to biological treatment but continue to be symptomatic from their dysthymia (13, 14). For the most part, however, treatment today continues to be predominantly in the form of psychological and social interventions.

PARANOIA
Nature of Paranoid Symptoms

A wide range of paranoid symptoms can occur in elderly persons. In some cases, the paranoid symptoms and behaviors occur for the first time in late life, and in other situations they are a continuation of an illness or personality type which developed much earlier in life. Paranoid symptoms can occur in isolation from other psychiatric symptoms, or they can occur as part of another illness such as depression, dementia, etc.

The criteria for "paranoid disorder" in DSM-III are shown in Table 6.7. A paranoid disorder can be further categorized either as paranoia when the symptoms have been present more than 6 months or as acute paranoid disorders when symptoms have been present less than 6 months. The category of a typical paranoid disorder is used in some cases.

Paranoid symptoms can be associated with other illnesses. For example, it is quite common for patients with Alzheimer's disease to have paranoid delusions at some point in their illness. This usually occurs relatively early in the course of a progressive illness such as Alzheimer's. It is easy to imagine that, when a patient loses things, it is less emotionally devastating to blame a thief than it is to recognize one's own failing memory. As with depressive symptoms which are also associated with Alzheimer's disease, patients characteristically stop their paranoid delusions as the illness progresses, and their memory becomes increasingly impaired.

While paranoid personality is a diagnosis in DSM-III, such personality disorders usually have a very pervasive sense of distrust and suspiciousness, and the symptoms characteristically begin early in life. In other cases paranoid symptoms can develop for the first time in late life when certain personality types encounter stresses associated with aging. A case example from an ambulatory geriatrics evaluation clinic illustrated an interplay of rigid, demanding personality with normal stresses and losses of late life to present a striking paranoid disorder.

Mr. Jones, an 81-year-old man, had been married to the same wife for 61 years. He came to the clinic insisting on blood tests to prove that none of their three children were his. He was convinced his wife had been unfaithful

Table 6.7
Criteria for Paranoid Disorders, According to DSM-III[a]

1. Persistent persecutory delusions or delusional jealousy.
2. Emotion and behavior consistent with the delusional system.
3. Symptoms for at least 1 week.
4. None of the major symptoms of schizophrenia (e.g., bizarre delusions, incoherence, marked loosening of associations).
5. Hallucinations not prominent.
6. Symptoms not due to other illnesses such as organic mental disorder or affective disorder.

[a]Modified from American Psychiatric Association: *Diagnostic and Statistical Manual of Mental Disorders*, ed 3. Washington, D.C., 1980.

throughout the marriage and was accusing her of continuing infidelity. He would not let her out of his sight, and both husband and wife were being made miserable by his constant accusations. He would talk of nothing else either with his wife, their children, or the very few friends who would remain to talk with him.

The suspiciousness and accusations began one year previously after his wife was hospitalized for a cholecystectomy, but events over the previous 10 years set the stage for the accusations. Mr. and Mrs. Jones had never spent a night apart until his wife was hospitalized 10 years previously. During that lengthy hospitalization, Mr. Jones had an affair with a woman in her 30s. This was the only known episode of infidelity in the marriage. Three years prior to the current clinic contact Mr. Jones had prostate surgery and had been impotent since then. When his wife was rehospitalized one year ago, his impotence prevented a recurrence of the infidelity. Instead the husband accused his wife of the behavior he had shown 10 years earlier.

Both Mr. and Mrs. Jones were rigid, stubborn people unable to bend to accommodate each other. Mr. Jones had always been insensitive and self-centered. Although the tension between the two had been present to some extent throughout their 60 years of marriage, it had dramatically escalated during his accusations. Mrs. Jones would make efforts to ignore her husband's accusations until she could no longer contain herself and would then respond with intense anger. During these times, she would sometimes say things that her husband took as confirmation of her guilt, thus adding fuel to the fire.

In this case, there was one central overwhelming delusion. As is often the case in late life paranoid disorders, the delusions involved a person on whom the patient was extremely dependent and occurred in the context of the patient's difficulty in handling his decreasing control over his environment and his own health. Such disorders can be extremely difficult to treat.

Another case example also demonstrates the role of controlling the environment in paranoid symptoms. An elderly woman was brought to the doctor's office because she was accusing her family of trying to poison her. The woman had been living alone in the house in which she and her husband had lived for many years prior to his death some 10 years ago. With increasing age, she became frail and found it difficult to maintain the house by herself. She decided to sell the house and to move several hundred miles to live with a daughter and the daughter's family. The main possession the woman kept from her house was her car. She almost never drove the car, but it was important to her to keep as a symbol of independence. The patient was convinced that her family members were trying to kill her to take her money. During the interview, it became apparent that the patient's daughter was letting the teenage granddaughter drive the patient's car without discussing it with her. In this case, the simple intervention of suggesting that the patient be the one to give permission for the use of the car eliminated the symptoms.

In yet another case, a 75-year-old woman was brought to a psychiatrist's office because she had poured Clorox into the orange juice of a college student who was rooming in her homes. This woman had always lived alone, never married, and throughout her life had been somewhat reclusive and perhaps eccentric, though she had no former psychiatric history. Her symptoms were responsive to antipsychotic medications but appeared to be relatively independent of specific stresses or environmental circumstances.

The last case raises a diagnostic question which involves some controversy. It is not completely clear how to consider paranoid illnesses which have some features of schizophrenia and begin late in life. One of the criteria for the diagnosis for schizophrenia in the DSM-III is an onset of symptoms before age 45. In Europe and Great Britain, the term paraphrenia is used to describe late onset paranoid thought disorders which have many of the symptoms of the schizophrenia (5, 6). At any rate, it is clear that paranoid disorders in the elderly can exist on a continuum from relatively mild fear and suspicion to psychotic conditions with firmly held delusions and occasionally hallucination (18).

Etiology of Paranoid Symptoms in Late Life

As noted above, a number of illnesses, stresses, and predisposing personality types can contribute to the development of paranoid symptoms in the elderly. Another factor which has received a great deal of attention is sensory impairment, especially deafness. A number of studies have found a higher proportion of deaf patients in paranoid groups than in other illnesses. Interestingly, other sensory losses such as blindness have not been found to be associated with increased paranoia. One group has suggested that blindness has less of a tendency to promote paranoia, because blindness interferes most with relationships between human beings and inanimate objects while deafness raises barriers between human beings. While genetic factors are clearly important in development of schizophrenia in younger patients, it is much less clear whether there is a significant genetic component in late onset paranoid disorders.

Treatment of Paranoid Disorders

A very important principal in treating elderly paranoid persons is to help them maximize a sense of control over their environment. Many fears, such as those experienced by elderly housing project residents concerning theft of their monthly retirement checks, can be very realistic.

Antipsychotic medications are also important in controlling psychotic paranoid patients. The more closely the paranoid disorder resembles schizophrenia, the more positive is the response to antipsychotic medications.

When interacting with a paranoid patient it is important to avoid both challenging the person's delusions and agreeing with the delusions. Paranoid persons frequently show a rather ambivalent attitude toward seeking mental health assistance. While it is completely illogical to speak to a psychiatrist or another mental health specialist if the problem is someone stealing from you, many paranoid people are surprisingly willing to talk with mental health professionals. The mental health professional can focus attention on associated symptoms such as sleeplessness and anxiety, rather than discussing the delusions directly. Attention can then be directed to improving the situation by altering the environment and, in most cases, by the use of antipsychotic medication.

CONCLUSIONS

A holistic approach to health care is especially important when working with older patients, because medical, psychiatric, and social problems so frequently coexist. Psychiatric or social problems can impose significant limits on a person's ability to respond to or even follow a treatment plan aimed at a physical illness.

Several of the most common psychiatric illnesses affecting older persons have been reviewed in this chapter. It is important to remember that many of these illnesses (especially depression and mild dementia) may not be recognized by family or physician. Those professionals working closely with patients may be the first to identify potentially treatable psychiatric disorders.

References

1. American Psychiatric Association: *Diagnostic and Statistical Manual of Mental Disorders*, ed 3. Washington, DC, American Psychiatric Association, 1980.
2. Akiskal HL, Bitar AH, Puzantian VR, et al: The nosological status of neurotic depression. *Arch Gen Psychiatry* 35:756–766, 1978.
3. Avery D, Winokur G: The efficacy of electroconvulsive therapy and antidepressants in depression. *Biol Psychiatry* 12:507–523, 1977.
4. Blazer D, Williams CD: Epidemiology of dysphoria and depression in an elderly population. *Am J Psychiatry* 137:439–444, 1980.
5. Bridge TP, Wyatt RJ: Paraphrenia: Paranoid states of late life. I. European research. *J Am Geriatr Soc* 28:193–200, 1980.
6. Bridge TP, Wyatt RJ: Paraphrenia: Paranoid states of late life. II. American research. *J Am Geriatr Soc* 28:201–205, 1980.
7. Carroll BJ, Feinberg M, Greden JF: A specific laboratory test for the diagnosis of melancholia. *Arch Gen Psychiatry* 38:15–22, 1981.
8. Crowe RR: Electroconvulsive therapy—a current perspective. *N Engl J Med* 311:163–167, 1984.
9. Folstein MF, Folstein SE, McHugh PR: "Mini-mental State": a practical method for grading the cognitive state of patients for the clinician. *Psychiatry Res* 12:189–198, 1975.
10. Folstein MF, McHugh PR: Dementia syndrome of depression. In Katzman R, Terry RD, Bick K (eds): *Alzheimer's Disease: Senile Dementia and Related Disorders*. New York, Raven Press, 1978, p 87.
11. Gillis LS, Zabrow A: Dysphoria in the elderly. *South African Med J* 62:410–413, 1982.
12. Gwyther LP: *Care of Alzheimer's Patients: A Manual for Nursing Home Staff.* Chicago, American Health Care Association and Alzheimer's Disease and Related Disorders Association, 1985.
13. Keller MB, Lavori PW, Endicott J, et al: Double depression: two-year follow-up. *Am J Psychiatry* 140:689–694, 1983.
14. Keller MB, Shapiro RW: "Double-depression": superimposition of acute depressive episodes on chronic depressive disorders. *Am J Psychiatry* 139:438–442, 1982.
15. Kupfer DJ, Reynolds CF III, Ulrich RF, et al: EEG, sleep, depression and aging. *Neurobiol Aging* 3:351–360, 1982.
16. Kupfer DJ, Spikder DG, Coble PA, et al: Electroencephalographic sleep recordings and depression in the elderly. *J Am Geriatr Soc* 26:53–57, 1987.
17. Mace NL, Rabins P: *The 36 Hour Day.* Baltimore, The Johns Hopkins University Press, 1981.
18. Post F: *Persistent Persecutory States of the Elderly.* London, Pergamon Press, 1966.
19. Reifler V, Larson E: Coexistence of cognitive impairment and depression in geriatric outpatients. *Am J Psychiatry* 139:623–625, 1982.
20. Reisberg B, Ferris S, De Leon MJ, Crook T: The global deterioration scale for assessment of primary degenerative dementia. *Am J Psychiatry* 139:1136–1139, 1982.
21. Spar JE, La Rue A: DSM III can be used to diagnose depression in the elderly. *Am J Psychiatry* 140:844–847, 1983.
22. Weiner RD: The role of electroconvulsive therapy in the treatment of depression in the elderly. *J Am Geriatr Soc* 30:710–712, 1982.
23. Wells CE: Pseudodementia. *Am J Psychiatry* 36:895–899, 1979.

7 Pharmacology and the Aging System

MARY ELLEN BRANDELL
RICHARD R. BRANDELL
RICHARD HULT

Editor's Note

Pharmacology is the study of the interaction between a drug and the living system receiving that drug. Given the extent of the physiological changes associated with aging, coupled with increases in chronic health problems in the elderly, it is not surprising that there is growing concern about the use and abuse of drug therapy in this population. The authors of Chapter 7 bring to their text an exceptional diversity of training and experiences that allows them to approach the topic of pharmacology and the aging system from a holistic perspective. Topics addressed include: pharmacokinetic factors; basic drug classification; pharmacodynamic changes in the elderly; patterns of drug usage and drug interactions in the older adult, with associated interactional side effects; and other age-related factors influencing drug effects and compliance with drug therapy in the older population. This chapter serves several important functions for the professional with an elderly client base. First, the basic information about drug classifications and interactions should provide an ongoing reference source for the practicing clinician. Second, client behaviors in assessment or intervention situations may be influenced by current medications. Failure to recognize these effects may lead to misperceptions as to the client's potential or motivation to respond to therapeutic managements. Finally, many drugs or drug interactions have a direct influence on communicative behavior. Without a thorough understanding of the pharmacology of aging and the specific drugs being taken by an individual client, misdiagnosis is possible.

INTRODUCTION

The use of appropriate drug therapy with the elderly is of growing medical, social and economic concern. Although older persons (over the age of 65) currently constitute 12% of the population, they spend more than $3 billion annually on prescription and over-the-counter (OTC) drugs, an amount which is nearly 25% of the overall national expenditure for these items. Fisher (11) reported that the average older adult buys more than 13 prescription drugs a year.

Compared to the younger population, the elderly suffer more illnesses with longer periods of acute care and hospitalization. Hollister (17) reported that this results in a greater number of drugs taken and an increased frequency of adverse drug reactions. The elderly tend to rely on health care professionals and also on medication more than the younger population. They are more likely to treat rather than tolerate perceived health problems.

Most of the information regarding clinical pharmacology has been a result of drug studies with young adults. However, the surge of interest and involvement in the geriatric population among health care professions during the past decade has facilitated research in clinical pharmacology and the elderly.

Pharmacology is defined as the study of the interaction between a drug and the living system to which it is administered. Implicit in this definition is the recognition that the drug not only acts upon the system, but also the system acts upon the drug. While the drug, because of its chemical consistency, can be expected to act on the body in a predictable manner, the body is not constant, and functions as a dynamic system. Thus the body's actions upon the drug may vary, depending upon when the drug is administered and under what conditions. This principle becomes extremely important when one realizes that how the body acts upon a particular drug is a major determinant of how much drug will reach and remain at its site of action. It is important for speech-language pathologists, audiologists and other health care providers to have a fundamental understanding that drugs, particularly those designed to modify functioning in the central nervous system, may affect communication behavior and that the degree of effect is directly related to the amount of drug available for action.

The concept of changing body physiology as it ages has been presented in Chapter 4. This chapter will further expand that concept and explain why the quantity of drug action can be influenced by the human system's pharmacokinetic processes, focusing on how aging can alter these processes. In addition, related topics concerning drug pharmacokinetics in the elderly will be briefly discussed.

PHARMACOKINETICS: THE INTENSITY OF DRUG EFFECT AS A FUNCTION OF TIME

Pharmacokinetics is the study of those factors which determine the concentration and effects of a particular drug at its site of action at any selected time. The factors include the dosage and the dynamic bodily processes of absorption, distribution, metabolism, and excretion. Aging can exert a profound influence on these physiological processes and consequently upon how the body responds to the presence of drugs. It should be emphasized (40, 41, 46) that physiological aging does not necessarily parallel chronological aging. Individuals may vary broadly with respect to the chronologic process of aging and subsequently to any alterations in their responses to drugs.

Absorption

Absorption of drugs refers to the rate at which a drug is disseminated into the body. In order for drugs to have their intended therapeutic effect, they must be absorbed from the site of administration and distributed to the intended site of activity. They should not accumulate in the body to excessive levels. Absorption of drugs in the elderly has not been extensively studied.

The rate and extent of drug absorption may be altered by three factors: the aging process, disease states, and drug interactions. The aging process has an effect on the gastrointestinal tract

(39). Lower gastric acidity and slowed gastrointestinal motility in the digestive system of the elderly may be expected to affect the rate of drug absorption. A decrease in gastric acid secretion causes an increase in gastric pH (acidity) as well as a decrease in gastric emptying time. Changes in gastric pH and peristaltic activity may affect drug solubility and transit time according to Robinson (35), leading to a decrease in the extent of or delay in absorption.

Of all the maladies that afflict the elderly, gastrointestinal disorders seem to cause significant physiological and psychological problems. According to Mayersohn (25), the gastrointestinal tract is the most common region of chronic distress, but there have been few rigorous studies of absorption and its relationship to gastrointestinal disorders in the aged. Prolonged gastric emptying may account for the wide range of plasma concentrations and/or erratic therapeutic drug effects in the elderly population with Parkinson's disease.

The most prevalent cause of altered absorption in the elderly is due to drug interactions. The use of antacids decreases absorption of digoxin (cardiac regulator) and tetracycline (antibiotic). Antacids may increase the absorption of levodopa (antiparkinsonian) (22). The use and abuse of laxatives may also have an effect on the quality of a specific drug absorbed. Because most drugs are absorbed by passive diffusion, the effect of any alterations is probably not substantial. Oustander (30) has stated that changes in absorption rate are the least important of age-related alterations in pharmacokinetics. Other factors which may influence absorption (particularly in the elderly) include emotional state, body position (especially for bedridden patients), and type of diet.

Distribution

Individual total body weight remains fairly constant from young adulthood to age 70. However, aging results in significant changes in body composition. Between 25 and 70 years of age, the weight of adipose tissue more than doubles from 14 to 30% of total body weight. A 25 to 30% loss of lean body mass accompanies this aging process. Total body water decreases approximately 17% as a result of these changes. This factor can have profound effects on the distribution of both lipid- and water-soluble drugs (23). Changes in body composition are clinically significant because many drugs are dosed according to body weight.

A number of other age-related changes influence drug distribution. Cardiac output decreases with age. Less blood flows to organs that play important roles in drug metabolism, such as the liver and the kidneys. Age 30 marks the beginning of this decline, which proceeds at an annual rate of 1%. Steinberg (41) noted that plasma binding of drugs has received more attention than other variables influencing drug distribution. When plasma protein levels are decreased, a standard dose of a drug that is protein bound, such as warfarin (blood thinner), will yield more free drug available to the action site and produce more intense effects. In addition, a drug like aspirin would tend to displace warfarin. This drug displacement may produce excessive amounts of free warfarin, leading to undesirably high levels of anticoagulation.

Metabolism

Metabolism is the process whereby the body chemically alters a molecule so that it may be eliminated from the body (25). Age-related changes in drug metabolism are difficult to measure because of the variety of factors influencing liver functions. Hepatic blood flow to the liver, which is the primary site of drug metabolism, decreases 40 to 45% with the aging process (46). The liver mass, as a percentage of body weight, decreases with age after about 50 years. While there is variation in the rate of hepatic drug metabolism in healthy adults, aging tends to slow this process. Studies reported by Riedenberg (34) have indicated that the elderly metabolize drugs at one-third to one-half the rate of younger persons. Since standard liver function tests may not indicate decreased metabolic activity, a better understanding of this process in the elderly is needed.

Excretion

The kidneys are a major organ of drug elimination. Functional changes in the renal system accompany the aging process. Research by Rowe (36) has shown a 35% average decline in the filtration rate between the ages of 20 and 80 years. The effect of aging on renal excretion has been well documented in humans because excretion is easier to measure than absorption, distribution, or metabolism.

Renal functions can also be impaired by potential adverse effects of a number of chronic diseases. These diseases include: hypertension, diabetes, atherosclerosis, and congestive heart failure. Decrease in function as a result of these diseases limits the ability of the kidney to function effectively in the process of eliminating drugs from the body (20).

The application of pharmacokinetics and the alteration of drug disposition with age need to be understood by clinicians to insure improved drug therapy in the geriatric population. Clinicians should learn to be aware of behavior which may manifest itself as a result of medication and aging physiology.

DRUG CLASSIFICATIONS

The elderly are more susceptible to problems regarding drug therapy because of age-related changes in their individual drug pharmacokinetics (16). In the first portion of this chapter, it was reported that problems can be associated with any of the physiological pharmacokinetic processes: absorption, distribution, metabolism, or excretion. Drug absorption can be delayed or decreased because of chronic disease or drugs used to treat disease. Drug distribution can be altered by changes in body composition and blood circulation. Altered metabolism has significant effects on the elimination of various drugs. Changes in excretion profoundly influence how much of a particular drug will remain available in the body at the site of action. Therefore, initiation of changes of drug therapy in the elderly should be carefully considered and closely monitored.

There are additional factors unrelated to the aging physiology which can influence a drug's activity. Clinicians who are planning and conducting therapy programs should have some understanding of how particular drugs affect the body, regardless of age. Drugs can be categorized according to the effect they normally have on individuals. A basic awareness of a drug classification system will also provide a foundation for understanding how some drugs interact adversely and cause an undesirable effect. The drug classification chart in Table 7.1 includes the drug category, desired effect and examples of drugs which are most commonly prescribed for elderly persons (4).

Much of the information concerning the responsiveness in the elderly to drugs lacks scientific confirmation. However, some predictions can be made concerning the margin of safety of a number of drugs regularly used by the aged (47).

Pharmacodynamic Changes in the Elderly

Elderly patients experience enhanced response to numerous drugs that depress the central nervous system. Increased age-related

Table 7.1
Drug Classification

Category	Desired Effect	Drug
Antiepileptic	Prevent seizures	Dilantin
		Mysoline
		Depakene
Antidepressants	Mood elevation	Tegretol, Elavil
		Ascendin
		Triavil
Anxiolytics	Antianxiety	Valium
		Xanax, Halcion
Analgesics	Pain reliever	Tylenol with codeine
Antihypertensives	Lower blood pressure	Captopril
		Minipres
Sedatives	Drowsiness/sleep	Phenobarbital,
		Tuinal, Amytal
		Dalmane, Restoril
Stimulants	Central nervous system stimulant	Ritalin
	(minimal brain dysfunction)	
Anticoagulants	Blood thinner	Panwarfin
		Coumadin
Diuretics	Remove excess fluids	Dyazide, Lasix
		Hygroton, Diuril
		Maxizide
Cardiac drugs	Heart function	Lanoxin
		Procardia
		Cardizem, Isoptin
		Calan
Hypoglycemic agents	Treat diabetic disorders	Micronase
		Orinase
		Diabinese
Antiinfectives	Combat infection	Amoxicillin, Keflex
		Penicillin, Sulfas
Gastrointestinal	Calming GI tract	Donnatal
Psychotropic	Tranquilizer	Thorazine
		Stelazine
		Haldol
Antiarthritics	Combat pain and swelling	Indocin
		Clinoril

[a](Adapted from Brandell ME, Brandell RR: Drug interaction in medical management of speech and language impaired. Presented at the American Speech-Language-Hearing Association Convention, San Francisco, 1978).

sensitivity has been reported for sedatives. Many clinicians believe that sedative or barbiturate use in the elderly should be reserved for control of seizures. Elderly patients have reported a variety of symptoms, including confusion, ataxia, and slurred speech.

Other drugs such as antidepressants have produced incidents of confusion and disorientation in the elderly. Since the elderly are more susceptible to CNS depressants, if possible the patient should be made aware of possible drug effects. Sleep patterns in patients receiving CNS drugs should be monitored.

Other drugs can have adverse effects in older persons. There is a greater sensitivity to the anticoagulant effects of warfarin in the elderly (41). This increased anticoagulant response has been demonstrated to occur even in those patients taking a lower drug dosage. Warfarin is a drug often prescribed for post cerebrovascular accident (CVA) patients. Clinicians should carefully educate patients in their caseloads to refrain from those activities that may result in severe bruising while taking this drug. Elderly clients are also more susceptible to increased side effects of drugs in the diuretic classification. There is a pronounced potential for dehydration in hot weather or in patients who fail to drink sufficient quantities of fluid. Other potential drugs which may have adverse affects

Table 7.2
Adverse Drug Effects in the Elderly

Drug	Classification	Adverse Effect
Amytal	Sedative	Confusion
Clinoril	Antiarthritics	Visual impairment
Thorazine	Psychotropic	Involuntary movement
Dilantin	Antiepileptic	Ataxia

[a](Adapted from Weiner M: Pharmacologic and pharmacodynamic changes related to elderly patients. In: *Pharmacy Practice for the Geriatric Patient*. Carrbora, NC, Health Sciences Consortium Inc., 1985, p 10.

are listed in Table 7.2 along with the classification and expected behavior.

A few examples of drug classifications which can be responsible for adverse reactions in the elderly have been presented. Since response to specific drugs is unique in each person, especially in the aging process, every patient must be evaluated individually.

Adverse Drug Interaction: Prescription and Over-the-Counter Drugs

Many reports of drug interactions involve the concurrent use of a prescription with a nonprescription drug such as aspirin, antacids, antihistamines, or decongestants. When a physician questions a patient about the medication he or she takes, the patient will often neglect to mention nonprescription medications. Many patients take preparations such as antacids, analgesics, and iron supplements for long

periods or in such a routine manner that they do not consider them to be drugs.

Although many elderly persons will have their prescriptions filled in the local pharmacy, they often purchase nonprescription drugs elsewhere, making identification of potential problems extremely difficult for the pharmacist as well as the physician. Elderly individuals should be aware of the possibility of interactions between prescription drugs and over-the-counter medications that they buy on a regular basis. If a person is taking an anticoagulant such as warfarin, he or she should be cautioned against using aspirin at the same time. Tylenol could be substituted with effective results. Diabetics should be alerted to the fact that many cold remedies with decongestants may raise blood sugar levels.

Drugs of similar color and/or shape may cause confusion. A recent report from Hurd and Blevin (18) indicated that geriatric patients had problems discriminating between yellow and white and between green and blue tablets. Changing to a medication which has similar properties but a different color or shape may help to resolve this problem. A drug diary in which the elderly person records his or her medication schedule and checks off each medication as it is taken would also be helpful. Side effects can be entered in this diary and brought to the attention of the patient's physician.

Knapp and Knapp (21) compared the elderly with younger age groups in terms of nonprescription use for various conditions. Table 7.3 represents the data.

Their data indicate that a smaller proportion of the elderly than is observed in younger age groups self-medicate for the most common complaints. A larger proportion of the elderly reported self-medicating for other conditions.

Table 7.3
Use of Nonprescription Medication by Various Age Groups

Condition	Age				
	Under 30 (%)	30−39 (%)	40−49 (%)	50−64 (%)	65 and over (%)
Sore throat	67	57	54	44	43
Coughs	64	63	53	49	44
Sinus trouble	20	23	20	13	10
Head colds	65	60	54	46	38
Hay fever	12	12	8	5	4
Skin problems	17	9	8	6	5
Sleeplessness	4	7	6	8	6
Upset or acid stomach	52	51	47	40	37
Other	11	11	17	21	25

[a](Adapted from Knapp DA, Knapp DA: The elderly and non prescribed medication. *Contemp Pharmacol Pract* 3:85−90, 1980.)

Patterns of Drug Usage in the Elderly

Usage of drugs is high in ambulatory and institutionalized elderly individuals. Law and Chalmers (24) reported that in a general practice study, 87% of ambulatory patients 75 years of age or older were taking prescription drugs. Nearly 34% of those individuals were taking three or four drugs daily. Of 244 ambulatory, community-dwelling men and women over 60 years of age, 83% were taking two or more prescriptions or over-the-counter drugs. In a separate study of Medicare recipients (26), respondents were found to have an average of 10 prescription drugs in their possession. Among institutionalized persons, as many as 95% may be using drugs on a regular basis. A government survey indicates that nursing home residents take an average of 4 to 7 prescriptions each. Elderly ambulatory patients used cardiovascular drugs most frequently, followed by sedatives, antiarthritics, and gastrointestinal agents. Table 7.4 lists the most frequently prescribed drugs according to a survey by the National Center for Health Statistics (29).

In the National Ambulatory Medical Care Survey (NAMCS), individuals over 64 years of age used 20% more cardiovascular drugs than all other age groups combined. Their use of diuretics was 18% higher than that of the next largest group, those between 45 and 64. The NAMCS found Lasix (diuretic) and Lanoxin (cardiac regulator) to be the most commonly used drugs among all older respondents. Dif-

Table 7.4
Drugs Prescribed for Ambulatory and Institutional Elderly Patients According to Classification

Ambulatory Elderly Persons	
Drug Classification	%
Cardiovascular	61
Sedatives and tranquilizers	17
Antiarthritics	12
Gastrointestinal	11
Institutional (Nursing Home) Setting	
Psychotropic	61
Diuretics and antihypertensions	46
Analgesics	44
Cardiovascular	39
Antiinfectives	31

[a](Adapted from National Center for Health Statistics: The National Ambulatory Care Survey, United States, 1979, Summary. *Vital Health Stat Series* [13] 12066: 9, Sept 1982.)

Table 7.5
Male and Female Drug Use According to NAMCS

Drug	Percentage of Population
Males	
Inderal (excess fluid)	40.5
Digoxin (cardiac regulator)	38.1
Isodril (circulation)	28.8
Dyazide (blood pressure)	24.1
Aspirin (pain)	19.3
Hydrochlorothiazide (diuretic)	19.2
Hydrodriril (diuretic)	18.7
Prednisone (antiinflammatory)	10.0
Females	
Dyazide (lower blood pressure)	43.0
Inderal (excess fluid)	42.4
Aldomet (hypertension)	34.0
Vitamin B_{12} (increase red blood cells)	32.7
Digoxin (cardiac regulator)	29.5
Motrin (pain)	24.1
Insulin (diabetics)	22.7
Hydrochlorothiazide (diuretic)	22.0

[a](Adapted from National Center for Health Statistics: The National Ambulatory Care Survey, United States, 1979, Summary. *Vital Health Stat. Series* [13] 12066: 9, Sept. 1982.

ferences among males and females in drug usage were also noted, as shown in Table 7.5.

The results of the NAMCS survey support the results of a recent study of drug usage in an ambulatory geriatric population in Florida (15). Table 7.6 presents the percentage of elderly patients using specific drugs according to classification.

The latest Census Bureau figures project a steady 2.2% annual growth rate in the number of people over age 64. This group already ac-

Table 7.6
Survey of Drug Use in the Elderly

Drug Classification	% Use Among Elderly
Antihypertension	30
Analgesics	19
Antihenuratics	16
Cathartics	15
Diuretics	9
Hypnotics	9
Congestive heart failure drugs	8
Antiarhythmics	6
Anticoagulants	5

[a](Adapted from Hale WE, Marks RG, Stewart RB, et al: Drug use in a geriatric population. *J Am Geriatr Soc* 27:374–377, 1979).

counts for 40% of all prescription sales. Older females who are prescribed almost twice as many drugs as older males will continue to greatly outnumber males. The elderly are fast becoming a powerful force in the drug marketplace (9).

PHARMACOKINETICS: ADDITIONAL INFLUENCING FACTORS

The elderly present unique problems for the speech-language pathologist and audiologist and other health care providers, due to a greater incidence of chronic disease, unpredictable drug response, and other psychological and sociological problems that affect their perceptions of themselves and their general well-being. Comfort (7) reported that aging is often categorized as having two counterparts: senescence, a gradual aging of the body, and senility, which is normal aging complicated by a variety of conditions. The National Center for Health Statistics (29) has listed in order of importance complications that may limit activity of older adults and move them from senescence into a state of senility. Approximately 80% of the elderly, as opposed to 40% of those under 65, suffer from one or more of the following chronic conditions which appear in Table 7.7.

Each of these chronic impairments may influence communication and social conditions in the elderly population. Clinicians should be alert to whether or not behavioral changes are a sign of disease, drug interactions, or sociological changes. Additional factors which influence pharmacokinetics in the elderly include: life-style, nutrition, multiple drug use, and noncompliant behaviors.

Table 7.7
Chronic Conditions of the Elderly

Chronic Condition	% Elderly Population
Heart condition	17–22
Arthritis and rheumatism	20–33
Visual impairments	9–15
Hypertension (without cardiac involvement)	7–16
Mental nervous conditions	6–10.5
Impairment of the lower extremities and hips	5.4
Hearing impairments	22

ᵃ(Adapted from Pepper WH: *Care of the Aging Disabled and Handicapped.* Springfield, IL, Charles C Thomas, 1982.)

Life-Style

The life-style of the elderly individual clearly influences drug therapy. Many older persons lead active lives. However, there are those who become inactive as a result of a physical disability or a loss of purpose in life. Many older individuals are living alone because of the death of a spouse. Oustander (30) states that this type of life-style may result in either overdependence or underdependence on professional services. Recognizing the need for care is the first step toward successful therapy.

The increase in drug usage by the elderly highlights other special problems, according to a nationwide report by Dilger (10). Aging individuals cannot see or hear well, problems which contribute to misuse of medications. Poor eyesight makes it difficult to read labels and inserts in drug packages. Poor hearing may cause the older person to miss the message in verbal directions. Memory loss reduces the ability to comply with regimens that can include as many as 12 or more different medications.

Cigarette smoking affects the metabolism of younger and older persons in different ways. Elderly smokers may have a reduced rate of enzyme induction. The effects of alcohol on drug metabolism should also be considered (45). Many elderly individuals are unaware of the potential dangerous interactions which could result from mixing alcohol with drugs.

Gerhino (12) stresses that, although all drugs do not interact with alcohol, even moderate drinking can be harmful when accompanied by certain drugs. The most hazardous combination involves alcohol and a central nervous system depressant. This occurs because alcohol alters the metabolism and plasma levels of diazepam, a drug which accounts for 50% of all psychotropic drugs prescribed for the geriatric population. This combination can also cause serious psychomotor impairments. Nonprescription drugs such as cold remedies and sleeping aids may produce undesirable effects in combination with alcohol. Lamy and Beardsley conclude: "A little alcohol goes a long way in interfering with psychomotor and cognitive function in subjects of all ages, most profoundly in the elderly" (23, p 42).

Clinicians may wish to consider using a measure such as the *Index of Risk* (23) when evaluating the life-style of elderly patients. As shown in Table 7.8, the *Index of Risk* can be used as an indicator of elderly individuals who are least likely to adhere to recommendations concerning drugs and in most need of intervention. The life-style of the elderly person

Table 7.8
Index of Risk

Life-Style Characteristic	Risk
Age	Greater risk of adverse drug interaction as age increases
Sex	Females have more negative drug interaction
Living arrangement	Elderly adults living alone make more mistakes in drug dosage
Multiple providers	Multiple health care providers may cause overlapping treatments and distortion of communication
Multiple drug therapy	Multiple drug therapy may lead to an increase of drug errors and adverse drug interaction
Support system	Absence of family or friends can cause emotional and physical problems
Sensory disorders impairments can facilitate	Hearing and/or visual errors in verbal and written directions
Disability level	A severe impairment will result in more communication problems and more difficulty in adapting to therapy programs

[a](Adapted from Lamy PP, Beardsley RS: The older adult and the pharmacist educator. Am Pharm 5:41–47, 1982.)

should always be considered in monitoring any therapy program.

Nutrition

An individual's nutritional status has a major influence on drug effectiveness. The elderly patient should be aware that the potential effects of diet on drug therapy can be significant. The metabolism and toxicity of drugs are determined by diet. Posner (32) reported that one-third of elderly patients seen by physicians from a geriatric service were suffering from clinical or chemical malnutrition. Deficiencies such as vitamin D and B were not uncommon. Reasons for nutritional inadequacies include apathy, depression, limited physical activity, and dental problems. Appetite reduction can be caused by any of these conditions.

There are some elderly persons who buy considerably fewer food products when prices are high. The cost and preparation time for a daily diet of fresh vegetables and fruit also may be difficult for some individuals. The elderly are often unaware of the principles of good nutrition, which include the body's need for fiber. Some individuals rely on easy-to-prepare foods that are high in fat and carbohydrates with little protein value. For example, they may not recognize the need to limit intake of foods with a high concentration of sodium, sugar, and saturated fats. Steinberg (40) believes that the effects of nutritional imbalance may be incorrectly attributed to "aging." This misper-

ception will aggravate the cycle of nonspecific symptomatology and treatment. The problem is further compounded because older persons who often use multiple drugs also suffer the effects of drug-induced nutritional deficits (40).

The physical condition of many elderly persons is often near dehydration because many concomitants of aging reduce fluid intake. Reiss and McLean (33) list the following factors for consideration of how water affects the health of the geriatric population:

1. The aging process reduces the sensation of thirst so that fluids are not actively sought by the elderly.
2. Since many elderly persons are incontinent, they impose self-restrictions on their fluid intake.
3. The elderly eat fewer meals each day, which reduces opportunities for fluid intake from coffee, tea, milk, soft drinks, etc.
4. Many elderly persons are taking diuretics which deplete their body fluids. Since they are told that the diuretic gets rid of excess water, the patient often assumes that he/she should avoid or limit fluid consumption.

The older individual needs to drink from six to seven 8-ounce glasses of water daily to satisfy the physiological needs of the body and help facilitate good health. This will maintain good kidney flow and blood volume. The importance of water for older persons taking drugs is usually not considered by the person nor the health professional. Reiss and McLean (33) emphasize that water should be taken with all oral medication because, in order to be absorbed by the bloodstream, the medication must dissolve in the stomach or intestine. These are organs which do not contain large amounts of liquid. A 6- or 8-ounce glass of water will supply enough liquid to help the medicine dissolve quickly and work faster.

There are other reasons for being concerned about fluid intake in older persons. The esophagus of elderly patients is often bent. Water will prevent medication from becoming stuck in the esophageal folds. Drugs such as aspirin and tetracycline are irritating to the stomach. Water taken with these drugs will diminish or perhaps prevent irritation by dissolving and diluting them. In addition, the effect of a drug is influenced by the volume of fluid circulating in the body. Because the elderly have as much as an 18% decrease in total body water, reduced doses of some drugs are necessary to prevent side effects.

There are some medical reasons for restricting water intake in individuals. Excess fluid intake can cause water intoxication, a complication of having cancer that can produce a dilution of sodium in the blood serums. When a physician has restricted fluid consumption, the order should be enforced. However, water is extremely important to the well-being of the elderly person taking oral medication. Water has a medical use as an expectorant and as a moisturizer for dry skin. Water is a diuretic which flushes toxic wastes from the blood via the kidney. In dealing with elderly clients, it is imperative that they understand their need for adequate fluid intake and the positive benefits of water.

Multiple Drug Use

The increased use of medications predisposes elderly patients to a much greater risk of developing adverse reactions. An adverse drug reaction has been defined as an unintended effect of a drug given for therapeutic purposes (48). The elderly as a group have taken more drugs than other age groups, but their pattern of multiple drug use has expanded during the decade of the 1970s (1). The National Health Survey of 1973 found that the average number of prescriptions allocated to individuals 65 years and over was 13.7 (29). In 1978, the number had risen to 17.9. A survey conducted by the Department of Health, Education and Welfare showed the average number of prescriptions per patient each month in nursing homes was 6.1 with a range of 0 to 23 drug orders (44). Forty percent of those patients had seven or more prescription orders.

Table 7.9
Physical, Social, and Psychological Influences on Nutrition

Physical
Physical handicapping conditions
Influence of drugs
Chronic disease
Dental problems
Minimal or lack of physical activity
Arthritic condition
Impairment of taste or smell
Difficulty with excretion

Social
Financial limitations
Difficulty in food preparation for single person
Problems in adaptation to hospital or nursing home setting
Erroneous dietary beliefs

Psychological
Depression or emotional problems
Absence of socialization at meal time
Anorexia
Habitual eating preferences
Cultural tastes

ᵃ(Adapted from Natlow AB, Heslin JA; Psychosocial forces that affect nutrition and food choices. In Natlow AB, Heslin JA (eds): *Geriatric Nutrition.* Boston, CBI Publishing Co. 1980, p 197.)

Many elderly individuals have one or more chronic diseases that affect their nutritional needs. Other factors which influence dietary intake include processing, packaging, and storage of food. Natlow and Heslin (28) developed a list of physical, social, and psychological factors which they believe have a major influence on the nutritional status of the elderly population (see Table 7.9).

Elderly individuals are unique persons whose nutritional balance is determined by social, emotional, and habitual factors in their lives. An adequate nutritional balance is as important in the healthy elderly person as it is in the elderly individual who is ill. Over- or undernutrition can be harmful to individuals in this unique population.

Multiple Drug Therapy

Multiple drug therapy may bring about a drug interaction in a patient. A drug interaction refers to the sequelae attending simultaneous use of two or more drugs. The interaction may result in enhanced or diminished drug effects and may be either useful or harmful. This problem is compounded further by other factors which influence the body's response to drugs such as: age, race, weight, sex, body tempera-

Table 7.10
Potential Drug Interactions in the Elderly

Anticonvulsants (prevent seizures)			
Drug	Combined with	Interaction	Possible effects on the elderly
Hydrantoins (Dilantin) Primadone (Mysoline)	Anticoagulants Phenobarbital	Increased effect Increase effect of phenobarbital	Dysarthria Sedation; slurred speech; drowsiness; malaise
Drugs for Mental Disorders			
Thorazine (tranquilizer)	Librium (muscle relaxant)	Enhanced sedation	Drowsiness; listlessness; learning difficulty
Elavil (antidepressant) Librium, Valium (tranquilizer)	Diuretic (removal of excess fluid)	Increased diuresis	Dizziness; fever; inability to attend
Analgesics (For Pain)			
Aspirin	Phenobarbital or anticoagulants	Decrease of analgesia	Short attention span; distractibility
Meperidine (Demerol)	Phenothiazine tranquilizers (Compazine, Thorazine)	Additive effect	Sedation; blurred vision; slurred speech
Sedatives			
Phenobarbital (sedative)	Librium (muscle relaxant) or antidepressant	Additive effect	Drowsiness; listlessness; inability to attend effectively to task
Phenobarbital	Antihistamine cough or cold	Inhibit each other	Hyperactivity (maybe severe); distractibility; cough, cold would persist; middle ear pathology may result
Phenobarbital	Orinase (diabetes)	Potentiates phenobarbital	Increased drowsiness; lethargy; ability to concentrate on specific activity is diminished
Antihypertensives (Prevent Tension/Lower Blood Pressure)			
Reserpine	Amphetamines (Dexedrine)	Inhibits reserpine	Hypertension; distractibility; irritability; difficulty attending
Apresoline	Thiazide diuretics (Diuril, Esidrex)	Potentiates Apresoline	Hypotension; malaise; inability to concentrate

Table 7.10
Continued

Anticoagulants			
Coumadin (blood thinner)	Orinase (diabetes)	Enhances hypoglycemia	Increased drowsiness; slurred speech
Panwarin (blood thinner)	Aspirin	Prevents action of anticoagulant; slow healing process	Slow response rate; potential CVA

Stimulants (CNS)			
Ritalin	Tofranil	Inhibition of medications	Increased hyperactivity; reduces ability to attend to task
Dexedrine (CNS stimulant)	Resperine (high blood pressure)	Inhibits both drugs	Depression; potential CVA; lethargy
Ritalin (CNS stimulant)	Dilantin (antiepileptic)	Inhibits antiepileptic effect	Distractibility; seizures; slurred and dysarthric-like speech

[a](Adapted from Brandell, ME, Brandell RR: Effects of Drugs on Communicative Abilities of the Geriatric Population. Presented at the American Speech-Language-Hearing Association Convention, Washington, DC, 1985).

ture, disease, method of administration, and other physiological states. Table 7.10 contains a list of combinations of drug classification of commonly prescribed drugs for the geriatric population. Potential interactions and possible effects on behaviors are included (5).

Although some drug interactions develop unexpectedly and are impossible to predict, others are related to known pharmacologic actions of drugs and can be anticipated. With multiple drug regimens, the ability to predict the specific action of any given drug diminishes. Because of this, it is necessary to maintain complete current medication records for patients and to monitor and supervise drug therapy carefully so that problems can be prevented or detected at an early stage.

The Boston Collaborative Drug Surveillance Program (3) reported that for 83,200 drug exposures in 9,900 monitored patients, primarily in acute disease hospitals, there were 3,600 adverse reactions. A total of 234, or 6.9%, of the adverse reactions were attributed to a drug interaction. In most cases the interaction resulted from cumulative pharmacological effects, the most common problem being excessive central nervous system depression resulting from administration of two or more CNS depressants.

There is an increased risk of drug interactions in the elderly since many of them have at least one chronic illness. The types of diseases frequently experienced by geriatric patients may contribute to an altered drug action

(37). There also appears to be an increased sensitivity to the action of certain drugs with advancing age (19). Adverse drug reactions and interactions contribute to a considerable number of hospital admissions in the elderly population (6, 27).

Medication Compliance

Noncompliance with medication occurs when an individual: (a) fails to take drugs at specific times; (b) interrupts the sequence of treatment; (c) makes errors in doses or sequence; or (d) takes other drugs (2, 38). An early study in 1962 by Swartz et al (43) revealed that 59% of the geriatric population made one or more errors in their medications, but only 26% of these were potentially serious to their health. Omission of medication was the most frequent type of error, followed by inaccurate knowledge, errors in self-medication, incorrect dosage, and improper timing (43).

The impact of nonprescribed medication on compliance may be significant. In a survey conducted by Guttman (14), 69% of the persons sampled admitted to using nonprescription drugs, although 85% of these reported no medical problem in the use of these drugs. However, potential problems and adverse effects can be caused by the use of nonprescribed drugs along with prescribed drugs. Knapp and Knapp (21) noted that the elderly do not read the warnings which are printed on package labels of nonprescription medication. Reasons given for not reading warnings were that the words were too long, too technical, or too medical. According to Sumner (42) an elderly person may have problems with two or more of these factors at any given time. Sumner (42) listed guidelines for improving medication compliance in geriatric individuals. The guidelines include:

1. Compensate for physical disabilities by eliminating childproof containers. Easy-to-open packaging would be beneficial to the elderly.
2. Large print should be used for labels and written instructions.
3. Encourage a centralized record keeping system so that a regular review of the patient's medication regimen can be done.
4. If possible, a new drug should not be prescribed without stopping use of the current medication. The elderly patient should be encouraged to return the old drugs to the pharmacist or destroy them.
5. If possible, set up a twice daily schedule of dosage. Intermittent schedules are difficult for the elderly to follow.
6. Since elderly patients often have difficulty swallowing, liquid preparations instead of large capsules and tablets should be used when possible.
7. The treatment plan should be explained to the individual as well as a friend or relative of the geriatric patient. Reasons for prescribing the drug, expected effects, and potential side effects should be explained.
8. A periodic check of the type and amount of over-the-counter drugs taken on a regular basis should be done. Most elderly people do not consider them to be potentially hazardous.
9. Be sure that the elderly patient does not take medication prescribed for someone else.
10. The patient's therapeutic plan should be periodically reviewed to insure that he/she has the information and the motivation to adhere to the prescribed drug plan.

In a report prepared for the Administration on Aging, recommendations were made to health care providers for assisting the elderly in improving their compliance with any therapy (38). According to Weintraub (48), the final recommendation is one of the most important. It suggests that the patient take some responsibility for the appropriate administration of his/her medication. Weintraub (48) recommends that the patient become part of the therapeutic team, gathering data formally and adding it to the information obtained by the health care

professional team. The exchange of information is important since it leads to modification of the therapy plan to meet the needs of the individual. It also provides an opportunity for the physician as well as involved clinicians to learn more about the disease, the therapy, and the outcome of treatment. As a result of active participation by the elderly patient, he/she will be more likely to make appropriate compliance decisions with a potential decrease in adverse drug reactions.

Geriatric Pharmacotherapy Precautions

Whenever medication is needed by the elderly, the dose should be reduced by 20 to 70% (8). Dosage of all drugs should be calculated on the basis of lean body weight. Significant differences between the physiology of men and women, along with age, disease severity, and accompanying illnesses, should be considered. Age-related changes are gradual, and rate of change varies from one person to another. In order to insure safe and effective pharmacotherapy for geriatric persons, each patient should be considered as an individual (13). Before any changes are made in drug therapy, a complete history, including life-style, diet, and drug history, should be completed. A special note should be made concerning the use of over-the-counter drugs or "folk remedies." Communication between the physician and pharmacist should be encouraged.

When a new medication is prescribed, the pharmacist and/or physician should take time to discuss it with the elderly client. Particular emphasis should be placed on the fact that drugs can not only relieve distressful symptoms but also cause them. Any changes which may be associated with drug usage should be reported.

Monitoring drug therapy is an ongoing process that involves review of the patient's medical status as well as an assessment and evaluation of patient information. All essential patient information identified during a drug regimen review should be documented on a patient medical profile form, including the pharmacist's review of the patient's drug regimen. This profile can communicate pertinent information about his/her status to the other clinicians working on the health care team.

The concept of associating drug use with a corresponding diagnosis or disease state is sometimes known as the Problem Oriented Medical Recorder. An alternate designation is SOAP (Subjective, Objective, Assessment and Plans or recommendations format). The system was originally designed to aid physicians in solving medical problems and has been adapted by speech and language pathologists working with the elderly in hospitals and skilled care and home settings. By using the SOAP format in drug regimen reviews, clinicians can evaluate patient data and document significant findings in the same process.

CONCLUSION

The influence of age on the processes of absorption, distribution, metabolism, and excretion must be viewed as a risk factor in drug therapy in elderly persons. Dietary habits, smoking, and problems like alcoholism influence the effect of certain drugs and should be considered in initiating a treatment plan. An accurate and complete record of both the prescription and nonprescription medications a patient is taking should be obtained by the clinician or a designated member of the health care team prior to beginning or changing a therapeutic regimen. Drug interactions have resulted because one physician was not aware of medications prescribed by another physician or because the elderly patient did not consider over-the-counter medications important enough to mention.

Knowledge of the properties and the primary and secondary pharmacologic agents of the drugs used or being considered for use is essential if the potential for drug interaction is to be accurately assessed. Clinicians need to understand the action and use of each medication prescribed for their elderly patients, and the possible communication side effects of such medications. The extensive publicity that certain drug interactions have received may give the impression that these problems are well identified and can be avoided. However, much of the information regarding drug interactions is conflicting and incomplete. Caution is needed in evaluating and using the information available. The role of the clinician in utilizing behavioral observation techniques is extremely important.

As a member of the health care team, the pharmacist can be a valuable resource to speech-language pathologists and audiologists. Graduate programs should include more information on drug classification and interaction so that future clinicians will have a better understanding of this important area. A copy of the *Physicians' Desk Reference* (PDR) published by Medical Economics Company should be available in all training programs and speech and hearing clinics. The use of appropriate drug therapy is a growing medical, social, and economic concern. It is the responsibility of all speech and hearing clinicians to become informed of pharmacological and physiological problems which may be inherent in their elderly patients.

References

1. Anonymous: Out of pocket cost and prescribed medicines. In: *Vital and Health Statistics*, Series 10, No. 108, DHEW Pub. 74-1518. Washington, DC, U.S. Government, Printing Office, 1977, p 15.
2. Blackwell B: The drug defaulter. *Clin Pharmacol Ther* 13:841–845, 1972.
3. Boston Collaborative Drug Surveillance Program: Adverse drug interactions. *JAMA* 220:1238–1239, 1972.
4. Brandell ME, Brandell RR: Drug interaction in medical management of speech and language impaired. Presented at the American Speech-Language-Hearing Association Convention, San Francisco, 1978.
5. Brandell ME, Brandell RR: Effects of drugs on communicative abilities of the geriatric population. Presented at the American Speech-Language-Hearing Association Convention, Washington, D.C., 1985.
6. Carenasos G, Stewart RB, Cluff LE: Drug induced illness leading to hospitalization. *JAMA* 228:713–720, 1974.
7. Comfort A: *The Biology of Senescence*, ed 3. New York, Elsevier, 1978.
8. Cooper JW: Pharmacologic drug related problems in the elderly. In Devereaux MO, Andrus H, Scott CD (eds): *Eldercare: A Guide to Clinical Geriatrics*. New York, Grune & Stratton, 1981, p 216.
9. Dickinson JG: Elderly explosion should set off drug boom. *Drug Topics* 127:2–3, 1983.
10. Dilger JC: Elder-Care. *Drug Topics* 127:50–52, 1983.
11. Fisher CR: Differences by age group in health care spending. *Health Care Fin Ref* 1:65–90, 1980.
12. Gerhino PP: Complications of alcohol and drug therapy. *Consult Geriatr* 30:10–13, 1982.
13. Gomolin IH, Chapron DJ: Rational drug therapy for the aged. *Compr Ther* 9:7–17, 1983.
14. Guttmann D: Patterns of legal drug use by older Americans. *Addict Dis* 3:337–356, 1978.
15. Hale WE, Marks RG, Stewart RB, et al: Drug use in a geriatric population. *J Am Geriatr Soc* 27:374–377, 1979.
16. Henny HR: Altered drug effects in the elderly. *US Pharmacol* 10:41–50, 1985.
17. Hollister LE: Prescribing drugs for the elderly. *Geriatrics* 23:9–71, 1977.
18. Hurd PD, Blevin J: Aging and the color of pills. *N Engl J Med* 310:202–210, 1984.
19. Hussar DA: Drug interactions. In Osol A (ed): *Remington's Pharmaceutical Sciences*, ed 16. Easton, PA, Mark, 1980, p 741.
20. Jusko WJ, Weintraub M: Mycardial distribution of digoxin and renal failure. *Clin Pharmacol Ther* 16:449–455, 1975.

21. Knapp DA, Knapp DA: The elderly and non prescribed medication. *Contemp Pharmacol Pract* 3:85–90, 1980.

22. Lamy PP, Vestal RE: Drug prescribing in the elderly. *Hosp Pract* 1:111–118, 1976.

23. Lamy PP, Beardsley RS: The older adult and the pharmacist educator. *Am Pharm* 5:41–47, 1982.

24. Law R, Chalmers C: Medicines and elderly people: a general practical survey. *Br Med J* 1:565–575, 1976.

25. Mayersohn M: Fundamental principles of pharmacokinetics. In Conrad KA, Bressler R (eds): *Drug Therapy for the Elderly*. St. Louis, CV Mosby, 1982, p 3.

26. Mitham CJ: Physician prescribing habits: effects of medicare. *JAMA* 217:585–587, 1971.

27. Miller RR: Hospital admissions due to adverse drug reactions. *Arch Intern Med* 134:219–225, 1974.

28. Natlow AB, Heslin JA: Psychosocial forces that affect nutrition and food choices. In Natlow AB, Heslin JA (eds): *Geriatric Nutrition*. Boston, CBI Publishing Co., 1980, p 197.

29. National Center for Health Statistics: The National Ambulatory Care Survey, United States 1979, Summary. *Vital Health Stat Series* [13] 12066: 9, Sept. 1982.

30. Oustander JG: Drug therapy in the elderly. *Am J Intern Med* 95:711–727, 1981.

31. Pepper WH: *Care of the Aging Disabled and Handicapped*. Springfield, IL, Charles C Thomas 1982.

32. Posner BM: Reaching for the answers, *The Washington Post*, May 23, 1984, p 21.

33. Reiss R, McLean W: Water effects on medicinal needs of the elderly. *Pharmacol Times* 87:58–64, 1980.

34. Riedenberg MM: Drugs in the elderly. *Bull NY Acad Med* 56:703–714, 1980.

35. Robinson DS: The application of basic principles of drug interactions to clinical practice. *J Urol* 100:113–120, 1975.

36. Rowe JW: The effect of age on creative clearance in man: a cross-sectional and longitudinal study. *J Gerontol* 31:155–163, 1976.

37. Samiy AH: Clinical manifestations of disease in the elderly. *Med Clin North Am* 67:333–334, 1983.

38. Sherman FT, Mandel J: Aging and drug compliance. In: Center for Human Services. *Wise Drug Use for the Elderly: Role of the Service Provider*. Prepared for the Administration on Aging, Washington, D.C., No. 90-A-1353, 1979, vol 3, pp 17–22.

39. Steinberg GM: Drug usage and illness in elderly patients (part I). *Pharmacol Times* 49:96–101, 1984.

40. Steinberg GM: Drug usage and illness in elderly patients (Part II). *Pharmacol Times* 50:94–102, 1984.

41. Steinberg FV: The aging of organs and organ systems. In Steinberg FV (ed): *Case of the Geriatric Patient*, ed 6. St. Louis, CV Mosby, 1980, p 3.

42. Sumner R: Medication compliance in the geriatric patient. *Pharmacol Times* 51:96–101, 1985.

43. Swartz D, Wang M, Zeitz L, et al: Medication errors made by elderly, chronically ill patients. *Am J Publ Health* 52:2081, 1962.

44. U.S. Department of HEW: Physicians drug prescribing patterns in skilled nursing facilities. Monograph No. 2, 1976, p 15.

45. Vestal RE: Aging and ethanol metabolism. *Clin Pharmacol Ther* 21:343–354, 1977.

46. Vestal RE, Dawson J: *Handbook of the Biology of Aging*, ed 2. St. Louis, CV Mosby, 1984.

47. Weiner M: Pharmocologic and pharmacodynamic changes related to elderly patients. In: *Pharmacy Practice for the Geriatric Patient*. Carrbora, NC, Health Sciences Consortium Inc., 1985, p 10.

48. Weintraub M: Intelligent noncompliance with special emphasis on the elderly. *Contemp Pharmacol Pract* 3:85–95, 1980.

The Communication Status of Older Persons

III

8 The Effects of Aging on Auditory Structures and Functions

MICHAEL A. NERBONNE

Editor's Note

The preceding section of this text has provided basic information concerning the ways in which normal aging affects social, physiological, cognitive, and emotional functioning, as well as responses to medications. In this next section, we turn to a closer examination of communication changes associated with aging. Chapter 8 describes in considerable detail changes in auditory structures and functions in the older adult. Nerbonne begins with an overview of prevalence data, noting that current estimates of the extent of hearing loss in the elderly are probably conservative and inaccurate in reflecting actual hearing difficulties in daily communication. Terminological and research methodological problems are reviewed. The remainder of the chapter is subdivided into consideration of two topics: age-related alterations of the peripheral and central auditory systems, and auditory function and aging. Nerbonne concludes this discussion by suggesting that hearing loss is a major health problem among the elderly. Since problems in everyday speech perception are not adequately reflected in conventional audiologic tests, there is a need for additional laboratory and clinical research designed to develop more appropriate and comprehensive assessment procedures. In particular, we need to develop better ways to evaluate the degree of hearing handicap and the ways to best select a hearing aid to meet the individual older client's profiles of needs and handicaps.

Declines occurring in auditory function with age, commonly referred to as presbycusis, have been the subject of a multitude of investigations during the past century. This interest has been evident particularly in the past two decades. A major portion of the research conducted has centered around identifying the structural changes and etiologies associated with presbycusis and determining the impact that those changes have on auditory function in the elderly. This chapter will review and discuss information regarding these and other related topics in an attempt to summarize what is presently known about the effects of aging on the auditory process.

BASIC CONSIDERATIONS

Prevalence

The prevalence data available regarding hearing loss among the aging certainly indicate that the extensive attention given presbycusis in the past has been warranted. Although prevalence figures vary greatly (due in part to the type of data gathered, sampling techniques used, and how normal hearing is defined), they collectively indicate that an alarming proportion of the elderly have hearing loss. Using questionnaire survey data, a National Health Interview Survey established that 24% of persons between 65 and 74 years of age have a hearing impairment, while the prevalence for those 75 years of age and older is about 39% (111). Slightly higher rates emerge when audiometric data are used. When pure tone averages (500, 1000, and 2000 Hz) greater than 26 dB hearing level (HL) are used in defining hearing impairment, prevalence figures were determined to be approximately 30 and 48% for these same age groups (153). Using a conservative definition of hearing loss as threshold levels greater than 20 dB HL for at least one frequency from 500 to 4000 Hz, the prevalence of hearing impairment was estimated to be 83% for adults from 57 to 89 years old (94). Finally, prevalence figures among elderly nursing home residents are considerably higher than those found among the general elderly population. Using a pure tone average cutoff of 26 dB HL, 82% were found to have hearing loss. With a more liberal 40 dB HL cutoff criterion, the rate was still found to be 48% (127).

Given these prevalence data, it is not surprising to learn that hearing loss is one of the most common, if not the most common, health impairment among elderly Americans (97). In connection with this, it should be pointed out that most prevalence figures are based solely on considerations of hearing sensitivity and do not factor in speech understanding difficulties, which may be present with or without a significant decline in hearing sensitivity. Given the high prevalence of speech perception problems among the aged, it is likely that the available prevalence data represent a rather narrow and conservative estimate of overall hearing difficulties for communication purposes within this age group.

Terminology

Unanimity exists regarding the existence of hearing loss among the elderly, but there is considerable debate as to how to label this condition. In its purest form, it has been proposed that the term presbycusis be used when referring solely to the biological aging of the auditory mechanism. Thus, any hearing dysfunction which results would stem strictly from the process of aging alone. Rather than being linked exclusively to biologic aging, others have chosen to use the term presbycusis simply to refer to hearing loss that is associated with the elderly. In this context presbycusis may be the cumulative result of a number of factors which act collectively over a person's lifetime to produce a given amount of hearing impairment. In addition to biologic aging, other factors like noise exposure or ototoxicity might logically be involved.

No easy solution exists at the present time to the proper usage of the term presbycusis. However, as Marshall (85) suggested, most professionals elect to use presbycusis when referring to cases with progressive, bilaterally symmetrical sensorineural hearing losses that emerge relatively late in adulthood.

Research Methodologies

Most investigators have employed either a cross-sectional or longitudinal research design when studying the potential effects of aging on auditory function. In the cross-sectional approach, subjects are arranged in specific age groups, performance is measured, and comparisons are made between age groups to determine if performance differences exist with increasing age. This design has been used frequently and is useful in many types of age-related research. However, problems can arise when using the cross-sectional approach, as described by Bergman (11) and Corso (25). For instance, cohort effects can have a confounding effect on the variable study. Cohort effects refer to the fact that persons born at different times have experiences and influences that are unique to their generation. It is likely that subjects differing in age may also be different in a number of ways which, though seemingly subtle in nature, could influence performance.

The other technique, the longitudinal design, involves the evaluation of the same subjects on two or more separate occasions to measure any performance changes that might occur over time. While this approach is useful in gerontologic research, it is prone to selective bias (11). That is, long-term studies tend to attract individuals with above average intelligence, motivation, and better physical and mental health. However, even with these potential problems, the longitudinal design can be utilized effectively to evaluate numerous aspects of auditory processing as a function of age.

The cross-sectional and longitudinal research techniques, as well as other methods of investigation, are discussed in detail elsewhere (11, 26, 49), and the interested reader should consult one or more of these sources for further elaboration. Examples of various designs will be apparent in the research to be reviewed. The strengths and limitations of each design, as well as the appropriateness of the design for a given study, should be carefully evaluated.

Other methodologic issues raised in the literature can influence the outcome of investigations with the aged (85). The manner in which presbycusic hearing loss is defined, for instance, can be vitally important. Studies which evaluate auditory sensitivity among elderly subjects selected from modern society, for example, are more likely to obtain results which, in part, are affected to an unknown extent by hearing loss stemming from routine noise exposure. The age of the young and elderly subjects used in research is another variable which may influence the outcome of an investigation. No clear consensus exists as to when the adult ceases to be young and becomes elderly, and studies have used minimum age cutoffs to separate the two, ranging anywhere from 40 to 65 years of age. If a relatively low minimum age for elderly subjects is used, it may be less likely that the elderly subject group will perform in a significantly different manner than their younger counterparts. Equally important is the need to include a sufficient sample of subjects above 70 years old. It is felt that some aspects of auditory function may not be adversely affected by aging until persons are well into their 70s, if at all, and too many studies have been conducted with only a limited number of subjects beyond 70 years of age in their elderly subject pool.

Investigations of age-related declining speech perception must match as closely as possible the hearing sensitivity of the young and old subjects being evaluated. For instance, even minor differences in auditory sensitivity can influence speech perception (13, 55). This means that studies that have compared speech perception performance of young and elderly subjects having many thresholds within normal limits (≤25 dB HL) still have not matched subjects closely enough to rule out the potential influence of peripheral hearing sensitivity on speech perception differences found between the two groups. In the same vein, matching young and old listeners closely for hearing sensitivity, using a three-frequency pure tone average (500, 1000, and 2000 Hz), also does not insure sufficient control of this factor, due to the important role that hearing sensitivity at 3000 to 4000 Hz plays in speech recognition performance. Matching of hearing sensitivity must encompass a broader frequency range to include consideration of the 250 to 4000 Hz at a minimum in order to evaluate more adequately any speech perception differences which may result from the process of aging. Failure to do so may result in incorrectly concluding that aging does adversely affect auditory processing, when in fact differences in hearing sensitivity may have been the determining factor.

A number of other potentially important methodological variables have been identified in connection with research in auditory processing by the aged. These include the proper control of subjects' language background for investigations of speech perception (11), the possible influence of conservative response criteria used by elderly subjects on certain auditory tasks (85, 116), the use of elderly subjects residing in nursing homes to represent the population of older persons at large (127), and the potential for ear canal collapse to exaggerate the degree of hearing dysfunction experienced by the elderly (86, 114, 126). These variables, and numerous others, must all be carefully taken into consideration and controlled to a reasonable extent to permit an accurate assessment of auditory function among older adults. In the literature to be reviewed it will be apparent that some investigations have been more successful than others in accomplishing that.

AGE-RELATED ALTERATIONS OF THE PERIPHERAL AND CENTRAL AUDITORY SYSTEMS

Anatomic/Physiologic Changes

Peripheral Auditory System

Outer Ear. A number of subtle alterations which can occur in association with the structures of the outer ears of middle-aged and elderly adults have been noted in the literature. For instance, the epithelial layer of the outer ear, especially the pinna, experiences a loss of elasticity and resilience (33, 152). The pinna may therefore become harder and less flexible than is normally observed in younger individuals (26).

More visible changes can also occur. Weg (156) indicated that pigmentation "spots" sometimes are observed, and Senturia (134) has noted that excessive freckling of the auricle occurs on occasion as well. A tendency also exists for older persons, particularly males, to have an excess amount of course hair growth along the helix, antihelix, and tragus of the pinna (19, 109, 158). Additional changes occur with respect to the size of the pinna. Tsai et al (152) measured pinna dimensions on young and older individuals and found that length and breadth may increase by several millimeters with increasing age.

Similar structural alterations also occur within the external auditory meatus. The cartilaginous portion suffers a loss of elasticity and that, plus the general force of gravity, results in a narrowing of the outer portions of the canal (19, 82). Corso (26) reported that senile atrophy of the tissue lining the canal may interfere with the excretion of cerumen. Related to this, Perry (109) stated that older persons experience a decrease in the number of cerumen-producing glands present, with their cerumen tending to be somewhat drier. He also found that no significant relationship apparently exists between age and the color of cerumen. While excessive amounts of cerumen are frequently observed in elderly cases (72, 89), it is still unclear whether this is the result of an increase in the production of cerumen or the byproduct of other factors, such as inconsistent health care. Senturia (134) has pointed out that the epidermal tissues which line the external auditory meatus also can become dry to a pronounced extent in the elderly.

Middle Ear. The aging process can produce additional structural changes within the middle ear, with these changes being relatively varied and inconsistent to some extent. Maurer and Rupp (87) observed that the tympanic membrane may be more rigid and yet more translucent, making various landmarks associated with the ossicular chain more visible during an otoscopic examination. This translucent trait has been verified in work conducted by Rossenwasser (121), with Covell (27) also noting a thinning of the eardrum. A sclerotic thickening of the eardrum has been reported in some elderly cases having a history of chronic rheumatism or arthritis (19).

The ossicular chain and associated ligaments and muscles in particular appear to be susceptible to alterations linked with aging. Substantial evidence exists regarding the development of increased rigidity within the ossicular chain. Belal and Stewart (9) have noted that arthritic alterations, including fibrous and bony anklosis of ossicular articulations, are common. Ossification of the ossicles also has been mentioned frequently as a relatively common condition among the aged (44, 69, 128). In addition, evidence presented by Rossenwasser (121) indicates that atrophy of the ossicles does occur, especially at the malleoincudal and incudostapedial joints which articulate the malleus, incus, and stapes. Along with the atrophy linked to the ossicles, similar age-related degeneration and atrophy take place in the tensor tympani and stapedius muscles and ossicular ligaments which may adversely affect ossicular chain motion and the protective function afforded by the middle ear reflex (27, 76, 125).

Maurer and Rupp (87) pointed out that age-related atrophy and degeneration of muscle fiber throughout the body may manifest itself within the auditory system in a variety of ways, including Eustachian tube dysfunction. Maintenance of adequate Eustachian tube function, which is vital to the integrity of the middle ear cavity, depends primarily upon the actions of several muscles, including the tensor and levator veli palatini, the tensor tympani, and the salpingopharyngeal (52). If the actions of these specific muscles are impaired as the result of aging, then Eustachian tube efficiency may be reduced. Two separate investigations have explored this issue by means of electroacoustic immittance measurements, with Newman and Spitzer (100) finding some evidence to support age-related Eustachian tube dysfunction and Chermak and Moore (22) discovering no significant differences between young and older adult subject groups. Further investigation of the issue appears to be needed, using a subject pool with a greater percentage of older adults above the age of 70 years.

Inner Ear and Auditory Nerve. Evidence has existed for half a century which implicates the inner ear and auditory nerve as primary loci of structural changes that are directly linked with hearing impairment in the elderly (28, 124). Continued research and improvements in investigative techniques have provided us with an even fuller understanding of the effects which the aging process has on the sensorineural portion of the auditory system. While much remains to be discovered, at least two major age-related structural alterations involving the inner ear and auditory nerve consistently have been observed histologically:

1. Extensive atrophy and degeneration of the hair cells and numerous supporting structures within the cochlea, as well as the stria vascularis;
2. Reduction in the number of functional spiral ganglia and nerve fibers comprising the peripheral portion of the cochlear division of the auditory nerve.

Numerous investigators have noted the senescent alterations which occur within the inner ear. Crowe et al (28) and Saxen and von Friendt (124) were among the earliest to document the degeneration which occurs within the organ of Corti. Crowe, Guild, and Palvogt determined that the degenerative process typically begins and is concentrated in the basal portion of the cochlea. In the research of Saxen and von Friendt, severe atrophy was noted within the organ of Corti in more than one-half of the temporal bones of the 33 cases they examined. Similar findings concerning the structures of the organ of Corti consistently have been reported since that time (47, 64, 96, 128, 129).

Of particular relevance is the extensive degeneration and loss of outer and inner hair cells found most often in the most basal portion of the cochlea. Closely associated with this is the atrophy and flattening of support cells within the organ of Corti, such as pillar cells, Dieter's cells, and Hensen's cells (128). While usually appearing initially in the lower basal turn, Johnson and Hawkins (63) found clear evidence that in time the more apical portions of the cochlea can exhibit degeneration of sensory and support cells as well. These same investigators also found somewhat startling evidence which indicates that age-related hair cell deterioration actually can begin in infancy.

A decrease in the elasticity of the basilar membrane which can accompany aging was initially identified by Mayer (88). Further support for this was provided by Schuknecht (129). Mayer felt that the stiffening of the basilar membrane was relatively uncommon and due to calcification. Pathologic studies by Nomura (102) also have revealed that cholesterol and fat deposits occur in the basilar membrane which contribute to this stiffening as well.

Atrophy of the stria vascularis has likewise been found to occur frequently in older persons (64, 124, 128, 129). Age-related degeneration of this structure is viewed as particularly significant because of the vital role which the stria vascularis is suspected of playing in the production of endolymph and the maintenance of bioelectric and biochemical balances within the cochlea.

As established by a host of investigators (74, 115, 124, 128, 129, 132), a gradual loss of ganglion cells and nerve fibers occurs in the basal portion of the cochlea and along the auditory nerve. In fact, Rasmussen's research disclosed that an average of 2200 fewer fibers were present in the cochlear division of the eighth nerve of persons 44 to 60 years of age than in that of persons in younger age groups. This is not surprising in light of Brody's (17) conclusion that a gradual loss of neurons throughout the entire central nervous system begins early and continues throughout one's life.

Krmpotic-Nemanic (74) conducted a series of investigations which led her to conclude that aging is accompanied by progressive constriction of the cochlear blood supply and nerve fibers in the spiral tract, due to osteoid apposition. The process appears to begin prior to 20 years of age on the basal coil, with fibers on the periphery of the nerve bundles becoming atrophic first. This progressive buildup of bony "cuffs" can also affect the vascular system of the cochlea in much the same manner. The relevance of Krmpotic-Nemanic's findings will be discussed further later in this chapter, as it pertains to providing potential explanations for the structural alterations observed in the auditory system which occur as a consequence of aging.

Central Auditory System

Normal aging has associated with it a host of changes in the central nervous system. Brody's (17) research provided us with valuable insights regarding the extent to which certain portions of the cortex are altered with age. Brody found that a significant loss of neurons within the brain actually begins early and continues throughout one's life. In comparing neuronal counts from cases over 70 years of age with those from cases under 48, he determined that significantly greater loss of neurons occurred in certain structures within the cortex of the older group. Brody's findings have generally been substantiated in later investigations (4,

23), with Tomlinson and Henderson (150) finding as much as a 50% decrease in neurons in some cortical areas for older adults.

In addition to a loss of neurons within specific areas of the cortex, it appears that a significant degree of cortical atrophy takes place with increasing age (90). In association with this, Smith and Sethi (138) and Dekaban and Sadowski (29) have demonstrated substantial reductions in overall brain weight for older subjects.

Other potentially important alterations include an accumulation of lipofuscin in the cytoplasm of neurons within the central nervous system (16), and a significant decrease in cerebral blood flow in some elderly cases (135). Finally, a decrease in brain wave activity was reported with increased age, particularly in the left hemisphere (138, 154).

Given all of these changes, it is not surprising that the central auditory pathway is also adversely impacted upon by the aging process. In fact, Brody's (17) findings suggest that portions of the central auditory system, particularly the superior temporal gyrus (which includes Herschel's gyrus), experience some of the greatest losses in neurons found in any of the other areas of the cortex. However, while portions of the auditory cortex appear especially vulnerable, the brain stem may sustain somewhat less of a loss of neurons as a consequence of aging (154).

While Hansen and Reske-Nielson (47) felt that the major alterations in the central auditory system resulting from aging occur in the cortex to a greater extent than in the ascending pathways, Kirikae et al (68) have provided evidence to indicate that the effects of aging within the central auditory system may be more diffuse. Their histopathologic study disclosed substantial atrophy and degeneration of neural tissue throughout the brain stem, including the ventral cochlear and superior olivary nuclei, inferior colliculus, and medial geniculate body. These observations have been supported by others as well (63, 130).

Types of Presbycusis

Based on his own investigations and the research of others regarding the structural alterations commonly observed throughout the auditory system, Schuknecht (128–130) chose to categorize four distinct forms of pathology which occur with advanced age.

Sensory Presbycusis

Schuknecht felt that this form of presbycusis was characterized by epithelial atrophy and degeneration of hair cells and supporting cells within the organ of Corti. While damage may be distributed diffusely throughout the cochlea, Schuknecht emphasized that alterations typically were concentrated in the basal coil. As a result, the hearing loss associated with sensory presbycusis is, according to Schuknecht, confined primarily to the higher frequencies. Figure 8.1 illustrates both the audiologic and histologic findings typically found.

Neural Presbycusis

This type was described by Schuknecht as involving a gradual reduction in the population of first-order neurons within the cochlea, as well as additional neuronal losses throughout the auditory pathway. Schuknecht reported that the loss of neurons has little effect on hearing

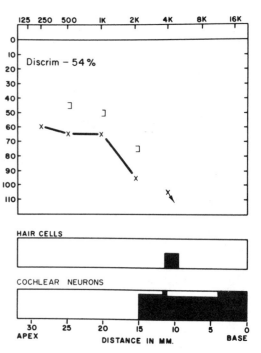

Figure 8.2. Neural presbycusis. This patient experienced bilateral progressive hearing loss, worse in the left ear, during the later years of life and died at the age of 75. Histological study of the left ear shows a severe loss of cochlear neurons in the basal 15 mm of the cochlea. (From Schuknecht HF: *Pathology of the Ear.* Cambridge, MA, Harvard University Press, 1974.)

sensitivity until the number of functional neural units remaining is significantly reduced (Fig. 8.2). However, a more severe disruption in speech perception is commonly observed. Because of the attrition of nerve cells within the brain stem and auditory cortex, included in Schuknecht's neural presbycusis, Johnson and Hawkins (63) recommended labeling this condition as "central presbycusis."

Strial (Metabolic) Presbycusis

Schuknecht noted that atrophy of the stria vascularis is relatively common among older individuals and appears most often in the middle and apical turns of the cochlea. He reported that the degeneration of the stria vascularis may lead to a potential disruption in the chemical and electrical balance within the inner ear, due to its apparent role in producing the positive DC potential of the scala media and the production of endolymph. Cases with strial presbycusis often yield relatively flat audiograms, as shown in Figure 8.3.

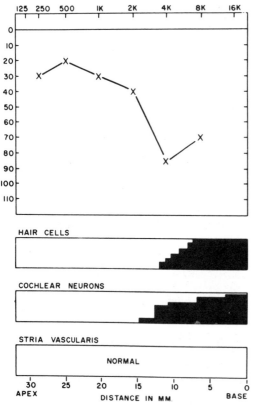

Figure 8.1. Sensory presbycusis. Abrupt high-tone hearing loss (bilateral, symmetrical) in a 79-year-old man. There is severe atrophy of the organ of Corti with loss of hair cells and cochlear neurons at the basal end of the cochlea. (From Schuknecht HF: *Pathology of the Ear.* Cambridge, MA, Harvard University Press, 1974.)

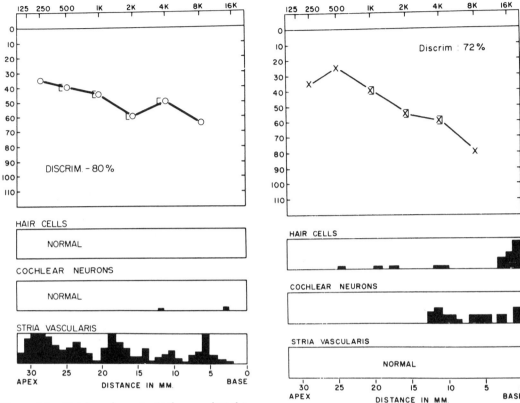

Figure 8.3. Strial presbycusis. At the age of 68 this woman had bilateral symmetrical hearing losses exhibiting flat threshold patterns with relatively good speech discrimination scores. She died at the age of 72. Histological studies show severe patchy atrophy of the stria vascularis throughout the cochleae, most severe in the apical regions. (From Schuknecht HF: *Pathology of the Ear*. Cambridge, MA, Harvard University Press).

Figure 8.4. Cochlear conductive presbycusis. Audiometric studies at the age of 66 show this man to have bilateral sensorineural hearing loss. He died at the age of 68. Both ears show slight loss of hair cells and cochlear neurons in the basal ends of the cochleae, but these changes are inadequate to explain the hearing loss. (From Schuknecht HF: *Pathology of the Ear*. Cambridge, MA, Harvard University Press, 1974.)

Cochlear Conductive (Mechanical) Presbycusis

This form of presbycusis was reserved by Schuknecht for those cases with a disorder in the motion mechanics of the cochlear duct. Shrinkage of the spiral ligament and changes in the stiffness and mass of the basilar membrane occur without appreciable alterations in the sensory and neural structures of the cochlea. Additional modification of the middle ear mechanics are also associated with this form of presbycusis. According to Schuknecht, hearing loss often emerges in middle age and usually produces a gradual decrease in sensitivity, with more hearing loss in the high frequencies than for lower frequencies (see Fig. 8.4).

To determine the incidence of these four types of presbycusis, Schuknecht and his associates (131) examined temporal bone specimens of 160 ears. Their resulting incidence data are shown in Table 8.1, and indicate that strial presbycusis is the most frequently encountered form, followed closely by neural presbycusis. Sensory presbycusis was found less than any other form, with about a 12% incidence rate.

In connection with this, Corso (26) observed that Schuknecht's four presbycusis types rarely occur in an isolated, pure form. Rather, sensory and neural degeneration often coexist, or atrophy of the stria vascularis may be present along with hair cell degeneration. However, Schuknecht's classification system is still felt by many to be a useful means of describing the general patterns in which the process of aging affects the peripheral and central auditory systems.

Table 8.1
Incidence of Four Types of Presbycusis

Type of Presbycusis	Ears	Individuals	%
Sensory	21	12	11.9
Neural	51	31	30.7
Strial	52	35	34.6
Inner ear conditions	36	23	22.8
Total	160	101	100.0

[a]From Schuknecht HF, Watanuki K, Takahaski T, Belal A, Kimura R, Jones D, Ota C: Atrophy of the stria vascularis, a common cause for hearing loss. *Laryngoscope* 84:1777–1821, 1974.

Potential Etiologies of Presbycusis

As discussed earlier, presbycusis is sometimes referred to as the biological aging of the auditory system. When it is defined in this rather restricted manner, the potential causes of presbycusis include a number of intrinsic factors, such as vascular alterations (47, 74, 83), genetic makeup (79, 130), and the generalized effects of cellular aging (96, 130). However, presbycusis is also the term used by many when referring to the auditory dysfunction associated with old age, and the number of potential contributors to presbycusis as it is used in this context is considerably greater. In addition to the list of intrinsic etiologies mentioned above, several extrinsic factors are also thought to be involved, including diet (119, 139, 140), noise exposure (24, 25, 39), and toxic drugs (125).

Clearly, the etiologies of hearing loss associated with aging are heterogeneous, with factors related to the physiology of the aging process and the cumulative effects of exposure to a number of potentially harmful agents during one's lifetime being involved collectively. This has made it difficult to analyze the precise manner in which any one particular etiology of presbycusis affects the auditory system in isolation. Despite this, numerous investigations have made important contributions toward describing the many apparent etiologies of age-related hearing impairment.

Intrinsic Etiologies

The role which the vascular system plays in creating presbycusis has received considerable attention on the part of investigators. Hansen and Reske-Nielsen (47) conducted histologic examinations of 12 aging individuals and found reduced blood supply to the organ of Corti and other important structures of the cochlea, as well as the internal meatus. This condition was thought to be brought about by a thickening and hardening of the walls of the general vascular system, which is termed arteriosclerosis. Likewise, Jorgensen (64) found increased thickening of the capillary walls associated with the stria vascularis that occurred with advancing age. This process was particularly pronounced for cases with generalized arteriosclerosis, and appears to be exacerbated further in adult cases with diabetes (130). Makashima (83) also found that the amount of narrowing of the internal auditory artery was highly correlated with atrophy of the spiral ganglia and hearing loss. These findings are consistent with those of Kimura (67), who conducted animal experiments in which vascular flow to the inner ear was controlled. Occlusion of the inferior cochlear vein in guinea pigs produced severe damage to outer hair cells and atrophy of the stria vascularis, as well as in the vestibular apparatus.

A particularly significant series of investigations regarding vascular abnormalities was completed under the direction of Krmpotic-Nemanic (74), who examined 2600 temporal bones from cases ranging in age from newborns to 90 years old. She found progressive opposition or growth of bone and dense connective tissue in the bottom of the internal auditory canal in the area of the spiral tract, starting at the basal coil. Because of the buildup of bony material, the diameter of the channels in the spiral tract through which nerve bundles pass from the inner ear is reduced. This creates an increasing degree of compression and constriction of the nerve fibers of the cochlea, as shown in schematic fashion in Figure 8.5, which can result in their atrophy. Krmpotic-Nemanic also reported that in, advanced age, the apposition of connective tissue and bone around the arteries in the fundus also occurs. These "cuffs" compress the arteries, which can decrease or disrupt the flow of blood to the inner ear. This may be responsible for age-related atrophy occurring within the stria vascularis and in the hair cells. It was Krmpotic-Nemanic's view that most of the types of presbycusis identified and described by Schuknecht (128, 129) could be explained by the effects of this process.

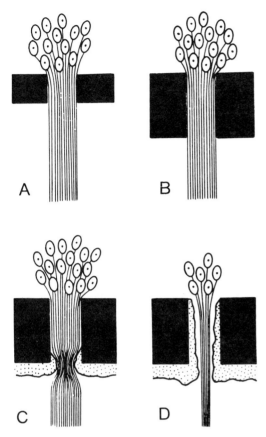

Figure 8.5. Progressive states of osteoid opposition in region of basal part of spiral tract. (From Krmpotic-Nemanic J: A new concept of the pathogenesis of presbycusis. *AMA Arch Otolaryngol* 93:161–166, 1971. Copyright 1971, American Medical Association.)

The etiology of presbycusis may be linked, in part, to genetics as well. Schuknecht (130) noted that several genes may work collectively to determine the rate at which specific individuals age. The time of onset and rate of aging in general and in specific systems of the body (such as the auditory system) vary widely. There may be, then, among a portion of the population a genetic predisposition to aging which results in more pronounced physiologic effects, including age-related alterations within the auditory mechanism. This same view has been expressed by Gerber and Mencher (37), who feel that a genetic component exists to presbycusis. What is sometimes referred to as "early presbycusis" in some individuals actually occurs as the result of a genetically based susceptibility to the hearing loss which accompanies aging. Schuknecht (130) presented case study evidence suggesting that atrophy of the

stria vascularis may, to some extent, be genetically predetermined, since it has a tendency to occur in several members of a given family.

Lowell and Paparella (79) provided further evidence regarding the genetic link with presbycusis. In a retrospective study in which audiometric data were analyzed, they found evidence to support the notion that some cases initially diagnosed as being presbycusic actually may have sensorineural hearing loss that emerges in middle age, and which stems from familial or genetic etiology. These cases had audiometric patterns which were distinct from cases whom the authors isolated as pure presbycusic cases (i.e., age-related hearing impairment).

Biologic aging occurs at all levels of the organism and manifests itself within the auditory system in a number of ways. Schuknecht (130) describes the atrophy and sharp reduction in the number of sensory and neural cells within the inner ear and neural pathway which naturally occurs over time in connection with an inability of certain cells in the body to reproduce. For example, Rassmussen (115) found 2200 fewer neural fibers in the cochlear division of the auditory nerve in persons from 44 to 60 years of age than in that of persons in younger age groups. Brody (17) has determined that up to half of the neurons in the auditory cortex are lost by 75 years of age.

Along with the loss of sensory and neural cells, an accumulation of a yellow-brown pigment called lipofuscin occurs in the cytoplasm of all epithelial cells within the inner ear with advancing age. Lipofuscin also accumulates throughout portions of the central auditory nervous system. Although it is presently not known if lipofuscin has an adverse effect on cell function, it appears to be a reliable measure of age-related central nervous system alterability (16). Schuknecht (130) felt that the buildup of lipofuscin may reflect exhaustion of enzymatic activity that leads to decreased cell function. However, others do not feel that lipofuscin has any significant negative effect on cell function (73).

Extrinsic Etiologies

Diet has been suspected for some time to be a potential cause of presbycusis. This was reinforced by the work of Rosen and his colleagues (118) with the Mabaan tribesmen in the Sudan. The elder Mabaans were found to have much better high frequency hearing sensitivity than their counterparts in modern society. In attempting to explain this, Rosen found among other things, that the Mabaans live on a diet of natural foods, consisting mostly of vegetables—that is, a diet quite low in fats.

To explore the potential link between fat breaks in the diet and presbycusis, Rosen and Olin (119) controlled the amount of saturated fat patients received at two mental hospitals in Finland. Evaluation of serum cholesterol levels, cardiac ischemia, and hearing sensitivity were done periodically for 5 years. Patients in the hospital where saturated fats were drastically reduced were found to have significantly less serum cholesterol in their blood than the patients in the other hospital, where a normal, high saturated fat diet was followed. Likewise, patients receiving a low fat diet also had reduced blood coagulability, and their prevalence of ischemic changes was lower as well. Therefore, a potentially close relationship was demonstrated between the degree of saturated fat in the diet of the subjects of Rosen and Olin and the amount of serum cholesterol, cardiac ischemia, and coronary heart disease observed. The hearing testing done on the patients after 5 years revealed that air conduction thresholds were better at all test frequencies in the group receiving the low fat diet. Rosen and Olin felt that the amount of fat in the diet was directly responsible for the differences found between the two subject groups in vascular/coronary measures and hearing sensitivity.

In a related investigation involving 444 cases with various types of inner ear disorders, Spencer (139, 140) found that nearly half (46.6%) had significant hyperlipoproteinemia (HLP), a condition which accompanies abnormally high serum cholesterol and triglyceride levels and is closely linked with atherosclerosis. As discussed by Gilad and Glorig (38), HLP also is thought to affect vascular circulation to the inner ear, producing hearing loss and other related symptoms. The inner ear effects appear much earlier in time than advanced coronary artery disease. Thus the onset of inner ear symptoms may serve as a warning sign for future coronary heart disease. Dietary restrictions, such as limiting those foods with high levels of saturated fats, can be effective in treating HLP. A substantial number of Spencer's cases also experienced improvements in hearing sensitivity, decreased episodes of dizziness, and other associated symptoms when cholesterol levels were reduced.

While the connection between high fat diets, atherosclerosis, and sensorineural hearing loss appears strong, not all the evidence available supports this. Lowry and Issacson (80), for example, found a lower incidence of lipoproteinemia in 100 presbycusic patients than would normally be present in cases of similar age and sex. Clearly, further investigation of the influence of diet-related variables on hearing function is needed before a full understanding of its potential influence will be known.

While Rosen felt that the fat-free diet of the Mabaans partially explained the minimal age-related hearing loss they possessed, he also was convinced that the relatively noise-free society in which the Mabaans lived contributed as well. It was Rosen's contention, as well as that of others (39, 40), that the cumulative effect of daily noise exposure that occurs in conjunction with living in modern society results in a degree of hearing loss that is added onto the auditory impairment caused by physiologic aging and other related factors. Glorig and Nixon (40) proposed use of the term "sociocusis" when referring to the auditory effects of exposure to nonoccupational noise over a lifetime, to more accurately distinguish it from the physiologic aspects of age-related hearing loss, or presbycusis.

Attempts have been made in urban populations to screen out individuals with a history of significant noise exposure when evaluating the relationships between age and hearing sensitivity. Corso (24, 25) selected subjects with no significant occupational or environmental/recreational noise exposure, and found that these subjects had auditory thresholds that were substantially better than those of similar age groups that were not screened with regard to noise exposure. Likewise, auditory threshold data were obtained by the National Institute for Occupational Safety and Health (NIOSH) (98) with persons screened for noise exposure. NIOSH's data were compared with similar data from the 1965 National Health Survey (153), where subjects were not excluded with a history of exposure to noise. The NIOSH mean threshold values were consistently more acute at test frequencies of 2000 Hz and higher for all comparable age groups. These comparisons demonstrate that routine exposure to noise throughout one's life does contribute to the total age-related declines observed in hearing sensitivity.

Presbycusis also appears to be impacted on by the intake of a wide variety of ototoxic drugs. The potential harmful effects of certain medications on the auditory system of the general population, particularly on the inner ear, have been well documented (12, 30, 113). The probability of drug-induced ototoxicity in advancing age is relatively high, due in part to: (a) the excessive volume of medication utilized in the treatment of acute and chronic disorders in the elderly; and (b) the fact that many older individuals seem more susceptible to drug ototoxicity (12). As with other extrinsic factors like noise, the sensorineural hearing loss caused by the intake of one or more of the many harmful medications is merely added to the auditory impairment associated with the biologic aspects of aging. Further information on drug effects in the elderly is found in Chapter 7 of this text.

AUDITORY FUNCTION AND AGING

Thus far information has been reviewed which establishes that numerous age-related structural alterations commonly occur within the auditory mechanism, and that several potential etiologies may be linked with these changes. In addition, a body of knowledge has been gathered regarding how these alterations affect the auditory performance of the elderly, and the next section will review some of the major conclusions reached in this regard. As will become immediately evident, the diversity seen in the structural modifications associated with the aging auditory mechanism is paralleled in the many ways in which the hearing abilities of this age group are affected.

Hearing Sensitivity

The decreases in hearing sensitivity seen with advancing age have been investigated extensively since the early work of individuals such as Zwaardemaker (162) and Bunch (18). The many investigations which followed (8, 24, 25, 41, 42, 69) have provided further documentation concerning the typical progression in hearing loss which takes place. Spoor (141) pooled normative data from several separate investigations concerned with quantifying the decreases found with advancing age, and Lebo and Reddell (77) later converted those cumulative data to the current American National Standards Institute (ANSI) audiometric norms (2). The resulting composite pure tone sensitivity curves for men and women as a function of age are shown in Figure 8.6. In general, hearing sensitivity decreases rather systematically with age, with the earliest and most pronounced decrement occurring in the higher frequencies. Only minimal decreases in sensitivity are observed for frequencies at or below 1000 Hz. The loss of hearing is generally bilateral and symmetrical. Men initially experience hearing loss earlier in life than women, and collectively possess more loss of hearing at virtually every age.

Considerable variability exists, however, in the hearing sensitivity of individual older per-

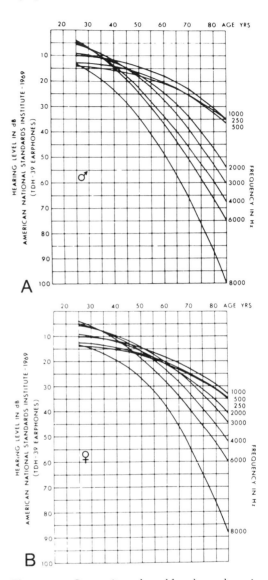

Figure 8.6. Composite male and female presbycusis curves (re: ANSI-1969). (From Lebo CP, Redell RC: The presbycusis component in occupational hearing loss. *Laryngoscope* 82:1399–1409, 1972.)

sons. This is due, in part, to the type of etiology involved and the severity and site(s) of the structural alterations involved within the auditory system.

Recognizing that several etiologies may act collectively, attempts have been made to specify the degree to which etiologies like physiologic or biologic aging and exposure to noise each contribute to the overall loss in hearing sensitivity found with age. Corso (24, 25), for example, carefully screened out those cases with a history of significant noise exposure and compared the average hearing sensitivity values of the relatively noise-free age groups with those of similar age groups made up of individuals with a background of exposure to noise. While decreases in hearing sensitivity still were found in the relatively noise-free subjects as a function of age, their thresholds were consistently better at 2000 Hz and above than all of those of the corresponding age groups having a history of exposure to noise. Similar findings occurred in the National Institute for Occupational Safety and Health (98) study discussed previously. Thus, physiologic aging and noise, as well as other potential etiologies, act collectively to produce the overall decrease of hearing observed with advancing age. Corso's data from subjects screened for a history of noise exposure may represent the best approximation available at the present time of the effects of physiologic aging alone on auditory sensitivity (75).

As discussed earlier, Schuknecht (129) characterized each of his four major types of presbycusis as having a relatively distinct form of hearing loss from an audiometric viewpoint. According to Gacek and Schuknecht (34), the configuration of the typical audiogram associated with the forms of presbycusis approximates those shown in Figure 8.7. Although considerable variation exists in the individual configuration of the thresholds of cases with the same type of presbycusis, Gacek and Schuknecht felt that the major forms of presbycusis could be characterized as follows. (a) Sensory presbycusis results in a sharp loss in the high frequencies. (b) Neural presbycusis produces rather modest decreases in hearing sensitivity relative to the adverse effects on speech perception. (c) Strial presbycusis often causes a generally equal loss of hearing for all frequencies. (d) Cochlear conductive presbycusis produces a gradually increasing loss of sensitivity from low to high frequencies.

Histologic and audiologic findings led Hansen and Reske-Nielsen (47) to suggest that cases with significant degeneration within the central portion of the auditory system had an abnormal amount of low frequency hearing loss. Hayes and Jerger (51) later investigated this and confirmed Hansen and Reske-Nielsen's earlier contention that excessive low frequency sensitivity loss is linked with age-related central pathology. Figure 8.8 illustrates the audiometric configuration Hayes and Jerger associated with central involvement.

Given these typical patterns, however, it should be noted once again that the classic presbycusic types do not generally occur alone, making it rather difficult (and ill-advised) to predict which form of presbycusis a given case may have based solely on the configuration of

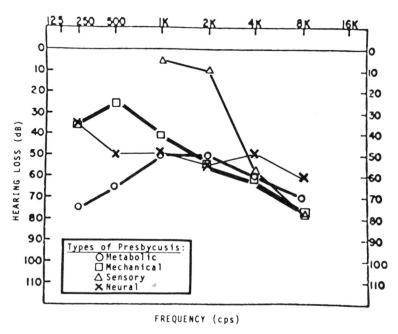

FREQUENCY (cps)

Figure 8.7. Representative audiograms for four types of presbycusis. (Data from Gacek RR, Schuknecht HF: Pathology of presbycusis. *International Audiology* 8:199–209, 1969.) (Figure from Corso JF: *Aging Sensory Systems and Perceptions.* New York, Praeger, 1981.)

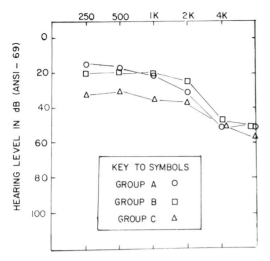

Figure 8.8. Average audiograms for three groups of elderly subjects categorized by "central aging effect." Elderly subjects with substantial central effects (Group C) show poorer low-frequency sensitivity than elderly subjects with peripheral effects (Group A) or intermediate peripheral-control effects (Group B). (From Hayes D, Jerger J: Low frequency hearing loss in presbycusis: a central interpretation. *Arch Otolaryngol* 104(1):9–12, Copyright 1979, American Medical Association.)

pure tone thresholds plotted on an audiogram. Prediction is further complicated by the high degree of variability in the severity of age-related alterations within the auditory mechanism from person to person and the fact that numerous etiologies other than those strictly associated with Schuknecht's four presbycusic types may in all likelihood have had an adverse effect on hearing thresholds as well. Suga and Lindsay (145) presented evidence demonstrating the lack of consistency between histologic findings regarding damage to the auditory system and the resulting audiometric configuration.

Air-Bone Conduction Differences

Because of the notion that presybcusis was strictly a sensorineural disorder, very little attention was given initially to the possible existence of any conductive abnormality associated with age-related hearing loss. However, the work of Glorig and Davis (39) provided evidence that structural changes within the outer and middle ears of aged persons can affect pure tone results. Testing subjects from 25 to 80 years of age, Glorig and Davis found substantial air-bone gaps at 2000 and 4000 Hz in the older subjects, and attributed their presence to middle ear involvement. Subsequent investigation

by Glorig and his colleagues (101) confirmed the original findings. Milne (93) also found air-bone gaps at 1000 and 4000 Hz in a high percentage of cases from 62 to 90 years old, which he attributed to ossicular abnormalities.

Other research has produced conflicting results. Sataloff et al (123) tested 55 men and women between 62 and 82 years of age and did not find any differences between air and bone conduction sensitivity. Other studies (9, 31) have found evidence of arthritic changes in the ossicular joints with age, but concluded that these do not have an effect on hearing sensitivity.

Randolph and Schow (114) have explored another potential contributor to the reported conductive component to presbycusis, the potential for ear canal collapse as a result of the pressure applied to the outer ear by earphones. They found a rather alarming prevalence of ear canal collapse of 36% in a group of listeners from 60 to 79 years old. In a related study, Schow and Goldbaum (126) reported an even higher prevalence among elderly nursing home residents. The results of these two studies are relevant in at least two respects. First, the high incidence of ear canal collapse in older individuals may explain, at least in part, why some studies may have found air-bone gaps in older listeners. Secondly, because ear canal collapse results in increased loss of hearing by air conduction, those studies in which hearing sensitivity was evaluated as a function of age may have produced data which overestimate the amount of hearing loss in the older age groups.

This prompted Marshall et al (86) to explore this issue further. Air and bone conduction pure tone thresholds were obtained for 147 ears from subjects ranging in age from 19 to 87 years. None of the individuals in the 60 and older group produced audiometric results clearly indicative of ear canal collapse. All cases with air-bone gaps were explained by other factors, including test-retest variability, excessive cerumen, or variant forms of middle ear abnormalities. Even though only three subjects in the study were over 70 years of age, the outcome of the investigation suggests that the overall incidence of ear canal collapse among the elderly may not be as high as that indicated previously. Further investigation appears warranted with a large sample of subjects 70+ years of age.

Immittance

A number of investigators have attempted to determine if any systematic age-related changes occur in results obtained with the subtests which make up the immittance test battery. Of primary interest has been the relationship between age and the compliance or admittance of the middle ear. Jerger et al (61) found that age did seem to have some degree of influence on acoustic impedance values, with compliance decreasing steadily with an increase in age beyond about age 40. Other studies (1, 14, 99) have found similar results, although the amount of decrease observed has not always been significant statistically. In contrast, Thompson et al (147) found no systematic change in admittance with aging. Collectively, these studies indicate that while structural modifications occur within the middle ear system in advanced age, they do not appear to manifest themselves in sharp shifts in acoustic impedance/admittance. However, since many of the studies have not included an adequate number of subjects over 70 years of age, future research should focus on older cases to get a more comprehensive view of the influence of aging on acoustic immittance.

Information gathered via the immittance battery has also been shown to be informative in evaluating Eustachian tube function in the elderly. Concern for Eustachian tube malfunction in this age group is based primarily on the documented atrophy and degeneration of neural and muscular tissues discussed earlier. Initially some concern about Eustachian function was noted (Nerbonne and colleagues, unpublished observations) when it was found that 17% of a sample of elderly patients exhibited abnormal negative middle ear pressure values. In a follow-up investigation by Newman and Spitzer (100), in which a tympanometric swallow procedure outlined by Williams (159) was employed to assess Eustachian tube function in young and old subjects, findings somewhat suggestive of hypofunction of the aged Eustachian tube were obtained. Chermak and Moore (22) conducted another investigation concerning this issue, utilizing both young and old (60 to 75 years of age) subjects. Using an adaptation of the Williams procedure made by Seifert et al (133), Chermak and Moore found no support for the contention that Eustachian tube function among the aged is impaired. However, it should be noted that the subjects in the latter study were considerably younger than those used in the other two investigations.

As suggested earlier, the effects of aging on various aspects of the auditory mechanism may not have the same timetable. Thus, adequate samples of individuals in their 70s and 80s may be necessary before some alterations in function produce abnormal test results. Future research is warranted concerning the effects, if any, which the aging process has on function of the Eustachian tube.

A number of investigations have also evaluated acoustic reflex performance in the elderly, with conflicting results emerging. Jepsen (53) and Jerger et al (61) observed a systematic decline in the acoustic reflex threshold with advancing age. Jerger et al (58) later confirmed this for acoustic reflexes triggered with pure tones, but found that reflex thresholds for white noise did not change with age. Other investigations which have carefully matched young and old subjects in hearing sensitivity (46, 136, 160) have generally found no significant differences in reflex thresholds between the two age groups for pure tones of 2000 Hz and lower. However, the elderly have been found to have elevated reflex thresholds for pure tones about 2000 Hz and for broad band noise. Thompson et al (148) found no significant changes in acoustic reflex thresholds for pure tones (500 to 2000 Hz) or high-pass filtered white noise stimuli with increasing age. They did find that the growth of the acoustic reflex decreased with advancing age, which was confirmed in a later study by Wilson (160). In a carefully controlled investigation using young and old subject groups matched for degree of hearing loss, Hall (45) also found a systematic decrease in both ipsilateral and contralateral reflex amplitude with increasing age. He noted that the decrease in reflex amplitude was markedly worse for males. Finally, limited information concerning the potential effect of aging on acoustic reflex decay suggests that advanced age does not produce greater amounts of decay than are usually observed with younger cases with similar hearing impairment (91).

The influence which age has on acoustic reflex thresholds will complicate further attempts to make predictions concerning degree of hearing loss based on reflex threshold data. While much remains to be done in applying various approaches for predicting hearing loss with the aged, Margolis and associates (84) have suggested that predictive procedures may prove effective if a low-pass noise is utilized as the wide band stimulus, rather than broad band noise.

Speech Perception

The speech perception abilities of the elderly have been investigated extensively. Numerous studies have gathered data which collectively demonstrate a rather systematic decline in the ability to perceive speech stimuli with advancing age. One of the earliest efforts in this regard was made by Gaeth (35). The speech recognition abilities of 27 subjects ranging in age from 43 to 70 were measured by Gaeth using the PB-50s. He found unusually poor performance in some elderly subjects which was unexpected on the basis of pure tone findings. This prompted Gaeth to label this condition as "phonemic regression." His early work has been followed up by many others, and the next section will attempt to review some of the major findings pertaining to speech perception by the elderly.

Perception of Undistorted Speech in Quiet

The fact that decreases in speech perception occur as a function of age should not come as a surprise. Speech perception has been shown to be closely associated with the degree of hearing loss present for listeners of all ages (55, 107). Consequently, decrements in hearing sensitivity observed in the aged will produce corresponding difficulty in the perception of speech. The many investigations of speech perception in this age group have attempted, with a variety of methological approaches, to ascertain the extent to which decreases in speech recognition performance are linked with aging per se, as well as with the peripheral loss of hearing older persons experience.

Pestalozza and Shore (110) measured speech recognition in a sample of subjects 60 years of age and older. They found numerous cases in which poor speech recognition occurred even though the degree of hearing loss was only mild, and found no significant relationship between the amount of hearing loss or configuration of the audiogram and speech recognition performance. Pestalozza and Shore concluded that the results supported Gaeth's contention regarding phonemic regression, and implied that the poor speech recognition of the elderly is associated with corresponding degenerative changes occurring in the spiral ganglia and auditory fibers.

Goetzinger and associates (43) used 90 subjects between 70 and 89 years of age with sensorineural hearing loss, and found systematic declines in speech recognition with age. Some of their older subjects exhibited much poorer performance than younger subjects with similar audiograms. However, predictable decreases in speech recognition generally occurred with increased hearing loss as well. It was concluded that decreases observed in speech perception among the aged are due to generalized damage occurring throughout the auditory system.

Harbert et al (48) compared speech recognition among elderly listeners with that of those having normal hearing or congenital sensorineural hearing loss. The presbycusic subjects as a group had worse mean word recognition scores than either of the other groups. Age and degree of hearing loss were both correlated weakly with speech recognition within the elderly listeners.

Punch and McConnell (112) measured speech recognition at 10 to 40 dB sensation levels (SLs) with two groups of older subjects from 69 to 82 years of age. One group of subjects had minimal hearing loss, while the other group possessed mild-to-moderate sensorineural impairments. Some decrease in speech perception was noted for the elderly group with minimal hearing loss, relative to scores routinely associated with young listeners with normal hearing. Punch and McConnell found considerably more decreases in their hearing impaired elderly subjects.

Using young and elderly subjects with matched audiograms, Luterman et al (81) found that the elderly had worse speech perception. Kasden (65) also compared speech recognition with young and aged subjects matched for degree of loss and slope of the audiogram. Unlike Luterman et al, Kasden found no significant difference between the two age groups at presentation levels from 10 to 50 SL. Rintelmann and Schumaier (117) also used young and old subjects with comparable degrees of hearing loss and demonstrated a significant age-related decrease in speech recognition, using the NU-6s. Because of previous research concerning the inability of the W-22s to consistently separate normal from impaired listeners (21), Rintelmann and Schumaier suggested that the differences found between young and old listeners in their study may have been related to the use of the more difficult NU-6s. However, in a later study Surr (146) used the NU-6s and tested 100 subjects ranging in age from 30 to 90 years with sensorineural hearing losses matched for degree and slope. Surr did not find any meaningful decreases in word recognition performance as a function of age.

In an extensive investigation of speech perception as a function of age, Jerger (55) obtained PB Max scores with over 2000 patients from 6 to 89 years of age. His data in Figure 8.9 demonstrate a decline in PB Max, beginning with those in their 30s, which become pronounced in persons over 60 years old. When hearing loss was held constant across all age groups, as shown in Figure 8.10, Jerger found that speech recognition scores still showed consistent declines with advancing age. The sharpest reductions

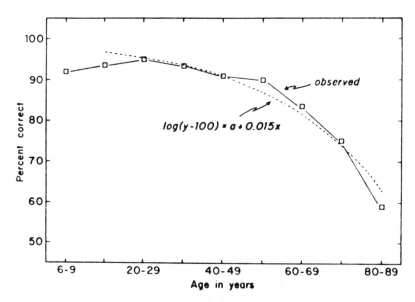

Figure 8.9. Average PB Max as a function of age averaged across PTA—2162 patients; 4095 ears. PTA, 0–69. (From Jerger J: Audiological findings in aging. *Adv Otorhinolaryngol* 20:115–124, 1973.)

in speech perception occurred when the degree of hearing loss exceeded 40 dB HL pure tone average (PTA) in patients over 60 years of age. Jerger's data indicate further declines in speech perception with age that cannot be linked exclusively with a loss of hearing sensitivity.

Using a large sample of cases with flat sensorineural hearing losses, Bess and Townsend (13) also found minimal declines in speech rec-

ognition with age for those with mild hearing loss and pronounced reductions when hearing loss became more severe. In a later study, Townsend and Bess (151) compared speech recognition performance of young and old subjects with mild sensorineural hearing loss. No significant differences were found between the two age groups. Because word recognition performance was more closely correlated with

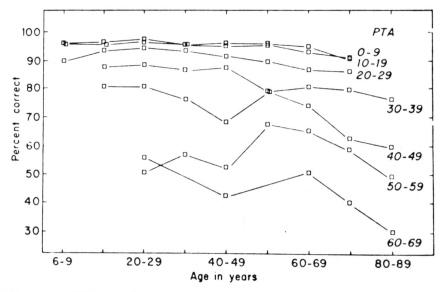

Figure 8.10. Average PB Max as a function of age with hearing loss (PTA) held constant. (Note the systematic decline in PB max with advancing age.) (From Jerger J: Audiological findings in aging. *Adv Otorhinolaryngol* 20:115–124, 1973.)

degree of loss rather than age, Townsend and Bess felt that the amount of hearing impairment may be more important than the factor of age in determining the decreases observed in speech perception with the elderly.

In summary, the decrease observed in speech perception with age is well documented, but the basis for the reduction appears complex. Peripheral involvement, as best manifested in decreases in hearing sensitivity on the audiogram, clearly plays a part, but considerable evidence also is available supporting the additional contribution of central factors to decreases in speech perception associated with the elderly.

Perception of Degraded Speech

Early investigations concluded that conventional speech perception testing with undistorted material generally was not effective in revealing difficulties in speech perception that usually accompany central auditory dysfunction. However, it has been demonstrated that, when the listening situation is made more difficult, speech perception is often reduced sharply. A number of approaches have been employed to increase the difficulty of the listening task, including frequency and temporal alterations of the speech signal, the inclusion of a competing signal or reverberation, and the use of high presentation levels. While originally developed for use in the assessment of

other forms of brain stem and auditory cortex disorders, their applications have been extended to include evaluation of the elderly to provide a more sensitive means of determining the speech perception capabilities of this particular age segment.

Altering the temporal features of speech has been shown to present a difficult perceptual task for older listeners. In an early study, Calearo and Lazzaroni (20) presented sentence material approximately 2½ times faster than the normal rate. Young subjects experienced no decrease in the perception of this material, but older listeners experienced a sharp reduction in performance. Stitch and Gray (143) presented phonetically balanced word lists that had been time compressed by 36, 46, and 59%, respectively, to four different subject groups arranged on the basis of age and type of hearing loss. They found that the elderly subject groups with normal hearing sensitivity and with sensorineural hearing loss both experienced substantially greater decrements in perception than corresponding groups made up of young listeners as the rate of compression of the speech stimuli increased.

These findings were confirmed further by Konkle et al (71). Using four progressively older groups of subjects with similar hearing sensitivity, they found, as shown in Figure 8.11, that intelligibility for the NU-6s decreased as a function of increasing subject age and time compression and decreasing sensation level of the material. All four of the older subject groups

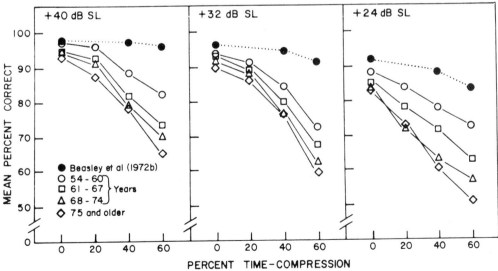

Figure 8.11. Mean percentage correct scores for the four age groups at each condition of time compression and sensation level. The Beasley et al data for 24 and 32 dB SL and 40 dB SL are shown for comparison purposes. (From Konkle D, Beasley D, Bess F: Intelligibility of time-altered speech in relation to chronological aging. *J Speech Hear Res* 20:108–115, 1977, © 1977, American Speech-Language-Hearing Association, Rockville, Maryland.)

experienced much reduced word recognition scores with increasing rates of time compression when compared with the performance of young listeners (6, 7). These findings were confirmed in an investigation reported later by Bergman (11) which compared speech perception of young and old subjects with speech material time compressed 50%.

The perception of filtered speech appears to diminish with advancing age. Kirikae et al (68) used low pass filtered monosyllabic speech material with young and old subjects with normal hearing sensitivity through 1000 Hz and found reduced recognition scores in the older age group. Bergman (11) demonstrated that filtering speech above 2000 Hz sharply reduced speech perception in older listeners compared to the performance of young subjects with normal hearing. Other investigators have presented low and high pass filtered speech simultaneously to the right and left ear in a dichotic listening task, and have found similar decreases in speech perception with age (10, 48, 108). However, a study by Kelly-Ballweber and Dobie (66), conducted with young and old subjects with closely matched audiograms, found no significant differences between age groups with a binaural synthesis listening task. Additional research is needed with the elderly to evaluate dichotic speech perception when hearing sensitivity is more tightly controlled.

Older listeners have been shown to perceive speech less effectively than young listeners when listening in the presence of competing signals. Comparisons of speech perception in noise or with a competing speech signal as a function of age have been done using normal hearing subjects (104, 137) and those with varying degrees of hearing impairment (32, 57). While exceptions have been noted in some presbycusic subjects (50), the speech perception of most elderly individuals is more adversely effected by noise than is normally observed in younger persons. Leskowitz and Lindstrom (78) suggest that this may occur in part because of an increased upward spread of masking among presbycusics.

Performance of the elderly with the Staggered Spondaic Word (SSW) Test has been investigated. While poorer results have been found in both raw (R) and corrected (C-SSW) scores with advancing age, it appears that a portion of the declines may be attributed to increasing amounts of peripheral hearing loss (3), at least for cases up to 70 years old. Further declines in SSW performance for subjects older than that may reflect both peripheral and central aging factors.

Another factor known to adversely affect speech perception is reverberation. While this is the case for all listeners (95), studies by Bergman (10) and Nabelek and Robinson (95) have demonstrated further decreases with age in the ability to perceive reverberant speech. This decline starts in the 4th decade of life, even before the onset of hearing loss.

The presentation level of speech material also influences the perception of speech by the elderly. Using the performance versus intensity (PI function) approach suggested by Jerger and Jerger (59) for identifying cases with certain retrocochlear disorders, Gang (36) found excessive reduction in speech recognition scores, or rollover, as the presentation levels were increased beyond the level where PB Max occurred. The degree of rollover in the PI function was significantly correlated with age, with older subjects demonstrating more severe rollover. Gang attributed the decrease observed at high presentation levels to neural degeneration within the brain stem or temporal lobe concomitant with the aging process.

It is apparent that making the listening task more difficult is likely to produce a larger reduction in speech perception than is observed with young individuals with similar hearing sensitivity. However, considerable variability exists from one person to the next in the resulting decrement, and the numerous methods for increasing the difficulty of the listening conditions do not produce the same degree of perceptual declines. Thus, while considerable information has been gathered regarding aging and the perception of speech, much remains to be done in this area.

Other Auditory Tests

The degree of auditory adaptation present is routinely measured by means of a variety of tone decay tests or Bekesy audiometry. Using the Carhart tone decay procedure with 90 men and women between 60 and 90 year of age, Goetzinger and co-workers (43) found no significant adaptation in any age groups, with only a few subjects demonstrating an appreciable amount of tone decay. Harbert et al (48), using a test of tone decay, also found no abnormal amounts of adaptation with 50 cases between the ages of 60 and 85. Willeford (157) reported finding a relatively small number of elderly subjects with excessive amounts of adaptation while using the Carhart tone decay procedure. Jerger and Jerger (60), however, found significant amounts of adaptation in 10 adult cases with a suprathreshold technique for assessing tone decay. They inferred that age may have contributed to the excessive adaptation found, as six of the subjects were over 60 years of age and the remaining four were between 43 and 56.

Jerger (54) used sweep frequency Bekesy audiometry with several hundred subjects, including 44 diagnosed cases of presbycusis, and found only two elderly cases that displayed any excessive adaptation. Harbert et al (48) also found no evidence of abnormal amounts of adaptation with most of the elderly subjects in their investigation. In those few cases in which excessive adaptation was found, it was usually confined to the high frequencies. Thus, although some older individuals may display abnormal adaptation, it is apparent that most presbycusics generally exhibit only minimal amounts.

Loudness perception and the influence of recruitment have been evaluated in the elderly with conventional loudness balance tests. Pestalozza and Shore (110) used the monaural loudness balance test with 24 subjects 60 years of age or older. They found considerable variability in the degree of recruitment exhibited, with 50% of the elderly not showing any recruitment. Goetzinger et al (43) employed the monaural and alternate binaural loudness test with subjects from 60 to 90 years of age, and found a somewhat higher prevalence of recruitment than Pestalozza and Shore noted. Of the 120 total ears tested, 34 showed complete recruitment; 57 showed incomplete recruitment; and the other 29 ears showed no recruitment. In another related investigation Harbert et al (48) used the monaural loudness balance test and found recruitment in less than 30% of a group of subjects over the age of 60. Collectively, these investigations imply considerable variation among presbycusics in the degree of recruitment present.

The Short Increment Sensitivity Index (SISI) has also been utilized to evaluate auditory function of elderly listeners. Jerger et al (62) found considerable variation in the SISI scores obtained with presbycusic cases and concluded that SISI scores among presbycusics are difficult to predict. Other studies (70, 161) have, however, found SISI scores with presbycusics which are more consistent with other forms of cochlear pathology.

It appears that test results suggestive of disruption of loudness perception are relatively common among persons with presbycusis. However, enough inconsistency exists to prevent us from making assumptions regarding this aspect of audition among elderly individuals.

Performance by the elderly on the Masking Level Difference (MLD) Test for pure tone and spondee stimuli has been investigated to quite an extent. In general, it has been found that the MLD values obtained with groups of older individuals are somewhat reduced for both types of stimuli relative to the results associated with younger adults (15, 103, 105, 149).

Auditory brainstem response (ABR) audiometry has definite utility in auditory assessment for cases across a wide age range, including the elderly. In establishing the applicability of this electrophysiologic procedure with the aged, a number of investigators have examined the effects of aging on wave V latency. Beagley and Sheldrake (5) grouped subjects from 11 to 79 years of age by decade. All subjects had normal hearing except for slight sensorineural hearing loss in the high frequencies for the older subjects. No significant changes in latency were found with increased age. A similar study by Jerger and Hall (56) with subjects from 25 to 55 years of age matched for gender and possessing normal hearing revealed a 0.2-millisecond increase in the latency of wave V in the older subjects. An even greater increase in wave V latency (0.4 millisecond) for older male subjects was found by Kelly-Ballweber and Dobie (66), when compared with results obtained from a group of young males matched for degree of hearing loss. Investigations by Rosenhamer et al (120) and Stockard and Stockard (144) both failed to demonstrate any significant alteration in ABR wave latency when comparing responses of older subjects with those for young adults. Overall, these findings suggest that current wave V latency normative values used for cases from 3 years of age on into adulthood for auditory brainstem response audiometry may not be appropriate for use with the elderly.

To provide further information regarding the auditory problems of presbycusis and to compare a number of diagnostic tests in terms of sensitivity, ease of administration, and other related issues, Otto and McCandless (105) completed an investigation with 30 elderly subjects and 30 young subjects with relatively matched, mild-to-moderate sensorineural hearing losses. An additional group of 30 young adults with normal hearing also were included. Concise data on subject performance were reported on each of the following tests: the Metz Test (92); acoustic reflex decay; PI function (NU-6); synthetic sentence identification (PI function at 0 MCR); time-compressed speech (NU-6 at 60% compression); tone decay; the Suprathreshold Adaptation Test (STAT); the Short Increment Sensitivity Index (SISI) Test; and a digit span test.

Using the Metz test and a liberal criterion of abnormality, 97% of the elderly subjects were found to present evidence of recruitment. Using a more stringent criterion, 80% were found to have recruitment. This high incidence in the elderly group contrasts with the relatively low percentage of cases with recruitment reported by previous investigations using a loudness balance task (48, 110). Tone decay test results also suggested more adaptation in the elderly group than those in either of the younger groups. Twenty percent of the elderly had 20 dB or greater amounts of tone decay. The STAT and acoustic reflex decay tests, however, produced negative results with nearly all of the older subjects.

The elderly exhibited only minimal phoneme regression and speech recognition rollover with the NU-6s. However, 30% had excessive rollover with the SSIs. PB Max scores for the SSIs also fell sharply among the elderly with increasing age. Results for the SISI revealed that the young sensorineural subjects consistently detected more of the 1 dB increments than the elderly. However, mean scores for the elderly group were positive (60% or higher) at 2000 and 4000 Hz when moderate-to-severe hearing loss was present.

Although the performance of the older subject group with time-compressed speech was reduced, it was not significantly different from the performance of the young sensorineural listeners. Data from the digit span test were significantly different for the young and old hearing impaired groups, suggesting a reduction in short-term memory with aging.

In a companion study, Otto and McCandless (106) reported on the result of auditory brainstem response testing with the same 90 subjects used in the previously discussed investigation. It was determined that the absence and lack of clarity found in the elderly for early waves, particularly I and II, were related to both hearing loss and aging. Otto and McCandless also observed isolated instances of delay in wave V latency among older subjects, although group mean latency times for the elderly were not significantly different from their young counterparts.

Thus, Otto and McCandless' results indicate considerable variability in audiometric test results among elderly cases. Some tests, such as the SSIs, appear more sensitive than others in revealing breakdowns within the auditory system. This finding is consistent with the results of a longitudinal case study recently reported with an elderly subject (142) which also demonstrated the utility of the SSIs in revealing declines in central auditory function. Otto and McCandless concluded that extensive site of lesion testing with the elderly can be crucial in determining candidacy for a hearing aid and other management issues.

CONCLUSIONS

The prevalence data available regarding presbycusis make it clear that hearing loss is a major health problem among the elderly at the present time. Given the demographic information related to longevity and population trends for the next few decades, it is also clear that the magnitude of the problem will accelerate further in the years to come. Health care professionals must respond by becoming more knowledgeable regarding hearing loss in the aged and by developing more effective service delivery systems to serve the increasing needs of this segment of the population.

Actually, the prevalence figures probably underestimate the proportion of older persons with hearing problems, due to our rather myopic approach in the past of using auditory sensitivity as the sole measure of hearing loss in the surveys that have examined hearing as a function of age. Because speech perception is disrupted by the process of aging to a greater degree than would be expected from the loss observed in hearing sensitivity, accurate measures of hearing function for communication purposes in the elderly require the use of more comprehensive assessment tests and criteria. The current data therefore represent a conservative estimate of the problem. This is especially true in light of evidence which indicates that aging produces a reduction in cognitive function (122) that undoubtedly contributes as well to the overall auditory processing declines found with the aged. Certainly, further research must be conducted to determine more completely the nature and extent of the role which cognition has in audition for listeners of all ages, including the elderly.

While there was a time when age-related hearing loss was thought to stem strictly from structural damage within the inner ear, it is now evident that the effects of aging on the hearing mechanism are global. Virtually every major division of the auditory system can experience a number of significant changes. The generalized nature of presbycusis changes for the elderly group can be attributed, in part, to the diverse nature of the etiologies suspected to be involved. However, on a case-by-case basis, the structural changes can be and often are quite individualized and variable in regard to severity and locale. Thus, while one instance of presbycusis may be due primarily to sensory cell degeneration within the cochlea, another may involve neural atrophy within the auditory cortex, with only minimal alterations within the peripheral division.

Because of the diversity of the damage associated with presbycusis, the audiological results obtained with the aged are highly variable. While declines in hearing sensitivity occur with age, the degree and configuration of the hearing loss experienced varies considerably from person to person. It is also evident that, while decrements in speech recognition performance in the elderly may parallel the degree of loss in hearing sensitivity, a substantial portion of the aged experience a disproportionate amount of difficulty in perceiving speech, particularly when the difficulty of the listening task is increased. Inconsistency in the results obtained with site of lesion tests simply is a consequence of the widespread and variable alterations which the aging process. The diversity associated with presbycusis presents a special challenge to the audiologist, since each elderly case is potentially different and requires that test selection and administration be individualized and comprehensive.

While some conventional audiologic tests are appropriate for use with the elderly, there is need for new tests and procedures to be developed which are more effective in describing the nature of an older person's peripheral and central auditory function and which provide more relevant information concerning rehabilitation, particularly the appropriateness of hearing aids. To accomplish this, additional research is needed to provide us with a further understanding of a number of important issues, including the effects of aging on the auditory mechanism, how specific structural changes effect auditory function, and the role of cognition in auditory processing. Thus, a more thorough understanding of presbycusis will ultimately make it possible for us to more adequately meet the needs of the elderly in future years.

References

1. Alberti P, Kristensen R: The compliance of the middle ear: its accuracy in routine clinical practice. In Rose D, Keating L (eds): *Mayo Foundation Impedance Symposium*. Rochester, Minn, Mayo Clinic Foundation, 1972.
2. American National Standards Institute. *American National Standards Specifications for Audiometers* (ANSI S3.6—1969). New York, American National Standards Institute, 1970.
3. Arnst DJ: Staggered Spondaic Word Test performance in a group of older adults: a preliminary report. *Ear Hear* 3:118–123, 1982.
4. Ball MJ: Neuronal loss, neurofibrillary tangles and granulovacuolar degeneration in the hippocampus with aging and dementia: a quantitative study. *Acta Neuropathol* 37:111–118, 1977.
5. Beagley HA, Sheldrake JB: Differences in brainstem response latency with age and sex. *Br J Audiol* 12:69–77, 1978.
6. Beasley D, Forman B, Rintelmann W: Perception of time-compressed CNC monosyllables by normal listeners. *J Aud Res* 12:71–75, 1972.
7. Beasley D, Schwimmer S, Rintelmann W: Intelligibility of time-compressed CNC monosyllables. *J Speech Hear Res* 15:340–350, 1972.
8. Beasley W: Generalized age and sex trends in hearing loss. In: *Hearing Study Series Bulletin No. 7*, National Health Survey. Washington, DC, U.S. Public Health Service, 1938.
9. Belal A, Stewart TJ: Pathological changes in the middle ear joints. *Ann Otal Rhinol Laryngol* 83:159–167, 1974.
10. Bergman M: Hearing and aging. *Audiology* 10:164–171, 1971.
11. Bergman M: *Aging and the Perception of Speech*. Baltimore, University Park Press, 1980, p 82.
12. Bergstrom L, Thompson P: Ototoxicity. In Northern J (ed): *Hearing Disorders*. Boston, Little, Brown, 1984, p 119.
13. Bess FH, Townsend TH: Word discrimination for listeners with flat sensorineural hearing loss. *J Speech Hear Disord* 42:232–237, 1977.
14. Blood I, Greenburg M: Acoustic immittance of the ear in the geriatric person. *J Am Aud Soc* 2:185–187, 1977.
15. Bocca E, Antonelli A: Masking level differences: another tool for the evaluation of peripheral and cortical defects. *Audiology* 15:480–487, 1976.
16. Bondareff W: The neural basis of aging. In Birren J, Schaie K (eds): *Handbook of the Psychology of Aging*. New York, Van Nostrand Reinhold, 1977, p 50.
17. Brody H: Organization of the central cortex. III. Study of aging in human cerebral cortex. *J Comp Neurol* 102:511–556, 1955.
18. Bunch CC: Age variations in auditory acuity. *Arch Otolaryngol* 9:625–626, 1929.
19. Calavita FB: *Sensory Changes in the Elderly*. Springfield, IL, Charles C Thomas, 1978, p 35.
20. Calearo C Lazzaroni A: Speech intelligibility in relation to the speed of the message. *Laryngoscope* 67:410–419, 1957.
21. Carhart R: Problems in the measurement of speech discrimination. *Arch Otolaryngol* 82:253–260, 1965.
22. Chermak GD, Moore MK: Eustachian tube functions in the older adult. *Ear Hear* 2:143–147, 1981.
23. Colon EJ: The elderly brain—a quantitative analysis in the cerebral cortex in two cases. *Psychiatr Neurol Neurochir* 75:261–270, 1972.
24. Corso JF: Aging and auditory thresholds in men and women. *Arch Environ Health* 6:350–356, 1963.
25. Corso JF: Age and sex differences in pure-tone thresholds. *Arch Otolaryngol* 77:53–73, 1963.
26. Corso JF: *Aging Sensory Systems and Perceptions*. New York, Praeger, 1981, p 79.
27. Covell W: Histologic changes in the aging cochlea. *J Gerontol* 7:173–177, 1952.

28. Crowe S, Guild S, Palvogt L: Observations on pathology of high-tone deafness. *Bull Johns Hopkins Hosp* 54:315, 1934.

29. Dekaban AS, Sadowsky D: Changes in brain weights during the span of human life: relation of brain weight to body heights and weights. *Ann Neurol* 4:345–356, 1978.

30. Duvall AJ, Wersall J: Site of action of streptomycin upon inner ear sensory cells. *Acta Otolaryngol* 57:581–598, 1964.

31. Enholm B, Belal A: Senile changes in the middle ear joints. *Ann Otol Rhinol Laryngol* 83:49–54, 1974.

32. Findlay RC, Denenberg LJ: Effects of subtle midfrequency auditory dysfunction upon speech discrimination in noise. *Audiology* 16:252–254, 1976.

33. Fowler EP: The aging ear. *Arch Otolaryngol* 40:475–480, 1944.

34. Gacek RR, Schuknecht HF: Pathology of presbycusis. *Int Audiol* 8:199–209, 1969.

35. Gaeth J: A study of phonemic regression in relation to hearing loss. Ph.D. dissertation, Evanston, IL, Northwestern University, 1948.

36. Gang RP: The effects of age on the diagnostic utility of the rollover phenomenon. *J Speech Hear Disord* 41:63–69, 1976.

37. Gerber SE, Mencher GT: *Auditory Dysfunction.* Houston, College-Hill Press, 1980, p 168.

38. Gilad O, Glorig A: Presbycusis: the aging ear (Part II). *J Am Aud Soc* 4:207–217, 1979.

39. Glorig A, Davis H: Age, noise, and hearing loss. *Ann Otolaryngol* 70:556–571, 1961.

40. Glorig A, Nixon H: Hearing loss as a function of age. *Laryngoscope* 27:1596–1610, 1962.

41. Glorig A, Roberts J: Hearing levels of adults by age and sex, United States, 1960–1962, *Public Health Service Publication*, N. 1000, Series 11, No. 11. Washington, DC, U.S. Public Health Service, DHEW, 1965.

42. Glorig A, Wheeler D, Quiggle R, Grings W, Summerfield A. 1954 Wisconsin State Fair Hearing Survey. Monograph, American Academy of Ophthalmology and Otolaryngology, 1957.

43. Goetzinger C, Proud G, Dirks D et al: A study of hearing in advanced age. *Arch Otolaryngol* 73:662–667, 1961.

44. Goodhill V: Bilateral malleal fixation and conductive presbycusis. *Arch Otolaryngol* 90:107–112, 1969.

45. Hall JW: Acoustic reflex amplitude. I. Effects of age and sex. *Audiology* 21:294–309, 1982.

46. Handler SD, Margolis RH: Predicting hearing loss from stapedial reflex thresholds in patients with sensori-neural impairment. *Trans Am Acad Ophthalmol Otol* 84:425–431, 1977.

47. Hansen CC, Reske-Nielsen E: Pathological studies in presbycusis. *Arch Otolaryngol* 82:115–132, 1965.

48. Harbert F, Young I, Menduke H: Audiologic findings in presbycusis. *J Aud Res* 6:279–312, 1966.

49. Hayes D: Central auditory problems and the aging process. In Beasley DS, Davis GA (eds): *Aging: Communication Processes and Disorders.* New York, Grune Stratton, 1981, p 258.

50. Hayes D, Jerger J: Aging and the use of hearing aids. *Scand Audiol* 8:33–40, 1979.

51. Hayes D, Jerger J: Low-frequency hearing loss in presbycusis. *Arch Otolaryngol* 104(1):9–12, 1979.

52. Holmquist J: Eustachian tube anatomy and physiology. *J Am Aud Soc* 2:115–120, 1977.

53. Jepsen O: Middle-ear muscle reflexes in man. In Jerger J (ed): *Modern Developments in Audiology.* New York, Academic Press, 1963.

54. Jerger J: Bekesy audiometry in the analysis of auditory disorders. *J Speech Hear Res* 3:275–287, 1960.

55. Jerger J: Audiological findings in aging. *Adv Otorhinolaryngol* 20:115–124, 1973.

56. Jerger J, Hall J: Effects of age and sex on the auditory brainstem response. *Arch Otolaryngol* 106:382–391, 1980.

57. Jerger J, Hayes D: Diagnostic speech audiometry. *Arch Otolaryngol* 103:216–222, 1977.

58. Jerger J, Hayes D, Anthony L et al: Factors influencing prediction of hearing level from acoustic reflex. *Monogr Contemp Audiol* 1:1–20, 1978.

59. Jerger JF, Jerger S: Diagnostic significance of PB word functions. *Arch Otolaryngol* 93:573–580, 1971.

60. Jerger J, Jerger S: A simplified tone decay test. *Arch Otolaryngol* 101:403–407, 1975.

61. Jerger J, Jerger S, Mauldin L: Studies in impedance audiometry. I. Normal and sensorineural ears. *Arch Otolaryngol* 96:513–523, 1972.

62. Jerger J, Shedd J, Harford E: On the detection of extremely small changes in sound intensity. *Arch Otolaryngol* 69:200–211, 1959.

63. Johnson LG, Hawkins JE: Sensory and neural degeneration with aging, as seen in microdissections of the human inner ear. *Ann Otolaryngol* 81:179–183, 1972.

64. Jorgensen MB: Changes of aging in the inner ear. *Arch Otolaryngol* 74:56–62, 1961.

65. Kasden SD: Speech discrimination in two age groups matched for hearing loss. *J Aud Res* 10:210–212, 1970.

66. Kelly-Ballweber D, Dobie R: Binaural interaction measured behaviorally and electrophysiologically in young and old adults. *Audiology* 23:181–194, 1984.

67. Kimura RS: Cochlear vascular lesions. In De Lorenzo AJ (ed): *Vascular Disorders and Hearing.* Baltimore, University Park Press, 1973, p 100.

68. Kirikae I, Sato T, Shitara T: A study of hearing in advanced age. *Laryngoscope* 74:205–220, 1964.

69. Klotz R, Kilbane M: Hearing in an aging population. *N Engl J Med* 266:277–280, 1962.

70. Konig E: Audiological tests in presbycusis. *Inst Audiol* 8:240–259, 1969.

71. Konkle D, Beasley D, Bess F: Intelligibility of time-altered speech in relation to chronological aging. *J Speech Hear Res* 20:108–115, 1977.

72. Kopra LL: Modifications of traditional techniques for assessment of the elderly client. In Hull RH (ed): *Rehabilitative Audiology.* New York, Grune & Stratton, 1982, p 322.

73. Kormenday CG, Bender AD: Chemical interference with aging. *Gerontologia* 17:52–64, 1971.

74. Krmpotic-Nemanic J: A new concept of the pathogenesis of presbycusis. *AMA Arch Otolaryngol* 93:161–166, 1971.

75. Kryter KD: *The Effects of Noise on Man.* New York, Academic Press, 1970, p 119.

76. Leake C: Study of the components of deafness. *Geriatrics* 18:506–509, 1963.

77. Lebo CP, Reddell RC: The presbycusis component in occupational hearing loss. *Laryngoscope* 82:1339–1409, 1972.

78. Leskowitz B, Lindstrom R: Masking and speech-to-noise ratio. *Aud Deaf Educ* 6:5–8, 1979.

79. Lowell SH, Paparella MM: Presbycusis: What is it? *Laryngoscope* 87:1710–1717, 1977.

80. Lowry LD, Issacson SR: Study of 100 patients with bilateral sensorineural hearing loss for lipid abnormalities. *Ann Otolaryngol* 87:404–408, 1978.

81. Luterman DM, Welsh OL, Melrose J: Responses of aged males to time-altered speech stimuli. *J Speech Hear Res* 9:226–230, 1966.

82. Maglodery J: Neurophysiology of aging. In Birren J (ed): *Handbook of Aging and the Individual.* Chicago, University of Chicago Press, 1959, p 174.

83. Makishima K: Arteriolar sclerosis as a cause of presbycusis. *Arch Otolaryngol* 86:322–326, 1968.

84. Margolis RH, Popelka GR, Handler SD, Himelfarb M: The effects of age on acoustic-reflex thresholds in normal-hearing subjects. In Popelka G (ed): *Hearing Assessment with the Acoustic Reflex.* New York, Grune & Stratton, 1981.

85. Marshall L: Auditory processing in aging listeners. *J Speech Hear Disord* 23:226–240, 1981.

86. Marshall L, Martinez S, Schlaman M: Reassessment of high-frequency air-bone gaps in older adults. *Arch Otolaryngol* 109:601–606, 1983.

87. Maurer JF, Rupp RR: *Hearing and Aging: Tactics for Intervention.* New York, Grune & Srattion, 1979, p 39.

88. Mayer O: Das anatomische Substrat der Alterschwergorigkeit. *Arch F. Ohren-Nasen Kehlkopfh.* 105:1, 1920.

89. McCartney J, Alexander D: Geriatric audiology nursing home project: first year evaluation. Presented at the Annual Convention of the American Speech and Hearing Association, Houston, 1976.

90. McMenemey WH: The dementias and progressive diseases of the basal ganglia. In Blackwood H (ed): *Greenfield's Neuropathology.* London, Arnold, 1963, p 188.

91. Melcher JA, Peterson JL: The effect of age and hearing impairment on acoustic reflex decay. *ASHA* 14:465, 1972.

92. Metz O: Threshold of reflex contractions of muscles of middle ear and recruitment of loudness. *Arch Otolaryngol* 55:536–543, 1952.

93. Milne J: A longitudinal study of hearing loss in older people. *Br J Audiol* 11:7–18, 1977.

94. Moscicki EK, Elkins EF, Baum HM et al: Hearing loss in the elderly: an epidemiologic study of the Framingham Heart Study Cohort. *Ear Hear* 6:184–190, 1985.

95. Nabelek AK, Robinson PK: Monaural and binaural speech perception in reverberation for listeners of various ages. *J Acoust Soc Am* 71:1242–1248, 1982.

96. Nadol JB: The aging peripheral hearing mechanism. In Beasley DS, Davis GA (eds): *Aging: Communication Processes and Disorders.* New York, Grune & Stratton, 1981, p 67.

97. National Center for Health Statistics: Prevalence of selected impairments, United States, 1977. *Vital Health Stat* [10], No. 134, 1981.

98. National Institute for Occupational Safety and Health: Criteria for a recommended standard—occupational exposure to noise, Report HSM 73-11001. Cincinnati, NIOSH, 1972.

99. Nerbonne M, Bliss A, Schow R: Acoustic impedance values in the elderly. *J Am Aud Soc* 4:57–59, 1978.

100. Newman CW, Spitzer JB: Eustachian tube efficiency of geriatric subjects. *Ear Hear* 2:103–107, 1981.

101. Nixon J, Glorig A, High W: Changes in air- and bone-conduction thresholds as a function of age. *Ann Otol Rhinol Laryngol* 74:288–298, 1962.

102. Nomura Y: Lipidosis of the basilar membrane. *Acta Otolaryng* 69:352–357, 1970.

103. Olsen WO, Noffsinger D, Carhart R: Masking level differences encountered in clinical populations. *Audiology* 15:287–301, 1976.

104. Orchik DJ, Burgess J: Synthetic sentences identification as a function of the age of the listener. *J Am Audiol Soc* 3:42–46, 1977.

105. Otto WC, McCandless GA: Aging and auditory site of lesion. *Ear Hear* 3:110–117, 1982.

106. Otto WC, McCandless GA: Aging and the auditory brainstem response. *Audiology* 21:466–473, 1982.

107. Owens E, Benedict M, Schubert E: Consonant phoneme errors associated with pure tone configurations and certain types of hearing impairment. *J Speech Hear Res* 15:308–322, 1972.

108. Palva A, Jokinen K: Presbycusis V. Filtered speech test. *Arch Otolaryngol* 70:232–241, 1970.

109. Perry ET: *The Human Ear Canal.* Springfield, IL, Charles C Thomas, 1957, p 26.

110. Pestalozza G, Shore I: Clinical evaluation of presbycusis on the basis of different tests of auditory function. *Laryngoscope* 65:1136–1163, 1955.

111. Punch JL: The prevalence of hearing impairment. *ASHA* 25:27, 1983.

112. Punch JL, McConnell F: The speech discrimination function of elderly adults. *J Aud Res* 9:159–166, 1969.

113. Quick CA, Fish A, Brown C: The relationship between cochlea and kidney. *Laryngoscope* 83:1469–1482, 1973.

114. Randolph L, Schow R: Threshold inaccuracies in an elderly clinical population: ear canal collapse as a possible cause. *J Speech Hear Res* 26:54–58, 1983.

115. Rasmussen A: Studies of the VIIIth cranial nerve of man. *Laryngoscope* 50:67–83, 1940.

116. Rees JN, Botwinick J: Detection and decision criteria for the detection of tones in noise. *J Gerontol* 26:133–136, 1971.

117. Rintelmann WF, Schumaier D: Five experiments on speech discrimination utilizing CNC monosyllables (N.U. Auditory Test No. 6)

Experiment III: Factors affecting speech discrimination in a clinical setting: List equivalence, hearing loss, and phonemic regression. *J Aud Res*, Suppl 2:12–15, 1974.

118. Rosen S, Bergman M, Plester D, et al: A presbycusis study of a relatively noise-free population in the Sudan. *Ann Otolaryngol* 71:727–743, 1962.

119. Rosen S, Olin K: Hearing loss and coronary heart disease. *Arch Otolaryngol* 82:236–243, 1965.

120. Rosenhamer HJ, Linstrom B, Lundborg J: On the use of click-evoked electric brainstem responses in audiological diagnosis. II. The influence of sex and age upon the normal response. *Scand Audiol* 9:93–100, 1980.

121. Rosenwasser H: Otitic problems in the aged. *Geriatrics* 19:11–17, 1964.

122. Salthouse TA: *Adult Cognition*. New York, Springer-Verlag, 1982.

123. Sataloff J, Vassolo L, Menduke H: Presbycusis: air- and bone-conduction thresholds. *Laryngoscope* 75:889–901, 1965.

124. Saxen A, von Friendt H: Pathologic und klinik der Altersschwerhorigkeit. *Acta Otolaryngol* (Suppl. 23):1–85, 1937.

125. Schow RL, Christensen JM, Hutchinson JM, Nerbonne MA: *Communication Disorders of the Aged*. Baltimore, University Park Press, 1978, p 79.

126. Schow RL, Goldbaum D: Collapsed ear canals in the elderly nursing home population. *J Speech Hear Disord* 45:259–267, 1980.

127. Schow RL, Nerbonne MA: Hearing levels among elderly nursing home residents. *J Speech Hear Disord* 45:124–132, 1980.

128. Schuknecht HF: Presbycusis. *Laryngoscope* 65:402–419, 1955.

129. Schuknecht HF: Further observation on the pathology of presbycusis. *Arch Otolaryngol* 80:369–382, 1964.

130. Schuknecht HF: *Pathology of the Ear*. Cambridge, MA, Harvard University Press, 1974, p 392.

131. Schuknecht HF, Watanuki K, Takahashi T et al: Atrophy of the stria vascularis: a common cause for hearing loss. *Laryngoscope* 84:1777–1821, 1974.

132. Schuknecht HF, Woellner R: Experimental and clinical study of deafness from lesions of the cochlear nerve. *J Laryngol* 69:75–97, 1955.

133. Seifert M, Seidemann M, Givens G: An examination of variables involved in tympanometric assessment of eustachian tube function in adults. *J Speech Hear Disord* 44:388–396, 1979.

134. Senturia B: *Diseases of the External Ear*. Springfield, Il, Charles C Thomas, 1957, p 50.

135. Shock NW: Physiology of aging. *Sci Am* 26:100–110, 1962.

136. Silman S: The effect of aging on acoustic reflex threshold. *J Acoust Soc Am* 66:735–738, 1979.

137. Smith RA, Prather WF: Phoneme discrimination in older persons under varying signal-to-noise conditions. *J Speech Hear Res* 14:630–638, 1971.

138. Smith BH, Sethi PK: Aging and the nervous system. *Geriatrics* 30:109–115, 1975.

139. Spencer JT: Hyperlipoproteinemia in the etiology of inner ear diseases. *Laryngoscope* 83:639–678, 1973.

140. Spencer JT: Hyperlipoproteinemia in inner ear disease. *Otolaryngol Clin North Am* 8:483–492, 1975.

141. Spoor A: Presbycusis values in relation to noise induced hearing loss. *Int Audiol* 6:48–57, 1967.

142. Stack BA, Jerger JF, Fleming KA: Central presbycusis: a longitudinal case study. *Ear Hear* 6:304–306, 1985.

143. Stitch T, Gray B: The intelligibility of time-compressed words as a function of age and hearing loss. *J Speech Hear Res* 12:443–448, 1969.

144. Stockard JE, Stockard, JJ: Recording and analyzing. In Moore EJ (ed): *Bases of Auditory Brain-Stem Evoked Responses*. New York, Grune & Stratton, 1983, p 682.

145. Suga F, Lindsay J: Histopathological observations of presbycusis. *Ann Otol Rhinol Laryngol* 85:169, 1975.

146. Surr, RK: Effect of age on clinical hearing aid evaluation results. *J Am Aud Soc* 3:1–15, 1977.

147. Thompson D, Sills J, Recke K, Bui D: Acoustic admittance and the aging ear. *J Speech Hear Disord* 22:29–36, 1979.

148. Thompson D, Sills J, Recke K, Bui D: Acoustic reflex growth in the aging adult. *J Speech Hear Res* 23:405–418, 1980.

149. Tillman TW, Carhart R, Nicholls S: Release from multiple maskers in elderly persons. *J Speech Hear Res* 16:152–160, 1973.

150. Tomlinson BE, Henderson G: Some quantitative cerebral findings in normal and demented old people. In Terry R, Gershon S (eds): *Neurology of Aging*. New York, Raven Press, 1976, p 211.

151. Townsend TH, Bess FH: Effects of age and sensorineural hearing loss on word recognition. *Scand Audiol* 9:245–248, 1980.

152. Tsai HK, Chou FS, Cheng TJ: On changes in ear size with age, as found among Taiwanese-Formosans of Fukienese extraction. *J Formosan Med Assoc* 57:105–111, 1958.

153. United States Health Examination Survey: Hearing levels of adults by age and sex in the United States, 1960-1962, Publication 1000, Series 11, No. 11, Washington, DC, U.S. Public Health Service, DHEW, 1965.

154. Valenstein E: Age-related changes in the human central nervous system. In Beasley DS, Davis GA (eds): *Aging: Communication Processes and Disorders*. New York, Grune & Stratton, 1981, p 91.

155. Wang HS, Obrist WD, Busse EW: Neurophysiological correlates of the intellectual function of elderly persons living in this community. *Am J Psychiatry* 126:1205–1212, 1970.

156. Weg R: Changing physiology of aging: normal and pathological. In Woodruff D, Birren J (eds): *Aging: Scientific Perspectives and Social Issues*. New York, D. Van Nostrand, 1975, p 235.

157. Willeford JA: The geriatric patient. In Rose DE (ed): *Audiological Assessment*. Englewood Cliffs, NJ, Prentice-Hall, 1971, p 309.

158. Willeford JA: The geriatric patient. In Rose DE

(ed): *Audiological Assessment.* Englewood Cliffs, NJ, Prentice-Hall, 1978, p 304.

159. Williams PS: A tympanic swallow test for assessment of Eustachian tube function. *Ann Otol Rhinol Laryngol* 84:339–343, 1975.

160. Wilson R: The effects of aging on the magnitude of the acoustic reflex. *J Speech Hear Res* 24:406–414, 1981.

161. Young IM, Harbert F: Significance of the SISI test. *J Aud Res* 7:303–311, 1967.

162. Zwaardemaker H: The range of hearing at various ages. *J Psychol* 7:10–28, 1894.

9 Changes in Speech Production and Linguistic Behaviors with Aging

BARBARANNE J. BENJAMIN

Editor's Note

Chapter 9 serves as a companion piece to Chapter 8, in that it provides a comprehensive review of the literature concerning normal changes in speech and language functioning in older adults. Benjamin begins by reminding the reader of the methodological problems in research in this area, noting particularly the linguistic impact of age cohort effects and the inadequacy of chronological age as an index of aging. The next section examines speech characteristics of older persons, exploring anatomic and physiological changes and their acoustic and perceptual correlates. The author concludes that changes in the speech mechanism and in speech output may not significantly detract from communication intelligibility. However, these same changes produce identifiable "older" voices and speech patterns which may contribute to stereotypical listener expectations (as described further in Chapter 10). The final section of Chapter 9 reviews the linguistic characteristics of normal aging. Benjamin first explores the potential effects of neurological and cognitive changes upon linguistic behaviors, followed by a more specific discussion of research on the linguistic parameters of phonology, morphology, syntax, semantics, and pragmatics. She concludes by noting that more research is needed concerning all aspects of linguistic functioning, but particularly the phonologic, morphologic, and pragmatic parameters. The need to examine both partners in the communication interaction is also stressed.

Subtle changes in speech and language behavior distinguish older adults from different aged speakers. Typically, research on communication development is limited to descriptions of behavior in children, but abilities in speech production and language use continue to evolve throughout adulthood. Adult-oriented research has focused primarily on normal young adult speakers or on the speech and language patterns of adults who exhibit disorders affecting the ability to communicate. While the speech and language abilities of normal older speakers have not been studied as extensively, significant contributions have been made.

Changes which occur in the speech production and language behavior of typical older adults are examined in this chapter. The first division of the chapter describes changes in speech production, including changes in anatomical structure and functioning which alter the acoustic output we perceive as speech. The second division concerns changes in linguistic characteristics that accompany the normal aging process.

Before undertaking an overview of research findings, however, we must recognize the lim-

itations of research concerning changes in normal older adults. Primarily descriptive, investigations of speech and language behaviors in the elderly are complicated by limitations in generalization due to various intrinsic characteristics of older subjects and to methodological restrictions. For instance, identification of unique commonalities within groups of older speakers is difficult because of the wide range of individual differences. Differences in physical condition and health-related factors contribute to increased variability within the older age group, and older adults are less likely to be similar in attitude, behavior, and physiology than are groups of younger speakers. Even performance is more variable with increasing age (35).

In addition, research methodology, designed to investigate the effects of aging on speech and language processes, also contributes to problems in identifying characteristics which differentiate and are common to older adult speakers. Both cross-sectional and longitudinal studies are contaminated by age cohort effects.

An age cohort is a group of people born during a particular period who experience similar events as they age. Age cohort effects are intrinsic differences which are common to an age group. These age cohort effects are due to unique societal events experienced by individuals of a particular age group at similar chronological ages. Persons from other age cohorts may experience the same societal events but experience them at different stages of life, resulting in different perceptions or impacts. For instance, a 65-year-old male in 1988 has experienced the Depression as a child, fought in World War II, raised a family during the 1950s and 1960s, and witnessed the pervasive influence of the telephone, automobile, and television. These societal milestones have left an indelible mark on today's "senior" citizen. On the other hand, a child born only 25 years later saw World War II through the eyes of a child, witnessed the Vietnam conflict and protest as a young adult, and has seen the development of television, rocketry, and nuclear power. The age at which these events were experienced provides a commonality for persons of an age cohort and subtly distinguishes them from persons of other age cohorts.

Age cohort effects limit the ability to generalize current descriptions of older adult speech and language to the communicative productions of future generations. Pervasive industrial pollution, noise contamination, societal attitudes, and other factors influencing cohort effects severely limit generalizations from today's 65-year-old speakers to individuals who became 65 during the remainder of this century. Continued updating of research data is mandatory.

A final methodological concern is the use of chronological age as the major criterion for identifying age groups. Although chronological age is the most reliable definition of age group, other definitional criteria may be valid. Alternative methods for establishing age groups may be provided by: physiological aging which may differentiate the healthy older adult from the older adult who is ill or in poor physical condition (107); perceived age based upon listener judgement, with this approach being particularly valuable in attempts to identify perceived vocal characteristics of normal aging (112); and the individual's own perception of, and feelings toward, age. Since self-report of health is significantly correlated with more objective measures of health status (see ref. 78), self-perception may also be a valid index of aging for sociological and communication research.

With these cautions in mind, the following review of literature must be viewed as preliminary in nature and subject to change as our data base increases. The remainder of the chapter explores typical changes in speech and language which occur with normal aging. These

nonpathological changes are identified so that they might be contrasted with characteristics indicative of pathological conditions addressed in Chapter 11.

SPEECH CHARACTERISTICS OF NORMAL ELDERLY PERSONS

The myoelastic aerodynamic theory of speech posits a causal relationship between the acoustic signal and the structure and functioning of the speech mechanism. Measurable changes in the structure of and the relationships among the components of the speech system are reflected in changes in the acoustic signal. As the human body undergoes typical anatomic and physiological changes associated with advancing age, alterations are expected in the speech patterns of normally aging persons.

In the following section, typical physical changes which affect the speech mechanism with age are described. These anatomic and physiological changes are thought to contribute to the typical vocal characteristics associated with the older voice. The second section examines acoustic characteristics of older speech. A description of perceptual and objective parameters of normal older adult speech is necessary before pathological conditions affecting older persons' communication can be adequately assessed.

Anatomic and Physiological Changes in the Speech Mechanism

Each subsystem of the speech mechanism undergoes anatomic and physiological changes resulting from the normal process of aging. Although these typical changes affect individuals at various rates, all individuals can be expected to demonstrate anatomic changes as normal aging progresses (103). Briefly, we will examine typical changes affecting the neurological component, respiratory support, laryngeal valving, and supralaryngeal mechanism.

Neurological Foundation

The neurological network is the foundation of all motor movements, including speech. As a result, neurological changes associated with advancing age may be reflected in alterations in older adults' speaking characteristics.

For instance, total brain mass is reduced by 10 to 15% in the normal aged individual compared to the young adult (36, 140) with primary tissue loss occurring in the cortex. The superior portion of the temporal lobes and the precentral gyrus, areas of the cortex primarily responsible for speech behavior, are affected (22). Additional alterations in neurologic tissue are detailed later in this chapter and in Chapter 4. These changes as well as other pervasive changes in neuroanatomy may adversely affect speech production. Extensive changes result in pathological conditions such as those covered in Chapter 11, whereas normal changes may be linked to subtle characteristic alterations in older adult speech production detailed in this chapter.

Respiratory Support

Anatomic and physiological changes which accompany advanced aging affect the respiratory system. Calcification of rib cartilage and weakening of the respiratory muscles limit rib cage expansion and have a profound effect on respiratory effort (see ref. 64). In addition, loss of lung elasticity as well as changes resulting in a less flexible pleural membrane contribute to a reduction in respiratory efficiency (66). Decreased contractive force of respiratory muscles, tissue atrophy, rib cage stiffening, and narrow airway passages also contribute to reduced respiratory efficiency in the older population (89). Chapter 4 provides a more detailed description of these changes in the respiratory system.

Reduction in older individuals' respiratory efficiency is well documented. The most notable change in spirometric measurements is an accelerating reduction of vital capacity with advanced age (38, 65, 105); expiratory flow and expiratory volume are reduced (89) along with a significant decrease in intraoral air pressure (105). Residual volume, the air remaining in the lungs after forceful exhalation, is increased in older speakers, thus contributing to a reduction of air available for vital capacity maneuvers (83, 132).

Such changes in the respiratory abilities of older adults would be expected to reduce air volume available for speech production. Anatomic and physiologic changes affect maximum respiratory effort and are most noticeable in extreme speaking situations in which excessive sustained respiratory effort is necessary. However when severe, reduction in respiratory efficiency may adversely affect loudness and may result in a need for more frequent pauses to replenish the air supply for speech (66). Such severe restrictions of air supply are not typical of the normally aging adult but are most often exacerbated by pathological conditions.

Laryngeal Valving

The phonatory subsystem, comprised of the vocal folds and larynx, is affected by the normal aging process. Calcification or ossification of the larynx is extensive by age 65, with the thyroid and cricoid cartilages primarily involved (67, 103). The mucous membrane is discolored, and a reduction in submucosal connective tissue results in looseness of the membrane covering the vocal folds (see ref. 66). The general loss of elasticity of the laryngeal ligaments, reduced muscle strength, and atrophy of the intrinsic laryngeal muscles affects laryngeal functioning (66, 82). In older male larynges, marked atrophy is present with 67% of older males presenting a glottal gap; edema of the vocal folds is present in 74% of older female larynges and in 56% of older male larynges (56).

These extensive changes in laryngeal structure are associated with alterations in phonatory function such as reduction in glottal resistance (66). Glottal resistance, a measure of laryngeal valving efficiency, highlights the interdependence of the phonatory and respiratory systems. For example, glottal resistance might have been used by older adults to compensate for the effects of reduced respiratory support. With reduced glottal resistance superimposed upon diminished respiratory efficiency, older adults have fewer intact compensatory mechanisms available to overcome reduced efficiency.

Supralaryngeal Mechanism

Supralaryngeal structures of resonation are affected by the normal aging process. Longitudinal research shows a continued growth of the cranial-facial complex throughout life (61, 62). In addition, the larynx is lower in older adults (82). This results in a longer vocal tract (40), and subsequent changes occur to the resonating characteristics of the speech system. The potency of valving between and within resonating cavities is also modified by changes in muscle tonus and sensory innervation which affect all systems with advanced age. For example, general weakening and atrophy of muscles in the body is also present in the muscles which control the velopharyngeal mechanism in including or excluding the nasal cavities from the speech tract. The dimensions of the pharyngeal passages are altered, and the elasticity of the pharyngeal walls is reduced; these changes result in modification of the mechanism's resonating characteristics (see ref. 66). In addition, sensory innervation of the pharynx is reduced (42). Although sensory reduction does not directly affect physical structure, subtle changes in control may be related to reduction in sensory feedback.

The speech articulators are also subject to anatomic alterations with advanced age. By age 65, approximately 50% of Americans have lost their teeth (93); reduction in the bony structure of the oral cavity and gum retraction are also common (120). Changes in the size and shape of the oral cavity make estimation of tongue size difficult. While it does not appear that overall tongue size is significantly reduced (68), tonus and mass of the lingual muscles appear to be reduced with advanced age (30). There is some evidence that tongue thickness at rest is significantly less than that found in young adults (124).

Dysfunction of the suspensory muscle of the tongue is more prevalent in older men (7), and circumoral muscles may be less effective with age. These dysfunctions have been related to speech alterations as well as bite injury, regurgitation, choking, and drooling. In addition, the oral mucosa are thinner with less firm attachment to underlying structures (127). A decrease in salivary secretions has also been reported in older adults (68), although "dry mouth" is more often associated with disease or the side effects of medications (6).

Sensory discrimination within the oral cavity is generally reduced with advancing age (34). Oral form discrimination is significantly reduced in subjects over 70 years of age, and reductions in pressure, touch, and vibratory discrimination in the oral cavity have been documented (25). Reduced sensitivity results in reduced tactile feedback available to the older speaker (66). Such reductions in feedback may be linked to articulatory imprecision, but substantiating research is not available.

Although changes in oral structures and reductions in sensory perception occur with aging, older adults maintain normal neuromuscular control for swallowing (16). In noninvasive ultrasound imaging of oral functioning for sustained phonemes, differences in direction and extent of tongue displacement for the vowel /a/ occurred but not for /i/ or /k/. Researchers found no evidence that tongue function was affected by age for the static positions assumed by articulators for speech targets (93). Older speakers tended to use a more central placement, less anterior for /i/ and less posterior for /k/. This centralized placement may be perceived as imprecise articulation. More sensitive measures of continuous overlapping articulatory movements in continuous speech have yet to be examined.

Summary

Anatomic and physiological changes occur with normal aging. Such changes as muscle atrophy, reduction in muscle strength, and loss of elasticity affect respiratory support, laryngeal phonation, supralaryngeal movement, and the resonatory characteristics of the speech tract. These changes may be sufficient to alter the acoustic characteristics of the speaking voice, but studies directly linking anatomic changes and acoustic measures of older speech have not been attempted. Since the speech mechanism consists of a complex, interconnecting system, simple cause-effect relationships between minimal structural changes and subtle acoustic alterations are infrequent. At present, we can simply suggest that the total concatenation of anatomic changes due to advancing age produces identifiable older speech patterns. The next section describes the characteristic speech patterns of normal older adults.

Acoustic Characteristics of Older Adult Speech

Listeners use acoustic characteristics of speech to estimate a speaker's age. Listening to connected speech samples, judges differentiated young adult from older adult speakers 99% of the time and differentiated young and old speakers 78% of the time based on only sustained vowel productions (104). In assigning speakers to perceived age decades, judges provided correct estimates of age decade for 51.7% of White females and 50.0% of White males but were less accurate in estimating age decade for Black speakers (137).

In several studies, a person's physical condition had a stronger affect on vocal characteristics than did chronological age (106, 107). Thus, the voice of a middle-aged adult in poor health may be perceived as older than the voice of a "senior citizen" in excellent physical condition. The issue of physical condition aside, listeners generally are able to estimate age from voice samples. A strong correlation exists between perceived age and chronological age (113, 118). Listener ability to estimate age from voice samples depends upon general vocal characteristics which differentiate older speakers from young adult speakers. The typical acoustic characteristics of older speech follow.

Respiratory-Related Vocal Changes

The components of the speech production system are highly interactive, with the interconnection between the respiratory and phonatory systems particularly close. This close interconnection is apparent in the acoustic tasks designed to evaluate respiratory support for speech productions. For instance, maximum phonation time and loudness of voice involve components of both the respiratory and phonation systems. This section of the chapter will arbitrarily examine these two acoustic parameters (maximum phonation time and intensity/loudness measures).

Normal exhalation for speech primarily involves the passive forces of elasticity and recoil as the muscles of respiration control the gradual expiration of air from the lungs. Expelled air passes through the laryngeal structure, which acts as a valve and may provide resistance to the air flow. Such resistance at the laryngeal level supplements respiratory control efforts. As a result, the respiratory and laryngeal mechanisms are inseparably involved in the control of air flow for maximum length of phonation.

Maximum phonation time, affected by aging changes in both respiratory support and laryngeal efficiency, is reduced in older speakers. The ability to sustain vowels is significantly reduced in older speakers, with reductions up to 26% reported when older adults' vowel durations are compared with those of young adults (73, 105). The task of maximum phonation time taxes the limits of the speaking system. Consequently, reduced vital capacity associated with age affects the older adults' ability to perform this task.

The interdependency of respiratory and phonatory functioning also affects vocal intensity and resulting measures of perceived vocal loudness. Reduction of perceived loudness is often cited as a characteristic of older speakers (82). In perceptual investigations, judges indicated that reduced loudness discriminated older and younger voices (104) and that voices of older female speakers were significantly less loud compared to voices of older males or young adult speakers (10). Although reduced loudness was often a perceived characteristic of the older voice, reduced loudness was not found in the majority of elderly voices (137).

Objective confirmation of reduced loudness in older speaking voices has been inconsistent. Both maximum intraoral pressure and vowel intensity in decibels were significantly reduced in a speech task performed by older male and female speakers (105). In contrast, significant increases in vocal intensity differentiated male readers over age 70 from males of younger age groups on reading and impromptu speaking tasks (111). Differences in tasks may explain the contradictory results of these two studies,

but additional investigations into this aspect of older adult speech are necessary.

Phonatory Alterations

The frequency or pitch component of the older adult phonatory system has been most extensively studied. Trained listeners perceived lower pitch in the voices of older male speakers (50), and 7 of 10 judges identified lower pitch as an important vocal characteristic for differentiating older from younger speakers (104). In a more recent study, judges rated 63% of older adult voices as displaying normal pitch levels, with 23% judged as lower than normal and 13% as higher than normal (137). While lower pitch suggests an older speaker, not all older speakers exhibit lower pitch.

Although fundamental frequency of male voices was positively correlated with age (57), in most studies the relationship between perceived pitch and objective measures of fundamental frequency was often only of moderate strength. Other vocal quality factors may have contaminated perceptual ratings of pitch (9, 88, 137). These contaminating factors may explain the discrepancy between the perception of lower pitch in older speakers and the objective measurement of higher fundamental frequency in older male voices.

Objective measurement of speaking frequency has generally shown an increase in fundamental frequency with age for males (55, 90), but age changes in fundamental frequency of the female voice are less clear. Studies have indicated a slight lowering of fundamental frequency (40, 46, 116) or no significant change in fundamental frequency with age (11, 26, 85). Differences in task, control of concomitant speaker factors, and methods of measurement may have contributed to discrepant research findings. Obviously, any frequency changes in the older female voice are less extensive than those occurring in the older male voice.

Perceived phonatory characteristics of the older voice are not limited to pitch. Hoarseness was also perceived as a characteristic used to identify older male voices (2, 50, 104). However, in a separate study, only 27% of older voices were judged as hoarse or harsh with 67% of older speakers rated as using normal voices (137). Slight hoarseness in the voices of 20 older women with a mean age of 75 years was perceived by a panel of laryngologists and speech-language pathologists, but hoarseness was not perceived in older male voices (56). The pervasiveness of slight hoarseness in older voices is greater than expected in a younger population, but severe hoarseness is not characteristic of normal older speakers.

Spectral noise component and fundamental frequency fluctuations have been used as objective measurements of hoarseness (63). The spectral noise component in hoarseness is based on noise in formants 1 and 2 and high frequency noise (143). Fundamental frequency perturbation, a measure of fluctuations in adjacent cycles of vocal fold vibration, is the result of changes in the structure or mass of the vocal folds (79). In addition, variation in the amplitude of vocal fold vibrations has also been associated with hoarseness (31).

Although few studies of the spectral noise characteristics of older adult voices are available, spectral noise in vowels appears to be associated with the physical condition of the speaker rather than with chronological age (106). Compared to the literature on spectral noise, research examining variations in vocal fold vibration is extensive. Greater absolute fundamental frequency perturbation (139) and a significantly greater percent of perturbation (11) distinguished older voices from young adult voices. These objectively measured acoustic changes in older voices may contribute to the slight hoarseness perceived in the voices of certain older speakers.

In an extensive study of three age groups of speakers in good or poor physical condition, Ramig and Ringel found an increased percent of jitter associated with the physical condition of the speaker (107). Although a condition-age interaction was not significant, the greatest amount of jitter (fundamental frequency perturbation) was produced by the older adult speakers who were in poor physical condition. Amplitude variation (shimmer) was not significantly greater in speakers in poor physical condition. The Ramig-Ringel study highlights the need to evaluate the physical condition of the speaker rather than rely solely on chronological age. Differences in the physical condition of the subjects may be a significant factor contributing to the diversity of research findings and the high degree of individual differences found in older adult groups.

Other measures of fundamental frequency variation include an age-related change in pitch sigma or in standard deviation. Several studies identified a tendency for greater flexibility and an increase in the total frequency range of older male speakers (90, 91), with frequency stability decreasing with age (80). On the other hand, McGlone and Hollien found a slight decrease in pitch variability in older female speakers (54). In a rare longitudinal study, Endres and associates studied six speakers over a period of up to 20 years and reported that speakers lose their ability to vary fundamental frequency with increasing age (40).

Although the fundamental frequency range of older adults is restricted when compared to that of younger speakers (2, 19, 40, 105), Ramig and Ringel found that physical condition, rather than age, remained the critical factor (107). Although their physical condition/age interaction was not statistically significant, advanced age and poor physical condition tended to be associated with the greatest restriction of maximum frequency range. Since older adults as a group may include a greater number of individuals in poor physical condition, restriction of maximum frequency range is expected in unselected groups of older adults. The preceding factors were likely to have influenced early studies (2, 19, 40, 105).

Intonation, a prosodic feature of voice sensitive to nuances of emotion and semantics, is controlled at the laryngeal level. Intonational change in speaking and reading is not necessarily affected by reported reductions in total or maximum available frequency range. Studies indicate that older adults use a greater number of inflections than do young adult speakers. For example, older female speakers show an increase in the number of downward inflections (26). In a reading task, both older female and male speakers used a greater number of both upward and downward inflections, increased maximum inflectional change, and increased intonational ranges (10). Greater numbers of inflections and larger inflectional changes in reading tasks may be attributed to age-related physiological changes indicative of a reduction in neuromuscular control or, more likely, they may be associated with oral reading style differences due to age cohort effects.

Other phonatory characteristics have been identified through perceptual studies. Older sounding male and female voices were perceived as possessing laryngeal tension (74, 112) with older male voices displaying hypovalving and older female voices displaying hypervalving (9). These perceptual characteristics may be somewhat supported by changes in air volume use in the production of vowels and consonants (10). Reduction in air expenditure involves more than the phonatory component; complex interactions of the respiratory, phonatory, and, to some extent, articulatory systems are involved.

In summary, evidence of change in the phonatory component of older adult speech is available. Laryngeal functioning is sensitive to rather subtle changes in laryngeal structure, and these changes are reflected in alterations to the acoustic signal. Phonatory function is also highly sensitive to the physical condition of the speaker. Since changes in physical condition may be more common in older than younger adults, poorer physical condition may account for phonatory changes typically found in older speakers.

Resonance Changes

Few studies have explored the resonation characteristics of older adult voices, although Sedlackova and associates (cited in ref. 52) considered the "hollow" voice as the most common indicator of old age. Physiological changes in the resonating cavities due to atrophy of muscles, growth of the cranial-facial skeleton, and mucosa alterations may be responsible for this perception.

Another resonance characteristic to be considered is nasality. Objective measures of the sound pressure level ratio of nasal and nasal/oral scores indicated higher levels of nasalance in older readers (60). These alterations were weakly reflective of nasality associated with different types of velopharyngeal incompetency. Although the objective measure of nasalance was higher in older voices, nasality in nonpathological older speakers was not perceived as excessive (9).

Articulatory Modifications

The articulatory dimension of speech involves movement of supralaryngeal structures to produce acoustic signals which listeners hear as speech. Two particular dimensions of articulation, articulatory precision and rate of production, may be sensitive to advanced age. Each dimension has been investigated through different research paradigms.

Older speakers are considered less adept in articulating speech (33) than are young adults. Imprecise consonants were identified as a significant factor in prediction of age in male voices (65), and imprecise articulation was perceived as descriptive of older male voices in several investigations (2, 10, 50, 74). However, in a separate study, 74% of older speakers were judged normal in articulatory precision (137). The authors concluded that articulatory precision was not a significant problem for the normally aging population. Older female speakers have not been identified as producing imprecise articulation and may be more likely to use precisely articulated speech (10). In summary, perceived articulatory imprecision is not necessarily a consequence of normal aging but

may be sensitive to associated factors such as sex, dialectal variation, attitude, and training.

Objective measures of articulatory precision include acoustic factors which reflect movement of the articulators. Researchers have measured the acoustic dimensions of formant structure, vowel transition, and a laryngeally controlled articulatory dimension, voice onset time.

A longitudinal study determined a progressive decrease in the first formant of vowels which was attributed to progressive lengthening of the vocal tract with age (40). A cross-sectional study of 75 women in young adult, middle-aged and older adult groups also supported a significant decrease in the frequency of first formants (80), but significance was not attained in another cross-sectional study (34). The lowering of the larynx with age (18) and the increase in cranial-facial dimensions (61, 62) provide a convenient explanation for changes in formant frequency with age.

A tendency for greater dispersal of vowel formant ratios suggests increased variability in older speaker's vowel productions (12). In an investigation of repeated syllables, productions of older adult speakers showed greater variability in timing of adjacent syllables and on syllable amplitude measures (3). Less stability and control of repeated articulatory movements may be characteristic of older adult speech. These findings may be reflective of neurological changes and support Ryan and Burk's suggestion that older adult speech falls on a dysarthric-normal continuum (112).

Although voice onset time in single word tasks did not vary significantly with age (92, 128), separation between voiced and voiceless cognates decreased (12, 128). Some older adults used significantly shorter voice onset times in certain contexts (92), which may explain the significantly reduced voice onset times reported in one study (12). The reduced separation of voice onset times in cognates may contribute to perceptions of imprecise articulation in older speech.

In the speech productions of 65- to 84-year-old males, vowel transitions were reduced, and changes in plosive closure duration indicated the use of increased effort to produce the tense, voiceless cognate /t/ (34). A longer silent interval in plosives was supported in another study using a slightly different procedure (12). These subtle changes in the acoustic dimensions of articulated speech may be indicative of alterations in timing of motor movements by older adults. The result is not disordered speech but may contribute to subjective impressions of imprecise articulation in certain older speakers.

Voice onset time, length of transition, and duration of silent interval are measures of speed on a subphonemic level which alter the articulatory characteristics of speech. Slow rate of articulation has contributed to the perception of age in voice (112). A reduced speech rate had been identified by judges as indicative of age (50, 104), and 22% of 62 older speakers were rated as slower than normal in speaking rate (137).

Objective indices of slow speaking rate include maximum speed on diadochokinetic tasks as well as measures of speech rate during speaking or reading. The ability to produce rapid alternating movements during a diadochokinetic task was reduced in older speaking groups (3, 104), with only one study not obtaining statistically significant results (73). Reading rate was generally reduced with advanced age, with 32 to 62 year old speakers producing 172 words per minute, 65 to 79 year olds producing 138 words per minute, and 80 to 92 year old subjects producing 124 words per minute (90). Other determinants of speaking rate, such as educational level, visual acuity, and physical well-being have been considered in examining the speaking rate of older adults (137).

Objective measures of reduced speaking rates support the perception of slowness in the speech of older adults. General reduction in reaction time and speed of motion is reflected, to some extent, in the speech characteristics exhibited by older individuals. These changes may subtly alter the speaking characteristics of the older adult, but they do not result in extreme deviations such as phonemic substitutions.

Summary

Neurological, anatomic, and physiological changes occur with normal aging. These changes result in specific acoustic characteristics listeners identify as the older-sounding voice. To a great extent, the physical condition of the speaker influences listener estimation of speaker age based on voice. Since advancing age and poor physical condition are often associated, these factors interact to create the stereotypical older voice. It is often this image that is employed by judges when estimating speaker age from voice samples.

When the speech system is taxed, differences between older and young adult abilities are apparent. Although older adults have reduced vital capacities and cannot sustain a vowel as long as a young adult can, these differences need not be apparent in everyday communication.

The phonatory aspects of speech have been
most extensively studied in older adults. In general, the pitch of older male speakers rises, but pitch changes in older female speakers are less clear. There are indications of hoarseness due to increased jitter in older male voices, but the physical condition of the speaker is paramount. An older adult in good condition should not present a hoarse voice. Hoarseness is diagnostically significant and must not be dismissed as indicative of old age. In addition, normal older adults use a greater number of inflections and greater maximum inflections. Changes in inflection are also diagnostically significant, since adults with laryngeal pathologies produce reduced maximum inflections (51).

Although articulatory precision is not reduced in all older speakers, older males are often judged as producing imprecise articulation. Subtle alterations in articulatory timing may account for perception of imprecise articulation by certain older speakers. Such changes have suggested a neurological basis similar to dysarthria.

The changes described in the first half of this chapter deal only with the speech mode. Although these age-related speech changes subtly influence the delivery of the communicated message, the linguistic component of the message is also affected. The next section of the chapter examines important changes in the linguistic dimension of communication.

LINGUISTIC CHARACTERISTICS OF NORMAL AGING

This second half of the chapter examines changes in linguistic functioning which occur with advancing age. First, changes in the neurological basis of language are outlined. The complex relationships among cognitive functioning, memory, and language are important, since changes in both cognitive style and memory efficiency are often examined through linguistic tasks. The impact of these complex interrrelationships on everyday linguistic behavior is more subtle. The second part of the section explores changes in each of five parameters of language in detail.

Changes Related to Linguistic Functioning

Specific neurological changes which accompany aging may affect the linguistic productions of older persons. Brain weight decreases 11% between the ages of 25 and 96 years (4). Decline in neuronal density in the cerebral cortex is most extensive in the superior temporal gyrus and involves the precentral gyrus area, striata, and postcentral gyrus (22). These areas of the brain are primarily involved with speech and language abilities and changes are reflected in correlate changes in speech production and linguistic behavior.

In addition to a reduction in brain weight, changes in older brains include atrophy of dendrite length and reduction in the number of dendrite spines and branches. Subtle changes also occur in the biochemical dimension, with certain substances accumulating in neural tissue. While possible reductions in neurotransmitter metabolism, brain lipid content, and myelin may be associated with advanced age, extensive reductions are necessary before pathologies are observed (see ref. 117). Neuronal cell loss, neuritic plaque, and neurofibrillary tangles affect the hippocampal formation and are particularly widespread in older adults (see refs. 69 and 131). Neurofibrillary tangles, granulovacuolar changes, and neuritic plaque are present in the brains of intact aged persons, but extensive increases are necessary before a neuropathological condition such as dementia is evident (see refs. 69, 99, and 134). However, normal changes do occur in those neural areas involved in linguistic production or in the related abilities of cognitive function and memory.

Changes in cognitive style and memory can be reflected in linguistic alterations. Differences in cognitive functioning may be subtle, and the impact on language may be seen primarily in strategies used to decode messages, formulate associations, and select topics selected for expression. Memory is also critical for language use. The older adult must remember what has been said to participate effectively in communication situations. Factors such as attention, perceptual saliency, and relevance affect the establishment of memories and can be manipulated to facilitate reception of messages.

Numerous studies investigating cognitive functioning and memory in older individuals have identified changes in these basic processes which may be reflected in language comprehension and production of older individuals (29, 102, 119, 141). Age cohort effects, large individual differences among older adults, and a need for valid assessment of cognitive function across the life span have been demonstrated. Plasticity of intellectual ability, ability to perform at higher levels with practice or training, and increasing ability to synthesize and integrate information with advancing age are

supported by qualitative interpretations of the cognitive abilities of older adults (141).

Cognitive competence in older adults remains intact if sufficient time is provided in assessment tasks. Slowing of response and reaction time in older adults has been established, with estimates of 11 to 12% reduction, depending on the task, age, and the health of subjects (see refs. 14, 15, 53, and 114). These changes in speed have been associated with both peripheral and central nervous system processing (141). Longer latency and slower decision making may affect testing, but impact on daily functioning has not been proven.

Sensory memory (which is necessary for brief storage of information) and primary memory (which involves a small capacity for control and assimilation of information) are relatively unaffected by aging (101). Secondary memory, which involves greater length of retention, is modified in older adults. The processes of learning new information and retrieving it, vital to the establishment of secondary memory, are affected. Older adults can benefit from relevant memory enhancement strategies but are less likely to spontaneously generate and utilize mnemonic devices (44, 108). Reduced memory for longer discourse segments may affect comprehension skills for detail and verbatim recall, but use of this memory is sensitive to the person's familiarity with the material, to attention-directing instructions, and to personal organizational strategies. Older adults report increased memory failures, are overly sensitive to memory failures, and rely on memory aids in everyday situations (see ref. 101).

The relationship of changes in cognitive and memory processing to linguistic changes in older adults is difficult to establish due to limitations in current experimental design (see ref. 133). High correlations between poor language performance and poor performance on learning and memory tests support the interrelationship of cognition and memory with language. Demonstration of interactive change is critical since these processes are basic to successful communication (39).

This brief summary of changes in cognitive functioning and memory provides a basis for examining linguistic change. The remainder of this chapter explores typical changes in older adults' linguistic behaviors.

Direct Changes in Language Comprehension and Expression

Linguistic changes are examined by focusing on each of five commonly defined parameters of language: phonology, morphology, syntax, semantics, and pragmatics. Arbitrary decisions to include certain topics within particular parameters have been made, since the interrelationships among these five linguistic domains are extensive.

The Phonological Parameter

The phonological parameter is not limited to production of speech sounds but may also include perception of phonemes. Changes in the hearing mechanism (see ref. 32 and 98) result in a reduction of hearing acuity in groups of older adults (77, 110) which may affect phonemic perception (see Chapter 8 for a detailed examination of hearing ability in older adults). Speech discrimination in older adults is poorer than predicted by pure tone thresholds (32, 43), and competing noise, reverberation, and time compression have an adverse affect on the speech discrimination abilities of older adults (84, 96, 138). Few studies other than those involved with speech discrimination and the verbal transformation phenomenon (see refs. 27, 97) have investigated changes in the phonological parameter of language in the older adult.

Upon examining acoustic differences between older and young adult speech, researchers have attributed these differences to performance variables (12) rather than to changes in phonology. The underlying phonological competency of normal older adults between the ages of 68 and 82 years does not appear to deteriorate.

Changes in articulatory characteristics of older male speech appear to indicate deterioration of control, yet older female speakers are perceived as articulating with normal precision. Since a purely physiological explanation for differences in articulatory performance between older male and female speakers has proved to be insufficient, an explanation involving phonological use was developed (10). Female speakers generally use a more prestigious, more carefully articulated phonological variant than do males (121). The interaction of this more prestigious phonological variant with the inevitable physiological changes occurring with advanced age may provide a more complete explanation of the speech characteristics of older females. Older female speakers compensate for changes in speech by increasing laryngeal and articulatory muscle tension and adopting more carefully enunciated speech.

Our understanding of phonological changes with age is limited. Possible changes are obscured by performance factors which affect both comprehension and peformance.

The Morphological Parameter

There is a paucity of research on the use of morphemes by aged speakers. In an evaluation of grammatical form use, Kynette and Kemper found a reduction in percentage of correct tense morphemes with advanced age in samples of 50 consecutive utterances during interviews with older adults (75). With statistical removal of education and employment effects, age was significantly correlated with fewer different verb tenses used, fewer different grammatical forms, and reduced percentage of forms used correctly.

The Syntactic Parameter

The syntactic parameter has been more thoroughly investigated than have the previous linguistic parameters. Although different measurement indices have been used, qualitative changes in the syntactic behaviors of older adults do not appear sufficiently detrimental to adversely affect communication in daily life.

In comprehending syntax, older adults do not exhibit a decline in understanding of words or simple sentences. Although an early study did not find age differences in comprehension of syntactically complex sentences (135), more recent investigations have reported age-related reductions in comprehension of center-embedded and right-branching relative clauses (41) and later-developing syntactic structures (39). Such age-related reductions in comprehension of the syntactic component of the message may be affected by differences in attention, memory, education, and vocabulary levels. There is also evidence to suggest that middle-aged and older listeners, although they performed less well on comprehension tasks, utilized grammatical redundancy more frequently than did young adults (45). While older adults demonstrate reduced comprehension for complex syntactical forms in artificial tasks of linguistic ability, the affect of age-related changes in this parameter on daily communication is presumed to be minor.

In syntactic production, particular grammatical indices are more highly dependent upon semantic and pragmatic parameters. Thus, observed changes may be attributed to cognitive processes, semantic organization, or pragmatic sensitivity rather than changes in syntactic ability. For instance, older speakers have been found to produce a significantly greater number of ambiguous references and to use significantly less lexical variety in noun choice (133). Compared with middle-aged adults, older speakers used a similar proportion of pronouns in constructing simple narratives but produced significantly greater proportions of pronouns in complex narratives and self-generated narratives. These syntactic measures which depend upon semantic and pragmatic effectiveness demonstrated a decline with advanced age.

Linguistic performance of normal elderly adults between the ages of 75 and 93 was compared with that of young adults between 30 and 42 (39). Statistical analysis indicated an inverse relationship between syntactic performance and age. Errors were produced on complex prepositions, passive and possessive relations in reversible constructions, changes in subject-verb-object order, and other complex syntactic constructions heavily dependent on semantics.

In an investigation of spontaneous speech in an informal conversational interview, active, healthy 70- to 80-year-old adults used right-embeddings to preserve sentence length but did not produce high memory structures such as multiple embeddings, subordinate clauses, or participle subrelative clauses as frequently as did 50 to 60-year-old speakers (75). Most grammatical forms were used by both groups, with more frequent errors and less complex structures occurring in the speech of older adults. In an investigation of question strategies used in conversation, older speakers produced a greater number of tag questions and fewer intonated declarative form questions than did younger speakers (13).

The T-unit analysis, a measure of grammatical complexity, was used to analyze an uninterrupted 75-word sample of conversation from 62 subjects over 60 years of age (137). In contrast to previous research, the investigators found a significant reduction in the mean number of words in grammatically correct conversation. The number of clauses per T-unit and the number of words per clause did not attain statistical significance. Consequently, older adults' use of complex grammatical embedding did not increase with advanced age (137).

These findings are at odds with studies of the written discourse of older individuals. Obler et al (cited in ref. 96) found that healthy 60-year-olds used a greater number of words in written descriptions of action pictures than did 50-year-old subjects. The older group used a greater number of embedded sentences, used modified nouns more often, and used a higher verb-to-noun ratio. In a longitudinal study, analyses of 56 years of Emerson's written journal (cited in ref. 52) also supported the premise that verb-adjective ratios increase with increased age.

In conclusion, changes in the syntactic parameter of language occur with aging. Although a relationship between syntactic complexity and/or errors and communicative effectiveness may be posited, the impact of such syntactic alterations on the accuracy and effectiveness of daily communications has yet to be demonstrated. Nonetheless, several syntactic modifications commonly present in older adult speech suggest that the semantic component is sensitive to aging changes.

The Semantic Parameter

Changes in semantic memory, cognitive style, and speed of processing with advanced age interact to alter the semantic parameter of language. In this section, the semantic parameter is explored through studies of word associations, categorization abilities, and vocabulary retrieval. Factors contributing to differences in semantic usage are noted.

Episodic memory, which utilizes temporal or contextual information in encoding and retrieval, has been studied most extensively (see ref. 119). Evidence suggests that older adults encode new information with less elaboration, imagery, and organization (45, 101, 108, 141). This shallow encoding contributes to deficits in retrieving information from memory and may influence performance on certain linguistic tasks.

Semantic memory, organized by concept or semantic meaning, is modified with advancing age. For instance, associative processes, which are considered a reflection of the development of semantic categorization, change throughout the life span. Young children tend to use syntagmatic responses in which an attribute, relation, or other part of speech is associated with a noun. In contrast, older children and young adults demonstrate categorical associations through in-class or paradigmatic responses. In one study, older adults primarily used paradigmatic associations but produced a greater number of syntagmatic responses than middle-aged subjects (109). For example, the older subjects associated a verb with a concrete noun stimuli more often than other adult speakers (e.g., the stimulus "dog" might as readily elicit a syntagmatic response of "barking" as a paradigmatic response of "cat"). In addition, the same investigation found that older subjects tended to produce more idiosyncratic associations than did other adults.

Older adults also created fewer categories in free picture categorization tasks (70, 72). Using strategies similar to those used by young adults, older subjects primarily implemented categorical-inferential strategies, those strategies which are similar to paradigmatic associations. Older adults also used relational-thematic strategies about 25% of the time, compared to those young adults who used these strategies 13% of the time. Lovelace and Cooley did not find a significant relationship between syntagmatic associations and age (81) and suggested that this association ability may be more sensitive to vocabulary than age. Other factors, such as the individual's life-style, daily demands made on cognitive function, and personal cognitive style, may contribute to performance on associative tasks.

Subtle alterations of semantic memory have been reflected in a shift toward more syntagmatic and idiosyncratic associations (35), but the underlying semantic meaning of words appears to remain intact in older adults (21, 114). The ability to find a word in semantic memory was, to a great extent, preserved in older subjects (76).

Passive vocabulary which reflects lifelong learning of word meanings has been reported to be maintained or increased with age (21). However, active use of learned vocabulary was more susceptible to changes with advanced age in two studies (39, 101). Older adults were 42% slower than young adults in accessing categorical information; this suggests slower semantic assessment speed (100). Although significant changes in confrontational naming did not occur with age, response time increased (130), and more errors were made (20). Familiarity with the objects to be named resulted in a nonsignificant difference in latency (102). Thus familiarity must be considered in timing of naming tasks. On word retrieval tasks, the benefits that older speakers derived from phonemic cueing, production of associated in-class words, and use of circumlocution suggested that disassociation of word and concept does not occur (47). Although certain vocabulary skills were maintained or improved with advancing age, elderly individuals complained that they forgot more words as they became older (96).

On divergent retrieval tasks in which the speaker is asked to generate as many words as possible in a specified category, word fluency was reduced with advanced age (58, 125). However, the impact of slower reaction time on performance of this task must be considered. Since analysis of conversational speech resulted in significantly higher type-token ratios for aged adult speakers, compared with those of young adults (137), a more varied vocabulary usage in spontaneous speech may occur with age.

Verification of meaning in short paragraphs was reduced in older subjects only if a delay was imposed between the reading and verification tasks (8). In one study, older adults were less likely to recall auditorially presented materials (28), but this deficit was not observed with educated subjects in other investigations (86). Although both young and older adults differed in the precision of retained semantic content, both groups integrated abstract linguistic information into holistic ideas (136).

In summary, literature on the semantic component reflects changes in memory, word associations, and reaction time. Recognition of vocabulary and acquisition of vocabulary meaning does not decrease with advanced age (24), but quick word retrieval in both divergent and confrontational naming tasks is diminished.

The Pragmatic Parameter

The pragmatic parameter involves the use and alteration of linguistic behavior to communicate with others. Older adults effectively adapt messages and interact with others while adjusting to and compensating for changes in sensory acuity, reaction time, and central processing. Memory and cognitive style contribute to the selection of pragmatic strategies and changes in memory and cognition may be reflected in the pragmatic strategies used by older adults.

Few studies of older adult communication have specifically investigated traditional pragmatic behaviors such as requesting, protesting, commenting, greeting, etc. Investigation of these pragmatic functions evolved as supplementary considerations to analysis of older speakers' discourse. In this section, the topics of structural organization of larger discourse units and question strategies are seen as transcending classification as indices of pragmatic, syntactic, or semantic parameters. Consequently, these activities are arbitrarily examined in the larger context of pragmatics. Conversational regulators, topic selection and maintenance, and sensitivity to the communication partner are also considered as essential aspects of the pragmatic parameter.

The pragmatic parameter is sensitive to changes in memory and related cognitive processes. Possible differences in sensory deficits, educational level, cognitive considerations, and past experience result in greater linguistic variability in normal healthy older adults (1, 115). In addition, language usage is sensitive to age cohort effects and reflects social identification. Slang use and phonetic realization are often frozen during the 20- to 30-year age decade. Thus, they reflect age group identification and serve to distinguish groups by age-related vocabulary use (23).

First, in our exploration of pragmatics, we will consider the effects of memory and organizational strategies on the recall and retelling of narrative discourse. Studies of memory beyond the word or sentence level have focused primarily on the number of recalled story ideas, with older adults recalling fewer facts and ideas than did young adults (28, 48, 122). This reduced ability to recall orally presented material may arise from deficits at the time of acquisition of information during retention, since even recognition of the material was somewhat reduced (see ref. 29). For example, although a statistically significant difference in total prose recall was not found, older subjects in one study demonstrated differences in organization of material to be recalled (86). When using recall strategies, older adults also used more additions and distortions which may be reflective of organizational differences (122).

An investigation of linguistic production in three tasks (conversing, describing sequential procedures for daily tasks, and retelling narratives) found differences in the amount and type of information included in older speakers' discourse (133). Structural disorganization of material was reflected in reduced ratings of clarity and situational relevance of language in conversation, in fewer essential steps and less information conveyed in the sequenced procedure task, and in failure to provide setting information for narrative tasks. Lack of referential specificity, measured by inflated pronoun use and unwarranted presuppositions concerning setting information, contributed to perceived reduction of discourse effectiveness by elderly speakers. Older speakers answered fewer probe questions, more frequently failed to produce acceptable summaries, and took twice as long to produce a moral (133). In another investigation of discourse productivity, older adults produced fewer content units per minute than did young adults (144). In general, a progressive decrease of discourse effectiveness occurs with advanced age. Although both syntactic and semantic parameters are involved, pragmatic effectiveness is affected.

Questioning strategies also have an effect on the pragmatic parameter. Older adults are less efficient in their questioning strategies than are younger speakers. In a 20-question-type task, older adults used a greater number of hypothesis-testing questions, yet used fewer constraint-seeking questions which are useful in the elimination and identification of categories (37). Discourse analysis of conversations between married couples showed that older adults used a greater number of information-seeking questions than clarification questions, and that older adults used more expanded responses to informational questions and a greater number of minimal responses to clarification questions than do younger adults (13). Questioning skills of older adults reflect alterations in cognitive strategy and less complex questioning styles.

Such differences in recall, sustained verbal production tasks, or questioning strategies do not necessarily reflect older persons' pragmatic functioning in everyday situations. In conversations between previously unacquainted older adult dyads, use of conversational regulators remained intact. Turn-taking was orderly and precisely timed, with older speakers more adept at "latching" conversational turns one upon another without pause than were younger adults (17). Turn-taking was smooth and precise with no temporal gap occurring between 22% of speaking turns of older adults, compared with 15.2% precision placement or latching of conversational turns by college students. Even in nursing home settings, normal older adults switched and maintained conversational topics appropriately and followed turn-taking rules (59). Assertions were the primary speech act used in the nursing home setting (59).

Older adults used common experiences and events from the past to further their conversational discourse (17) with skillful juxtaposition of past and present providing multiple levels for association (18). Older persons were also skillful at integrating an element from the previous speaker's statement into the turn-taking sequence in order to shift topic. Thus, older speakers have greater topic resources available for conversational maintenance and topic change. The appropriate use of rich topic association enriches conversations (18), but inappropriate use may account for descriptions of older speaker's discourse as rambling.

Adaptation and sensitivity to the communication partner is central to the pragmatic parameter. Although early studies suggested that older adults were more dogmatic and less sensitive to the reactions of others, current research does not support a hypothesis of increased egocentricity with advanced age. Active older adults perceived others in complex terms and were adept at interpreting motives from subtle communications tactics (see ref. 94). For instance, 64- to 78-year-old speakers used different linguistic strategies to accommodate to different-aged listeners (87). With younger listeners, older speakers used fewer utterances, repetitions, and start overs. When speaking to older age peers, older adults used a greater number of and longer utterances. Such adaptations made by older speakers may reflect expectations based on age stereotypes or may be due to sensitivity to subtle feedback cues.

Fluency, a performance characteristic, affects the flow of discourse. Disfluency may be the result of motor speech disturbances, may reflect transient cognitive dysfunction such as word retrieval difficulty, or may indicate spontaneous discourse revision. Adapting to the communication partner through sentence revision suggests sensitivity to the pragmatic parameter of language. Such disfluencies in older adult speech have been arbitrarily classified within the inclusive pragmatic parameter.

Lack of smoothness and increased hesitation were identified as perceptual cues indicating older speech (104). Supporting this perception are studies which found that older adults produced a greater number of disfluencies than high school students (142) and than young adults (137). While 83% of older adults and 65% of younger adults exhibited interjections as the primary disfluency (137), the ratio of interjection to other types of disfluencies was not significantly different (142). In adults, the typical disfluency pattern does not appear to change significantly with age, although only 30% of young adults exhibited revision behavior while 56% of older adults revised their statements (137). These objective measures confirm the perception that older speakers produce less smooth speech.

The quality of discourse is also related to competence in daily life. Older adults who operated in a more demanding environment and engaged in a greater number of activities were judged as more competent (95). Although there existed wide variability between older individuals, Holland found that the accumulation of aging changes affected functional communication in daily life situations. A reduction in assessed performance on *The Communicative Abilities in Daily Living* occurred for normal subjects over the age of 65 years and for normal adults living in an institutional setting (54).

The reduction in communicative effectiveness examined above may reflect both cognitive changes with aging and modifications in the older adult's environment. Cognitive differences associated with aging have been discussed in the second section of this chapter dealing with the semantic parameter. In addition, typical modifications of the environment impact communication through changes in an older adult's social network with the onset of retirement (129). These typical life-style changes gradually result in modification of communication patterns. For instance, efficient transfer of information may become less important than comradery (133). As a result, the elaboration found in certain older adults' discourse may facilitate social interaction and reflect a high level of pragmatic skill.

In summary, older adults were less able to organize information for accurate recall in specific discourse tasks. Structural disorganization was reflected in their linguistic productions as well as in reduced specificity and increased reliance upon presupposed information. Analysis of less structured discourse in informal conversational settings provided more positive information concerning the pragmatic skills of older adults. Older adults excelled in latching conversational turns, used common past experiences for maintenance and change of topic, and were adept at adapting their communication to their communication partner. The pragmatic parameter, though altered, continues to be functional for older adults.

Summary

Linguistic changes with age are sensitive to memory differences, cognitive changes, and environmental necessities. Such factors affect the five linguistic parameters differently.

The phonological and morphological parameters have not been fully investigated. Sensory and performance variables obscure findings related to phonology, and studies of grammatical forms have not been sufficiently detailed to assess free and bound morpheme use directly. The syntactic parameter has been investigated more extensively. Although some reduction in comprehending complex sentences occurs with age, the impact on daily life is presumed to be minimal. Complex syntactic tasks which are dependent upon memory and/ or semantics are most sensitive to aging.

The semantic parameter, sensitive to cognitive style and memory, is affected by aging. Although the meaning of words is not lost with age nor do meanings become disassociated from words, older adults use a greater proportion of syntagmatic and idiosyncratic associations than do young adults. Older adults are highly sensitive to word-finding difficulties and can benefit from word retrieval strategies. They are less adept at quick word retrieval in divergent and convergent naming tasks but demonstrate semantic competence when diminished reaction time does not affect the task.

The pragmatic parameter is important for daily communication activities. Older adults recall fewer facts and produce less informative discourse in certain linguistic tasks. The lack of referential specificity and reliance on presupposed knowledge in these tasks does not appear to affect the older adult's daily communication ability. Investigations of informal conversation suggest that older adults are competent communicators who adapt to listener's needs and have a rich array of experiences to extend and maintain a conversation.

CONCLUSIONS

This chapter has examined changes in speech production and linguistic behavior which occur with age. Neurological changes such as reduced brain weight, decreased neural complexity, and increased neurofibrillary tangles and neuritic plaque affect motor speech production and linguistic behavior. Anatomic and physiological changes, as they become more extensive, are reflected in the speech characteristics of older adults.

Reduced vital capacity in older adults is one of the most stable findings in the gerontological literature. Reductions in expiratory measures such as maximum phonation time are common. Calcification or ossification, atrophy and reduced muscle strength, and loss of elasticity affect the functioning of the larynx. These changes commonly affect the older male voice by raising the fundamental frequency. Changes in the pitch characteristics of older females are more subtle, with slight or nonsignificant decreases in fundamental frequency occurring. Studies investigating the perception and objective measurement of loudness are contradictory. While older voices are often perceived as less loud, studies of objectively measured intensity have been inconsistent.

Other phonatory characteristics depend on vocal fold functioning. Although hoarseness is more prevalent in older speakers and jitter is significantly increased in groups of older adults, the physical condition of the speaker is the most important variable. A greater proportion of older (as compared with younger) adults are in poorer physical condition. This factor may account for previous research findings. Maximum frequency range is also sensitive to physical condition, whereas extent and number of inflections are sensitive to pathological changes and style of reading. Normal older adults use larger and greater numbers of inflections than do young adults and adults with laryngeal pathologies.

Lowering of the larynx with age, growth of the cranial-facial complex throughout life, and changes in muscle tonus affect the resonation characteristics of the speech tract. Although changes in resonation characteristics may be a common indicator of age, few studies have investigated resonance qualities in older adults.

Increases in nasalance, an objective measure of velopharyngeal competence, were not supported by increases in perceived nasality in older voices.

Changes in supralaryngeal functioning are most noticed by older adults and, therefore, are more likely to be under conscious control. Perceived articulatory precision is reduced in certain older male speakers but not in normal older female speakers. Increased variability and reduction in the timing of motor speech occurs with age. Slow rate of speech on diadochokinetic, reading, and speaking tasks also contributes to perception of age in voice.

In addition to such motoric and acoustic differences in older speech, changes in the parameters of language have been investigated. Neurological changes not only affect speech and language functioning but also affect the related processes of memory and cognitive style. Changes in these related processes are reflected in linguistic behavior.

Changes in sensory acuity and performance have obscured investigations of the phonological parameter, but deterioration of phonology does not appear to be age related. Investigation of the morphological parameter has been included within syntactical studies. When tasks involve memory, time, or semantics, syntactical differences occur. Comprehension of complex sentence forms is reduced; greater numbers of errors in producing complex constructions occur; and less complex syntax is spontaneously generated by older speakers (at least in some studies).

Changes in semantics reflect differences in education, attention, memory, and cognitive associations. Passive vocabulary does not decline with age, but differences in active vocabulary occur. Although older adults primarily use paradigmatic associations, they employ a greater proportion of syntagmatic associations, and use a greater proportion of relational-thematic strategies.

The pragmatic parameter is most important for successful communication. Reduced information, lack of referential specificity, and reliance on presupposed knowledge are apparent in discourse generated by older adults. Older adults use a greater number of pronouns, produce fewer content units per minute, and are less efficient in questioning. In actual conversations, older adults demonstrate skills in pragmatic effectiveness. Latched turn-taking in older adult conversations exceeds that of younger adults, and experiences from the past and present provide numerous associations to further or change conversational topic development. Sensitivity to the communication partner, linguistic adaptation, and revision of sentences indicate continued competence in the pragmatic parameter with advancing age.

Focus solely upon older adult behavior in a communicative interaction is misleading when examining the pragmatic parameter. The older adult is only one interactor in the communication situation. The other interactor, whether a young person or a peer, also contributes to the success or failure of communication.

Attitudes, expectations, and stereotypical images may color other communicators' interactions with older adults. Although inconsistent in findings, research has frequently identified negative attitudes toward older adults from naive listeners (10, 126) and from professionals (49, 71, 123). The attitudes of each partner affect his/her own communication behaviors as well as those of the other partner in the communication situation.

For interactors in a communication exchange, perception of age was the most productive aspect in listener attribution of personality characteristics to speakers (5). Older sounding female speakers were perceived as more reserved, inflexible, passive, and "out of it," and older male speakers were judged as inflexible (113). When listener's age and sex were considered, older female speakers were judged most negatively on an activity factor by older female listeners, most negatively on an intelligence-sincerity factor by older male listeners, and most negatively on a femininity factor by young female listeners (10). Young male listeners consistently responded most positively in rating older female voices on personality characteristics (10). These responses to the sound of the older voice have a potential for altering the communicative interaction. Artificial barriers to communication can occur when inappropriate expectations of older adult personality are involved.

Since successful communication depends on active participation of all participants, the contribution of both the older communicator and the other participants in the communicative interaction must be determined. It is tempting to examine the older communicator and the components of communication interactions in isolation, but human communication is a complex, interrelated process which cannot be simply understood. The following chapter explores these and related issues in detail.

References

1. Albert J: Language in normal and dementing elderly. In Obler L, Albert M (eds): *Language and Communication in the Elderly*. Lexington, MA, DC Heath, 1980, p. 145.
2. Amerman JD, Parnell MM: Clinical impressions of the speech of normal adults. Presentation at the American Speech-Language-Hearing Association Convention, San Francisco, 1985.
3. Amerman JD, Parnell MM: Oral motor precision in older adults. *J Natl Stud Speech-Language-Hearing Assoc* 10:56–66, 1982.
4. Appel FW, Appel EM: Intracranial variation in the weight of the human brain. *Hum Biol* 14:48–68, 1942.
5. Bassili JN, Reil JE: On the dominance of the old-age stereotype. *J Gerontol* 36:686–688, 1981.
6. Baum BJ: Normal and abnormal oral status in aging. In Eisdorfer C (ed): *Annual Review of Gerontology and Geriatrics*, vol. 4. New York, Springer Publications, 1984, p. 87.
7. Baum BJ, Boder L: Aging and oral motor function: evidence for altered performance among older persons. *J Dent Res* 62:2–6, 1983.
8. Belmore SM: Age-related changes in processing explicit and implicit language. *J Gerontol* 36:316–322, 1981.
9. Benjamin B: Acoustic, aerodynamic, and perceptual characteristics of geriatric speech. Ph.D. thesis, University Park, PA, The Pennsylvania State University, 1980.
10. Benjamin BJ: Dimensions of the older female voice. *Lang Commun* 6:35–45, 1986.
11. Benjamin BJ: Frequency variability in the aged voice. *J Gerontol* 36:722–726, 1981.
12. Benjamin BJ: Phonological performance in gerontological speech. *J Psycholinguist Res* 11:159–167, 1982.
13. Billens-Ivory S, Brandt JF: Pragmatic and linguistic aspects of spontaneous questions of healthy geriatrics. Presentation at the American Speech-Language-Hearing Association Convention, San Francisco, 1984.
14. Birren J: Toward an experimental psychology of aging. *Am Psychol* 23:124–135, 1970.
15. Birren J, Woods AM, Williams MV: Behavioral slowing with age: causes, organization, and consequences. In Poon LW (ed): *Aging in the 1980's: Psychological Issues*. Washington, DC, American Psychological Association, 1980, p. 293.
16. Blonsky ER, Logemann, JA, Boshes B, Fisher HB: Comparison of speech and swallowing function in patients with tremor disorders and in normal geriatric patients: a cinefluorographic study. *J Gerontol* 30:299–303, 1975.
17. Boden D, Bielby DD: The past as resource: a conversational analysis of elderly talk. *Hum Dev* 26:308–319, 1983.
18. Boden D, Bielby DD: The way it was: topical organization in elderly conversation. *Lang Commun* 6:73–89, 1986.
19. Bohme G, Hecker G: Gerontologische untersuchungen uber stimmumfang and sprechstimmlage. *Folia Phoniatr* 22:176–184, 1970.
20. Borod JC, Goodglass H, Kaplan E: Normative data on the Boston Diagnostic Aphasia Examination, Parietal Lobe Battery, and the Boston

Naming Test. *J Clin Neuropsychol* 2:209–215, 1980.

21. Bowles NL, Poon LW: Aging and retrieval of words in semantic memory. *J Gerontol* 40:71–77, 1985.
22. Brody H: Organization of the cerebral cortex. III. A study of the human cerebral cortex. *J Comp Neurol* 102:511–556, 1955.
23. Brown P, Levison S: Social structure, groups, and interaction. In Scherer KR, Giles H (eds): *Social Markers in Speech*. Cambridge, Cambridge University Press, 1979, p. 291.
24. Burk DM, Light LL: Memory and aging: the role of retrieval processes. *Psychol Bull* 90:513–546, 1981.
25. Canetta R: Decline in oral perception from 20 to 70 years. *Percept Mot Skills* 45:1028–1030, 1977.
26. Charlip WS: The aging female voice: selected fundamental frequency characteristics and listener judgments. Ph.D. thesis, Bloomington, IN, Purdue University, 1968.
27. Clegg J. Verbal transformation on repeated listening to some English consonants. *Br J Psychol* 62:303–309, 1971.
28. Cohen G: Language comprehension in old age. *Cogn Psychol* 11:412–429, 1979.
29. Cohen D, Wu S: Language and cognition during aging. In Eisdorfer C (ed): *Annual Rev Gerontol Geriatrics*, New York, Springer Publications, 1980, vol. 1. p. 71.
30. Cohen T, Gitman L: Oral complaints and taste perception in the aged. *J Gerontol* 14:294–298, 1959.
31. Coleman RF: Effect of waveform changes upon roughness perception. *Folia Phoniatr* (Basel) 23:314–322, 1971.
32. Corso J: *Aging Sensory Systems and Perception*. New York, Praeger Publications, 1981.
33. Critchley M: And all the daughters of musick shall be brought low: language function in the elderly. *Arch Neurol* 41:1135–1139, 1984.
34. Curtis AP, Fucci P: Sensory and motor changes during development and aging. In Lass N (ed): *Speech and Language: Advances in Basic Research and Practices*, New York, Academic Press, 1983, vol. 9. p. 153.
35. Davis GA: Effects of aging on normal language. In Holland AL (ed): *Language Disorders in Adults: Recent Advances*. San Diego, College-Hill Press, 1984, p. 79.
36. Dekaban AS, Sadowsky D: Changes in brain weights during the span of human life: relation of brain weights to body heights and body weights. *Ann Neurol* 4:345–356, 1978.
37. Denny NW, Denny DR: The relationship between classification and questioning strategies among adults. *J Gerontol* 37:190–196, 1982.
38. Dontas AS, Jacobs DR Jr, Corcondilas A, et al: Longitudinal versus cross-sectional vital capacity changes and affecting factors. *J Gerontol* 39:430–438, 1984.
39. Emery OB: Linguistic decrement in normal aging. *Lang Commun* 6:47–64, 1986.
40. Endres W, Bambach W, Flosser G: Voice spectrographs as a function of age, voice disguise,

and voice imitation. *J Acoust Soc Am* 49:1842–1848, 1971.
41. Feier CD, Gerstman LJ: Sentence comprehension abilities throughout the adult life span. *J Gerontol* 35:722–728, 1980.
42. Ferreri G: Senescence of the larynx. *Ital Gen Rev Oto-Rhino-Laryngol* 1:640–709, 1959.
43. Fisch L: Special senses: the aging auditory system. In Brocklehurst JC (ed): *Textbook of Geriatric Medicine and Gerontology*. New York, Churchill Livingstone, 1978, p. 276.
44. Fullerton AM: Age differences in the use of imagery in integrating new and old information in memory. *J Gerontol* 38:326–332, 1983.
45. Fullerton AM, Smith AD: Age-related differences in the use of redundancy. *J Gerontol* 35:729–735, 1980.
46. Gilbert HR, Weismer GG: The effects of smoking on the speaking fundamental frequency of adult women. *J Psycholinguist Res* 3:225–231, 1974.
47. Goodglass H: Naming disorders in aphasia and aging. In Obler LK, Albert ML (eds): *Language and Communication in the Elderly*. Lexington, MA, DC Heath, 1980, p. 37.
48. Gordon SK, Clark WC: Application of signal detection theory to prose recall and recognition in elderly and young adults. *J Gerontol* 29:64–72, 1974.
49. Green MG, Adelman R, Charon R, Hoffman S: Ageism in the medical encounter: an exploratory study of the doctor-elderly patient relationship. *Lang Commun* 6:113–124, 1986.
50. Hartman DE, Danhauer JL: Perceptual features of speech for males in four perceived age decades. *J Acoust Soc Am* 59:713–715, 1976.
51. Hecker M, Kreul EJ: Description of the speech of patients with cancer of the vocal folds. Part I. Measurements of fundamental frequency. *J Acoust Soc Am* 49:1275–1283, 1971.
52. Helfrich H: Age markers in speech. In Scherer KR, Giles H (eds): *Social Markers in Speech*. Cambridge, Cambridge University Press, 1979, p. 63.
53. Hicks LH, Birren JE: Aging, brain damage and psychomotor slowing. *Pyschol Bull* 74:377–396, 1976.
54. Holland AL: Working with the aging aphasic patient: some clinical implications. In Obler LK, Albert ML (eds): *Language and Communication in the Elderly*. Lexington, MA, DC Heath, 1980, p. 181.
55. Hollien H, Shipp T: Speaking fundamental frequency and chronologic age in males. *J Speech Hear Res* 15:155–159, 1971.
56. Honjo I, Isshiki N: Laryngoscopic and voice characteristics of aged persons. *Arch Otolaryngol* 106:149–150, 1980.
57. Horri Y, Ryan WJ: Fundamental frequency characteristics and perceived age of adult male speakers. *J Acoust Soc Am* 57:569, 1975.
58. Howard DV: Category norms: a comparison of the Bittig and Montague (1969) norms with the response of adults between the ages of 20 and 80. *J Gerontol* 35:225–231, 1980.
59. Hutchinson JM, Jensen M: A pragmatic evaluation of discourse communication in normal

and senile elderly in a nursing home. In Obler LK, Albert ML (eds): *Language and Communication in the Elderly*. Lexington, MA, DC Heath, 1980, pp. 59.

60. Hutchinson JM, Robinson KL, Nerbonne MA: Patterns of nasalance in a sample of normal gerontologic subjects. *J Commun Dis* 11:469–481, 1978.

61. Israel H: Age factor and the pattern of change in craniofacial structures. *Am J Phys Anthropol* 39:111–128, 1973.

62. Israel H: Continuing growth in the human cranial skeleton. *Arch Oral Biol* 13:133–137, 1968.

63. Isshiki N, Yanagihara N, Morimoto M: Approach to the objective diagnosis of hoarseness. *Folia Phoniatr* 18:393–400, 1966.

64. Jacobs-Condit L, Ortenzo ML: Physical changes in aging. In Jacobs-Condit L (ed): *Gerontology and Communication Disorders*. Rockville, MD, ASHA, 1984, p. 26.

65. Jalavisto E: The role of simple tests measuring speed of performance in the assessment of biological vigor: a factorial study in elderly women. In Welford A, Birren J (eds): *Behavior, Aging, and the Nervous System*. Springfield, IL, Charles C Thomas, 1965, p. 353.

66. Kahane JC: Anatomic and physiologic changes in the aging peripheral speech mechanism. In Beasley DS, Davis GA (eds): *Aging: Communication Processes and Disorders*. New York, Grune and Stratton, 1981, p. 21.

67. Kahane JC: A histomorphological study of the aging male larynx. Presented at the American Speech and Hearing Association Convention, Atlanta, 1979.

68. Kaplan H: The oral cavity in geriatrics. *Geriatrics* 26: 96–102, 1971.

69. Kemper T: Neuroanatomical and neuropathological changes in normal aging and in dementia. In Albert ML (ed): *Clinical Neurology of Aging*. New York, Oxford University Press, 1984, pp. 9–52.

70. Kogan N: Categorizing and conceptualizing styles in younger and older adults. *Hum Dev* 17:218–230, 1974.

71. Kosberg JI: The importance of attitudes on the interaction between health care providers and geriatric populations. In Kleinman MD (ed): *Interdisciplinary Topics in Gerontology*, Basel, A. Karger, 1983, vol. 17. p. 132.

72. Kramer DA, Woodruff DS: Breadth of categorization and metaphoric processing: a study of young and older adults. *Res Aging* 6:271–286, 1984.

73. Kreul EJ: Neuromuscular control examination (NMC) for parkinsonism: vowel prolongations and diadochokinetic and reading rates. *J Speech Hear Res* 15:72–83, 1972.

74. Kukol RJ: Perceptual speech and voice characteristics of aging male and female speakers. Ph.D. thesis, Wichita, KS, Wichita State University, 1979.

75. Kynette D, Kemper S: Aging and the loss of grammatical forms: a cross-sectional study of language performance. *Lang Commun* 6:65–72, 1986.

76. LaBarge E, Edwards E, Knesevich JW: Performance of normal elderly on the Boston Naming Test. *Brain Lang* 27:381–384, 1986.

77. Lebo CP, Reddell RC: The presbycusis component in occupational noise induced hearing loss. *Laryngoscope* 82:1399–1409, 1972.

78. Liang J: Self-reported physical health among aged adults. *J Gerontol* 41:248–260, 1986.

79. Lieberman P: Some acoustic measures of the fundamental periodicity of normal and pathological larynges. *J Acoust Soc Am* 34:344–353, 1963.

80. Linville SE, Fisher HB: Acoustic characteristics of women's voices with advancing age. *J Gerontol* 40:324–330, 1985.

81. Lovelace EA, Cooley S: Free associations of older adults to single words and conceptually related word triads. *J Gerontol* 37:432–437, 1982.

82. Luchsinger R, Arnold GT: *Voice-Speech-Language*. Belmont, CA, Wadsworth Publishing, 1965.

83. Lynne-Davies P: Influence of age on the respiratory system. *Geriatrics* 32:57–60, 1977.

84. Marshall L: Auditory processing in aging listeners. *J Speech Hear Dis* 46:226–240, 1981.

85. McGlone R, Hollien H: Vocal pitch characteristics of aged women. *J Speech Hear Res* 6:164–170, 1963.

86. Meyer BJF, Rice GE: Learning and memory from text across the adult life span. In Fine J, Freedle RO (eds): *Developmental Issues in Discourse*. Norwood, NJ, Albex, 1983, pp. 291–306.

87. Molfese VJ, Hoffman S, Yuen R: The influence of setting and task partner on the performance of adults over age 65 on a communications task. *Int J Aging Hum Dev* 14:45–53, 1981–1982.

88. Moran MJ, Gilbert HR: Selected acoustic characteristics and listener judgments of Downs syndrome voice. Presented at the American Speech-Language-Hearing Association Convention, San Francisco, 1978.

89. Morris, JF, Koski A, Johnson LD: Spirometric standards for healthy, nonsmoking adults. *Respir Dis* 103:57–67, 1971.

90. Mysak ED: Pitch duration characteristics of older males. *J Speech Hear Res* 2:46–54, 1959.

91. Mysak ED, Hanley TP: Aging process in speech: pitch and duration characteristics. *J Gerontol* 13:309–313, 1958.

92. Neiman GS, Klich RJ, Shuey EM: Voice onset time in young and 70-year-old women. *J Speech Hear Res* 26:118–123, 1983.

93. Nizel NE: *Nutrition in Preventive Dentistry: Science and Practice*. Philadelphia, WB Saunders, 1981.

94. Norris JE, Rubin KH: Peer interaction and communication: a life span perspective. In Lass N (ed): *Life Span Development and Behavior*, New York, Academic Press, 1984, vol. 6, p. 355.

95. North AJ, Ulatowsak HK: Competence in independently living older adults: assessment and correlations. *J Gerontol* 36:576–582, 1981.

96. Obler LK, Albert ML: Language and aging: a neurobehavioral analysis. In Beasley DS, Davis GA (eds); *Aging: Communication Processes and*

Disorders. New York, Grune & Stratton, 1981, p. 107.

97. Obusek CJ, Warren RM: A comparison of speech perception in senile and well preserved aged by means of the verbal transformation effect. *J Gerontol* 28:184–188, 1973.

98. Oyer H, Kapur Y, Deal L: Hearing disorders in the aging: effects upon communication. In Oyer H, Oyer E (eds): *Aging and Communication.* Baltimore, Univeristy Park Press, 1976, p. 175.

99. Petit TL: Neuroanatomical and clinical neuropsychological changes in aging and senile dementia. In Craik FIM, Trehub S (eds): *Aging and Cognitive Processes: Advances in the Study of Communication and Affect,* New York, Plenum Press, 1982, vol. 8, p. 1.

100. Petros TV, Zehr HD, Chabot RJ: Adult age differences in accessing and retrieving information from long-term memory. *J Gerontol* 38:589–592, 1983.

101. Poon LW: Differences in human memory with aging: causes and clinical implications. In Birren J, Schaie K (eds): *Handbook of the Psychology of Aging.* New York, Van Nostrand Reinhold, 1985, p. 427.

102. Poon LW, Fozard JL: Speed of retrieval from long-term memory in relation to age, familiarity, and lateness of information. *J Gerontol* 33:711–717, 1978.

103. Pressman JJ, Keleman G: *Physiology of the Larynx.* Rochester, MN, American Academy of Ophthalmology and Otolaryngology, 1970.

104. Ptacek PH, Sander EK: Age recognition from voice. *J Speech Hear Res* 9:273–277, 1966.

105. Ptacek PH, Sander EK, Maloney WH, Jackson C: Phonatory and related changes with advanced age. *J Speech Hear Res* 9:353–360, 1966.

106. Ramig LA: Effects of physiological aging on vowel spectral noise. *J Gerontol* 38:223–225, 1983.

107. Ramig LA, Ringel RL: Effects of physiological aging on selected acoustic characteristics of voice. *J Speech Hear Res,* 26:22–30, 1983.

108. Rankin JL, Collins M: Adult age differences in memory elaboration. *J Gerontol* 40:451–458, 1985.

109. Riegel KF: Changes in psycholinguistic performance with age. In Talland GA (ed): *Human Behavior and Aging: Recent Advances in Research and Theory.* New York, Academic Press, 1968, p. 239.

110. Ruben R, Kruger B: Hearing loss in the elderly. In Plum F (ed): *The Neurology of Aging.* Philadelphia, FA Davis, 1983, p. 123.

111. Ryan WJ: Acoustic aspects of the aging voice. *J Gerontol* 27:265–286, 1972.

112. Ryan WJ, Burk KW: Perceptual and acoustic correlates of aging in the speech of males. *J Commun Dis* 7:181–192, 1974.

113. Ryan EB, Capadano HL: Age perceptions and evaluative reactions toward adult speakers. *J Gerontol* 33:98–102, 1978.

114. Salthouse TA: *Adult Cognition: An Experimental Psychology of Human Aging.* New York, Springer, 1982.

115. Sarno M: Communication disorders in the elderly. In Williams F (ed): *Rehabilitation in*

the Aging. New York, Raven Press, 1984, p. 161.

116. Saxman J, Burk K: Speaking fundamental frequency characteristics of middle aged females. *Folia Phoniatr* 19:167–172, 1967.

117. Selkoe D, Kosik K: Neurochemical changes with aging. In Albert ML (ed): *Clinical Neurology of Aging.* New York, Oxford University Press, 1984, p. 53.

118. Shipp T, Hollien H: Perception of the aging male voice. *J Speech Hear Res* 12:703–710, 1969.

119. Smith AD, Fullerton AM: Age differences in episodic and semantic memory: implications for language and cognition. In Beasley DS, Davis GA (eds): *Aging: Communication Processes and Disorders.* New York, Grune and Stratton, 1981, p. 139.

120. Silverman SJ: *Degeneration of Dental and Orofacial Structures. Orofacial Function: Clinical Research in Dentistry and Speech Pathology.* ASHA Reports No. 7, Washington, DC, American Speech and Hearing Association, 1972.

121. Smith PM: Sex markers in speech. In Scherer KR, Giles H (eds): *Social Markers in Speech.* Cambridge, Cambridge University Press, 1979, p. 109.

122. Smith SW, Rebok GW, Smith WR, Hall SE, Alvin M: Adult age differences in the use of story structure in delayed free recall. *Exp Aging Res* 9:191–195, 1983.

123. Soloman K, Vickers J: Attitudes of health workers toward old people. *J Am Geriatr Soc* 27:186–191, 1979.

124. Sonies BC, Baum BJ, Shawker TH: Tongue motions in elderly adults: initial in situ observations. *J Gerontol* 39:279–283, 1984.

125. Spreen O, Benton A: *Neurosensory Center Comprehensive Examination for Apahsia.* Victoria, British Columbia, University of Victoria, 1969.

126. Stewart MA, Ryan EB: Attitudes toward younger and older adult speakers: effects of varying speech rates. *J Lang Soc Psychol* 1:91–109, 1982.

127. Squier CA, Johnson NW, Hopps RM: *Human Oral Mucosa.* London, Blackwell Scientific Publications, 1976.

128. Sweeting PM, Baken RJ: Voice onset time in a normal-aged population. *J Speech Hear Res* 25:129–134, 1982.

129. Tamir LM: *Communication and the Aging Process.* New York, Pergammon Press, 1979.

130. Thomas JC, Fozard JL, Waugh NC: Age-related differences in naming latency. *Am J Psychol* 90:499–509, 1977.

131. Tomlinson BE, Henderson G: Some quantitative cerebral findings in normal and demented old people. In Terry RD, Gershon S (eds): *Neurobiology of Aging.* New York, Raven Press, 1976, p. 183.

132. Turner JM, Mead J, Wohl ME: Elasticity of human lungs in relation to age. *J Appl Physiol* 25:664–671, 1968.

133. Ulatowska HK, Cannito MP, Hayashi MM, et al: Language abilities in the elderly. In Ulatowska HK (eds): *The Aging Brain: Communication in the Elderly.* San Diego, CA, College-Hill Press, 1985, p. 125.

134. Valenstein E: Age-related changes in the human central nervous system. In Beasley DS, Davis GA (eds): *Aging: Communication Processes and Disorders.* New York, Grune and Stratton, 1981, p. 87.

135. Walsh DA, Baldwin M: Age differences in integrated semantic memory. *Dev Psychol* 13:509–514, 1977.

136. Walsh DA, Baldwin M, Finkle TJ: Age differences in integrated semantic memory for abstract sentences. *Exp Aging Res* 6:431–443, 1980.

137. Walker VG, Hardiman CJ, Hedrick DL, Holbrook A: Speech and language characteristics of an aging population. In Lass N (ed): *Speech and Language Advances in Basic Research and Practice.* New York, Academic Press, 1981, vol. 6, p. 143.

138. Whitbourne S: *The Aging Body.* New York, Springer-Verlag, 1985.

139. Wilcox KA, Horri Y: Age and changes in vocal jitter. *J Gerontol* 35:194–198, 1980.

140. Wisniewski HM, Terry RD: Neuropathology of the aging brain. In Terry RD, Gershon S (eds): *Neurobiology of Aging.* New York, Raven Press, 1976, p. 265.

141. Woodruff DS: A review of aging and cognitive processes. *Res Aging* 5:139–153, 1983.

142. Yairi E, Clifton NF: Disfluent speech behavior of preschool children, high school seniors, and geriatric persons. *J Speech Hear Res* 15:714–719, 1972.

143. Yanagibara N: Significance of harmonic changes and noise components in hoarseness. *J Speech Hear Res* 10:531–5541, 1967.

144. Yorkston KM, Beukelman DR: An analysis of connected speech samples of aphasic and normal speakers. *J Speech Hear Disord* 45:27–36, 1980.

10 Interpersonal Communication Patterns and Strategies in the Elderly

BARBARA B. SHADDEN

Editor's Note

Earlier chapters have examined aspects of normal aging and various specific changes in speech-language-hearing functions observed in older adults. In Chapter 10, an attempt is made to synthesize this information within the context of the Communication and Aging Model, by highlighting the interactive nature of communication. The chapter begins with a brief discussion of the multidisciplinary nature of research concerning aging and communication; a lack of consistent focus and the relative dearth of literature in this area are noted. The potential communication effects of social, physiological, and cognitive/emotional changes associated with aging are then summarized. Particular emphasis is placed on the influence of attitudes and expectations upon patterns of interpersonal relationship. It is suggested that a major source of communication breakdown may be the failure of participants to engage in appropriate or adequate perspective-taking or speech style accommodation, due to preexisting stereotypes. The next chapter section focuses upon patterns of communication in interactions involving health care providers and older individuals. Possible causes for communication breakdown in these settings are identified. The chapter concludes with a description of research needs, with special attention to key variables that must be manipulated or controlled. The author suggests that any of the communication problems targeted in this chapter may already be in existence when an older individual attempts to cope with one or more of the specific communication disorders described in Chapter 11.

Communication was defined earlier in this text as the sending and receiving of both verbal and nonverbal messages between two or more individuals within a specific social and physical context. A Communication and Aging Model was proposed as a mechanism for developing a sound theoretical foundation for understanding the effects of aging on communication processes *and* the manner in which communication can serve as a tool in meeting the social, emotional, and service needs of the elderly. Hopefully, this foundation has been established in the preceding chapters. Since Chapter 9 concludes with a discussion of the pragmatic aspects of linguistic functioning, one might very well wonder why a separate chapter on interpersonal communication is necessary.

A quick review of the Communication and Aging Model provides a partial answer to this question (see Fig. 10.1). While the resources and deficits associated with both aging and communication have been explored in this text,

the central interaction between these two elements of the model has not been described. In particular, we have not fully examined the manner in which aging creates needs or stresses affecting communicative behavior, or the extent to which communication attributes may actually represent adaptive or coping responses. In other words, we need to begin to understand the influence of the total aggregate of speech-language-hearing changes on communicative interactions.

This understanding is important for several reasons. Our knowledge of the factors contributing to communicative behavior in older adults influences our clinical interactions with elderly clients. This same knowledge allows us to both design more effective interventions for communicatively disordered individuals and to provide better education, counseling, and support for their significant others. The need for communication interventions for older individuals *without* a specific speech-language

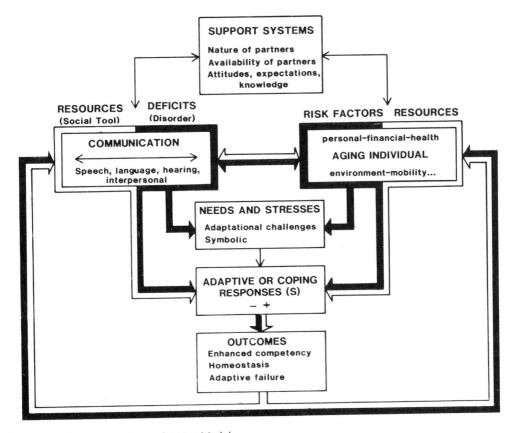

Figure 10.1 Communication and Aging Model.

or hearing impairment can also be evaluated more comprehensively. Finally, a basic understanding of the dynamics of communication in aging can provide a much-needed framework for systematic research in this area.

Given the breadth and complexity of communication topics, this chapter is rather arbitrarily subdivided into four main sections. The first section reviews sociocultural, physiological, and cognitive/emotional aspects of aging and speculates about their probable influence upon communicative behavior. When available, appropriate research data are included. The second chapter section addresses issues of ageism, the attitudes and stereotypes related to aging and the elderly, and their effects upon interpersonal behaviors. In the third section, much of the literature concerning communicative interactions and the elderly is discussed, with particular emphasis upon health care settings. Some of the more common recommendations concerning communicating with an older client are included here. Finally, an overview of basic research needs is presented. Before proceeding with this discussion, however, some

brief comments about the available research literature are appropriate.

PROBLEMS IN COMMUNICATION AND AGING RESEARCH

A number of years ago, Lubinski (60) provocatively entitled an article "Why So Little Interest In Whether or Not Old People Talk . . .?" The problem is not so much that there is no interest in communication, but rather that communication is not *specifically* targeted in most investigations. Certainly, much of the social gerontological literature does address issues that involve communication (60), and there are frequent reports of the paucity of communication opportunities in certain settings (7, 42, 45, 107). The problem, therefore, is that the presence and influence of communication is so pervasive that few researchers or theorists have bothered to focus in on the communication domain itself. In effect, it is taken for granted.

In addition, as noted in Chapter 1, the multidisciplinary nature of both the communications and gerontology fields results in a lack of clear or consistent perspective guiding research efforts (13). The available data base is fragmentary and difficult to organize into a coherent picture of the communication status of the older person. Research emphases vary from profession to profession and investigator to investigator. The most common emphases in current publications include: (a) interpersonal communications theories; (b) mass media communications as they affect the elderly or reflect society's images of aging; (c) language behaviors in normal older adults (particularly discourse characteristics); (d) behaviors of communicatively impaired adults; (e) communication characteristics in dementia; (f) communicative interactions between older persons and professionals; and (g) communication dynamics in specific settings, particularly long-term care facilities. One particular problem in research with older adults is that studies of normal communicative behavior may be biased because of the use of volunteers who represent a more affluent, educated, and articulate subgroup of the elderly.

It should be obvious that such disparate research emphases can only result in a relatively piecemeal accumulation of data concerning communication and aging. For this reason, the remainder of this chapter will focus on fairly broad topics that allow some interface of the communication and gerontology literature (13). By examining basic subdivisions of the aging process, it should be possible to speculate about the effects of various changes on communication.

POTENTIAL EFFECTS OF AGING ON COMMUNICATION

Sociocultural Changes

The social realities of aging are well documented (cf. 2, 33, 39, 50, 61, 94, 103). They include:

1. Median incomes below the national average and fixed incomes in times of escalating daily living and health care costs;
2. Considerably more women than men, with at least half of the women being widowed;
3. Major alterations in life roles due to retirement, shifts in family status (e.g., parent to grandparent), and loss of status or membership in previous professional or social groups;

4. Frequent physical relocation, either within or outside the home community, due to changes in family size and needs, reduced income, or diminished resources for managing the home environment (although only 5% are institutionalized);
5. Geographical dispersal of the family and friends;
6. The increasing occurrence of the death of age peers, whether family members or friends;
7. Increased leisure time, although some older persons have reduced capability to enjoy previous leisure activities.

While this list provides only a cursory overview of some of the more salient sociocultural facts of aging, the implications of these changes should be obvious. One major concern is the isolation of the older population from the rest of society (43). As life roles and social status shift, and relocation to retirement facilities occurs, we begin to find enclaves of the elderly in settings not broached by younger individuals.

These physical moves, along with other social aspects of aging, may produce significant changes in life-style along with high levels of stress. Lieberman and Tobin (57) note that, within one year after a group of older persons changed residence, one-half were dead, physically impaired, or psychologically deteriorated. Thus the adaptational challenges involved in relocation, coupled with perceptions of loss and increased awareness of the fact of life's termination, may be sufficient to undermine the physical or mental health of the older person. Isolation, physical relocation, and the death or geographic dispersal of friends and family can also be assumed to alter the size and composition of available social support networks (85). Yet social interaction, social support networks, and life satisfaction have been shown to be significant predictors of maintenance of health and utilization of services (30, 82). It is not surprising that two of the most frequent topics in the gerontological literature are support networks and life satisfaction (see portions of Chapter 19, and refs. 15, 16, 74, and 97).

What does all of this mean for communication? Isolation, restriction of social contacts to age peers, and general reductions in support networks obviously alter the frequency and nature of interpersonal communication opportunities available to the older person. Thus, both the satisfaction inherent in such contacts and the tool use of communication behaviors may be affected. Unfortunately, there are limited data concerning the specific effects of these changes on communication. Using the Communication and Aging Model in Figure 10.1, we can speculate that at least some older individuals will develop various coping or adaptive strategies to overcome potential deficiencies in social contacts.

A number of the communication attributes described in the study presented in Chapter 2 might be understood as adaptive strategies. For example, the older person's perceived dominance of conversations, unwillingness to select topics of interest to the partner, garrulousness, rambling style, and failure to take another's perspective may simply be ways of maintaining control of the communication event and thus prolonging social contact. It was also suggested that some older persons create major social events out of minor contacts with community service people like the bank teller or postman. Runnebohm (75) has indicated that similar behavior may also be seen in health care interactions when the older individual desires or even demands that the helping professional assume an active role in the elderly client's social network. Physical reaching out and inappropriate demands for attention in nursing home settings may be expressions of such needs (24).

The degree to which social skills in general become altered with advanced age has received some discussion in the gerontology literature. Furnham and Pendelton (37) reported that older adults experienced a higher incidence of social anxiety across 40 hypothetical situations than their younger counterparts. However, Shonfield (83) concluded that social skills may actually improve during the adult years, showing decline only in cases of severe sensory or mental impairment. It is probable that social skills deteriorate most obviously in institutional settings (101).

The communication effects of living environments, particularly retirement residences or nursing homes, cannot be ignored. Kastenbaum (47) suggests that special environments for frail or impaired elderly tend to confirm and intensify social isolation. In addition, many such environments are activity limiting because of design or programming flaws (52). Withdrawal and passivity might be anticipated. In turn, the time spent alone by older adults has been shown, in some circumstances, to be associated with low affect and low arousal (55). A cycle of negative social interaction may be established.

The reader should review carefully the various social gerontological theories of aging presented in Chapter 3. Each of these approaches has implications for understanding the social impact of aging in general and the particular strategies being utilized by a specific client.

Physiological Changes

The physiological changes associated with aging have been described in great detail in Chapter 4 (see also refs. 48, 79, 80, 104). It is sufficient to note here that a generalized loss in efficiency tends to occur in all physical systems with increasing age. Even those organ systems involved in the basic bodily functions of sleeping, eating, and elimination may be affected. The body's ability to heal itself declines progressively, and there is a concurrent increase in the incidence of chronic and multiple health problems. Not surprisingly, generalized chronic fatigue is reported by 70% of older persons, second only to pain as a daily symptom (64).

These generalized physiological changes are among those first noted by adults as they move through middle age into old age. The effects upon interpersonal communication tend to be relatively indirect. Sensory limitations, health problems, or mobility restrictions may reduce the frequency and variety of activities that are either pleasurable or accessible. The result can be increased isolation and disengagement in social contacts. An understandable preoccupation with physical or health problems may also lead to a kind of self-absorption that is not likely to enhance communicative interactions. These same physical and/or health problems can create anxiety and fear. Chronic fatigue may drain away resources needed to engage in quality relationships. High levels of drug usage and frequent drug interactions increase the likelihood of medication-related decrements in communication behavior due to sensory, motor, or cognitive side effects (see Chapter 7).

Physiological aging may also have a more direct impact on communication processes. Reduced visual acuity restricts the older adult's ability to take advantage of the nonverbal cues provided by other persons and the environment. Ironically, this may occur at a time when nonverbal abilities in general begin to decline (78) and when nonverbal signals of support and relating are most needed (3, 41).

Changes in motor speech behavior were described in Chapter 9. While Benjamin notes that there is no clear evidence that these speech changes disrupt communication, alterations in vocal output in particular may affect the conveying of subtle emotional and content nuances. In addition, age-related changes in speech production are readily identifiable by listener. The extent to which they may trigger negative evaluative listener responses is discussed in more detail in the section of this chapter called "The influence of attitudes and stereotypes on interpersonal interactions."

Finally, the nature and effects of presbycusic hearing loss are well documented elsewhere in this text (see Chapters 8, 13, 14). Of particular interest is the fact that hearing impairment creates major situational barriers to communication (60). Pastalan (70) notes that both hearing and visual sensory impairments lead to a sense of insulation from the surrounding world, complicated by feelings of vulnerability. Uncertainty when social and physical cues were inaccessible was reported to lead to fear, anger, despair and embarrassment, as well as increased fatigue. Common adaptive responses were reduced social contacts, preoccupation with bodily sensations, and increased time spent in fantasy.

Even when the degree of measurable hearing loss is minimal, older adults may experience other auditory phenomena that reduce their ability to rely on acoustic information in communication settings (108). For example, the ability to maintain and reorient auditory selective attention was reduced in older, as compared with younger, subjects in one study (69). Binaural auditory analysis and synthesis problems (the "cocktail effect") were described in another investigation (105). Clearly, major difficulties in communications involving groups of people might be anticipated, with predictable adaptive strategies.

Cognitive and Emotional Changes

Cognitive changes associated with aging have been described in Chapter 5, followed in Chapter 6 by a brief overview of common emotional and psychiatric disturbances found in the elderly. Only a few selected topics will be highlighted here.

Personal Responses to Cognitive Decline

While there remain many unanswered questions concerning changes in various cognitive dimensions across the life span, it is clear that at least some skills show declines with advanced age. In addition, a number of older adults fear cognitive decline (with its implications of senility) more than any other aspect of the aging process. Anxieties about real or imagined cognitive deficits may lead to withdrawal from social communicative situations where the deficits might be revealed. Self-image, and thus the image one presents to the world, may suffer. Others may also shape their communications

to their perceptions of the cognitive level of a particular older person. If those perceptions are stereotypical (e.g., the person is expected to be confused, with poor memory skills), the level of the communication may be highly inappropriate.

Life Stage Review

A number of writers have advocated a life cycle perspective in examining personality growth and change in old age (10, 20, 35). Within this perspective, the developing human being is seen as passing through various stages which are dominated by a particular need or particular outlook on life. Datan (20) describes the critical dimensions of human experience in this process as attachments to others, activity, and the sense of self. Regardless of one's theoretical approach, however, most writers accept the fact that old age is, or should be, a time for life review (10). In life review, the older individual engages in a process of contemplative examination of his life to date, with efforts to integrate observed patterns and experiences into a meaningful whole that gives validity to the fact of the individual's existence. The reminiscence groups described in Chapter 20 attempt to facilitate this process.

From a communication point of view, the older person's conscious or unconscious engagement in this process may be perceived socially as a kind of egocentrism or narcissism (20, 58, 59, 65). For example, a life review perspective would predict that the older individual would make frequent communicative references to the past, would be less concerned about others' evaluations in the present, and would also be preoccupied with charting and accepting aspects of the current aging process. A kind of introspective quality to communication behaviors might be anticipated, since the functions being served in any particular conversation may be different from those served socially or emotionally at other points in the life span. Interestingly, some of these same patterns form the substrate for many common stereotypes concerning the communication behaviors of the elderly.

Depression and Stress

There is some controversy concerning whether or not depression is found more commonly in older adults than in other age groups. Feinson (32) reviewed a number of studies in which limited evidence for higher than normal levels of emotional dysfunction was found in older persons. In his own work, only measures of anxiety differentiated age groups. Sinnott (90) also examined somatic and nonsomatic symptoms of poor mental health in older men and women. Despite the fact that the majority of participants were symptom free, many did voice complaints about depression or stress. Hyer and colleagues (44) reviewed the literature pertaining to life changes and stress in the elderly. They concluded that older persons remain active agents of adaptive change even in the later years. The antecedents of coping laid down in early and middle adulthood prove effective in predicting coping strategies in old age. In fact, they suggest that we may observe excessive levels of stress only in frail elderly individuals.

Despite studies like these, depressive symptoms are the most common complaint of the elderly (cf. 56). Typical symptoms of depression include poor appetite, weight loss, psychomotor retardation, and constipation, along with emotional characteristics of apathy, withdrawal, hypochondriasis, self-depreciation, agitation, delusions, and confusion. Many of these symptoms are also associated with dementia, creating patient fears of admitting his problems and physician problems in differential diagnosis. The prevalence of somatic symptoms often creates confusion for the elderly patient in accepting the diagnosis of or treatment for depression (34). It has been proposed that a new diagnostic label—"the depression syndrome of the elderly"—be utilized in order to avoid the connotations of mental illness.

Many authors also continue to explore the nature of stress and stress responses in the elderly. Lieberman and Tobin (57) note that the major life crises affecting the elderly are events involving loss (symbolic stress) and situations that disrupt customary modes of behavior or environments (adaptational challenges). Like others, they believe that perhaps the single most important variable in stress management is a sense of mastery or control over one's life (66). One major factor that may interfere with perceived locus of control is a fear of aging itself. In one study (49), fear of aging was negatively correlated with subjective well-being. Schonfeld and colleagues (82) also note that one's sense of control can mitigate against the negative effects of stressors, inadequate environments, and depression. In fact, Thorson and Thorson (98) suggest that loss of control should be added to existing stress scales, since it is highly predictive of reactions to stressful events.

Clearly depression and stress responses are highly individualized. From a communication point of view, however, depressed or highly stressed persons tend to be operating with limited emotional reserves. They present with low affect, little energy, and reduced motivation to interact socially. Their partners may perceive them as uninteresting, difficult to relate to, confused, or generally unworthy of the time and effort involved in establishing and maintaining an interpersonal relationship. Communication breakdown is likely to occur.

Linguistic Changes

Although there have been studies of verbal learning and memory in the elderly for many years, comprehension strategies and pragmatic or communicative uses of language have only been examined more recently. Of particular interest have been various discourse strategies involved in organizing conversational flow and content and in information-seeking. Research findings are summarized in Chapter 9, and will not be duplicated here. Perhaps the best single summary is that there is no consistency in the data available at the present time.

Elderly individuals have been described as using more total words but fewer total sentences in discourse (due to an increased frequency of embedded clauses), as producing more dysfluencies, and as more talkative than younger persons (possibly due to disinhibition related to changes with age in the frontolimbic system or in Wernicke's area) (7, 67, 68, 96). The efficiency of discourse has been questioned (102, 111). Differences in comprehension and recall skills and strategies have been noted in a number of studies, although these are not always supported (17, 18, 31, 36, 63, 81, 95, 102). There has been considerable speculation concerning whether or not the neurologic substrate for language changes with advanced age (21, 96).

Ulatowksa and colleagues (102) have concluded that there is a positive relationship between communicative competence and functional capacity for daily living. However, they note that cognitive factors are not sufficient to explain observed changes in discourse and comprehension. They suggest instead that three variables should be considered: (a) the linguistic elements of semantics and pragmatics; (b) changes in the social functions that older persons assume as they become sidetracked from the mainstream of social activities; and (c) sensory impairments and their associated compensatory adjustments. Primary semantic/pragmatic changes appear to relate to lower ratings of social relevance, reduced information communicated in discourse, and alterations in presuppositional behaviors. Changes in social functions may relate to the fact that the older person is under less pressure to communicate efficiently. Thus interactions without any agenda (except perhaps social camaraderie) may become more common. In such interactions, what one says and how one says it are less important than the simple fact of interacting.

The conclusions of Ulatowska and her colleagues are intrinsically appealing in that they target the influence of societal and environmental factors upon the communication strategies adopted by any individual older person. The Communication and Aging Model in Figure 10.1 would also predict considerable individual variability in communicative style, depending upon the degree to which intrinsic and extrinsic aspects of aging have reduced or modified the older individual's resources. Discrepant research findings may be attributed to the fact that these age change factors have not been fully controlled.

Ulatowska et al (102) specifically note that more research is needed concerning the effects of the expectations of others regarding the older person as a communicator. The following section explores issues of attitudes, stereotypes, and expectations in greater detail.

THE INFLUENCE OF ATTITUDES AND STEREOTYPES ON INTERPERSONAL INTERACTIONS

In 1953, Tuckman and Lorge (100) shocked researchers and public alike with their compelling evidence of society's negative stereotypes concerning aging and the elderly. With subsequent investigations, it became apparent that unfavorable beliefs and attitudes regarding the elderly were extremely prevalent (4, 9). Older individuals themselves were reported to subscribe to similar conceptual views of other older persons. This cluster of stereotypes and myths came to be known as ageism. As reviewed in Solomon (91) and Davis and Holland (22), subsequent research established that ageism pervaded the health professions. Working with older clients was undervalued. Perceptions of general capabilities and rehabilitation potential of older persons were negative; at times, even the value of lifesaving measures was questioned.

More recently, the concept of pervasive negative stereotyping of older persons has been challenged (51, 62), either on procedural grounds (110) or because it is believed that society's attitudes are changing (99). Schonfield (84), for example, reviewed the terminological confusions created by such concepts as myths, attitudes, beliefs, and stereotypes. He concluded that the prevalence of ageism has been exaggerated to the point that it has become difficult to develop and maintain an honest and realistic appraisal of age-related changes and behaviors. In fact, Kalish (46) suggests that we are seeing a "new ageism," particularly among service providers. This new ageism is reflected in the attitudes and behaviors of those persons who deny any negative stereotypes and publicly decry ageism while still adopting a paternalistic, protective stance towards the elderly.

Regardless of current trends, however, the problem of negative valuation of old age and older people is undoubtedly still with us. If so, it may act as one of the major barriers to effective communication for the elderly. Ageism, or its newer counterpart, can interfere with interpersonal interactions on two levels.

On one level, negative attitudes and stereotypes act as barriers to social relations because they keep us from seeing the individual clearly. If one perceives older adults as rambling, disoriented, dependent, egocentric, or uninteresting, one will avoid any interactions with such persons. A considerable body of research exists to suggest that the mere fact of age does, in fact, lead to stereotypical responses, and these responses occur even when the only information available is a photograph or a fragment of a tape-recorded speech sample (87). For example, Ryan and Capadano (76) demonstrated that when undergraduate college students listened to matched speech samples from old and young speakers, the older adults were judged as more reserved, passive, out-of-it, and inflexible. Other judgments from speech alone include viewing the older person as less desirable, competent, benevolent, or healthy. Ironically, the stimulus attributes in the older person's voice and/or speaking patterns may be sufficient to elicit communication-interfering negative evaluations. Both frequency and quality of social interactions can be expected to suffer.

One interesting complication in this picture is provided by various investigations of what happens when one disconfirms expectations. Disconfirmation of expectations occurs when a person behaves in a manner inconsistent with a given stereotype. Several studies suggest that presenting a hypothetical older person in an atypical manner leads to artificially inflated positive evaluations of that individual (19). In contrast, similar disconfirmation of expectations regarding younger persons leads to negative evaluative responses. Disconfirmation of expectancy regarding communication has been explored by varying speech rate and message effectiveness (77, 93). These findings may account for the fact that positive attitudes may be held regarding a particular known older person, despite negativism about the elderly in general.

On a second level, the prevalence of stereotypes about aging, whether positive or negative, may have a more specific effect on the nature of communication behaviors produced. Effective communication depends heavily on the degree to which the communication partners are able to share each other's social realities and decenter (5). The term decentering refers to the process of listener perspective-taking (23). The degree to which one can take another's perspective in framing a message is largely responsible for the success or failure of the message transmission. Perspective-taking skills begin to develop in childhood and continue to acquire sophistication into adolescence (109). Presumably, young and middle-aged adults are capable of assuming the other's point of view.

Whether or not one chooses to engage in such perspective-taking, however, is dependent upon one's motivation to communicate with a particular partner. This motivation may be reduced or modified if the partner is an older individual who is not valued highly. It has also been suggested that there is a decline in the older adult's ability to decenter in social interactions, associated with a possible increase in egocentrism (40, 58, 59). Labov (53) suggests that older men lose their motivation to engage in style shifting when their concern for power relationships disappears (associated with retirement). A loss of need for or interest in perspective-taking might explain some fairly common stereotypes of the garrulous, conversationally dominant, self-preoccupied older individual.

Perspective-taking is also dependent upon the accuracy of one's perceptions of the other individual. If one attempts to frame a message in terms of a stereotypical image of the communication partner's perspective, a breakdown in communication may occur. For example, persuading grandfather to contribute to the purchase of a new car by reminding him of his own youth can be an attempt on the grandson's part to take the older person's perspective. His assumptions, however, may be stereotypical ones—"Old people like to talk about the past"—that are inappropriate to this particular family member.

Attitudes and negative expectations also affect speech style accommodations, a process similar to the perspective-taking described above. Giles (38) postulates that one's selection of speech style, code, or register is a direct reflection of one's perceptions of the communication partner and one's motivation to communicate. By trying to adapt one's manner of speaking to the listener's speech style, a desire to communicate is signaled. A failure to engage in speech accommodation signals a lack of motivation to engage in social interaction.

Speech style consists of both content and noncontent dimensions. The content components include: dialect/accent; vocabulary; length of utterance; lexical diversity; syntax; and word retrieval. Noncontent components emcompass: vocal pitch; vocal intensity; vocal quality; rate of speaking; pauses; intonation; and fluency.

When a mother reduces the length and complexity of her utterances in speaking to her 2-year-old child, appropriate speech style accommodation can be said to occur. When the same woman reduces the length and complexity of her utterances and raises her vocal intensity in speaking to an older stranger in the grocery store, speech style accommodation has also occurred. However, accommodation has been made to a stereotypical image of a slightly confused, hearing-impaired elderly individual with a reduced memory span. The appropriateness of this accommodation is not known, and the older stranger may well be offended by the resulting child-like tone. Conversely, a failure to appropriately adapt to the needs of a hearing-impaired older person suggests disinterest in the communication exchange.

It is interesting to note that the fairly consistent descriptions in Chapter 2 of the ways in which others communicate with older persons almost invariably reflected the stereotypical type of speech style accommodation. Several respondents in fact expressed awareness that an automatic "old people" talking mode was not necessarily appropriate to any specific older individual.

As with listener perspective-taking, it is not clear whether or not older persons engage in appropriate style shifts dependent upon the listener. Molfese et al (65) examined this question by asking 12 older adults to provide directions for following a map route to age peer or non-age peer partners. It was reported that the older subjects did adopt different communication strategies, depending upon the age of the partner; age peer communications were characterized by greater length, more frequent restarts, and more exact repetitions. The fact that the older partners did experience more difficulty following the directions suggests that this speech style accommodation was appropriate and reflected flexibility on the part of the older subjects.

Clearly, a failure to engage in either listener perspective-taking or appropriate speech style accommodation can result in communication failure (73). As Dowd suggests, "Human behavior tends to be oriented towards the expectations of other people" (27, p 48). Communication becomes the medium of exchange through which these expectations and perceptions are exchanged, and a kind of vicious cycle evolves. The initial power differential between older and younger conversational participants establishes a negative interactive pattern which becomes part of the new reality for both participants. Each subsequent interaction is colored by the previous negative history. The active, involved older adult with many resources can ultimately modify negative labels and renegotiate the communicative exchange. The older individual with few resources, however, can do little to interrupt the pattern of power imbalance. Dowd concludes that it is not surprising to find many disadvantaged elderly demonstrating apparently paranoid perceptions of those around them.

Much of the preceding discussion has been speculative in nature. Further research is needed to explore adequately the effects of attitudes and stereotypes upon communication behaviors of all age groups. It is useful, however, to turn next to consideration of patterns and problems in communicative interactions, particularly in service delivery.

PATTERNS AND PROBLEMS IN COMMUNICATIVE INTERACTIONS INVOLVING HEALTH CARE PROVIDERS

While all aspects of communicative interactions involving the elderly are of interest, much of the literature has focused on the role of communication in the interface of the health professional and his services with the older individual and his needs. Clearly no form of service delivery can be effective until aged and professional individuals develop strategies for communicating with each other. As Blazer (6) suggests, misunderstandings between client and physician may lead to behavior patterns that are maladaptive and nontherapeutic for the client and frustrating for the physician.

Problems in Communication Interactions and Environments

The gerontological literature is replete with references to problems in health professional/older person communications in service delivery or in institutional settings. In one pilot study, Shadden (88) noted that both communication disorders professionals and older persons perceive communication difficulties in the service delivery interaction, although the reasons for such difficulties varied, depending upon the perspective of the respondent. Some specific communication patterns were described in more detail in Chapter 2 of this text.

Pratt et al (72) reported that the fourth highest-ranked area of difficulty described by pharmacists working with older clients was poor communication; 20% of those interviewed indicated that this was the primary problem. Interestingly, at least one higher-ranked problem area in their study, noncompliance, may also be seen as indirectly reflecting poor communication. Specifically, as Dengiz and colleagues (25) have suggested, physician/patient noncongruence in perceptions fosters ineffective communication and thus carries the risk of long-term noncompliance with treatment programs.

In other instances, the critical role of interpersonal communication and the possibility of deficiencies in this arena are simply assumed. In an investigation of health professional interactions with older persons, Adelson and colleagues (1) began with the premise that quality of service is linked integrally with quality of interpersonal interactions. They measured interactions behaviorally through a checklist containing primarily communication-enhancing behaviors. Some indirect support for their premise can be found in a recent study by Elliott and Hybertson (28), in which positive attitudes about the provision of nursing care to elderly patients were shown to be correlated with factors reflecting the patients' level of social and interpersonal functioning. Negative attitudes were correlated with impaired ability to hear, among other factors.

A number of studies have considered communication patterns and messages in particular settings. For example, Lubinski (60) examined staff and resident perceptions of communications in a long-term care setting. Residents reportedly noted that spoken communications were limited in quantity, frequently meaningless and disparaging, and constrained by situational and logistical barriers. Other studies have indirectly alluded to inadequacies in communication interactions in institutional settings (7, 42, 45, 107).

Larson and colleagues (54) explored staff-resident communication in a nursing home through questionnaires and personal interviews. Favorable evaluations of staff interactional behaviors were found to be related to a series of attitudes, including rejection of the notion that the nursing home resident is "different" from others and support for developing close personal relationships with residents. Negative staff evaluations were associated with staff attitudes of "sorrow" for the patient who is placed in a nursing home and/or staff expectations that patients should be happy, thankful, and cooperative.

Sigman (89) presents a series of observations about communication behaviors based on analyses of conversational patterns at two homes for the elderly. He highlights two critical avenues for investigation. First, patterns of talking may serve an important role in constructing social relationships within the institutional environment, in defining ". . . . the status of the people with whom they interact, with whom they avoid interaction, and their own relative ranking or prestige" (89, p 152). Choices of communication behavior are particularly important in defining "we/they" patterns, in which "we" are normal and alert, and "they" are helpless and senile. Second, Sigman emphasizes the importance of the ideological assumptions held by institutional caregivers, noting that many see their charges as nonpersons. As a result, passivity and dependence are encouraged, and verbal initiative is discouraged. The latter observations relate back to Larson's findings reported earlier (54) and are echoed in other studies suggesting institutionalized elderly are viewed as categories or labels, not persons (cf. 8, 14).

One of the most detailed set of studies of caregiver/elderly communications in a nursing home was reported by Caporael and colleagues. In the first study, nurse's aides and older residents of a health care facility participated in an exploration of the paralinguistic aspects of communications to the elderly (11). Three basic types of communications were identified: (a) "baby talk" (comprising 22% of the caregivers' utterances); (b) nonbaby talk addressed to older residents; and (c) normal adult conversation addressed to other caregivers. College students' judgments of the presence of baby talk appeared heavily dependent upon the presence of high pitch and wide pitch variability (accounting for 61% of the variance). The baby talk messages were judged as more comforting than nonbaby talk, which was perceived as somewhat arousing and irritating. Caporael (11) speculated that baby talk may be used to convey nurturance and affection, whereas nonbaby talk may reflect an "institutional" register promoting negative responses.

In the second study, an attempt was made to explore further the actual judgments of caregivers and care receivers concerning the qualities of these paralinguistically different speech styles (12). Institutionalized older judges with lower functional abilities were disposed to like the baby talk more than judges with relatively high functional skills. Caregivers were asked to predict which clients would like particular speech forms and which forms might be most effective for certain clients. Invariably, those older adults with lower social ratings were predicted to like baby talk best and to benefit most from its usage.

Caporael's work represents one of the few systematic attempts to define the nature of communications to the elderly and the factors influencing choice of communication style and reception of that style. Thus it is interesting that her findings provide some support for the speculations concerning attitudes offered earlier in this chapter. Caregivers appeared to be modifying their communications based on a stereotype of the elderly (through either institutional or baby talk registers). This type of modification can hardly be considered fine tuning or healthy speech accommodation, since it suggests a lack of responsivity to either the individual or the moment. In addition, the use of baby talk may contribute to infantilization, a process of encouraging dependency and childlike behavior in the older adult (26).

Recommended Strategies for Communicating with Older Clients

In view of these various concerns about inadequacies in communicative interactions between professionals and older clients, it is not surprising to find that techniques for effective communication with the elderly have received attention in the literature of a number of professions. Pfeiffer (71), for example, highlights the importance of verbal and nonverbal communication signals, cautioning that ignoring these signs in the earliest contacts may have a negative impact on all subsequent aspects of service delivery. Similarly, in a description of the medical counseling process, Schwartz (86) emphasizes the physician's critical role, first in "hearing" the older person's message and, second, in communicating distinctly so he can be heard and unambiguously understood.

Steel (92) notes multiple health problems, vision or hearing impairments, and memory restrictions that may interfere with history-taking and communication of treatment messages. Other general sources of breakdown in communicating with institutionalized elderly are described by Weinberg (106) as: the question-and-answer conversational paradigm; the values conflict between an older person and a conversational partner; and the partner's failure to understand the dilemma of the institutionalized elderly. Like Schwartz, Weinberg recommends really listening to the older individual, with particular emphasis upon allowing life review to occur. He also suggests that we improve our skills at receiving the hidden messages or latent content of the older person's communications.

Two of the most comprehensive discussions of professional/elderly communications have been provided by Epstein (29) and Blazer (6). Epstein suggests we must consider all elements contributing to communication, including voice, body language, the visual experience (e.g. dress), touch, and overt or covert status symbols displayed in the service setting. In particular, we must become more sensitive to our own discomfort with aging and the elderly as well as with any emotions of helplessness, frustration, or hostility that we may project. We must anticipate that a client's fears of aging (49) may lead to communicative and interpersonal behaviors such as concealment of evident symptoms, accusatory statements, loquaciousness, denial of realities, and self-centeredness.

Many of these same concerns are addressed in Blazer's (6) discussion of the client and clinician variables that may influence communicative interactions. Client variables include: anxiety; sensory deprivation; cautiousness; unrealistic views of the professional and his/her roles; a preoccupation with persistent themes (e.g., somatic concerns, loss reactions, life review, loss of control, and death); increasing isolation; and stereotypes of the young. Clinician variables include: stereotypes and negative expectations related to aging; a failure to view the individual holistically; and specific verbal and nonverbal language patterns.

Among Blazer's many recommendations for effective communication with the elderly, the importance of reading and sending appropriate nonverbal cues deserves further attention. In particular, touch has been described as an important tool for enhancing social interaction in the elderly, particularly those with some form of dementia. DeLong (24), for example, notes that nursing home residents try to bring others closer to them with touch. Touch broaches the personal space of an individual, thus potentially communicating important information to the confused or nonresponsive older person. Hollinger (41) described a study in which selective use of touch during communication interactions increased the frequency and duration of verbal responses. Touch is also believed to establish trust and a positive emotional climate with Alzheimer's patients (3).

The increase in publications concerning "how to" communicate with the older client is encouraging, in that it suggests greater awareness of the need for productive communicative

interactions and of the factors that potentially interfere with this process. However, one caveat must be offered. In our efforts to clarify the barriers to communication that may be present, we must avoid contributing to a stereotypical view of the elderly as a homogeneous, rather than heterogeneous, group. That risk will continue to exist until our research questions and methodologies have been refined sufficiently to define communicative behaviors in the elderly more accurately.

RESEARCH NEEDS

Almost 10 years ago, Lubinski (60) stated that more research is needed concerning communicative interactions in institutions, from the perspectives of both caregivers and older persons. Phrased more broadly in terms of communicative interactions in general, that statement is equally valid today. We continue to know very little about the actual patterns of interaction that occur when an older partner is involved, and even less about the factors that define the particular patterns that are present at any given time. What is needed is a program of research in which an older person, a conversational partner, and task variables are systematically manipulated in order to measure actual communication behaviors *and* perceptions of the interaction. A brief synopsis of key variables is provided below.

1. Older Person Variables—residential setting, health, presence of age decrements in sensory or motor skills, education, socioeconomic status, sex, age, marital status, extent and perceived quality of social support network, premorbid communication skills;
2. Conversational Partner Variables—age, education (general level and specific knowledge of aging), role relationship to older person, frequency of contacts with older persons in general, attitudes and expectations regarding the elderly in general, and specific older communication partners;
3. Interaction Variables—task (complexity, memory demands, naturalness or artificiality), degree of personal investment in the communicative exchange, setting, known or unknown partner, measurement procedures, availability, and accuracy of information concerning the communication partner;
4. Communication Behaviors of Interest—degree and nature of speech accommo-

dation (content and noncontent), syntactic complexity and accuracy, lexical selection, fluency, turn-taking skills, topic introduction and maintenance behaviors, management of communication breakdown and repair strategies, communication style, comprehension skills and sources of comprehension breakdown, presuppositional behaviors, relevance or appropriateness of behaviors;

5. Associated Measures of Interest—perceptions of both communication partners with respect to each other's personality and communication traits (including measures of the perceived adequacy, value, and pleasantness of the interaction); also measures of the older person's level of cognitive, emotional, linguistic, and sensory functioning (as needed).

All of the variables and measures identified above pertain to analyses of actual interactions, whether real or contrived. This should not minimize the obvious need for ongoing research concerning specific speech-language-hearing changes associated with aging (as described in Chapters 8 and 9). In addition, longitudinal studies of communicative behavior must be initiated and maintained. Without such longitudinal data, it will remain difficult (if not impossible) to determine the extent to which an observed behavior reflects a change over which the older individual has no control, an adaptive or compensatory strategy, or simply a preexisting communication pattern.

CONCLUSIONS

This chapter has reviewed some of the more common aspects of aging and the elderly that may influence communicative behaviors, including separate consideration of the potential effects of ageist attitudes and expectations on interpersonal interactions. Problems in communications between health professionals and older persons have been described, and frequently cited recommendations for enhancing such interactions have been provided. Research needs have been summarized.

Many of the observations made in this chapter are purely speculative. They arise out of an understanding of the dynamics of aging and the components of communicative behavior, as captured in the Communication and Aging Model. No apology is offered for these digressions into hypothesis and conjecture. There is simply very little research available to confirm or deny some of our most commonly accepted

perceptions of communicative interactions with older persons. Hopefully, the reader will be encouraged to pursue his/her own investigations of the topics presented here.

There can be no doubt, however, that some older individuals will display changes in communicative behavior that can be traced to the aging process, or to strategies designed to facilitate adaptation to life changes associated with aging. We must not lose sight of this reality as we move on to consider specific communication disorders in Chapter 11.

References

1. Adelson R, Nasti A, Sprafkin JN, Marinelli R, Primavera LH, Gorman BS: Behavioral ratings of health professionals' interactions with the geriatric patient. *Gerontologist* 22:277–281, 1982.
2. American Association of Retired Persons: *A Profile of Older Americans: 1985.* Washington, DC, American Association of Retired Persons, 1985.
3. Bartol MA: Nonverbal communication in patients with Alzheimer's disease. *J Gerontol Nurs* 5:21–31, 1979.
4. Bennett R, Eckman J: Attitudes towards aging: a critical examination of recent literature and implications for future research. In Eisdorfer C, Lawton MP (eds): *The Psychology of Adult Development and Aging.* Washington, DC, American Psychological Association, 1973, p 79.
5. Blakar RV: An experimental method for inquiring into communication. *Eur J Soc Psychol* 3:415–425, 1973.
6. Blazer D: Techniques for communicating with your elderly patient. *Geriatrics* 33:79–84, 1978.
7. Brown A: *Nurses, Patients, and Social Systems.* Columbia, MO, University of Missouri Press, 1969.
8. Brubaker D, Barresi T: Social workers' levels of knowledge about old age and perceptions of service delivery to the elderly. *Res Aging* 1:213–232, 1979.
9. Butler R: Overview on aging. In Usdin G, Hofling CK (eds): *Aging: The Process and the People.* New York, Brunner/Mazel, 1978, p 1.
10. Butler R: The life review: an interpretation of reminscence in the aged. In Neugarten BL (ed): *Middle Age and Aging.* Chicago, University of Chicago Press, 1968, p 486.
11. Caporael LR: The paralanguage of caregiving: baby talk to the institutionalized aged. *J Pers Soc Psychol* 40:876–884, 1981.
12. Caporael LR, Lukaszewski MP, Culbertson GH: Secondary baby talk: judgements by institutionalized elderly and their caregivers. *J Pers Soc Psychol* 44:746–754, 1983.
13. Carmichael CW: Communication and gerontology: interfacing disciplines. *West Speech Commun* 40:121–129, 1976.
14. Ciliberto DJ, Levin J, Arluke A: Nurses' diag-

nostic stereotyping of the elderly. *Res Aging* 3:299–310, 1981.

15. Cohen CI, Rajkowski MPH: What's in a friend? Substantive and theoretical issues. *Gerontologist* 22:261–266, 1982.

16. Cohen CI, Teresi J, Holmes D: Social networks, stress, adaptation, and health. *Res Aging* 7:409–431, 1985.

17. Cohen G: Language comprehension in old age. *Cogn Psychol* 11:412–429, 1979.

18. Cohen G, Faulkner D: Memory for discourse in old age. *Discourse Processes* 4:253–265, 1981.

19. Crockett WH, Press AN, Osterkamp M: The effect of deviations from stereotyped expectations upon attitudes toward older persons. *J Gerontol* 34:368–374, 1979.

20. Datan N: Star-crossed love: the developmental phenomenologies of the life cycle. In Rowles GD, Ohta RJ (eds): *Aging and Milieu*. New York, Academic Press, 1983, p 29.

21. Davis GA: Effects of aging on normal language. In Holland AL (ed): *Language Disorders in Adults: Recent Advances*. San Diego, College-Hill, 1984, p 79.

22. Davis GA, Holland AL: Age in understanding and treating aphasia. In Beasley DS, Davis GA (eds): *Aging: Communication Processes and Disorders*. New York, Grune & Stratton, 1981, p 207.

23. Delia J, Clark RA: Cognitive complexity, social perception, and the development of listener-adapted communication in six-, eight-, ten-, and twelve-year-old boys. *Commun Monogr* 4:326–345, 1977.

24. DeLong AJ: The microspatial structure of the older person. In Pastalan LA, Carson DH (eds): *Spatial Behavior of Older People*. Ann Arbor, MI, University of Michigan Institute of Gerontology, 1970, p 68.

25. Dengiz AN, Rakowski W, Hickey T: Congruence of health and treatment perceptions among older patients and primary care providers. Presented at the Gerontological Society Convention, Boston, 1982.

26. Dolinsky EH: Infantilization of the elderly: an area for nursing research. *J Gerontol Nurs* 10:12–19, 1984.

27. Dowd JJ: *Stratification among the Aged*. Monterey, CA, Brooks/Cole, 1980.

28. Elliott B, Hybertson D: What is it about the elderly that elicits a negative response? *J Gerontol Nurs* 8:568–571, 1982.

29. Epstein L: Issues in geropsychiatry. In Obler LK, Albert ML (eds): *Language and Communication in the Elderly*. Lexington, MA, Lexington Books, 1980, p 139.

30. Evans LK: Maintaining social interaction as health promotion in the elderly. *J Gerontol Nurs* 5:19–21, 1978.

31. Feier CD, Gerstman LL: Sentence comprehension abilities throughout the adult life span. *J Gerontol* 35:722–728, 1980.

32. Feinson MC: Aging and mental health: distinguishing myth from reality. *Res Aging* 7:155–174, 1985.

33. Fischer CS: *To Dwell among Friends*. Chicago, University of Chicago Press, 1982.

34. Fogel BS, Fretwell M: Reclassification of depression in medically ill elderly. *J Am Geriatr Soc* 33:446–448, 1985.

35. Freud S: *Civilization and Its Discontents*. New York, WW Norton, 1961.

36. Fullerton AM, Smith AD: Age-related differences in the use of redundancy. *J Gerontol* 35:729–735, 1980.

37. Furnham A, Pendleton D: The assessment of social skills deficits in the elderly. *Int J Aging Hum Dev* 17:29–38, 1983.

38. Giles H: Social psychology and applied linguistics. *ITL: Rev Appl Linguist* 35:27–40, 1977.

39. Haak LA: A retiree's perspective on communication. In Oyer HJ, Oyer EJ (eds): *Aging and Communication*. Baltimore, University Park Press, 1976, p 17.

40. Helfrich H: Age markers in speech. In Scherer KR, Giles H (eds): *Social Markers in Speech*. Cambridge, Cambridge University Press, 1979, p 63.

41. Hollinger LM: Communicating with the elderly. *J Gerontol Nurs* 12:9–13, 1986.

42. Hoyer W, Kafer R, Simpson S, et al: Reinstatement of verbal behavior in elderly mental patients using operant procedures. *Gerontologist* 14:149–152, 1974.

43. Hutchinson JM, Jensen M: A pragmatic evaluation of discourse communication in a nursing home. In Obler LK, Albert ML (eds): *Language and Communication in the Elderly*. Lexington, MA, Lexington Books, 1980, p 59.

44. Hyer L, Barry J, Tamkin A, McConatha D: Coping in later life: an optimistic assessment. *J Appl Gerontol* 3:82–96, 1983.

45. Jones D: Social isolation, interaction and conflict in two nursing homes. *Gerontologist* 12:230–234, 1972.

46. Kalish RA: The new ageism and the failure models: a polemic. *Gerontologist* 19:398–402, 1979.

47. Kastenbaum R: Can the clinical milieu be therapeutic? In Rowles GD, Ohta RJ (eds): *Aging and Milieu: Environmental Perspectives on Growing Old*. New York, Academic Press, 1983, p 3.

48. Kenney RA: *Physiology of Aging: A Synopsis*. Chicago, Yearbook Medical Publishers, 1982.

49. Klemmack DL, Roff LL: Fear of personal aging and subjective well-being in later life. *J Gerontol* 39:756–758, 1984.

50. Knox AB: Adult development. In Beasley DS, Davis GA (eds): *Aging: Communication Processes and Disorders*. New York, Grune & Stratton, 1981, p 3.

51. Kogan N: Beliefs, attitudes, and stereotypes about old people: a new look at some old issues. *Res Aging* 1:11–36, 1979.

52. Koncelik JA: Human factors and environmental design for the aging: aspects of physiological change and sensory loss as design criteria. In Byerts TO, Howell SC, Pastalan LA (eds): *Environmental Context of Aging*. New York, Garland STPM Press, 1979, p 107.

53. Labov W: *The Study of Nonstandard English*. Urbana, IL, National Council of Teachers of English, 1970.

54. Larson CE, Knapp ML, Zuckerman I: Staff-resident communication in nursing homes: a factor analysis of staff attitudes and resident evaluations of staff. *J Commun* 19:308–316, 1969.

55. Larson R, Zuzanek J, Mannell R: Being alone versus being with people: disengagement in the daily experience of older adults. *J Gerontol* 40:373–381, 1985.

56. Lazarus LW, Davis JM, Dysken MW: Geriatric depression: a guide to successful therapy. *Geriatrics* 40:43–53, 1985.

57. Lieberman MA, Tobin SS: *The Experience of Old Age: Stress, Coping, and Survival.* New York, Basic Books, 1983.

58. Looft WR: Egocentrism and social interaction across the life span. *Psychol Bull* 78:73–92, 1972.

59. Looft WR, Charles DC: Egocentrism and social interaction in young and old adults. Presented at the Gerontological Society Meeting, San Francisco, 1970.

60. Lubinski RB: Why so little interest in whether or not old people talk: a review of recent research on verbal communication among the elderly. *Int J Aging Hum Dev* 9:237–245, 1978-1979.

61. Maddox GG: The social and cultural context of aging. In Usdin G and Hofling K (eds): *Aging: The Process and the People.* New York, Brunner/Mazel, 1978, p 20.

62. McTavish DG: Perceptions of old people: a review of research methodologies and findings. *Gerontologist* 11:90–101, 1971.

63. Meyer B, Rice GE: Information recalled from prose by young, middle, and old adult readers. *Exp Aging Res* 17:253–286, 1981.

64. Mitchell CA: Generalized chronic fatigue in the elderly: assessment and intervention. *J Gerontol Nurs* 12:19–23, 1986.

65. Molfese V, Hoffman B, Yuen R: Influence of setting and task partner on the performance of adults over age 65 on a communicative task. *Int J Aging Hum Dev* 14:45–53, 1981.

66. Molinari V, Niederehe G: Locus of control, depression, and anxiety in young and old adults: a comparison study. *Int J Aging Hum Dev* 20:41–52, 1985.

67. Obler LK: Narrative discourse style in the elderly. In Obler LK, Albert ML (eds): *Language and Communication in the Elderly.* Lexington, MA, Lexington Books, 1980, p 75.

68. Obler LK, Albert ML: Language and aging: a neurobehavioral analysis. In Beasly DS, Davis GA (eds): *Aging: Communication Processes and Disorders.* New York, Grune & Stratton, 1981, p 107.

69. Panek PE, Rush MC: Simultaneous examination of age related differences in the ability to maintain and reorient auditory selective attention. *Exp Aging Res* 7:405–416, 1981.

70. Pastalan LA: Sensory changes and environmental behaviors. In Byerts TO, Howell SC, Pastalan LA (eds): *Environmental Context of Aging.* New York, Garland STPM Press, 1979, p 118.

71. Pfeiffer E: Handling the distressed older patient. *Geriatrics* 34:24–29, 1979.

72. Pratt CC, Simonson W, Lloyd S: Pharmacists' perceptions of major difficulties in geriatric pharmacy practice. *Gerontologist* 22:288–292, 1982.

73. Rubin KH, Brown IDR: A life span look at person perception and its relationship to communicative interaction. *J Gerontol* 30:461–468, 1975.

74. Rundall TG, Evashwick C: Social networks and help-seeking among the elderly. *Res Aging* 4:205–226, 1982.

75. Runnebohm S: Patterns of interpersonal communication with the elderly. Presented at the Arkansas Speech-Language-Hearing Association Convention, Little Rock, AR, 1981.

76. Ryan EB, Capadano HL: Age perceptions and evaluative reactions toward adult speakers. *J Gerontol* 33:98–102, 1978.

77. Ryan EB, Johnston DG: The influence of communicative effectiveness on evaluations of younger and older adult speakers. Presented at the Gerontological Society Convention, San Antonio, 1984.

78. Sasanuma S, Itoh M, Watamori TS, Fukuzasa K, Sakuma N, Fukusako Y, Monoi H: Linguistic and nonlinguistic abilities of the Japanese elderly and patients with dementia. In Ulatowska HK (ed): *The Aging Brain: Communication in the Elderly.* San Diego, College-Hill, 1985, p 175.

79. Schmall VL: Growing older: sensory changes, Pacific Northwest Extension Publication 196. Portland, OR, Oregon State University, 1980.

80. Schmall VL: Physical change and aging. Portland, OR, Oregon State University, 1978.

81. Schmitt JF, McCroskey RL: Sentence comprehension in elderly listeners: the factor of rate. *J Gerontol* 36:441–445, 1981.

82. Schonfeld L, Garcia J, Streuber P: Factors contributing to mental health treatment of the elderly. *J Appl Gerontol* 4:30–39, 1985.

83. Schonfield D: The variety of social skills: remarks by discussant. *Int J Aging Hum Dev* 17:39–42, 1983.

84. Schonfield D: Who is stereotyping whom and why? *Gerontologist* 22:267–271, 1982.

85. Schulz R, Rau MT: Social support through the life course. In Cohen S, Syme L (eds): *Social Support and Health.* New York, Academic Press, 1984, p 321.

86. Schwartz AN: Counseling: listening with the third ear. *Geriatrics* 35:95–102, 1980.

87. Sebastian RJ, Ryan EG, Abbott AR: Social judgments of speakers of different ages. Presented to the Midwestern Psychological Association Convention, Detroit, 1980.

88. Shadden BB: Communication process and aging: information needs and attitudes of older adults and professionals (grant report). Washington, DC, American Association of Retired Persons, 1982.

89. Sigman SJ: Conversational behavior in two health care institutions for the elderly. *Int J Aging Hum Dev* 21:137–154, 1985.

90. Sinnott JD: Stress, health, and mental health symptoms of older men and women. *Int J Aging Hum Dev* 20:123–132, 1985.

91. Solomon K: Social antecedents of learned help-

lessness in the health care setting. *Gerontologist* 22:282–287, 1982.

92. Steel RK: A clinical approach to communication with the elderly patient. In Obler LK, Albert ML (eds): *Language and Communication in the Elderly*. Lexington, MA, Lexington Books, 1980, p 133.

93. Stewart MA, Ryan EB: Attitudes toward younger and older adult speakers: effects of varying speech rates. *J Lang Soc Psychol* 1:91–109, 1982.

94. Streib GF: Changing roles in later years. In Kalish RJ (ed): *The Later Years: Social Applications of Gerontology*. Monterey, CA, Brooks/Cole, 1977, p 69.

95. Surber JR, Kowalski AH, Pena-Paez A: Effects of aging on the recall of extended expository prose. *Exp Aging Res* 10:25–28, 1984.

96. Taylor OL: Some generalizations on language and aging. Presented at the Conference on Gerontology and Communication Disorders, American Speech-Language-Hearing Association, Rockville, MD, 1983.

97. Tesch S, Whitbourne SK, Nehrke MF: Friendship, social interaction and subjective well-being of older men in an institutional setting. *Int J Aging Hum Dev* 13:317–327, 1981.

98. Thorson JA, Thorson JR: How accurate are stress scales? *J Gerontol Nurs* 12:21–24, 1986.

99. Tibbitts C: Can we invalidate negative stereotypes of aging? *Gerontologist* 19:10–20, 1979.

100. Tuckman J, Lorge I: Attitudes toward old people. *J Soc Psychol* 37:249–260, 1953.

101. Twining TC: Social skill, psychological disorder, and aging. *Int J Aging Hum Dev* 17:7–13, 1983.

102. Ulatowksa HK, Cannito MP, Hayashi MM, Fleming SG: Language abilities in the elderly. In Ulatowska HK (ed): *The Aging Brain: Communication in the Elderly*. San Diego, College-Hill, 1985, p 125.

103. U.S. Bureau of Census: *Demographic and Socioeconomic Aspects of Aging in the United States*, Current Population Reports, Series P-23, No. 138. Washington, DC, U.S. Government Printing Office, 1984.

104. Wantz MJ, Gay JE: *The Aging Process: A Health Perspective*. Cambridge, Winthrop Publishers, 1981.

105. Warren LR, Wagener JW, Herman GE: Binaural analysis in the aging auditory system. *J Gerontol* 33:731–736, 1978.

106. Weinberg J: What do I say to my mother when I have nothing to say? *Geriatrics* 29:155–159, 1974.

107. Weinstock C, Bennett R: Problems in communication to nurses among residents of a socially heterogeneous nursing home. *Gerontologist* 8:72–75, 1968.

108. West RL, Cohen SL: The systematic use of semantic and acoustic processing by younger and older adults. *Exp Aging Res* 11:81–86, 1985.

109. Wiig EH, Semel E: *Language Assessment and Intervention for the Learning Disabled*, ed 2. Columbus, OH, Charles E. Merrill, 1984.

110. Wingard JA, Health R, Himelstein S: The effects of contextual variation on attitudes toward the elderly. *J Gerontol* 37:475–482, 1982.

111. Yorkston KM, Beukelman DR: An analysis of connected speech samples of aphasic and normal speakers. *J Speech Hear Disord* 45:27–36, 1980.

11 Communication Disorders in the Elderly

JOHN D. TONKOVICH

Editor's Note

Compared to the general population, older individuals are at high risk for the development of specific hearing or speech-language disorders. In many instances, these disorders are superimposed upon other changes in communicative functioning described in the preceding chapters. In Chapter 11, Tonkovich reviews the most common forms of communication impairment found in the elderly, including stroke-related communication impairments (primarily aphasia and right hemisphere communication deficits); communication disorders in dementia; motor speech disorders; laryngectomy; and hearing loss. The discussion of hearing loss is restricted to prevalence comments because of the more extensive presentation in Chapter 8. For each of the other disorders, data are provided (when available) concerning prevalence, etiology, communication characteristics, and associated problems. The reader should pay close attention to descriptions of the manner in which chronological age influences the nature and severity of a disorder or its rehabilitation prognosis. Tonkovich concludes this chapter by pointing out the need for improved gerontological training in the field of communication disorders in order to enhance the quality of service provision and meet anticipated manpower needs in coming years.

INTRODUCTION

It is generally accepted that across age groups, approximately 1 in 10 individuals suffers from a speech, language, and/or hearing disorder. For some populations, the incidence is much higher. Any of us who have ever been in a nursing facility could attest to the fact that the incidence of communication disorders in this institutionalized population approaches nine out of ten individuals. A rather high incidence of communication disorders exists for the non-institutionalized elderly as well. In fact, it has been estimated that the incidence of hearing loss in the elderly ranges from 20 to 97% (78), and that perhaps 1,000,000 elderly individuals or more suffer speech and/or language disabilities. With improvements in health care, changes in life-style, and better health maintenance techniques, individuals are now surviving longer than they did several decades ago. With this increased longevity comes an increased susceptibility to communication disorders.

Debilitating conditions which may result in communication disorders can occur in all elderly individuals, regardless of race, socioeconomic status, or educational background. The prevalence of communication disorders rises sharply with increasing age, reflecting the greater frequency of occurrence of conditions such as stroke, cancer, and dementing illness.

In this chapter, we will examine some of the major illnesses encountered by the elderly, and their concomitant communication disorders. The incidence of stroke will be provided, along with a discussion of the types of communication problems seen in patients following left hemisphere and right hemisphere strokes. Next, there will be a summary of conditions which may result in reversible dementing states, as well as an examination of those conditions which result in chronic irreversible dementing states. In the following two sections, disorders affecting speech production in the elderly will be addressed: those neurological disorders which result in so-called "motor speech disorders" (31) and those requiring surgical removal of the larynx. Finally, there will be a brief discussion of incidence data regarding hearing loss in the elderly.

One issue not addressed in this chapter is that of environmental changes which may adversely affect an elderly individual's opportunities for communication. Holland, for instance, noted differences in communicative performance between institutionalized patients and those who lived at home (42). Widowed individuals who live alone may not experience the frequency of communicative interactions they did in younger years. Elderly individuals who become communicatively deprived in late adulthood may indeed have communication problems, whether or not they are labeled as specific communication disorders. Clearly environmental influences may also compound a communicatively disordered older individual's social interactional problems (see Chapters 10 and 18 for further discussion of these issues).

STROKE AND COMMUNICATION IMPAIRMENTS IN THE ELDERLY

Overview

The term "stroke" refers specifically to disorders resulting from an impairment of blood circulation in the brain. A synonymous term, cerebrovascular accident (CVA), is also commonly used. The use of the term CVA implies an etiology which is vascular in origin and distinguishes it from other brain disorders which are not related to circulation but may have stroke-like symptomatology (60). Stroke is one of the major causes of death in the United States. However, it has been noted that the incidence of stroke has been declining over the past 50 years (98), primarily as a result of life-style changes, early recognition of patients with a predisposition to stroke, and appropriate preventative interventions.

Stroke is recognized primarily as a disorder of aging, with incidences higher for older age groups. Kurtzke (49) noted that, for individuals under the age of 50, the incidence is less than one per 1,000 population annually. By age 70, the incidence climbs to nearly 10 per 1,000, and by age 80, incidence is approximately 20 per 1,000. Stroke incidence figures led Metter (60) to infer that, for a population of 230 million people at any given time, approximately one million will be living after suffering a stroke, while 250,000 to 500,000 will suffer a stroke annually, and 125,000 to 250,000 will subsequently die from stroke-related causes.

Stroke is the major medical condition underlying a number of communication disorders. It is the most common cause of aphasia, and may result in a variety of other cognitive-language disturbances and motor speech disorders. Communication disturbances associated with stroke are related primarily to location and size of lesion. Effects are also apt to be cumulative, in that individuals who suffer more than one stroke typically will demonstrate a more complex array of communicative impairments than they did following the initial CVA.

In the following sections, we will focus on two major communicative impairments which commonly result from CVA—aphasia (resulting from left hemisphere lesions) and communication impairments resulting from right hemisphere damage. While CVA is often an underlying cause of dementia and of dysarthric speech, these two disorders will be addressed later in the chapter.

Aphasia

Aphasia (dysphasia) refers to a reduction in language reception, expression, and/or usage as a result of brain damage. It most commonly results from strokes involving the left cerebral hemisphere, although *crossed aphasia* (an aphasic condition in right-handed individuals following right hemisphere damage) has been reported in as many as 10% of all aphasic patients (15). Aphasia may result from other disorders, such as closed head injury, brain tumors, chronic subdural hematoma, and multiple sclerosis. In these conditions, patients do not follow homogeneous recovery patterns and may often show increased communicative difficulties over time.

Methodological issues in aphasia research have perpetuated a controversy regarding how aphasia is classified. Some investigators have viewed aphasia as a unitary disorder and as a reduction of available language which crosses all modalities. Others have identified several types of aphasia, with distinguishable symptom complexes which vary as a function of site of lesion. This controversy has added confusion about how to interpret aphasia research findings, and the issue of whether or not to classify aphasia has been addressed recently by several investigators (3, 22, 80, 99).

In clinical practice, most speech-language pathologists tend to try to classify aphasia, assuming perhaps that such classifications afford important diagnostic, prognostic, and treatment implications. A summary of some widely used aphasia classification systems is presented in Table 11.1

The four category system for classifying aphasia developed by Weisenberg and McBride (95) is a useful one, although it is often misused in clinical practice. Weisenberg and McBride's original notion that patients exhibited *predominantly expressive* and *predominantly receptive* aphasia has often been implemented incorrectly as *expressive aphasia* and *receptive aphasia*, implying some level of intact ability in the opposite language dimension. It has been well established that aphasic individuals whose primary communicative deficit is expressive

Table 11.1
Some Widely Used Aphasia Classification Systems

Weisenburg and McBride (1935): Aphasia Classification System
  Predominantly receptive
  Predominantly expressive
  Amnesic
  Expressive-receptive
Schuell (1964): Aphasia Classification System
  Group 1—Simple aphasia
  Group 2—Aphasia with visual involvement
  Group 3—Aphasia with sensorimotor impairment
  Group 4—Aphasia with scattered findings compatible with generalized brain damage
  Group 5—Irreversible aphasic syndrome
  Minor Syndrome A—Aphasia with partial auditory imperception
  Minor Syndrome B—Mild aphasia with persisting dysarthria
Wepman and Jones (1966): Aphasia Classification System
  Pragmatic aphasia
  Semantic aphasia
  Syntactic aphasia
  Jargon aphasia
  Global aphasia
Goodglass and Kaplan (1972): Aphasia Classification System
  Nonfluent Aphasias
    Broca's aphasia
    Global aphasia
    Transcortical motor aphasia
  Fluent Aphasias
    Wernicke's aphasia
    Anomic aphasia
    Conduction aphasia
    Transcortical sensory aphasia
    Alexia with agraphia
  Pure Aphasias
    Aphemia (subcortical motor aphasia)
    Pure word-deafness (subcortical sensory aphasia)
    Pure alexia (pure word-blindness)
    Pure agraphia
  Callosal Disconnection Syndromes
    Unilateral tactile aphasia
    Unilateral agraphia and apraxia
    Hemioptic aphasia
Benson (1972): Syndromes of Aphasia
  Perisylvian Aphasia Syndromes   Nonlocalizing Aphasia Syndromes
    Broca aphasia   Anomic aphasia
    Wernicke aphasia   Global aphasia
    Conduction aphasia   Alexia
  Borderzone Aphasia Syndromes   Parietal-temporal alexia
    Transcortical motor aphasia   Occipital alexia
    Aphasia of anterior cerebral artery   Frontal alexia
      infarction   Agraphia
    Transcortical sensory aphasia   Related Syndromes
    Mixed transcortical aphasia   Aphemia
  Subcortical Aphasia Syndromes   Pure word deafness
    The aphasia of Marie's quadrilateral   Apraxia of speech
      space   Nonaphasic misnaming
    Thalamic aphasia
    Striatal aphasia
    Aphasia from white matter lesions

also experience some receptive language deficits, and vice versa. Weisenberg and McBride's system, while useful for distinguishing aphasia types in a rudimentary way, is limited in that the four aphasia categories do not correspond to lesion sites, nor do they differentiate aphasia symptom complexes adequately.

Schuell's (79) classification system for aphasia is unique in that, while it presumes a unitary aphasic condition, discrete categories of aphasia are based on severity. Simple aphasia represents the least severe type of aphasia and irreversible aphasic syndrome the most severe form. Prognosis for recovery from aphasia was presumed to follow a similar pattern, in that individuals with simple aphasia were capable of complete recovery and those with irreversible aphasic syndrome had limited recovery potential. Schuell's aphasia types were derived from patient cluster groups identified during standardization of her *Minnesota Test for Differential Diagnosis of Aphasia*. While potentially useful for categorizing aphasic patients by severity, this system has not been used widely in clinical practice or research.

In recent years, perhaps as a result of technological advances such as CAT scans and magnetic resonance imaging techniques, the classification systems of Goodglass and Kaplan (37) and Benson (9) have become popular in clinical and research use. The focus of the Goodglass and Kaplan system is fluency of verbal output, while Benson's system focuses primarily on the locus of the lesion. Nevertheless, certain common aphasic syndromes occur in both systems.

Broca's aphasia, associated with lesions involving the third frontal convolution, is a nonfluent aphasia. It is typified by agrammatism, restricted vocabulary, and apractic speech, while auditory comprehension is generally well-preserved. Reading comprehension is only mildly affected, but writing is usually at least as severely impaired as speech. Wepman and Jones (96) referred to this type of aphasia as syntactic aphasia. Patients with Broca's aphasia have been observed to show greater than average amounts of recovery and more rapid recovery rates than patients with other types of aphasia (46). Approximately 20% of all aphasic patients exhibit this type of aphasia (88).

Wernicke's aphasia, attributable to lesions of the first temporal gyrus, is a fluent aphasia characterized by impaired auditory comprehension, and fluently articulated by neologistic verbal output, in the context of relatively well spared syntactic structure and prosody. Patients with Wernicke's aphasia experience substantial naming deficits, impairment of word and

sentence repetition, and reading and writing deficits. Wepman and Jones labelled this syndrome pragmatic aphasia (96). Approximately 15 to 20% of all aphasic patients have Wernicke's aphasia (88).

Conduction aphasia is a fluent aphasia resulting from lesions involving the arcuate fasciculus and/or supramarginal gyrus. Its chief characteristics are infrequent yet fluent speech, near normal auditory comprehension, and difficulty with word and sentence repetition. On repetition attempts, conduction aphasic patients often experience literal paraphasia (difficulty choosing and sequencing phonemes), and these literal paraphasic errors repeatedly occur during spontaneous speech. Persons with conduction aphasia have demonstrated a considerable degree of recovery and rapid recovery rates (46). Approximately 5 to 10% of all aphasic patients have this type of aphasia (10).

Two less frequently occurring syndromes are transcortical sensory aphasia and transcortical motor aphasia, both characterized by remarkably intact repetition skills and impaired auditory comprehension, the former with fluent and paraphasic speech, and the latter with nonfluent speech and largely intact confrontation naming. Lesions associated with transcortical sensory aphasia have been localized to an area posterior to Wernicke's area around the anterior boundary of the occipital lobe (30), and this syndrome occurs in about 2% of aphasia patients (88). Lesions producing transcortical motor aphasia occur in the region anterior to and superior to Broca's area, and this syndrome also occurs infrequently.

Two aphasic syndromes which are not readily localizable are global aphasia and anomic or semantic aphasia (9, 96). Global aphasia is the most frequent type of aphasia, occurring in 20 to 25% of all aphasic patients (88). Patients with global aphasia show severe impairment across all language modalities, sparse, meaningless verbalizations and little comprehension. It is not unusual to observe this condition immediately post onset, with speech-language symptoms more closely resembling another aphasic syndrome as recovery occurs (13, 46). Anomic aphasia represents approximately 8% of the total number of cases of aphasia (88). Patients with this aphasic syndrome show difficulties primarily in confrontation naming and in word finding in spontaneous speech. Speech is characteristically fluent and circumlocutionary as patients attempt to say something specific, while auditory comprehension is well-preserved. Many aphasic patients following treatment and with recovery present a clinical picture of anomic aphasia. Research findings have indicated that both global aphasic and anomic aphasic patients show the smallest amount of recovery and the slowest rates of recovery on the *Western Aphasia Battery* (46), although it has been noted that anomic aphasic patients have high initial performances on this test, leaving little room for improvement (32).

A number of other aphasic syndromes have been identified, including aphasias resulting from lesions involving subcortical structures such as the thalamus (62, 90), the internal capsule and putamen (29, 68), and the caudate (16). Some so-called "pure aphasias," syndromes in which a single language modality is impaired, have also been described in the literature and include pure word-blindness (alexia-without agraphia), pure word-deafness, and aphemia (in which only oral expression is impaired). Both the subcortical and the pure aphasias occur rarely relative to those aphasic syndromes previously described.

It should be noted that, because elderly aphasic patients may be experiencing concomitant aging-related deficits in communication skills and may have more complicating medical conditions than younger patients, the clinical pictures they present may not always resemble the clinical syndromes of aphasia described here. For that reason, when patients fail to fall into one of the classically defined aphasic syndromes, speech-language pathologists often use more generic labels such as *mixed aphasia* to classify the aphasic syndrome. It is considered good clinical practice to describe the aphasic symptoms observed, even if a classification label is utilized.

In summary, a variety of aphasia classification systems have been proposed. Some systems are based on severity of aphasia, while others presuppose relationships between the type of language deficits and site of lesion. No one system for classifying aphasias is superior to any other, as long as the aphasic symptoms are adequately and accurately described. In the next section, age-related findings relative to aphasia will be provided.

Aphasia in the Elderly

There have been conflicting reports in the literature about age of onset of aphasia and its influences on recovery. It was previously assumed that older aphasic patients could improve with therapy, but the gains would not be as dramatic as for younger aphasic patients (78). The findings of a number of studies were interpreted to support this notion that age was an important predictor of recovery for aphasic patients (61, 75, 89). A more contemporary point of view is that age itself is not a strong predictive variable of recovery from aphasia. Age was not found to be a significant factor in studies exploring the relationship between age and spontaneous recovery from aphasia (46, 77). In fact, in an investigation of spontaneous recovery from aphasia, Culton demonstrated that older aphasic subjects improved more than the younger ones (24). Similarly, there has been no significant relationship demonstrated between age of onset and amount of recovery in treated patients in several recent studies (5, 44, 70, 76). Because of the potential interference of many conditions associated with aging, Davis has cautioned that we cannot rule out age as a predictor of recovery, but it may not be as important a factor as it was once believed to be (32).

While age of onset may not have strong predictive value relative to the amount of recovery from aphasia, it has been demonstrated to be an important influence on the type of aphasia observed (42, 69). In general, there seems to be a trend toward more pronounced disturbances of comprehension with increasing age in aphasic patients. Holland (42) investigated the relationship of age to type of aphasia and observed that Wernicke's aphasic patients were significantly older than Broca's and anomic aphasic patients. Global aphasic patients were also significantly older than anomic aphasic patients. She postulated that these findings implied a relationship between language deficit and cognitive function at the far end of the life span, and cautioned that great care should be taken in differentially diagnosing aphasia, particularly as it related to cortical dementia and atrophy. Output is similar in both Wernicke's aphasia and cortical dementia.

Holland (42) also commented that the world view of younger clinicians is often imposed on the much different world view of elderly aphasic patients. She suggested that many older aphasic individuals consequently are treated against their wishes because clinicians think they need therapy. Holland suggested that this was a gross clinical error which dehumanized patients and wasted time. In all rehabilitation efforts, we should be mindful of the fact that some patients do not desire treatment, and it is important to respect these wishes.

In summary, age of onset of aphasia may play a minor role in predicting recovery, although it is not, by itself, a potent prognostic indicator. There does appear to be a relationship between age and type of aphasia, in that there seems to be a trend toward aphasic syndromes with more pronounced auditory comprehension impairments (i.e., global aphasia, Wernicke's aphasia) as a function of increasing age. Finally, we should be careful in preserving the dignity of elderly aphasic patients in our rehabilitation efforts, as we may not share their perceptions about what is important.

Aphasic impairments have been widely studied, and incidence data and aging effects have been documented. Communication impairments associated with right hemisphere lesions are somewhat more elusive. It is only recently that they have received much attention in clinical and research interventions. In the next section, a description of the types of communication problems which have been identified in right hemisphere-damaged patients will be provided.

Right Hemisphere Communication Impairments

While a number of motor and neurobehavioral sequelae resulting from right hemisphere damage have been described and subjected to research investigation, communication disturbances resulting from lesions to the right hemisphere went largely unnoticed and ignored until the past decade or so. Speech-language pathologists, by and large, did not treat patients with right hemisphere CVAs unless they exhibited severely dysarthric speech. Because patients with right hemisphere damage typically could express their needs in fully grammatical sentences, they were not referred for speech-language pathology services. While these patients were often noted to have copious verbal output, speech language pathologists prior to the mid 1970s were not accustomed to working on communicative disorders that were not deficits in word retrieval or syntactic structure. The patients themselves did not seek speech-language pathology advice, partly because of the indifference toward their own illness sometimes associated with right hemisphere lesions and mostly because they could talk.

As interest in pragmatic aspects of communication has evolved in the last 10 years or so, however, a new role for the speech-language pathologist has emerged. Not only is treatment geared toward remediating deficits in language structure, but clinicians have become acutely aware of the need to intervene with patients who show adequate language structure, but inadequate language function. Difficulties right hemisphere damaged patients have with the subtle nuances of communicative behavior consequently are being remediated by many speech-language pathologists.

Communicative deficits in right hemisphere damaged patients are often highlighted on tasks requiring engagement in conversational speech. Myers (64) noted that, as the level of abstract-

ness of a task increases, right hemisphere damaged patients are more likely to demonstrate: (a) difficulty organizing verbal information meaningfully and efficiently; (b) impulsive, poorly thought out statements characterized by tangential and related, but unnecessary detail; (c) difficulty distinguishing between important and unimportant information; (d) problems in assimilating and utilizing contextual information; (e) literal interpretations of figurative language; (f) overpersonalization of external events; and (g) reduced sensitivity to the communicative situation and the pragmatic aspects of communication. Other communicative impairments which have been reported for right hemisphere damaged patients include inappropriate jocularity, confabulatory output, and nonprosodic or flat delivery (35); embellishment (82); impaired ability to use prosodic cues in conveying and/or interpreting emotional tone (72); impaired propositionality and distorted presuppositions (51); and disturbed nonverbal communication, conversational initiation disorders, poor eye contact, turn-taking disturbances, and topic maintenance disruptions (19).

Further complications to the observed clinical picture in right hemisphere damaged individuals are posed by additional symptoms which may interfere with communicative appropriateness. Among these are hemispatial neglect (38), anosognosia (denial of illness) (25), disturbances of facial expression (33), disturbances of facial and voice recognition (86, 91), topographical disorientation (58), and a variety of neuropsychiatric disorders (2, 25).

Lesion sites and incidence data regarding right hemisphere communication impairments are not available to date. It has been noted that, since the right cerebral hemisphere is more diffusely organized than the left, it it not often easy to correlate narrowly defined deficits with highly specific lesions (65). Several symptoms which have been observed in right hemisphere damaged patients have been localized to gross regions of the hemisphere, and these symptoms will now be discussed.

Hemispatial neglect, while sometimes occurring as a result of left hemisphere lesions, is typically more severe in patients with right hemisphere damage. Patients with this symptom fail to recognize, attend to, and orient to stimuli presented to the side of space contralateral to the site of lesion. While this condition has been observed as a result of frontal, parietal and subcortical damage, it is usually more pronounced and persistent subsequent to damage to the parietal lobe (59, 92). In right hemisphere damage, patients may show left hemispatial neglect, characterized by inattention to stimuli presented to the left of midline. This neglect

Table 11.2
Several Concomitant Attitudes Patients with Anosognosia May Display Relative to Their Paretic Limbs[a]

Condition	Manifestations
Anosodiaphoria	Patient minimizes the extent of paresis and jokes about paretic limb(s) (e.g., "I left my arm in occupational therapy—it likes being down there").
Somatophrenia	Patient attributes ownership of the paretic limb(s) to another person (e.g., "That's Joe Wrigley's arm anyway").
Misoplegia	Patient expresses overt hatred of the limb (e.g., "I hate my hand and want to trade it in").
Anosognosic Overestimation	Patient exaggerates the strength of the limb.

[a](Adapted from Cummings JL: Neurological syndromes associated with right hemisphere damage. In Burns MS, Halper AS, Mogil SI (eds): *Clinical Management of Right Hemisphere Dysfunction*. Rockville, MD, Aspen Systems Corporation, 1985, p 7.)

syndrome may create a variety of problems, including difficulty in reading and writing; spatial disorientation and poor alignment of letters in copying tasks; failure to orient to auditory and/or tactile stimuli presented on the left side; lack of detail on the left side of drawings; and written arithmetic errors resulting from poor spatial alignment of numbers on paper. It is not uncommon to observe patients with left hemispatial neglect bumping into furniture and/or walls in their attempts to move about the environment.

Anosognosia or denial of illness often accompanies left hemispatial neglect. Anosognosia may range in severity from a total denial of deficits (i.e., left hemiparesis, left visual field disturbances) to an underestimate of the severity of the disorder. Most commonly, anosognosia results from lesions involving the right parietal lobe (25). Table 11.2 summarizes several concomitant attitudes that patients with anosognosia may display relative to their paretic limbs. A related condition which has been observed in some patients is the belief that an additional limb has been attached on the paralyzed side (94). These forms of anosognosia interfere with normal communication interaction, and may impede speech-language rehabilitation efforts. It has been noted that rehabilitation attempts with patients who demonstrate left hemispatial neglect and anosognosia may be unsuccessful (38), since patients are not convinced they have deficits in the first place. However, some clinical reports have documented successful rehabilitation of these patients (34).

Production of emotionally driven prosody has been attributed to anterior lesions in the right hemisphere (72), while patients with right parietal lobe lesions have been reported to fail in comprehension of such prosodic elements (25). Facial recognition disturbances have been associated with posterior lesions in the right hemisphere (25). These symptoms also impede communicative interactions.

In summary, right hemisphere lesions give rise to a number of communication disorders, as well as associated deficits which may interfere with normal communicative interactions. The nature and theoretical underpinnings of these disorders are not thoroughly understood, as neurological organization in the right hemisphere makes localization of these symptoms difficult. We might, however, predict that patients with posterior (in contrast to anterior) lesion in the right hemisphere might display more serious complexes of communication-related behaviors. Incidence data are not available, and there have been few investigations of communicative functions of right hemisphere damaged patients to date. Myers (66) has addressed the urgency of systematic data collection about communication impairments in this population. No doubt there will be important research findings in the coming years regarding right hemisphere damaged patients, and relationships between aging and right hemisphere symptoms might be established.

The sequelae of cerebrovascular accidents are varied. Communicative disturbances associated with left hemisphere lesions are fairly well-defined, and most can be attributed to specific lesion sites. Communicative disturbances associated with right hemisphere damage are more subtle and less clearly defined, with fewer identifiable sites of lesion. It should not be inferred that communication disorders resulting from right hemisphere lesions are less serious disturbances than those associated with left hemisphere lesions, as Kozy and Tarvin (48) have addressed some of the needs family members have in coping with these disabilities. Not only families, but elderly patients themselves must cope with the limiting communication disabilities they suffer following a CVA.

COMMUNICATION DISORDERS IN DEMENTIA

Overview

It comes as no surprise that speech-language pathologists have been reluctant to become involved in the management of communicative disorders resulting from dementing illnesses. Patients with dementing illnesses have poor prognoses for recovery and typically do not demonstrate much potential for favorable rehabilitation outcomes or new learning. In addition, Medicare and other third party reimbursers generally have not been supportive of speech-language therapeutic interventions for dementia patients. For these reasons, the literature regarding communicative management strategies for dementing patients is sparse. Specific intervention considerations for dementing individuals are found elsewhere in this volume (see Chapter 17).

In the following sections of this chapter, a review of the major causes of reversible dementia and irreversible dementia will be presented. Incidence and prevalence figures will be provided when these are available. Finally, communication symptoms associated with dementing illnesses will be described, as well as typical courses of progression.

Dementia is a phenomenon which is often, though not always, associated with old age. It is commonly characterized by gradual and progressive deterioration of memory, intellect, judgment and orientation, accompanied by increasing lability and shallowness of affect. In the past several decades, it has become clear that some chronic dementing conditions that have lasted several months to a year may be partly or completely reversible. For this reason, it is imperative that the dementing patient undergo a thorough medical differential diagnostic examination (see Chapters 6 and 17). Bayles (7) advised that, while speech-language pathologists may play an important role in identifying individuals with reversible dementia, irreversibility of the syndrome should not be presumed without a thorough review of the patient's case history and medical examination findings. Speech-language pathologists may only be involved in intervention for those with irreversible dementia, but it is important to understand reversible causes of the condition nonetheless.

Reversible Causes of Dementia

A number of reversible causes of dementia have been identified, including drug toxicity, depression, visual and hearing disorders, metabolic and endocrine disorders, normal pressure hydrocephalus, intracranial masses, infection, and arteriosclerotic complications. Patients with dementias resulting from the aforementioned causes may exhibit decreased mental functioning until some medical, psychiatric/psychologic or surgical intervention causes the symptoms to subside or reverse. A discussion of the major reversible causes of dementia follows.

Drug Toxicity

Burks (17) noted that, while individuals over age 65 comprised only approximately 10% of the population, these same individuals consumed 25% of all prescription drugs. Excessive drug ingestion may result in dementia symptoms in older individuals. Even small amounts of drugs may induce these symptoms in older elderly persons, especially those who are undernourished, those who have significantly reduced kidney function, and those with arteriosclerosis. Table 11.3 provides a partial listing of medications which may produce symptoms of dementia (for more detail on drug effects, see Chapter 7).

Psychotropic agents are often used in the treatment of manic-depressive illness, and psychoactive drugs such as lithium carbonate and haloperidol may cause dementia symptoms. Antihypertensive drugs such as diuretics may cause dehydration and subsequent mental confusion. Levodopa (antiparkinsonian) and indomethacin (antiarthritic) may also result in diminished mental function (20). In drug-induced dementias, the toxic effects are often reversible by discontinuation of the drug.

Depression

A number of emotional and psychiatric disorders may produce dementia symptoms as well. Patients with these disorders may exhibit marked social withdrawal, confusion, hypochondriasis, delusions of persecution, and hostile behavior. A class of depressions known as retarded depression has often been cited as a major psychiatric cause of reversible dementia. According to Cummings and Benson (26), patients with retarded depressive dementia are

Table 11.3
A Partial Listing of Medications Which May Produce Symptoms of Dementia

1. Antibiotics
     Chloramphenicol
     Griseofulvin
     Penicillin
     Polymyxins
     Sulfonamide
2. Anticholinergic Compounds
3. Anticonvulsant Drugs
     Barbiturates
     Ethosuximide
     Phenytoin
4. Antihypertensive Agents
     Diuretics
     Methyldopa
     Propanolol hydrochloride
5. Psychotropic Agents
     Haloperidol
     Lithium carbonate
     Phenothiazines
     Tricyclic antidepressants
6. Other Agents
     Amphetamines
     Anticholinergic compounds
     Antidiabetic agents
     Bromides
     Digitalis
     Disulfiram
     Ergot
     Levodopa
     Oral contraceptives
     Steroids

a(Adapted from Cummings JL, Benson DF: *Dementia: A Clinical Approach.* Boston, Butterworth, 1983.)

apt to show symptoms of psychomotor slowing, bent posture, bowed head, and slow whispered speech, as well as latency of response, forgetfulness, disorientation, impaired attention and poor abstraction abilities.

The dementia associated with retarded depression often progresses more rapidly and is shorter in duration than other more degenerative types of dementia. Patients will typically show impaired word-list recognition, cognitive deterioration, reduced memory, depressed affect, and awareness of cognitive deficits. Careful differential medical diagnosis is imperative, as dementias resulting from depression and other psychiatric disorders may be treatable with psychotherapy and/or medications. Table 11.4 summarizes some of the signs and symptoms associated with depressive dementia, distinguishing it from more insidiously degenerative dementia. Although depressive dementia has been noted occasionally in younger patients, it is generally atypical of early or midlife, and occurs most often in the elderly (23).

Visual and Hearing Disorders

Elderly individuals with markedly reduced vision and hearing may display symptoms of dementia, such as disorientation, poor memory, difficulty with new learning and increased speech irrelevance. The introduction of prosthetic aids (e.g., corrective lenses, amplification) to vision and hearing and/or multimodal sensory inputs may reduce or reverse the dementia symptoms.

Metabolic and Endocrine Disorders

A number of metabolic conditions may give rise to reversible dementias, as prolonged or recurring interruptions of vital metabolic substrates result in intellectual impairment. Examples of metabolic disturbances which might cause reversible dementias are anoxia; encephalopathies resulting from kidney, liver, or pancreas disorders; electrolyte imbalances,

Table 11.4
Clinical Signs and Symptoms Which Differentiate Depression and Dementia

Depression	Dementia
Rapid onset; causally linked	Slow, ill-defined onset
Typically rapid progression of symptoms	Typically slow progression of symptoms
Preoccupation with deficits	Minimal awareness of deficits
Complaints regarding symptoms	Cover up and/or denial of symptoms
Often worse in morning, better as day goes on	Worse later in day or when fatigued
Vegetative symptoms (e.g., loss of appetite, insomnia) common	Vegetative symptoms absent or negligible
Speech comprehension and production generally intact	Speech comprehension and/or production disturbances noticeable

particularly relative to serum sodium concentrations; and vitamin deficiencies, particularly of thiamine, cyanocobalamin (B_{12}), niacin, and folic acid.

Endocrinopathies, such as those resulting from abnormal functioning of the thyroid, parathyroid, adrenal or pituitary glands may also result in reversible dementing conditions. Restoration of cerebral oxygenation, fluid-electrolyte imbalancing, and dietary and hormonal supplements may be prescribed by the patient's physician for reversing those dementing conditions arising from metabolic and endocrine origins.

Normal Pressure Hydrocephalus

The dementia resulting from normal pressure hydrocephalus is not particularly common, but it is treatable. This phenomenon is characterized by a gradual enlargement of brain ventricles in conjunction with normal cerebrospinal fluid pressure, and often follows previous head trauma, meningitis, or subarachnoid hemorrhage (20). Surgical shunting of the cerebrospinal fluid from the ventricular space to the peritoneal space, the atrium of the heart, or the pleural cavity serves to reverse the dementia symptoms.

Intracranial Masses

Intracranial masses may give rise to a number of dementia symptoms, depending on their size, speed of growth, and location. When medically possible, they are treated with combinations of surgical removal, chemotherapy, and/or radiotherapy on the basis of their location and nature, and the symptoms subside or reverse accordingly.

Infection

Pneumonia, tertiary syphilis, encephalitis, and meningitis, particularly in elderly individuals, may result in reversible dementia symptoms. Medical interventions often can reverse the dementing condition associated with these infections.

Arteriosclerotic Complications

In arteriosclerosis, blood flow to the brain is impeded. As a result, insufficient oxygen and nutrients reach the brain tissue, leading to reductions in intellectual and memory functions. Chronic arteriosclerosis may eventuate in transient ischemic attacks or cerebrovascular accidents, which in turn may lead to more chronic and irreversible dementing states. In early stages of dementia arising from arteriosclerosis, symptoms can often be reversed through surgery or through drug therapies, such as those involving vasodilators.

Given the large number of potential causes of reversible dementia, a careful and thorough medical examination is essential. Heston and White (39) have commented on the effects of incomplete medical examination, in that a less than thorough examination may result in months of suffering from a treatable illness. Those individuals with reversible dementing conditions will often have excellent prognoses for recovery and for restoration of intellectual and memory functions to within normal limits. Those with irreversible dementias, in contrast, face progressive deterioration of intellectual and memory functions, followed by a fatal end. It is this latter group of patients that the speech-language pathologist will likely encounter in most medical and health care facilities (7). A discussion of some of the causes of irreversible dementing conditions follows.

Major Irreversible Dementia Producing Diseases

In recent years, considerable media attention has focused heavily on the most common dementing illness, Alzheimer's disease. Alzheimer's disease accounts for approximately half of the cases of dementia at any age and an estimated 20 to 30% of the population who live to their mid-80s. A number of other conditions may result in irreversible dementias as well: multiinfarct dementia; Parkinson's disease; Huntington's disease; Pick's disease; Creutzfeldt-Jacob disease; and Binswanger's disease. In the following sections, we will focus attention on these disease processes.

Alzheimer's Disease

A number of methodological and diagnostic obstacles have precluded the determination of accurate incidence and prevalence figures for Alzheimer's disease. Cummings and Benson (26) reviewed seven previous dementia studies and reported Alzheimer's disease as accounting for from 22% (43) to 57% (87) of the dementia patients in individual studies. Despite this wide range, it is clear that Alzheimer's disease is the most prevalent cause of irreversible dementia.

Alzheimer's disease is a medical diagnosis of exclusion, based on the absence of other identifiable source of dementia. In autopsy, brains of individuals with dementia of Alzheimer's type (DAT) show pronounced atrophy, especially in the temporoparietal and anterior frontal regions (26), and characteristic neurofibrillary tangles, senile plaques and granulovascular degeneration. Sim et al (84) noted that, during early phases of DAT, individuals demonstrate remarkably well-preserved personality and social behavior as intellect deteriorates insidiously. Given these preserved functions, individuals are often able to continue working and participating in social activities, while the extent of their dementia goes unnoticed. As the disease progresses, personality, memory, and intellectual functions become diminished.

Early onset of irreversible recent memory deficits in DAT often tends to be associated with a shorter duration of illness (39). When onset of these deficits occurs between ages 55 and 70, there is an increased duration of illness and an average survival period of approximately 8.5 years. When the onset occurs at more advanced ages, the duration of illness and subsequent survival period decrease.

Multi-infarct Dementia

Dementia resulting from multiple infarctions (often in individuals with a history of chronic hypertension or arteriosclerosis) differs from DAT. Approximately 20% of all dementing patients have this type of dementia, and it has been proposed that another 15% of dementing patients have DAT and multi-infarct dementia concurrently (85). Age of onset of multi-infarct dementia is typically between 50 and 70 years, with an average age of 66 years, and it appears more commonly in men than women (20).

Patients with multi-infarct dementia are not as homogeneous in their symptoms and courses of illness as those with DAT. Because symptoms and courses relate to the number and extent of brain lesions present, which vary widely, individuals with multi-infarct dementia follow no typical course. Multi-infarct dementia patients typically have a history of previous strokes, abrupt onset of mental deterioration and an uneven and erratic decline in functioning. Since both cortical and subcortical structures are involved, these patients display a wide variety of symptoms, ranging from amnesia, visuospatial deficits and aphasia from cortical lesions, to memory impairment and psychomotor retardation stemming from subcortical lesions.

Onset of multi-infarct dementia is rapid, with over 50% of cases occurring acutely in the form of a sudden attack of confusion. There is usually a gradual intellectual loss, and memory impairment associated with multi-infarct dementia tends to be inconsistent rather than complete. In other words, patients may be unable to remember one minute and then regain total capacity the next. Individuals with multi-infarct dementia also may have inconsistent insight regarding their problems as well as inconsistent judgment skills (20).

Binswanger's Disease

Binswanger's disease is characterized by multiple infarcts of the white matter in the cerebral hemispheres and deterioration of subcortical myelin. The dementia associated with Binswanger's disease is slowly progressing; it occurs in individuals between the ages of 50 and 65 (20). It has been demonstrated (71) that the brains of Binswanger's disease patients on CT scan show dramatically enlarged ventricles as well as multiple lucencies identifying infarctions in the hemispheric white matter.

Parkinson's Disease

Parkinson's disease is a degenerative neurological disorder of unknown etiology, which results from a deficiency of the neurochemical inhibitor substance released in the basal ganglia. Its salient characteristics are exaggerated tone, slowness and limited range of movement, cogwheel rigidity, and masklike facial expression (20, 31). The prevalence of Parkinson's disease in the population is approximately one per 1000 (26), and incidence figures of between 500,000 and 1,000,000 cases in the United States have been cited (78), with between 25,000 and 43,000 new cases identified each year. The typical age of onset of Parkinson's disease is between ages 50 and 65, with a mean duration of illness of 8 years, although some individuals may live much longer. Death is usually attributable to aspiration pneumonia, urinary tract infections or some unrelated condition affecting the elderly such as cancer or heart disease (40, 57, 81). Irreversible dementias occur frequently in patients with Parkinson's disease, approaching 50% of all patients, although incidence figures in different studies have been reported to range from 3 to 93% of Parkinson's disease patients (12).

It has been noted that the occurrence of dementia in Parkinson's disease becomes more prevalent and increases in severity as the disease progresses (63). With the disease progression, Parkinson's disease patients also are more likely to demonstrate decreased performance on cognitive and memory tasks on neuropsychological test batteries (56). Examinations of a number of Parkinson's disease patients have led several investigators to suggest that two varieties of the disease exist—one essentially a motor disorder without dementia, involving only subcortical structures, and a second variety characterized by both motor dysfunction and dementia, and involving both cortical and subcortical changes (14, 36, 52).

Huntington's Disease

[handwritten margin note: DYSARTHRIA AS WEll]

Huntington's disease is a heredity disease characterized by atrophy of subcortical structures such as the caudate, globus pallidus, and putamen. Its onset is typically in middle age, and it progresses to death within 10 to 20 years of onset (20). Patients with Huntington's disease display incessant and uncontrollable choreic movements and a concomitant progressive dementia.

Huntington's disease occurs in 40 to 70 individuals per million (41, 67), and has equal likelihood of occurrence in males and females (26). Impaired verbal fluency and memory disturbances are observed early in the course of the disease (21). Unlike patients with DAT, who can retain and recall remote information in early stages of dementia, Huntington's disease patients have as much difficulty with recall of remote as well as recent information (1). As the disease progresses, patients with Huntington's disease experience increasing difficulties with organization and sequencing of language and with naming tests that require retrieval of low frequency words (45).

Pick's Disease

Pick's disease is a progressive neurological disease of unknown etiology, with an estimated age of onset of 55.4 years and an average survival rate of seven years (39). Post-mortem examination of brains of patients with Pick's disease reveal atrophy primarily of the anterior portions of the frontal and temporal lobes (20).

Early symptomatology observed in patients with Pick's disease includes personality changes characterized by a loss of tact and concern, impaired judgment, and a decline in recent memory (20, 26). As the disease progresses, deterioration of language, memory, and cognitive skills is observed, and patients may become totally mute in final stages of the disease (27).

Creutzfeldt-Jakob Disease

Creutzfeldt-Jakob disease is a rare, progressive neurological and dementing disorder. It is believed to arise from infectious disease attributable to a virus (39). The onset of Creutzfeldt-Jakob disease typically begins in the fourth or fifth decade of life, and it is usually distinguishable from other irreversible dementias by its relatively rapid course. Death often occurs within 9 to 12 months following onset (20). In Creutzfeldt-Jakob disease there is a degeneration of cortical tissues, which in addition to dementia, is manifested as alterations in consciousness, myoclonus, cerebellar disturbances, and sensory and visual impairments (78).

Korsakoff's Disease

Korsakoff's disease results from chronic alcohol abuse; it is characterized by cortical atrophy. Associated with this disease is a dementia often referred to as an alcoholic dementia. It has been estimated that 3% of alcoholic hospital inpatients and approximately 7% of all patients admitted to the hospital for dementia have this form of irreversible dementia (28, 54). Alcoholic dementia is more apparent in older than in younger patients, and it appears earlier and with a shorter history of alcohol abuse in women that in men (28).

Symptoms of the dementia associated with Korsakoff's disease are mild and either nonprogressive or slowly progressive. They include decreased memory skills, confabulation, psychomotor retardation, circumstantiality, poor attention, disorientation, and an inability to retain new information (20, 50, 53). Apparently a source of controversy in the literature, some investigators suggest that there are not sufficiently convincing data for a dementia associated with alcoholic damage to exist (20), possibly because of the mild, minimally progressive nature of the condition.

A review of the *major* irreversible dementia-producing illnesses has been provided, although dementing states have been described for a number of other medical conditions. As expected, etiologically different dementias have characteristically different communication symptoms, reflecting the very different neurological disease processes associated with each medical diagnosis. Unfortunately, longitudinal data regarding the progression of communication deterioration associated with each diagnostic category do not exist to date. However, some preliminary information is available concerning how some dementing individuals differ in communicative behavior. In the next section, we will explore some ways in which different dementing patients differ from one another, as well as how they are similar, relative to communication skills.

Dementia and Communication

Because of individual subject differences within each dementing illness category, it is difficult to isolate the symptoms which typify the dementia associated with these categories. Some investigators have attempted to dichotomize dementias according to cortical and subcortical types (26). Unfortunately, because of individual differences among patients, consistent communicative behavior profiles are somewhat tenuous. Further, a lack of longitudinal studies of dementing individuals to date limits our knowledge about the order of communication deterioration as a particular disease process progresses.

A preliminary attempt to provide evidence for differences in communication behavior across dementia groups was provided in Bayles (6). Her study compared the performance of dementing individuals with Alzheimer's disease, Parkinson's disease, and Huntington's disease with the performance of normal individuals on a battery of neuropsychological and language tests. Some interesting findings emerged. In general, Alzheimer's disease patients performed more poorly than other individuals and normals. They differed significantly from Parkinson's disease patients on confrontation naming. They also performed significantly poorer than Huntington's disease patients on the *WAIS Block Design* subtest, the *Mental Status Questionnaire*, and on confrontation naming. Huntington's disease patients performed poorer than Parkinson's disease patients on two measures of pragmatic behavior, one requiring them to select the most appropriate utterance for a particular context and another requiring them to judge the literality of an utterance.

Another experimental finding of interest was that all dementing individuals demonstrated some common areas of difficulty, in spite of etiological differences. Dementing subjects showed the following: decreased receptive vocabulary abilities on the *Peabody Picture Vocabulary Test*; difficulty comprehending meanings of ambiguous sentences; decreased ability to provide verbal descriptions of common objects; and a decreased ability to identify a speaker's intent when provided with the utterance context. While these latter findings are not revolutionary, they provide some support for the notion that there may be common threads to the communication deterioration seen in dementia, regardless of etiology.

Bayles and her colleagues (8), in fact, addressed some of these common threads in a description of communication changes which occur subsequent to dementia. Behavioral descriptors were provided for dementing individuals in early, middle and advanced stages of their illness. This kind of interpretation has a great deal of clinical as well as practical utility.

According to these investigators, mildly demented individuals showed only subtle changes in communication. They were apt to be labile, socially withdrawn, and distractible; they might exhibit subtle overall intellectual deterioration and disorientation to time. These patients might demonstrate failing memory for recent events and difficulty remembering names, and might frequently misplace objects. Speech in these patients was apt to be fluent, with brief pauses before nouns and an increase in revisions and sentence fragments. They might have some word finding difficulties and might demonstrate increased use of automatisms and cliches. A mild loss of desire to communicate might be noticed, as well as occasional disinhibition. Oral discourse might often be characterized as vague and empty, and these individuals might have occasional irrelevancies in conversation. Syntax, phonology, and verbal repetition skills would likely be intact.

Patients with moderate dementia would demonstrate more obvious communication breakdowns. These patients were likely to display shallow affect, generalized intellectual deterioration and disorientation for time and place. Memory deficits would now be prominent, especially recent memory, and the patient would probably be unable to form new memories. Speech would be hypofluent, with perseveration, pauses, intrusions, sentence fragments and revisions. Patients at this stage would have significantly reduced vocabularies, characterized by verbal paraphasias in discourse, and semantic and visual errors on visual confrontation naming. Pragmatic aspects of language would be disrupted, characterized by declining sensitivity to context, diminished eye contact, lack of conformity to conversational rules and egocentricity. Discourse would be characteristically disjointed, with a decline in propositional language. A reduction in syntactic complexity and completeness would be likely, and phonological aspects of language and verbal repetition skills would continue to be generally intact.

In advanced dementing stages, individuals would tend to be oblivious to the environment and others, and might sometimes display agitation. They would show global failure of intellectual functions and be disoriented for time, place and person. There would be a global failure of all memory. Speech would be either fluent and melodic, with frequent pauses, or nonfluent with prolonged hesitations. Pragmatic aspects of language would be disturbed, and patients would not adhere to conversational rules or maintain eye contact or social awareness, and would be unable to form purposeful communicative intentions. Organization and relevance of discourse would be severely diminished, although these individuals might occasional formulate appropriate word combinations. Jargon would not be uncommon, reflecting phonologic and semantic deterioration, and patients might be echolalic.

While these descriptors may not hold for every dementing patient, they can serve as a useful framework for determining progression of the communication disorder in dementia. With increased longevity of our population and an increasingly older population, the need for better understanding of the communication disorders arising from dementia will be urgent in the very near future. Longitudinal studies are needed, as well as studies which examine whether any intervention attempts alter the course of communication deterioration.

In summary, a variety of illnesses and conditions may give rise to dementia in the elderly. Some of these dementias are reversible, so that thorough case history and medical examination of patients is essential. The majority of irreversible dementia producing diseases are fatal, and our understanding of communication disorders associated with the various etiologies is limited at this time. Suggestions for the clincal assessment and management of dementing patients are provided elsewhere in this volume (see Chapter 17).

MOTOR SPEECH DISORDERS

Two classes of speech disorders often referred to as motor speech disorders are observed in elderly individuals. These are dysarthrias and apraxia of speech (31). Dysarthria is a condition stemming from neurological damage which results in muscle weakness and/or involuntary movements and consequently slurred speech. Apraxia of speech is a condition resulting from neurological damage in which speech is disturbed in the absence of neuromuscular involvement of the articulators. Extensive incidence/prevalence data for these two classes of speech disorders are not available, but because they arise from conditions usually associated with aging, they are speech disorders which typically have their onset later in life. A dis-

cussion of the characteristic symptoms and neurogenic bases of these disorders follows.

Dysarthrias

Darley et al (31) popularized the notion that dysarthria types could be distinguished on the basis of their auditory perceptual characteristics, reflecting the site(s) of lesion associated with their origins. Six classes of dysarthria were subsequently identified, based on examination of audiotaped samples of a variety of dysarthric speakers: flaccid; spastic; ataxic; hypokinetic; hyperkinetic; and mixed.

Flaccid dysarthrias stem from damage to lower motor neurons. Conditions which may result in flaccid dysarthria include bulbar palsy (especially when the last four or five cranial nerves are involved) stemming from CVAs, tumors, trauma, congenital factors and viral infections as well as myasthenia gravis. Speech characteristics of flaccid dysarthria often include consonant imprecision, breathy voice quality, hypernasality, and/or audible inhalation.

Spastic dysarthrias stem from damage to upper motor neurons. They can be caused by multiple lesions in both cerebral hemispheres (pseudobulbar palsy), arising from a number of disorders such as tumors, trauma, infections, degenerative diseases, vascular disturbances, and most commonly, CVAs. Salient perceptual features of this type of dysarthria include what has been referred to as "strained-strangled phonation" (31) and consonant imprecision. In a number of bilaterally damaged patients, spastic dysarthria is accompanied by emotional lability during speech efforts.

Ataxic dysarthria is caused by damage to the cerebellum. This damage has been attributable to CVAs, tumors, toxic and metabolic disorders (especially alcohol effects), and encephalitis (31, 78). The characteristics of ataxic dysarthria include irregular articulatory breakdown, irregular changes in rate and rhythm during speech attempts, inappropriate stress, staccato-type syllabification of polysyllabic words, and burst of vocal effort. The irregular changes in rate are highlighted when ataxic dysarthric patients are asked to repeat syllables on alternate motion rate tasks.

Hypokinetic dysarthria, attributable to extrapyramidal damage, is typically the dysarthric condition seen in Parkinson's disease patients. Patients with hypokinetic dysarthrias speak in a monotone, with limited pitch and loudness variability. Other characteristics which are often observed include breathiness, harshness, and inappropriate silences. Accelerated speech rate resulting in a blurring of speech is not uncommon in these patients, and it is usually most apparent on alternate motion rate tasks of syllable repetition.

The hyperkinetic dysarthrias also stem from damage to the extrapyramidal system, and are characterized by abnormal, random, involuntary movements of the articulators. Two subgroups of hyperkinetic dysarthria have been identified (31): quick hyperkinetic dysarthrias and slow hyperkinetic dysarthrias. The quick variety can be found in disorders typified by myoclonic jerks, tics, chorea, and ballism (78). Perceptual characteristics are likely to include imprecise consonants, variable rate, prolonged interword or intersyllabic intervals, inappropriate silences, harsh voice, and sudden, uncontrolled loudness variations. In addition, patients with chorea may exhibit involuntary tongue and/or lip smacks during the speech attempts. Quick hyperkinetic dysarthrias, despite the implications of the name, are also typified by decreased rate of speech. Slow hyperkinetic dysarthrias are associated with athetosis, dyskinesia, and dystonia. Speech characteristics often include imprecise consonants and distorted vowels, harsh, strained-strangled voice, slow rate, and difficulty maintaining phonation. This latter symptom is highlighted when the patient is asked to sustain phonation of "ah."

Because some neurological diseases affect more than one site, and because the resulting dysarthria involves multiple symptoms, a category of mixed dysarthria exists. Mixed dysarthria is associated with several neurological conditions, including amyotrophic lateral sclerosis (ALS), multiple sclerosis (MS), and Wilson's disease. In ALS, a progressive and fatal degenerative neurological disease, both upper and lower motor neurons are involved in the disease process. Not surprisingly, patients with ALS demonstrate a mixed dysarthria consisting of both flaccid and spastic components (31). The resulting speech is typically slow and labored with a growling quality to it. On syllable repetition, the patient's tendencies to voice unvoiced consonants and to speak at an extremely slow rate are highlighted. Dysarthrias associated with multiple sclerosis patients generally vary widely within this group. Flaccid, ataxic and spastic components are commonly noted, relative to the neurological progression of the illness. A mixed dysarthria has also been noted in Wilson's disease (11), a neurological condition stemming from a disorder of copper metabolism. The dysarthria associated with Wilson's disease includes hypokinetic, ataxic and spastic components.

Apraxia of Speech

It is beyond the scope of this chapter to provide evidence for the several points of view about apraxia of speech (also known as verbal apraxia). This disorder has been referred to in the literature as a motor speech disorder (31), a more central aphasic impairment of the phonologic system (55), and most typically a mixture of both. Apraxia of speech often accompanies Broca's aphasia, which is not surprising since both are attributable to lesions involving the third frontal convolution in the left hemisphere (Broca's area). While it may exist in a pure form, the disorder most commonly is seen in association with aphasia. However, the controversy about this disorder has continued from the mid-1970s to the present time.

Apraxia of speech is characterized by variable articulatory patterns, disturbed prosody, oral struggle behavior, and inappropriate phonemic sequencing (31). Typically, patients may have no articulatory disturbances during the production of automatic phrases or rote sequences, but inconsistent articulatory errors in volitional speech.

The motor speech disorders occur primarily in the elderly, despite the fact that adequate incidence estimates are not available. The dysarthrias and apraxia of speech are often amenable to speech-language treatment, and even patients of advanced age are usually able to develop compensatory techniques to improve the intelligibility of their speech during the course of speech-language treatment.

LARYNGECTOMY

Another speech disorder encountered by a number of elderly persons is caused by cancer of the larynx, which necessitates surgical removal of the larynx (laryngectomy). Cancer of the larynx afflicts mostly elderly individuals, and it has been reported the mean age at which patients must undergo laryngectomies is 62 (47). Seventy-five percent of all males with cancer of the larynx are over 55 years of age (4), and men are more susceptible to the disease than women (83). It has been estimated that 8100 men and 1100 women per year will be diagnosed as having cancer of the larynx in the United States (83).

When the larynx is removed, individuals are rendered speechless as a result of the lack of vocal folds. Breathing takes place through a permanent tracheostoma in the neck which allows for the exchange of air from the lungs. A variety of postsurgical speech options are available for the laryngectomized person. He or she may choose to use any one of a number of artificial larynges, which serve as sound sources for speech production. Some of these devices provide sound generation held at the neck, while others provide intraoral sound generation. Patients who use these devices articulate as they did prior to surgery, except that air from the lungs no longer serves as the medium for sound generation. A number of other patients utilize esophageal speech for communicative purposes postoperatively. In this method of speech production, individuals must learn to speak on belched air, which is trapped in the esophagus. The vibration source for esophageal speech is provided by the pharyngoesophageal (PE) sphincter muscles. In recent years, successful use of tracheoesophageal puncture techniques and a variety of corresponding prosthetic devices have facilitated esophageal speech production in laryngectomized individuals.

In a survey of 2730 laryngectomized persons, 13% responded that they did not speak at all, 11% spoke entirely with the aid of an artificial larynx, 70% used esophageal speech exclusively and 6% utilized a combination of artificial larynx and esophageal speech, depending on context. It should be noted that psychological adjustments to laryngectomy are often difficult for older individuals, who concurrently face other medical problems, the loss of friends and loved ones, and their own mortality. Also, many individuals with cancer of the larynx must undergo additional surgery for cancers which may attack other articulatory structures such as the tongue and jaw. For these latter patients, speech rehabilitation potential is often poor, and they must learn to rely on nonoral means of communication such as writing or electronic communication devices.

HEARING LOSS IN AGING

Unlike other communication disorders associated with aging, hearing impairment is both a natural concomitant of the normal aging process and a specific source of communication deficit. While hearing loss in aging is discussed in depth elsewhere in this volume, a brief discussion of prevalence figures can provide some insight into the magnitude of this communication disorder in the elderly population. Presybcusis, the hearing loss associated with aging, progresses with increasing age. It is typified by a bilateral sensorineural hearing loss, especially in the higher frequencies. It has been estimated that nearly one-half of all Americans with hearing impairments are 65 years of age and older (74). According to Rupp (73), prevalence figures for handicapping hearing loss among the elderly fall between 10 and 90% with institutionalized elderly demonstrating poorer audiologic findings than their noninstitutionalized peers.

Given these data, one cannot help but consider that a number of the previously mentioned speech-language and cognitive disturbances in older patients are accompanied by hearing loss as well. Not only are these individuals limited in their expressive communication attempts, but receptive communication may be impaired as well. A more thorough review of hearing impairments in the elderly has been presented in Chapter 8.

SUMMARY AND CONCLUSIONS

In this chapter we have examined a number of conditions which may render an older individual handicapped with respect to communication. Whether the problem involves speech, language, cognition, or hearing, the elderly individual with communication impairment must make dramatic alterations in his/her lifestyle. Because many adult onset communication disorders are related to specific disease processes and illnesses, older persons who have survived may confront increased susceptibility to debilitating illnesses and communication disorders with each additional year of survival. Fortunately, some communication disorders in aging are remediable and/or reversible; with rehabilitation efforts, many communicatively impaired elderly persons may resume normal or nearly normal communicative behaviors. For those with irreversible conditions and/or conditions which are progressively degenerative, there is no hope for restored communication abilities.

Holland (42) has suggested that most professionals lack experience with aging, and consequently do not have a good understanding of the aging process. We have been adolescents, and thus we appreciate that experience, but the concept of aging and of being elderly is not well understood. This notion should not be forgotten in our rehabilitation efforts with the communicatively impaired elderly. Older clients should be treated with respect and dignity. As we attempt to provide "appropriate" intervention, we should make every effort not to impose our desires and expectations on people who have their own desires and expectations.

As our population becomes increasingly older over the next several decades, there will no doubt be a corresponding increase in the incidence of communication disorders. University training programs should begin to modify their curricula to include more course work and practicum experiences with communication disorders associated with aging, in order to meet future manpower needs. Further, additional research in the area of communication disorders in the elderly is urgently needed, particularly in the areas of treatment outcomes incidence. Increased knowledge about the communicatively disordered older adults and increased sensitivity to their needs will only serve to improve the quality of life for these persons in the years to come.

References

1. Albert MS, Butters N, Brandt J: Patterns of remote memory in amnesic and demented patients. *Arch Neurol* 38:495–500, 1981.
2. Alexander MP, Stuss DT, Benson DF: Capgras' syndrome: a reduplicative phenomenon. *Neurology* 29:334–339, 1979.
3. Aten J, Darley F, Duffy J, Holland A, Ulatowska H, Wertz RT: Panel: Aphasia with and without adjectives. In Brookshire RH (ed): *Clinical Aphasiology Conference Proceedings*. Minneapolis, BRK Publishers, 1983, p 186.
4. Barclay THC, Rao NN: The incidence and mortality rates for laryngeal cancer from total cancer registries. *Laryngoscope* 85:254–258, 1975.
5. Basso A, Capitani E, Vignolo L: Influence of rehabilitation on language skills in aphasic patients. *Arch Neurol* 36(4):190–196, 1979.
6. Bayles KA: Language and dementia. In Holland AL (ed): *Language Disorders in Adults: Recent Advances*. San Diego, College-Hill Press, 1984, p 209.
7. Bayles KA: Management of neurogenic communication disorders associated with dementia. In Chapey R (ed): *Language Intervention Strategies in Adult Aphasia, ed 2*. Baltimore, Williams & Wilkins, 1986, p 462.
8. Bayles KA, Tomoeda CK, Caffrey JT: Language and dementia producing diseases. *Communicative Dis Aud Cont Educ J* 7:131–146, 1982.
9. Benson DF: *Aphasia, Alexia, Agraphia*. New York, Churchill-Livingstone, 1979.
10. Benson DR, Sheramata WA, Bouchard R, Segarra JM, Price D, Geschwind N: Conduction aphasia. *Arch Neurol* 28:339–346, 1973.
11. Berry WR, Darley FL, Aronson AE, Goldstein NP: Dysarthria in Wilson's disease. *J Speech Hear Res* 17:169–183, 1974.
12. Boller F: Mental status of patients with Parkinson's disease. *J Clin Neuropsychol* 2:157–172, 1980.
13. Boller F, Kim Y, Mack JL: Auditory comprehension in aphasia. In Whitaker H, Whitaker HA (eds): *Studies in Neurolinguistics, Volume 3*. New York, Academic Press, 1977, p 1.
14. Boller F, Mizutani T, Roessmann V, Gambetti P: Parkinson disease, dementia and Alzheimer disease: Clinicopathological correlations. *Ann Neurol* 7:329–335, 1980.
15. Branch C, Milner B, Rasmussen T: Intercarotid sodium amytal for the lateralization of cerebral speech dominance. *J Neurosurg* 21:399–405, 1964.
16. Brown JW, Perecman E: Neurological basis of language processing. In Chapey R (ed): *Language Intervention Strategies in Adult Aphasia, ed 2*. Baltimore, Williams & Wilkins, 1986, p 12.
17. Burks TF: Autonomic agents. In: Levinson AJ (ed): *Neuropsychiatric Side Effects of Drugs in the Elderly*. New York, Raven Press, 1979, p 69.
18. Burns MS: Language without communication: The pragmatics of right hemisphere damage. In Burns MS, Halper AS, Mogil SI (eds): *Clinical Management of Right Hemisphere Dysfunction*. Rockville, MD, Aspen Systems Corporation, 1985, p 17.
19. Burns MS, Halper AS, Mogil SI: Diagnosis of communication problems in right hemisphere damage. In Burns MS, Halper AS, Mogil SI (eds): *Clinical Management of Right Hemisphere Dysfunction*. Rockville, MD, Aspen Systems Corporation, 1985, p 29.
20. Butler RN, Lewis MI: *Aging and Mental Health*. New York, A Plume Book, 1983.
21. Butters N, Sax D, Montgomery K, Tarlow S: Comparison of the neuropsychological deficits associated with early and advanced Huntington's disease. *Arch Neurol* 35:585–589, 1978.
22. Caramazza A: The logic of neuropsychological research and the problem of patient classification in aphasia. *Brain Lang* 21:9–20, 1984.
23. Cavenar JO, Maltbie AA, Austin L: Depression simulating organic brain disease. *Am J Psychiatry* 136:521–523, 1979.
24. Culton GL: Reaction to age as a factor in chronic aphasia in stroke patients. *J Speech Hearing Dis* 36:563–564, 1971.
25. Cummings JL: Neurological syndromes associated with right hemisphere damage. In Burns, MS, Halper AS, Mogil SI (eds): *Clinical Management of Right Hemisphere Dysfunction*. Rockville, MD, Aspen Systems Corporation, 1985, p 7.
26. Cummings JL, Benson DF: *Dementia: A Clinical Approach*. Boston, Butterworth, 1983.
27. Cummings JL, Duchen LW: The Klüver-Bucy syndrome in Pick disease. *Neurology* 31:1415–1422, 1981.
28. Cutting J: Alcoholic dementia. In Benson DF, Blumer D (eds): *Psychiatric Aspects of Neurologic Disease*, vol 2. New York, Grune & Stratton, 1982, p 149.
29. Damasio AR, Damasio H, Rizzo M, Varney M, Gersch F: Aphasia with nonhemorrhagic lesions in the basal ganglia and internal capsule. *Arch Neurol* 39:15–20, 1982.
30. Damasio H: Cerebral localization of the aphasias. In Sarno MT (ed): *Acquired Aphasia*. New York, Academic Press, 1981, p 27.

31. Darley FL, Aronson AE, Brown JR: *Motor Speech Disorders.* Philadelphia, WB Saunders, 1975.

32. Davis GA: *A Survey of Adult Aphasia.* Englewood Cliffs, NJ, Prentice-Hall, 1983.

33. DeKòsky ST, Heilman KM, Bowers D, Valenstein E: Recognition and discrimination of emotional faces and pictures. *Brain Lang* 9:206–214, 1980.

34. Diller L, Weinberg J: Hemi-inattention in rehabilitation: the evolution of a rational remediation program. In Weinstein EA, Friedland RP (eds): *Advances in Neurology,* New York, Raven Press, 1977, vol 18, p 63.

35. Gardner H, Hamby S: The role of the right hemisphere in the organization of linguistic materials. Presented to the International Neuropsychology Symposium, Dubrovnik, Yugoslavia, 1979.

36. Garron DC, Klawans HL, Narin F: Intellectual functioning of persons with idiopathic parkinsonism. *J Nerv Ment Dis* 154:445–452, 1972.

37. Goodglass H, Kaplan E: *The Assessment of Aphasia and Related Disorders.* Philadelphia, Lea & Febiger, 1972.

38. Heilman KM: Neglect and related disorders. In Heilman KM, Valenstein E (eds): *Clinical Neuropsychology.* New York, Oxford University Press, 1979, p 268.

39. Heston LL, White JA: *Dementia: A Practical Guide to Alzheimer's Disease and Related Illnesses.* New York, WH Freeman, 1983.

40. Hoehn MM, Yahr MD: Parkinsonism: onset, progression, and mortality. *Neurology* 17:427–442, 1967.

41. Hogg JE, Massey EW, Schoenberg BS: Mortality from Huntington's disease in the United States. *Adv Neurol* 23:27–35, 1979.

42. Holland AL: Working with the aging aphasic patient: some clinical implications. In Obler LK, Albert ML (eds): *Language and Communication in the Elderly: Clinical Therapeutic, and Experimental Issues.* Lexington, MA, Lexington Books, 1980, p 181.

43. Hutton JT: Results of clinical assessment for the dementia syndrome: Implications for epidemiologic studies. In Mortimer JA, Schuman LM (eds): *The Epidemiology of Dementia.* New York, Oxford University Press, 1981, p 62.

44. Keenan JS, Brassell EG: A study of the factors related to prognosis for individual aphasic patients. *J Speech Hear Dis* 39:257–269, 1974.

45. Kennedy J, Fisher J, Shoulson I, Caine E: Language impairment in Huntington disease. *Neurology* 31 (2):81–82, 1981.

46. Kertesz A, McCabe P: Recovery patterns and prognosis in aphasia. *Brain* 100:1–18, 1977.

47. King PS, Everill WF, Peirson GA: Rehabilitation and adaptation of laryngectomy patients. *Am J Phys Med* 47: 192–203, 1968.

48. Kozy MC, Tarvin GA: Working with families. In Burns MS, Halper AS, Mogil SI (eds): *Clinical Management of Right Hemisphere Dysfunction.* Rockville, MD, Aspen Systems Corporation, 1985, p 97.

49. Kurtzke J: Epidemiology of cerebrovascular disease. In: *Cerebrovascular Survey Report for Joint Council Subcommittee on Cerebrovascular Disease,* NINCDS, Rochester, MN, Whiting Press, 1980.

50. Lee K, Hardt F, Moller L, Haubek A, Jenson E: Alcohol-induced brain damage and liver damage in young males. *Lancet* 2:759–761, 1979.

51. Lemon PG, Burns MS, Lehner LH: Communication deficits associated with right cerebral brain damage. Presented to the American Speech-Language-Hearing Association, Atlanta, 1979.

52. Lieberman A, Dziatolowski M, Kupersmith M, Sorby M, Goodgold A, Korcin J, Goldstein M: Dementia in Parkinson disease. *Ann Neurol* 6:355–359, 1979.

53. Lishman WA: Cerebral disorder in alcoholism: syndromes of impairment. *Brain* 104:1–20, 1981.

54. Marsden CD, Harrison MJG: Outcome of investigation of patients with presenile dementia. *Br Med J* 2:249–252, 1972.

55. Martin AD: Some objections to the term apraxia of speech. *J Speech Hear Dis* 39:53–64, 1974.

56. Matthews CG, Haaland KY: The effect of symptom duration on cognitive and motor performance in parkinsonism. *Neurology* 29:951–956, 1979.

57. McDowell FH, Lee JE, Sweet RD: Extrapyramidal disease. In Baker AB, Baker LH (eds): *Clinical Neurology.* New York, Harper & Row, 1978, p 1.

58. McFie J, Piercy MF, Zangwill OL: Visual-spatial agnosia associated with lesions of the right cerebral hemisphere. *Brain* 7 3:167–190, 1950.

59. Mesulam MM: A cortical network for directed attention and unilateral neglect. *Ann Neurol* 10:309–325, 1981.

60. Metter EJ: Medical aspects of stroke rehabilitation. In Chapey R (ed): *Language Intervention Strategies in Adult Aphasia,* ed 2. Baltimore, Williams & Wilkins, 1986, p 141.

61. Mitchell J: Speech and language impairment in the older patient. *Geriatrics* 13:467–476, 1958.

62. Mohr JP, Walters WC, Duncan GW: Thalamic hemorrhage and aphasia. *Brain Lang* 2:3–17, 1975.

63. Mortimer JA, Pirozzolo FJ, Hansch EC, Webster DD: Relationship of motor symptoms to intellectual deficits in Parkinson disease. *Neurology* 32:133–137, 1982.

64. Myers PS: Treatment of right hemisphere communication disorders. In Perkins WH (ed): *Language Handicaps in Adults.* New York, Thieme-Stratton, 1983.

65. Myers PS: Right hemisphere communication impairment. In Chapey R (ed): *Language Intervention Strategies in Adult Aphasia,* ed 2. Baltimore, Williams & Wilkins, 1986, p 444.

66. Myers PS: Right hemisphere impairment. In Holland AL (ed): *Language Disorders in Adults: Recent Advances.* San Diego, College-Hill Press, 1984, p 177.

67. Myrianthopoulos NC: Huntington's chorea. *J Med Genet* 3:298–314, 1966.

68. Naeser MA, Albert MS, Kleefield J: New methods in the CT scan diagnosis of Alzheimer's disease: examination of white and gray matter mean CT density numbers. In Corkins S, Davis KL, Growdon JH, Usdin E, Wurthman RJ (eds): *Alzheimer's Disease: A Report of Progress in Research.* New York, Raven Press, 1982, p 63.

69. Obler LK, Albert ML, Goodglass H, Benson DF: Aging and aphasia type. *Brain Lang* 6:318–322, 1978.

70. Rose C, Boby V, Capildeo R: A retrospective survey of speech disorders following stroke, with particular reference to the value of speech therapy. In Lebrun Y, Hoops R (eds): *Recovery in Aphasics.* Amsterdam, Swets & Zeitlinger, 1976, p 89.

71. Rosenberg GA, Kornfeld M, Stovring J, Bicknell JM: Subcortical arteriosclerotic encephalopathy (Binswanger): computerized tomography. *Neurology* 29:1102–1106, 1979.

72. Ross ED: The aprosodias. *Arch Neurol* 38: 561–569, 1981.

73. Rupp RR: Speech input processing, hearing loss, and aural rehabilitation with the elderly. In Obler LK, Albert ML (eds): *Language and Communication in the Elderly: Clinical, Therapeutic, and Experimental Issues.* Lexington, MA, Lexington Books, 1980, p 159.

74. Rupp, RR: Understanding the problems of presbycusis. *Geriatrics* 25:100–107, 1970.

75. Sands E, Sarno MT, Shankweiler D: Long-term assessment of language function in aphasia due to stroke. *Arch Phys Med Rehabil* 50:202–207, 1969.

76. Sarno MT: Recovery and rehabilitation in aphasia. In Sarno MT (ed): *Acquired Aphasia.* New York, Academic Press, 1981.

77. Sarno MT, Levita E: Natural course of recovery in severe aphasia. *Arch Phys Med Rehabil* 52:175–178, 186, 1971.

78. Schow RL, Christensen JM, Hutchinson JM, Nerbonne M: *Communication Disorders of the Aged: A Guide For Health Professionals.* Baltimore, University Park Press, 1978.

79. Schuell HM: *Differential Diagnosis of Aphasia with the Minnesota Test.* Minneapolis, University of Minnesota Press, 1965.

80. Schwartz MF: What the classical aphasia categories can't do for us and why. *Brain Lang* 21:3–8, 1984.

81. Selby G: Parkinson's disease. In Vinken PJ, Bruyn GW (eds): *Diseases of the Basal Ganglia, Handbook of Clinical Neurology.* New York, American Elsevier, 1968, vol 6, p 173.

82. Senner-Hurley F, Lefkowitz N: Stroke: Speech-language rehabilitation. In Logigian M (ed): *Adult Rehabilitation: A Team Approach for Therapists.* Boston, Little Brown, 1982, p 275.

83. Silverberg E: Cancer statistics. *Ca-Cancer J Clin* 27:26–41, 1977.

84. Sim M, Turner E, Smith WT: Cerebral biopsy in the investigation of presenile dementia. I. Clinical aspects. *Br J Psychiatry* 112:119–125, 1966.

85. Tomlinson BE: The pathology of dementia. In Wells CE (ed): *Dementia*, ed 2. Philadelphia, FA Davis, 1977, p 113.

86. VanLancker DR, Canter GJ: Impairment of voice and face recognition in patients with hemispheric damage. *Brain Cogn* 1:185–195, 1982.

87. Victoratos GC, Lenman JAR, Herzberg L: Neurological investigation of dementia. *Br J Psychiatry* 130:131–133, 1977.

88. Vignolo LA: Afasia. In *Enciclopedia Medica Italiana*, vol 1. Firenze, Edizioni Scientifiche, 1973, p 845.

89. Vignolo LA: Evolution of aphasia and language rehabilitation. *Cortex* 1:344–367, 1965.

90. Wallesch C, Kornhuber H, Brunner R, Kunz T, Hollerbach B, Suger G: Lesions of the basal ganalia, thalamus and deep white matter: differential effects on language functions. *Brain Lang* 20:286–304, 1983.

91. Warrington EK, James M: An experimental investigation of facial recognition in patients with unilateral cerebral lesions. *Cortex* 3:317–327, 1967.

92. Watson RT, Heilman KM: Thalamic neglect. *Neurology* 29:690–694, 1979.

93. Watts RF: Total rehabilitation of laryngectomees. *Laryngoscope* 85: 671–673, 1975.

94. Weinstein EA, Kahn RL, Malitz S: Delusional reduplication of parts of the body. *Brain* 77:45–60, 1954.

95. Weisenberg TH, McBride KE: *Aphasia.* New York, Commonwealth Fund, 1935.

96. Wepman JM, Jones LV: Studies in aphasia: classification of aphasic speech by the noun-pronoun ratio. *Br J Dis Commun* 1:46–54, 1966.

97. Wertz RT: Language disorders in adults: State of the clinical art. In Holland AL (ed): *Language Disorders in Adults: Recent Advances* San Diego, College-Hill Press, 1984, p 1.

98. Whisnant JP: The role of the neurologist in the decline of stroke. *Ann Neurol*, 14:1–7, 1983.

99. Whitaker HA: Two views of aphasia classification. *Brain Lang* 21:1–2, 1984.

Age-Related Concerns in the Management of Communication Disorders

IV

12 Considerations for the Practitioner with Older Clients

E. PHILIP TRAPP

THEA SPATZ

Editor's Note

Chapter 12 introduces the final section of this text in which management of the communicatively disordered older person is explored in greater detail. It is appropriate, therefore, that authors Trapp and Spatz urge us to stop for a moment and take stock of our own personal and professional understanding and biases as they relate to aging and the elderly. Many of the themes and concerns presented in Chapter 12 echo earlier comments, particularly the discussion of ageism and its potential effects on older individuals and clinicians. Other concerns point towards subsequent chapters in which assessment and intervention accommodations to the characteristics of aging and the elderly are discussed at length. Problems of depression and adjustment to loss are mentioned briefly here, preparing the reader for the recurrence of these themes in Chapter 19 on significant others. Chapter 12 concludes on an extremely positive note. Stressing the holistic approach to clinical management of older clients, Trapp and Spatz propose that interventions should be guided by optimism resulting from recognition of the elderly individual's potential for learning, for assuming active control of his/her life, and for personal growth.

The demographic phenomenon of 20th century America is the rise in the number of our aged. Because of decreased rate in fertility, increased rate in longevity, and stricter immigration laws (the young tend to immigrate more than the old), we are growing older at a positively accelerated rate. The pace should continue until the end of the World War II baby boom (year 2025). We have 7 times as many elderly today as in 1900 and can expect 10 times as many by the end of the century. The aged have doubled since 1950 and should double again in 40 years, to pass the 50 million mark. Within the aged population, the 75-and-older group has become the fastest growing segment, increasing three times faster than the 65 to 75 group in just the past decade (5). For an even more vivid graphic, each day 5000 people turn 65, and 3600 people over 65 die, adding 1400 people daily to the swelling ranks of the aged. People celebrating their 65th birthday can expect an active life well into their 80s. The meaning of these statistics for providers of services is self-evident: Caseloads will become more and more skewed with senior citizens. Few providers are ready to deal with the implications of this reality.

HISTORICAL PERSPECTIVE

Our government lacks a comprehensive national policy on aging. Further, the programs we have tend to stigmatize, segregate, and depersonalize the elderly and reduce them to dependency status, which only magnifies the problem. Correcting the situation calls first for a marked change of attitude in society, among service providers, and among the elderly themselves.

Historically, society has shown little involvement in the affairs of the aged (16). Universities ignored courses in gerontology, and medical schools offered minimal or no training in geriatrics. The few research studies published in the field were fraught with flawed methodologies, giving rise to spurious generalizations. Several of our popular myths on aging can be traced to these studies. The early workers in mental health generally considered the aged high risks for therapy. Many still do, and so a major proportion of the 10 to 20% estimated to have serious mental health problems (percentages depending on criteria used) go unattended.

The White House Conferences on the Aged were the first concerted efforts to raise public consciousness. The first conference, held in the early 1960s, led to the health packages of Medicare and Medicaid; the second conference, held in the early 1970s, led to the formation of the National Institute on Aging (NIA), the major research arm of the aged; the last conference, held in the early 1980s, devoted itself primarily to the development of strategies to cope with the threatening cuts in budget. Thus far, the programs for the aged have suffered least compared with most other domestic programs.

We have made some measurable progress. We now have over 60 Federal laws dealing with the elderly in the areas of income maintenance, employment, health care, taxes, housing, consumer affairs, and social service (9). Gerontological courses are becoming more available in the universities. Medical schools are increasing their geriatric training. Gerontological journals have doubled in number over the past decade, and the emerging research studies reflect more sophisticated designs. Gerontological research centers are expanding. The Veterans Administration is increasing its support of research on the aged, and NIA operated on a budget of about $40 million last year. Still, that is but a fraction of what it should be. A rule of thumb in industry is to allocate 3% of assets into research to maintain competitive viability. If we apply this formula to the $55 billion old-age health enterprise, NIA should approximate a $1 billion budget.

AGEISM

It is small wonder that we have been dragging our feet. Ours is an Oil-of-Olay society that dreads the thought of growing old and does all in its power to delay the inevitable. Although the focus of this chapter is on clinician-client relationships, neither enter into it from a vacuum. Each brings into the relationship elaborate social conditioning. Clinicians must be attuned to and perceptive of the broader social value system if they wish to sharpen understanding and improve the quality of the intervention process.

Society looks upon the aged much as it looked upon schizophrenia at the turn of the century. Schizophrenia, then called dementia praecox, was seen as a progressively deteriorating, irreversible disease. The prognosis was hopeless; the condition, incurable. In the same vein, old age today is viewed as a hopelessly deteriorating, incurable disease. The elderly who do not see themselves fitting the pattern consider

themselves the exception, never suspecting the rule.

Robert Butler, former director of NIA, labels this jaundiced perspective "ageism" (1). "Isms" (racism, sexism) draw heavily on the stereotype. They strive to make members of a class alike, overlooking the fact that individual differences are endemic to human nature. This makes possible absurd generalizations such as "all females are labile," "All blacks are indolent," and "All old people are rigid." People are clumped into preconceived pigeonholes.

We have all seen the charts on infant motor development in baby books. They graph the monthly progression of motor skills preceding walking, the highlight of the neonatal year. The sequence is orderly, stable, and highly predictable: normal infants at 1 month do the following; infants at 2 months do the following; infants at 3 months do the following, etc. Ageism resorts to this chart-like conceptualization in describing the aging process. Normal people at 65 do the following, etc. So act your age! The behavior, in contrast to the infant's, is steadily regressive, culminating in senility—if one should live so long.

Typical of stereotypes in general, ageism is pejorative in its portrait of the aged. The elderly are rigid, unproductive, uncreative, petty, selfish, humorless, complaining, parasitic, reclusive, useless, cantankerous, unreliable, mind-wandering, confused. There are some old people, like some young people, who closely fit this description, but most do not. The pattern is more likely to be seen in those afflicted with a severe brain disease or entrapped in abysmal poverty. A healthy brain in a happy milieu should flourish to the end.

The key concept in characterizing old age is diversity. Heterogeneity in behavior is a direct function of aging, which means there is more variability among 60 year olds than 50 year olds, more among 70 year olds than 60 year olds, etc. This makes group norms of little value for individual prediction in the late years. The old standby that the best predictor of future behavior is past behavior has its highest utility for the aged. The coping skills displayed with life's earlier developmental tasks set the odds for successfully dealing with the stresses of old age.

Ageism is locked in with chronological age, not behavior. The 65th birthday marks the crossing of the line. An observer from outer space would be led to believe a cataclysmic metamorphosis had taken place in the human organism. The person is suddenly stripped of all major responsibilities and cast into social exile. A gala celebration (reflecting society's relief) is arranged to ostensibly reward long and loyal service. Overnight, the honoree has lost status, power, influence, income and, most devastating of all, self-esteem. How grandly we herald the golden years!

The special nature of 65 has an interesting origin. About 100 years ago, a frugal German government was searching for a suitable age to retire and pension government workers. On checking the actuary tables, they observed the attrition rate at age 65. (The same government scanning today's tables might have selected 80.) Since that time, the age began to take on its special meaning, which has now become engraved in stone.

On the other hand, we have no satisfactory criteria for realistically determining the onset of old age. A popular tendency among authorities in the field is to conceptualize the life span in terms of stages (6, 10, 11), each stage distinguishable by a core set of developmental tasks. The stages, however, are not self-evident and are more influenced by the author's theoretical orientation than by empirical findings. For example, Havighurst has six stages; Erickson, eight; Hurlock, ten. Further, the stages are not clearly individuated. Much overlap occurs among them in all of the models.

There might be a temptation to equate life's last stage with the post retirement years. Persons retired from the work force do share many common needs, values, and adjustments. The main difficulty with this objective criterion is the wide range of retirement ages among the diverse occupations. The criterion, for example, would combine young retired professional athletes and military personnel with physicians, lawyers, and self-employed businessmen who often do not retire until their very advanced years. The adoption of the retirement criterion would merely replace one set of problems with another.

For research purposes and for the analysis of demographic data, the age criterion appears to be the most convenient and practical measure available to identify the aged, which brings us full circle. The point of the discussion is to remind the clinician that, although the age measure is arbitrary and without empirical foundation, many people have aggrandized it, and some have even become traumatized by it.

In many clinicians, ageism betrays itself in a contrasting positive stereotype, stimulated perhaps from very early fond memories of an exceptionally wise, kind, loving, and generous grandparent. This form of ageism arouses compassion for the elderly and may be a primary motivating factor in career selection. Nevertheless, stereotypes, even when infused with benevolence, break down communication because they distort perceptions and are untrue to reality.

This stereotype, called "New Ageism" (12), tends to reinforce dependency. It can be seen in the clinician who becomes too involved in the client's support system (perhaps overreacting to the client's dwindling social network), or too active in making decisions for the client, or too inclined to overstructure the client's environment. The consequences increase feelings of uselessness and incompetency and bring on a loss of self-confidence, the conditions that foster the development of "learned helplessness" (18). Clinicians who are also likely to court this attitude are those whose work with the aged is supported by grants. Successful grantsmanship involves, in a large measure, the skill of convincing the granting agency that the population to be affected is deserving, is in need of the services, and would be in dire straits without the support. The dependency contingency is thus built into the grant justification. The clinicians, persuaded by the force of their own exaggerated appeal, are hoisted on their own petard.

On the surface, ageism and new ageism appear poles apart, yet their long-range effects dovetail. Both ultimately obscure individual differences in prescribing rigid standards of appropriate behavior; both reinforce the sickness-and-poverty model of aging; and both support the failure model in the implicit message given to the aged. The net result is defeatism, which is a damaging blow to self-growth and independence, a setback to a prime objective of the clinician-client relationship.

Ageism has contributed heavily to the confusion between normal and pathological aging. Because chronic illnesses and multiple handicaps are not uncommon among the elderly, cause and correlation get confounded. The aging process slips into becoming the cause of a given disease. Even physicians, with their intensive training in differential diagnosis, frequently lapse into this error. They will speak of a patient dying of old age, whereas, in truth, the patient died of a disease. To die truly of old age, the body cells must have reached the end of their capacity to regenerate. The so-called Hayflict limit, programmed genetically for each species, has been estimated as high as 150 years for *Homo sapiens* (14), although the more common estimate is in the 110 to 120 age range.

The story circulates of an octogenarian who visited his physician, complaining of a painful right knee. After the examination he was told that nothing could be done for him; his problem was old age. He would have to reconcile himself to the fact that his was an old knee. Whereupon, the old sage replied that by his calculations his left knee was approximately the same age, and it did not hurt. The moral of this story is that it is time we stop using age as a scapegoat.

There is substantial evidence that certain physiological and chemical changes do take place during the aging process, but their meaning is unclear. For one thing, the brain itself reaches maximum growth when a person is about age 20 and thereafter begins to shrink slowly in size, shedding off about 3 ounces by age 70. The shriveled-up knot, however, appears little the worse for wear. More recent gerontological studies report such things as plaque forming on the cortex and fiber bundles forming inside the nerve cells. Further, the number of neurotransmitters apparently decreases with age. No consistently adverse behavioral changes have as yet been correlated with any of these findings. We are coming to the general conclusion that the normal, healthy brain suffers little decline in function during the aging process. How the client uses his aging brain is another story.

Comfort (4) coined the expression "sociogenic aging" to describe that part of the total aging picture not accountable to biological changes. He is referring to the impact of folklore, prejudice, and misconceptions (the stuff of ageism) on the aging process. Comfort estimates that as much as 75% of the variance found among older persons can be attributed to sociogenic factors. He sees the problem as a classic example of the self-fulfilling prophecy. When people believe that on a fixed calendar date they will become "unintelligent, asexual, unemployable, and crazy," they will tend to act accordingly.

A common diagnostic error is to confuse the onset of senility with the effects of depression, malnutrition, or overmedication. The symptoms of all four conditions have much overlap, the crucial distinction being that all but senility are reversible states. The error can lead to tragic consequences.

RELEVANT AGING CONSIDERATIONS

The myths of ageism notwithstanding, the aging process does have its related concerns. Let us examine them briefly and look at the options available to clinicians.

Sensory acuity diminishes linearly with age, albeit with marked individual differences.

Seeing, hearing, smelling, tasting, and tactual discriminations—all follow a negative slope.

Clinicians should have well-lighted offices for their elderly clients. People of 70 need more than three times the light they had required at 20. But, intensity is only part of the problem. The most irritating visual problem for the majority of the elderly is glare. Thus, the light source should be spread evenly throughout the room rather than localized at one source. The use of three lamps with 100-W bulbs is much preferred to one lamp with a 300-W bulb. Sensitivity to the color spectrum is also uneven. The blue end is much more affected than the red end. Blues and greens slowly become indistinguishable. Thus, green carpets will tend to merge with ice-blue walls, causing the boundaries of the floor to blur. Boundaries also get blurred from intensely contrasting colors. A vibrantly green staircase rising against a hot-red wall is a hazard. Since depth perception worsens, steps and risers should never be of the same color.

Hearing loss is more than a simple matter of volume adjustment, which can easily be corrected with hearing aids or with people talking louder. Most often the problem is with frequencies. The upper frequencies, 2000 cycles and above, tend to fade out. Simply increasing vocal loudness may amplify the distortion implicit in loss of high frequency sounds. Background noises become increasingly irritating. They cannot be filtered out as efficiently as they once could. Clinicians should take measures to reduce outside noises, especially if their offices are on busy streets, and decorate their offices in ways to deaden vibrations.

Because the sense of smell and taste is weakening, foods begin to lost their pungent flavors. They taste bland and more alike. This accounts for some of the appetite problems noted as a common complaint of the elderly, and can become a major contributing factor to malnutrition. The use of stronger seasonings is suggested.

Fine muscular control suffers with age. Opening milk cartons, turning thin pages in books, and shuffling slick plastic cards are examples of tasks that get increasingly more difficult and frustrating.

Clinicians should also be aware of the importance of room temperature to client comfort. Circulatory and metabolic problems generally necessitate a higher room temperature.

The point that is stressed here is that although the sense organs do gradually deteriorate with age, the clinician, society, and the elderly themselves can do much to alleviate the condition and restore in the elderly a stronger sense of control over their environment.

The clinician needs to understand that there are important differences in the health problems of the young and the old. The young are afflicted primarily with acute diseases, ones that run short courses and usually respond quickly and positively to medication and surgery. In contrast, the old are afflicted with chronic diseases and disabilities, which have a long, nagging prognostic outlook. This fundamental difference definitely affects perspective. For example, when the young fall and suffer injury, their concerns are chiefly tied into direct recovery; the old, with ultimate consequences. Hence, the clinician's focus of attention with the elderly should be on the fears and anxieties related to long-range effects.

The major chronic diseases and disabilities affecting the elderly are heart disease, cancer, atherosclerosis, hypertension, osteoporosis, cirrhosis, diabetes, arthritis, and rheumatism. Although the weakening immunological system causes increased vulnerability to system breakdown, maladaptive behaviors also play a major role. Smoking, excessive drinking, improper diet, lack of exercise, overuse of medications, and poor safety precautions are common culprits. Most of the 10 leading causes of death today have their roots in behavior.

Smoking contributes to heart disease, cancer (lung, mouth, larynx, esophagus, bladder, kidney, and pancreas), accidents (most fatal household fires are caused by burning cigarettes or the matches used to light them), stroke, influenza, and pneumonia. Excessive use of alcoholic beverages contributes to cirrhosis, fatty liver disease, acute pancreatitis, alcoholic hepatitis, and cancers of the liver, esophagus, larynx, and mouth. Alcohol is a factor in half of all serious motor vehicle accidents, two-thirds of all other accidents among adults, half of all homicides, and one-third of all suicides. With over 3 million alcoholics among the aged, it ranks as the most serious of the drug abuse problems among that group (3).

Improper diet can lead to heart disease, high blood pressure, cancer, stroke, diabetes, gallbladder disease, gastrointestinal problems, osteoporosis, and dental caries. It is a major factor in obesity. Obese people are 10 times more likely to develop diabetes, 3 times as likely to have severe atherosclerosis, and 30% more likely to die of coronary heart disease. They are at higher risk for gallbladder disease, cancers of the uterus, breast, and colon, and arthritis of the weight-bearing joints. They tend to have higher levels of blood fat and secrete more cholesterol in their bile.

Lack of exercise decreases cardiorespiratory fitness, increases risk of heart disease, and lowers general well-being and morale (19). Exercise to improve strength and flexibility may reduce the disability associated with lower back pain and arthritis and may increase general mobility. Regular weight-bearing exercise and sufficient calcium intake may help prevent fractures by maintaining bone strength. A gradual, sensible program of exercise is healthy and not dangerous and can contribute to weight loss, improved appearance, more restful sleep, increased ability to cope with aging, and improved self-confidence (7).

The misuse and abuse of drugs is a common occurrence among the elderly. Constituting 12% of the population but consuming 25% of the prescribed drugs (excluding over-the-counter drugs), the elderly have adverse drug reactions three times more often than any other age group. Approximately one of seven hospitalized elderly are admitted for reasons of drug reaction. Over one-third of patients 75 and older take three to four different drugs daily. The error rate in taking drugs is about 60% for patients over 60 years old and increases markedly if more than three drugs are prescribed. Common factors contributing to these errors are poor communication between patient and physician on multiple drug therapies, complicated scheduling, adverse reactions, and inability to pay for drugs. The problem is further compounded when the recommended doses are based on data sampled from younger adults, which most often is the case. The elderly metabolize drugs slower than middle-aged people, so presumed safe dosages can have cumulative effects. Also, little is known about drug interactions, the major risk factor in polypharmacy. Clinicians should be particularly alert to potential drug problems with clients who are frail, in a more advanced stage of illness, of poor appetite and nutrition, having poor fluid intake, immobile, confused and forgetful, having multiple illnesses, or having improper supervision. The loss or gain of 10 pounds may change considerably the effect of a drug (8).

Poor safety precautions often precipitate accidents with the elderly. Injuries represent the fifth leading cause of death among people 65 to 75 and the sixth leading cause among those above 75. The chief causes of injury are falls, motor vehicle-related accidents, and burns. Home safety checks and a few behavioral guidelines can reduce significantly the number of injuries. The proper placement of furniture, rugs, and electrical cords in the home; adequate lighting; and appropriate interior decorating can make a big difference. Burns are most frequently caused by hot water, cooking-related fires, and smoking in bed. Hot water heaters should never be set above 120°F. Factors outside the home to be considered include the conditions of sidewalks and curbs and the temporary hazards of snow and ice. Auto-related injuries are compounded by the fact that less than 10% of the elderly use seat belts.

From the biological perspective, reaction time does slow down with aging; sensory judgments lose sharpness; and the body is less adaptable to extreme exposures of heat and cold, thus increasing the risk of hypothermia and other heat-related illnesses. Clients must learn to compensate for these realities.

The salience of environmental factors, habit patterns, and general life-style to the health and well-being of the elderly draws attention to the significance of the home visit as an assessment measure. The clinician can obtain much valuable diagnostic information about the client's needs and level of functioning with a visit to the home (20).

A general inspection of the home will at once betray problems with cleanliness, clutter, and hazards. Sometimes simple modifications of the home may make the client more comfortable and the environment safer. Attention should be given to heating, lighting, and ventilation to see that they are adequate. Medications should be checked, both prescriptions and over-the-counter (OTC) drugs. The containers should be inspected to determine if the labeled medications are truly present. A brief questioning about all the medications in use can be helpful. The kitchen should be carefully observed. Are nutritious and wholesome foods available in sufficient supply? Is the stove safe? For some clients an electric stove may be much safer than a gas stove with its open flame and requirement for matches. Individuals with pacemakers should not have a microwave oven.

It is desirable to have a competent family member or friend present during the visit. The intent is to have the visit flow easily and smoothly. The friend might be a social worker, cleric, or visiting nurse—someone the client is comfortable with (20).

Most families are open to suggestions on nutrition, exercise, and the general care and safety of the elder person. Suggestions should be written as well as verbal.

Depression strikes many of the aged. The loss of energy, a ubiquitous complaint among the elderly, is more often than not a symptom of depression. Some expend energy in maintaining denial of depression. Not all depression, of course, is pathological. It can at times be constructive, serving as a motivating force to cope with unpleasantries that otherwise might be avoided. The DSM-III, the standard classification system of mental disorders, recognizes normal grieving. How much actual depression is suffered by the elderly is difficult to quantify

because we lack a good, objective, valid measure. The established depression scales were either standardized on younger adults or were developed as rather short, subjective screening devices. Current assessment instruments are poor in differentiating depression in the elderly from brain disease. More recently developed instruments for research purposes are holding promise for clinical application (2).

Loss because of death within the family or among longstanding friends is a frequent cause of sadness and depression among the elderly. The loss of old friends is painful, and it weakens the support system, but no loss is as devastating as the death of a spouse or child. It can be as poignant as the gripping reality of one's own terminal illness. In fact, Kubler-Ross (15) describes the emotional stages in watching a close family member slowly die as paralleling the pattern of the dying person. Kubler-Ross's stage theory has been criticized on methodological and conceptual grounds (13, 17), and Kubler-Ross herself readily acknowledges that many of the dying do not go through the complete sequence of denial-anger-bargaining-depression-acceptance and that the stages are not always mutually exclusive (many people show elements of different stages at the same time). The model, nevertheless, is a useful guide for the clinician trying to cope with the issue of death and dying.

The vague uneasiness that some clinicians experience around the elderly may be rooted in their own unresolved anxieties over their own mortality. It is essential that they come to terms with their own anxieties if they aspire to aid their clients in resolving theirs. The female, because of usually marrying an older male and having the longer life expectancy (by 7 years), is most likely to have to face the lost spouse anxiety and the living-alone adjustment. The practitioner needs to be prepared to deal with these realities.

Dying itself has dramatically changed, and with it comes a new set of anticipatory worries and concerns. People seldom die in their homes, as in the "old days." Eighty percent of all deaths now take place in hospitals. In the hospital the death scene has moved to the intensive care ward, where time of death has become largely an administrative decision—when to pull the plug of the machine. Traditionally, death has been defined by the absence of vital signs such as heartbeat and respiration. Next, brain death had become the more sophisticated measure—the moment the EEG goes flat. Now, however, with mechanical respirators, electronic pacemakers, and parenteral nutrition, machines can do the work of the brain, heart, and lungs, and the patient can live for years with a flat EEG.

Debate rages over the legal and moral implications. It is not our purpose here to marshal arguments either pro or con but to alert the clinician that elderly clients are likely to have the need to discuss their feelings about this subject.

The trend seems to be toward voluntary, passive euthanasia, voluntary meaning with the patient's consent and passive meaning with the physician's cessation of treatment. The Euthanasia Society, growing in number from 400 to 50,000 in 4 years, has developed a "living will," giving the signer the freedom to be allowed to die without medical interference when the time comes. Of groups polled, the strongest opposition to euthanasia comes from the elderly. What they desire most from their doctors is honesty about their terminal illness, which is what they are least likely to get (polls indicate only about 20% of physicians will level with terminally ill patients). This deceit may be seen as yet another facet of ageism. The clinician should never underestimate the potential control clients have in matters of life and death. When given the facts and the opportunity to cast off irrational beliefs, older persons can influence significantly the will to live and the consequent timetables for departure. They can pull their own plugs, so to speak.

Not all painful losses, forerunners of depression, relate to the obituary column. Depression can occur over the perceived loss of status, influence, income, personal appearance, usefulness, self-esteem, and health. While many of these perceptions are realistically based, many are also derivatives of ageism. The feeling of usefulness may be considered a case in point. It is shattering to self-esteem, but should not be linked to the aging process. Many older citizens live highly useful and productive lives. Those who do not are often victims of poor retirement planning. Too many people enter old age with too little forethought. Retirement was blissfully equated with leisure, recreation, and travel. This life-style in a society conditioned on the work ethic wears thin quickly. The elderly need to get involved in a second career, one based not so much on pecuniary considerations as on self-growth potentials. This becomes the outlet for their creativity, the antidote for lost self-esteem. The clinician can play a major supporting role in this new venture.

CONCLUDING REMARKS

Several themes have run through the content of this chapter. Some were less explicit than others. For the summary we will restate them in a more concise, direct fashion.

First, diversity keynotes the behavior of the aged. Clinicians must shake loose from the notion of an old-age stereotype and recognize the heterogeneity in the needs, wants, interests, and capabilities of their elderly clients.

Second, the holistic approach provides the best and most efficient service to the aged. The elderly are biopsychosocial beings in the fullest sense of the word, and their requirements often necessitate an integrated, interdisciplinary plan. Each member of the team should know the inputs of the others to avoid canceling-out effects or, worse, incompatible instructions or interventions.

Third, optimism rather than pessimism should guide the development of treatment goals. A healthy brain is capable of new learning throughout the life span. Clinicians who promote holding patterns in their treatment programs are sadly shortchanging their elderly clients.

Fourth, the elderly can actively control much of their destiny. As they become more educated on such matters as nutrition, exercise, and lifestyle, they will be able to alter mental and physical states they had hitherto assumed to be irrevocably locked into the aging process. The clinician should be a catalyst in this movement toward increased self-governance.

Fifth, life's last stage, like all the previous stages, should be viewed as a period for further personal growth. For some, crushing disability, dire poverty, or ingrained negative conditioning will make progress unrealistic, but for the great majority the opening of new vistas is entirely possible. The clinician's role is to focus on the developments that free the elderly to pursue new goals. Some of the unique advantages of the elderly to keep in mind are:

1. The relief from the earlier binding responsibilities of growing children, of aging parents (in the many cases in which they are no longer living), and of those unstimulating 9 to 5 jobs.
2. The freedom from direct control of others. Older adults can be their own persons if they so wish. They need not fear that what they say or do might cost them a job or cause them to lose favor with their children, who seek to keep them within the boundaries of the restrictive parental role.
3. The availability of a large amount of discretionary time. The elderly have control over the use of much of their time and the activities they wish to pursue.
4. The motivation that comes in knowing the future is finite. This can encourage the

appropriate use of time, reestablishing priorities and learning to make the most of the passing minutes, and not get caught up in vain pursuits.

In a one-sentence summary, growth and development, not maintenance and repair, should spearhead the practitioner-client relationship.

References

1. Butler R: *Why Survive? Being Old in America.* New York, Harper & Row, 1975.
2. Brink T: *Clinical Gerontology: A Guide to Assessment and Intervention.* New York, Hawthorn Press, 1986.
3. Cohen S: Geriatric drug abuse. *Vista Hill Foundation Drug Abuse and Alcoholism Newsletter,* March 1975, p 4.
4. Comfort A: Age prejudice in America. *Soc Pol* 3:286–301, 1976.
5. Cutler NE, Harootyan RA: Demography of the aged. In Woodruff DS, Birren JE (eds): *Aging: Scientific Perspectives and Social Issues.* New York, Van Nostrand Reinhold, 1975.
6. Erikson EH: *Childhood and Society,* ed 2. New York, Norton, 1963.
7. Gilbert SB: Health promotion for older Americans. *Health Values: Achieving High Level Wellness* 10 (3):38–46, 1986.
8. Grahame-Smith DC, Aronson JK: *Oxford Textbook of Clinical Pharmacology and Drug Therapy.* Oxford, Oxford University, Press, 1984.
9. Harootyan RA: *Annotated Index of Federal Legislation Impacting on the Elderly.* Los Angeles, University of Southern California Press, 1977.
10. Havighurst RV: *Developmental Tasks and Education,* ed 3. New York, David McKay, 1972.
11. Hurlock EB: *Developmental Psychology,* ed 4. New York, McGraw-Hill, 1975.
12. Kalish RA: The New Ageism and the failure models: a polemic. *Gerontologist* 19 (4):398–402, 1979.
13. Kastenbaum R: Is death a life crisis? On the confrontation with death in theory and practice. In Datan N, Ginsburg LA (eds): *Life-span Developmental Psychology.* New York, Academic Press, 1975, p 128.
14. Kermis M: *The Psychology of Human Aging.* Boston, Allyn & Bacon, 1984.
15. Kubler-Ross E: *On Death and Dying.* New York, Macmillan, 1969.
16. Lowy L: *Social Work with the Aging.* New York, Harper & Row, 1979.
17. Schulz K, Aderman D: Clinical research and the stages of dying. *Omega* 52:137–143, 1974.
18. Seligman MEP: *Helplessness: On Depression, Development, and Death.* San Francisco, WH Freeman, 1975.
19. United States Public Health Service Association, Aging: *Aging and Health Promotion: Market Research for Public Education,* Contract No. 282-83-0105. Bethesda, MD, SRA Technologies, 1984.
20. Zebley III JW: Geriatric follow-up: what only a home visit can tell you. *Geriatrics* 41:100–104, 1986.

A Direct Services to the Communicatively Impaired Adult

13 Modifications in Hearing Assessment Procedures for Older Adults

CAROLYN A. RAIFORD

Editor's Note

Chapter 13 begins a series of five chapters devoted to exploration of "Direct Services to the Communicatively Impaired Older Adult." In this chapter, Raiford addresses the topic of assessment of hearing impairment in elderly clients. After considering the standard audiometric test battery, she points out a number of crucial age-related factors that must be considered in assessment. The major portion of the chapter explores the ways in which the standard test battery can be adapted or expanded to provide a more comprehensive and realistic evaluation of auditory function in the older client. One section of the text highlights the importance of scales which allow the client or family member to identify their perceptions of the degree of handicap imposed by the hearing loss and the specific situational and emotional problems created by hearing impairment. Particular emphasis is placed upon gathering data necessary for fitting of a personal hearing aid or selection of an assistive listening device. The importance of providing information and counseling immediately after the audiological evaluation is noted, and problems in the counseling situation are described. The unique situation of the bedfast patient is also discussed briefly. As with all subsequent chapters, Raiford has attempted to provide recommendations and guidelines concerning the ways to manage the special hearing assessment needs of the elderly.

Self-perceived hearing problems are reported to be the third most prevalent chronic disability in individuals over the age of 65 years (33). It should be clear, therefore, that hearing impairment warrants considerable research and clinical attention on the part of those professionals working closely with older clients. One of the most important components of clinical management of hearing disorders is the assessment process. Although great strides have been made in testing older adults in recent years, much additional work needs to be completed.

The basic purpose of any hearing test procedure is to obtain as much information as possible about the degree and type of hearing loss and the possible problems created by the loss. The standard audiological test battery provides very complete information about two of the above areas—the degree and type of loss. However, with any age population, this standard battery is not as effective in identifying or describing the problems created by the loss. In addition, elderly individuals present a unique cluster of social, psychological, and physiological characteristics that must be accommodated in testing.

The purpose of this chapter will be to discuss the applicability of standard testing procedures to audiological evaluation of the older patient and to suggest possible modifications or additions to current testing that may provide more complete information, not only about the hearing loss itself but also about the daily difficulties created by the loss. This latter type of information, while primarily important for rehabilitation purposes, often is not seriously evaluated in the basic hearing test battery. The reason for including this type of testing reflects a specific orientation toward diagnosis. It is not sufficient simply to gather information about the hearing loss; information that can be used in planning rehabilitation must also be obtained.

THE STANDARD AUDIOMETRIC TEST BATTERY

The standard test battery is defined as pure tone testing, including both air and bone conduction thresholds, and speech audiometry, including the speech reception threshold and word discrimination scores. These four measures have been carefully standardized on listeners for stimuli, intensity levels, and method of presentation and responses. The normative populations were subjects between the ages of 18 and 24 with no history of ear pathology.

The application of this battery of tests with its normative values and methodologies is made across all age groups. Modifications in the standardized procedures are only implemented in those instances in which a particular group of subjects is unable for some reason to carry out the prescribed methodology. The most common group for whom modifications are routinely made are children who, because of their level of physical and/or mental development, cannot respond appropriately. The literature is replete with suggestions for modifications in stimuli, methods of signal presentation, and methods of response to accommodate the special needs of these children (34).

For most adults, however, very little is required in terms of modifying test procedures. The exception to this may occur with individuals who have language problems or physical and/or mental disorders. Variations either in stimuli or response behaviors will be adopted to meet the particular needs of the individual. The basic intent, however, is to adhere as closely to the standardized procedures as possible. ·

The assumption in modifying test procedures is that there is some reason the individual cannot respond to the test battery in the standardized manner or that some problem is present that cannot be identified with such a battery. To justify the need for modification in evaluating the older patient, problems unique to this group must be identified.

RELEVANT CHARACTERISTICS OF OLDER ADULTS

Auditory Characteristics

Numerous studies have investigated the degree of loss and type of hearing loss associated with the aging process (7, 29, 33, 50). A comprehensive review of the research literature is provided in Chapter 8. Only a few salient observations will be summarized in this section.

The general findings indicate that a hearing loss may begin as early as the 4th decade of life and becomes increasingly greater with age (6, 11, 21). Hearing impairment occurs in both sexes but is greater in men than in women of comparable age (6, 11). Physiological studies indicate that the loss of hearing found in older adults is primarily associated with degenerative changes in cochlea. The presence of similar degenerative changes in the central auditory system have also been suggested, but the extent of these problems has not been clearly substantiated. We do not yet know the extent to which the aging process, per se, contributes to hearing loss in the elderly. The effects of environmental agents such as exposure to high levels of occupational or recreational noise, disease processes, or ototoxic drugs are difficult, if not impossible, to separate out from other aging processes (24).

The statistics on the number of older persons suffering from hearing loss are extremely variable. Percentages range from 20 to 45% (7, 25, 50). These figures are undoubtedly a gross underestimation of the extent of the problem. This underestimation is probably a function of averaging across age ranges and of a lack of systematic data gathering for older persons. Much more important data would be provided by statistics on individuals at the various age decades.

For example, in a recent survey of 1549 older persons, significant differences in degree of hearing impairment were reported for comparisons among the 60 to 69-year-old group, the 70 to 79-year-old group, and those over age 80 (15). The overall incidence of hearing impairment (pure tone averages above 25 dB in the better ear) was reported to be 61.9% for individuals over the age of 60. In our clinic, 80 to 85% of the clients over the age of 70 have a hearing loss which is considerable enough to interfere with communication. Percentages will also be equally high in any age group which suffers from severe medical problems such as heart, lung, kidney, and circulatory disorders.

Studies have also been concerned with determining any differences in auditory skills of older persons (as compared with young adults). One common finding is the older person's slower response time to auditory stimuli (28, 37). To accommodate this problem, audiologists have traditionally slowed the rate of stimulus presentation of both pure tone and speech stimuli. This modification is a simple one and in no way affects the standardization of the tests involved.

Another significant difference found in the auditory abilities of older patients is reduced speech discrimination skills. Gaeth (8) was one of the first investigators to identify an unusual drop in speech discrimination scores for subjects age 60 and older. He applied the terminology "phonemic regression" to his findings. Other investigators have continued to substantiate this phenomenon (1–3, 14, 18, 19, 38).

This problem has been reported for older subjects presented with stimuli ranging from sentences to monosyllables to nonsense syllables (4, 9, 12, 39). Even older subjects whose hearing thresholds fall within normal limits were found to have poorer discrimination scores than their younger counterparts (9, 12). These discrimination differences become even greater when speech is degraded in any manner. Older subjects were found to have even poorer speech recognition abilities than younger subjects with comparable loss when speech is presented in noise (9), is interrupted (12), or is reverberated (31, 32). Studies to determine the kinds of errors made by older subjects suggest that the problem is one of degree, not of kind.

An additional problem often found in older subjects is a reduced ability to process the temporal cues of speech (23). McCroskey and Kasten (28) showed a deterioration in the older person's ability to detect short silent intervals between pure tones. Another problem found is reduced ability to comprehend speech that is rate altered (23, 26, 43, 44) or subject to various types of reverberation (31, 32). However, these data are conflicting, and a clear determination of the nature and scope of this problem has not been made.

The presence of recruitment in older patients is commonly reported by audiologists clinically, but is difficult to support in formal studies. The ABLB, as the only direct test for recruitment, is frequently not usable with older clients because the typical presbycusis loss is bilaterally symmetrical. Use of the monaural loudness balance tests has yielded mixed results (38), but this may be due to the difficulty of the task involved (13).

The picture is clearer if indirect estimates for recruitment are used. Using such measures as the acoustic reflex threshold, reduced dynamic range, and short increment sensitivity index (SISI) scores, recruitment shows up as a problem but inconsistently (18, 35). The implications for successful hearing aid use make it important that this phenomenon be identified if possible.

The presence of deficiencies in central auditory processing skills in older subjects has been consistently reported. However, the type and extent of these problems is still not clearly known. The clinical tests that are used to identify central auditory processing problems in older patients were originally designed to identify specific lesions in the central auditory system (40).

Harbert (13), investigating binaural fusion of filtered monosyllables in older persons, found lower overall performance in all filtered conditions, but binaural performance remained consistently superior to monaural performance. Palva and Jokinen (36) also found that age had a significant influence on discrimination of filtered monosyllables when presented dichotically. Kelly-Ballweber and Dobie (22), however, found no differences with filtered spondees.

The masking level differences (MLD) test has also been used to assess aging effects on binaural analysis. Tillman et al (49) studied MLDs for spondees. While they report that binaural release from masking was found for all subjects, MLDs were reduced in the older subjects.

Other possible central effects have been reported. Willeford (55) found greater amounts of tone decay in his studies, while others found no differences at all (13, 49). Abnormal amounts of adaptation have been found with Bekesy-type audiometry (17). Differences among older subjects have also been found in dichotic performance (16).

Nonauditory Characteristics

Nonauditory characteristics of older persons also need to be taken into account during testing. Earlier portions of this text (cf. Chapters 3 through 7) have detailed many of the socioeconomic, cognitive, emotional, and physical changes that may accompany the aging process. Weinstein (54) has subdivided these into intrinsic and external factors.

Intrinsic factors must include consideration of any age-related decrements in performance. Among the most obvious are changes in sensorimotor functioning. For example, declines in visual acuity may limit the client's ability to take advantage of nonverbal cues in communication situations. Reduced vision may also interfere with the adequacy of the speech reading information obtained in supplementing auditory reception of speech. Movement impairments in the elderly must also be considered, including restricted range of motion, reduced fine motor coordination, slower response time, tremor, and specific health problems, such as arthritis. Motor dysfunction is of particular concern because of its influence on the independent use of hearing aids and other assistive listening devices. Possible declines in cognitive status must also be recognized since disorientation and memory impairment significantly reduce an older client's ability to manage a personal hearing aid. Even subtle changes in cognitive style and task-oriented behaviors can interfere with testing procedures.

Other intrinsic factors relate to physical and emotional health. The elderly are more prone to chronic health problems and generalized fatigue. Both of these factors will affect the audiological testing process and may limit the degree of effort and attention an individual is willing or able to expend in order to maximize hearing. Motivation to participate fully in an aural rehabilitation process may also be affected by acute or chronic depression, a condition that is fairly prevalent in the older population.

External factors, as defined by Weinstein (54), include social support systems, financial resources, and environmental conditions. The older client's social support system may be somewhat restricted or altered in comparison with that of earlier years in his/her life. If there are limited opportunities to communicate because of a lack of communication partners, the desire to seek professional assistance in managing a hearing loss may be reduced. Elderly members of the population also typically have fixed, frequently inadequate incomes. Chronic health problems may also reduce the financial resources available for audiological services and personal or environmental amplification devices. Finally, the older client's current physical and/or social environment may present major barriers to adequate hearing and communication. Unless these environmental problems are addressed, the most adequately fitted hearing aid and the best program of rehabilitation will be inadequate.

HEARING ASSESSMENT OF OLDER ADULTS: SOME RECOMMENDATIONS

Case History and Interview

A thorough case history should be obtained prior to the test session(s). This is generally done through the use of a preinterview questionnaire mailed to the patient before the appointment. A preinterview form is preferred, as it can be filled out at the patient's leisure, thus eliminating any time constraints imposed by the appointment itself. The completed form will provide the basis for follow-up questioning in the interview preceding actual testing.

Most clinics use a single case history form for all adults. Ideally, however, a form specifically oriented to the unique status and needs of older adults should be prepared. For example, this population will generally include retired individuals who may have living arrangements or social and recreational activities which are quite different from those of other adult age groups. Consequently their communication needs may also be quite unique to their age group and residential setting, and will direct future rehabilitation planning. The case history form should probe residential status, social and family contacts, and daily activities and interests. Other topic areas that should be considered for inclusion on this form are vision status, mobility restrictions, health problems, and medications. If possible, a few case history items should also explore the client's own perception of hearing handicap, the concerns of significant others, motivation to remediate the problem, and financial considerations. All of these can be pursued in greater detail either through the pretest interview or through the use of scales designed to assess perceptions of and attitudes toward one's hearing impairment. At least one case history form item should be designed to determine who referred the individual for evaluation and the reasons for referral. Many older clients are unwilling participants in the audiological evaluation. Their resulting resistance and lack of motivation are important factors to be considered in counseling and in making treatment decisions.

The format of the case history document should also be carefully considered. The use of large type is helpful to those persons with visual problems. As writing may be difficult for some, the use of as many checklists as possible is also recommended.

When necessary, the examiner should consider utilization of supplementary assessment tools that may be relevant to the needs of a particular client. For example, one of several available screening tools, such as the Mental Status Questionnaire designed to assess mental status, may be employed if level of cognitive functioning is questionable (54). If a patient already owns a hearing aid, a profile of hearing aid usage may also be of value (42, 53).

Attitude Scales

One of the most helpful sources of information for future rehabilitation is the use of attitude or perception scales. Several of these scales have been developed specifically for use with older adults. The patients' or family's perceptions about the problems created by their hearing loss or their attitudes toward the use of hearing aids or other amplification systems are extremely valuable in planning rehabilitation and in counseling. A review of the information found in these scales can also be helpful at the initial test session in determining strategies that may be needed in the interview and counseling periods.

A number of examples of self-reporting hearing handicap or performance scales are available in the literature. McCarthy and Alpiner (27) reported on the development of a scale of hearing handicap for family use, and Giolas and colleagues (10) developed a 158-item Hearing Performance Inventory (HPI) for adults of all ages. The HPI takes nearly an hour to administer in its entirety, but is subdivided into six problem areas reflecting everyday listening: (a) Understanding Speech; (b) Intensity; (c) Response to Auditory Failure; (d) Social; (e) Personal; and (f) Occupational. Responses to probe items are scaled from "Frequently" to "Almost Never."

Two scales more specifically developed for use with older adults include the Self-Assessment of Communication (SAC) of Schow and Nerbonne (46) and the Hearing Handicap Inventory for the Elderly (HHIE) of Ventry and Weinstein (51). The SAC, and its correlate version for significant others, consists of 10 questions probing experiences in various communication settings and feelings about communication. The HHIE consists of 25 items also exploring emotional and situational responses.

Attitude or self-perception scales can provide information critical to the rehabilitation process. In particular, they reveal the client's awareness and interpretation of the problems being experienced and suggest specific situations in which assistance is needed. This sit-

uational information in particular may shape decisions about the possible benefits of assistive listening devices and about needed environmental intervention. Knowledge of the degree of emotional distress being experienced by the client can also guide the audiologist in individual and family counseling.

Modifications in the Standard Test Battery

Several modifications in both pure tone and speech testing can be made to meet the special needs of the older patient. One of these has already been suggested. Slowing the rate of stimulus presentation of both pure tone and speech stimuli will obviate the older person's problem of slower response time. While this modification conflicts with the need to reduce the overall time of testing to avoid possible fatigue, the benefits may outweigh the costs.

Other ideal procedural modifications may also increase the time spent in testing. For example, repetition and simplification of testing instructions, along with extended opportunities for practice, may reduce confusion and increase self-confidence. Frequent verbal reassurances may also need to be provided. Because of fatigue, health problems, or general limitations in auditory attention span, the length of testing sessions may need to be reduced (even at the cost of scheduling an additional session to complete all procedures).

One area in which testing time can be shortened is in speech discrimination testing. The traditional discrimination test involves the presentation of 50 monosyllables to each ear. Most clinical audiologists routinely shorten this list to 25 words, but the effect of this modification on the accuracy of the discrimination score is not really known. A better and more accurate approach has been proposed by Runge and Hosford-Dunn (41). These authors found that only a limited number of words in each word list actually contribute to the overall discrimination score. They proposed rearranging the words in each list from most often missed to least often missed. Using their criteria, the lists have the potential of being shortened to only 10 words or, at most 25, without sacrificing the accuracy of the test.

The most important problem experienced by the older adult, that of significantly reduced speech discrimination ability, is only minimally addressed in the standard test battery. The only procedure that looks at this problem is the word discrimination test. The limitation of this test is that it fails to provide adequate information about the extent and type of problem. It will be necessary to add additional speech testing to fully probe speech discrimination abilities.

Additional Audiometric Tests

The additional audiometric tests recommended in this section are directed primarily toward probing the older person's speech discrimination abilities. As has been pointed out earlier, older clients tend to have greater problems in speech discrimination than those in other age groups. This interesting finding is true whether the older person has a hearing loss or not. For example, Gelfand (9) evaluated consonant recognition abilities in quiet and noise for normal listeners at decade age groups extending from 21 to 68 years of age. He found tht the older subjects consistently performed more poorly than the younger subjects. Gordon-Salant (12) evaluated discrimination of two age groups (21 to 33 and the 65 to 72) for natural and time/intensity altered consonant-vowel syllables (CVs). She too found that older subjects performed more poorly than younger subjects in all conditions.

The only test for speech discrimination in the traditional audiometric battery is the 50 word monosyllabic word list discussed earlier. We can generally be assured that most older patients will show some difficulty with this test. The test should probably be performed (preferably in the shortened, reorganized lists), as it provides the audiologist with useful statistical information. However, it does not make available information about the patient's ability to understand speech in context. For rehabilitation purposes, that latter piece of information may be far more important.

From a psychological point of view, these single-word lists often create a great deal of frustation for the patient. Patients have often interrupted me in the middle of testing to indicate that they understand the carrier phrase but not the word. Many become so frustrated or exasperated that they cease to cooperate with the testing procedures. If the single-word list is the only test used, the audiologist's credibility in counseling the patient about the kinds of communication problems he may be having is seriously impaired.

A better approach would be to include the use of other types of speech stimuli. The purpose of such testing would be to evaluate speech discrimination abilities in different types of speech contexts. Can the client respond to sentences or paragraphs? Can understanding be improved by cueing the subject matter? This type of information will be far more important in predicting success in the use of a hearing aid than the standardized discrimination test. The testing serves another purpose in that the patient can see for himself the problems he is having.

One example of this type of expanded speech discrimination testing is the Speech Perception in Noise (SPIN) Test developed by Kalikow et al (20). The SPIN test consists of low predictability (PL) and high predictability (PH) sentences against a noise background of multiple speakers. The client's task is to repeat the last word of the sentence. In one study, use of the SPIN sentences in both quiet and noise was found to discriminate subjects with normal hearing from those with hearing loss (52), although the SPIN measures did not predict results of hearing handicap scales with any accuracy.

Another piece of information needed is the effect on speech discrimination when visual cues (lipreading) are added to the auditory signal. While there are many misconceptions associated with lip reading and lip reading training (which will be dealt with in the next chapter), there is no doubt that speech discrimination can be significantly improved if both visual and auditory information can be used simultaneously (48). The presence or absence of improved discrimination with both visual and auditory cues is important in determining the need for future lip reading training.

One type of testing rarely investigated is the patient's use of binaural hearing. Psychoacoustic literature has clearly established the benefits of binaural over monaural hearing (47). Two of the most important benefits include an improved threshold and better discrimination of speech (5). Binaural hearing testing could be very helpful in determining the need for binaural versus monaural hearing aid fittings. While no clinical procedure has been developed that clearly demonstrates the superiority of binaural over monaural fittings, many hearing aid users have reported a significant improvement in speech discrimination with the binaural approach (30).

Another important test measure needed is the patient's threshold of discomfort. This measure serves two functions. It provides the audiologist with information about the range of usable hearing and serves as an indirect measure of recruitment. A reduced dynamic range severely limits the person's ability to use an aid. It certainly will dictate the choice of amplification system as well as the frequency response, maximum power output levels, and gain settings the audiologist must select in adjusting the aid.

The preceding discussion has intentionally avoided any more comprehensive review of the variety of audiological and psychoacoustic procedures that have been utilized with older individuals, since these are discussed extensively in Chapter 8. Some procedures have been primarily of research value, including examination of responses to time-compressed speech, filtered signals, speech in the presence of competing noise or other speech, and reverberation. Other procedures are a more familiar part of the clinical audiological battery. This latter category encompasses several tasks described in this section and includes measures of: auditory adaptation (e.g., tone decay, Bekesy), loudness perception and recruitment (e.g., SISI, monaural and alternate binaural loudness tests), auditory brain stem responses, and acoustic reflex decay.

Some of these measures may be able to provide important diagnostic data that can aid in the rehabilitation process. Others may be of greater value in the future when the dynamics of the aging auditory mechanism are better understood. Despite this chapter's emphasis on presbycusic hearing loss, however, it is important to remember that there may be other causes for the hearing impairment found in a particular older client. Just because an individual is elderly, we must not assume that any observed hearing impairment is a byproduct of the aging process. Any and all audiological procedures necessary for determination of an appropriate differential diagnosis can and should be utilized.

Counseling

Counseling is an ongoing process throughout assessment and rehabilitation procedures. Both the hearing impaired older adult and family members or significant others will require assistance in understanding the nature and degree of hearing loss, its consequences, all recommendations for rehabilitation, and possible strategies for coping with the interpersonal stresses created by the hearing impairment. One of the biggest problems encountered in testing the older client is the problem that brought him to the hearing test—his hearing loss. The communication problems created by the loss will be present during the pretest interview and during counseling following completion of audiometric procedures.

The hearing test generally begins with a pretest interview in which the audiologist will review and clarify the case history information. Following the testing, the results of the hearing test and the recommendations for rehabilitation must be discussed with the patient. Any major communication problems could seriously hinder the getting and/or giving of the information.

There is, of course, no easy answer to this problem. One solution is to bring a family member or friend into the interview/counseling setting. At least in this way, basic information and recommendations can be communicated. The use of an all-purpose amplification system, such as a speaking tube, is also very helpful if available.

The counseling session following the testing is most important. It is also a highly difficult situation. A great deal of information must be communicated, often in a short period of time. The degree and type of loss experienced by the patient must be explained, as well as the implications of this problem for speech understanding. The audiologist's recommendations for or against the need for amplification, and the reasons for these recommendations must be outlined. The need for any other types of rehabilitation, such as hearing aid orientation or lip reading and auditory training services, must be clarified.

It is quite probable that the client will understand and/or remember very little of the information provided at the initial counseling session. Because of this, it is important that relevant information be presented as often and in as many ways as possible. Obviously much of this information will be covered in the subsequent hearing aid evaluation and orientation sessions. It is very helpful if printed material can be given to the patient. Some excellent publications explaining the hearing test, the hearing aid, rehabilitation techniques, etc. are available. Another procedure which is extremely valuable is the use of videotapes, which can be shown to the patient and/or family at the clinic or, if a VCR is available to the patient at home, can be loaned to him.

The Special Case of the Nonambulatory Patient

A major problem in testing hearing with older patients is the individual who is nonambulatory. To obtain a valid hearing test, the test must be performed in a sound suite. This means that patients must be brought to the test facility. Wheelchair bound patients present no problems, as most test facilities have wheelchair access to both the clinic and to the sound suite. Those clients, however, who are "bedfast" create greater difficulties.

To compensate for this, many audiologists have agreed to compromise the accuracy of hearing testing by taking a portable audiometer to the patient's bedside. The only possible testing in this situation is pure tone audiometry. Speech audiometry, which is the most important type of testing for rehabilitation purposes, cannot be done in this environment. Yet, from this limited testing, hearing aids are recommended and fitted.

While the reasons for this type of compromised audiometry are understandable, the procedure does not appear acceptable (at least to this author). There is simply too much room for error in this form of testing, and the data obtained do not provide the audiologist with enough information to make adequate rehabilitation recommendations. Further, it is probable that many of these patients are not good candidates for personal hearing aids (45).

A different type of evaluation and subsequent rehabilitation can be proposed. The patient who is truly confined to a bed has very special and limited communication needs: talking to doctors/nurses, talking to family, watching television, etc. Most of these interactions are highly specific events and may take up only a limited part of the day. In these instances, a more productive approach would be to provide the bedfast patient with an assistive listening device (ALD). In this way an amplification system can be selected to meet a specific communication need and can be used as required by the situation. Assessment consists of a systematic analysis of the individual's environmental communication needs, based perhaps on a 24-hour inventory of the frequency and nature of communicative interactions, as well as the most common communication partners and settings. Such an inventory could be completed by primary caregivers whether family members or professional staff persons.

Other advantages of the assistive listening devices are that they are cheaper individually and can be used by several patients. They tend to be larger and thus easier for patients to handle. ALDs usually have better acoustic characteristics (broader frequency response, more gain and less distortion). They also avoid problems related to the reluctance of some older patients to wear a hearing aid. Further discussion of assistive listening devices is provided in Chapter 14.

There are always exceptions to the above recommendations concerning confined patients. If the patient is indeed alert, is active and wants amplification throughout the day, there is no reason why arrangements cannot be made for formal testing. Transportation by wheelchair or even by gurney can be arranged, and testing can be done in a suite in either of these conditions.

CONCLUSIONS

The assessment of hearing impairment in older adults can be a complex and, at times, difficult task. The unique auditory characteristics of various forms of presbycusis, coupled with intrinsic and extrinsic aspects of aging that may complicate testing and rehabilitation, present major challenges to the audiologist. Modifications in administration procedures used in the standard hearing test battery, along with selected specialized audiological tests, can provide data useful in determining the type and degree of hearing loss. However, current procedures are less adequate to the task of determining the communicative, social, and emotional problems created by the hearing loss. As a result, rehabilitation efforts may be hindered.

This chapter has discussed some of the major considerations to be addressed in assessing auditory functioning in older clients. Appropriate content for the case history form and preliminary interview was identified. The use of supplemental attitude or self perception of hearing handicap scales was strongly advocated. Recommendations were made for modifications in the administration procedures for the standard testing battery and for the use of additional testing strategies and tasks. General concerns were also noted as they relate to the process of providing a preliminary summary of evaluation findings and basic counseling.

With any form of communication impairment, the process of assessment is, or should be, inextricably linked to the development and ongoing maintenance of the rehabilitation program. Assessment and intervention exist on a continuum, and both processes should continue throughout the course of management of a particular client. Nowhere is this more evident than in the case of the hearing impaired older adult. In many instances, preliminary assessment data (both quantitative and qualitative) virtually dictate the selection of a personal hearing aid or assistive listening device. These same data should also target problems in management, whether they relate to intrinsic or extrinsic client factors.

The decision to address assessment issues only in this chapter establishes an arbitrary dichotomy in the assessment/treatment continuum. The reader is urged to consider Chapters 13 and 14 as a continuous unit. Chapter 14 will build upon material presented in this chapter in discussing current management strategies for the hearing impaired older adult. The focus continues to be gerontological. In other words, emphasis is placed upon understanding those unique aspects of the older person's situation that must be addressed in any rehabilitation program.

References

1. Bergman M: Hearing and aging. *Audiology* 10:164–171, 1971.
2. Bergman M, Blumfield V, Cascardo D, Dash B, Levitt H, Marguiles M: Age-related decrement in hearing for speech: sampling and longitudinal studies. *J Gerontol* 31:533–538, 1976.
3. Bergman M: *Aging and the Perception of Speech.* Baltimore, University Park Press, 1980.
4. Blumenfeld VG, Bergman M, Millner E: Speech discrimination in an aging population. *J Speech Hear Res* 12:210–217, 1969.
5. Breakey M, Davis H: Comparison of thresholds for speech: word and sentence test, receiver vs. field, and monaural vs. binaural hearing. *Laryngoscope* 59:236–250, 1949.
6. Corso JF: Age and sex differences in pure-tone thresholds. *Arch Otolaryngol* 77:53–73, 1963.
7. Fein DJ: Population data from the U.S. Census Bureau. *ASHA* 25:31, 1983.
8. Gaeth J: A study of phonemic regression in relation to hearing loss. Unpublished Ph.D. thesis, Evanston, IL, Northwestern University, 1948.
9. Gelfand SA, Piper N, Silman S: Consonant recognition in quiet and noise with aging among normal hearing listeners. *J Acoust Soc Am* 80:1589–1598, 1986.
10. Giolas T, Owens E, Lamb S, et al: Hearing performance inventory. *J Speech Hear Disord* 44:169–195, 1979.
11. Glorig A, Nixon JC: Distribution of hearing loss in various populations. *Ann Otol Rhinol Laryngol* 69:497–516, 1960.
12. Gordon-Salant S: Recognition of natural and time/intensity altered CV's by young and elderly subjects with normal hearing. *J Acoust Soc Am* 80:1599–1607, 1986.
13. Harbert F, Young IM, Menduke H: Audiologic findings in presbycusis. *J Aud Res* 6:297–312, 1966.
14. Hayes D: Aging and speech understanding. *Semin Hear* 6:147–158, 1985.
15. Hergenreder P, Schallenkamp KK, Pistulka LM, Swisher WE: The incidence of hearing loss among the geriatric population. Presented at the American Speech-Language-Hearing Association Convention, Detroit, 1986.
16. Inglis J, Caird WK: Age differences in successive response to simultaneous stimulation. *Can J Psychol* 17:98–105, 1963.
17. Jerger J: Bekesy audiometry in analysis of auditory disorders. *J Speech Hear Disord* 3:275–287, 1960.
18. Jerger J: Audiological findings in aging. *Adv Otorhinolaryngol* 20:115–124, 1973.
19. Jerger J: Hayes D: Diagnostic speech audiometry. *Arch Otolaryngol* 103:216–222, 1977.
20. Kalikow D, Stevens K, Elliott L: Development of a test of speech intelligibility in noise using sentence materials with controlled word predictability. *J Acoust Soc Am* 61:1337–1351, 1977.
21. Kelly LS: Hearing loss in the older person. *Hear J* 38:24–27, 1985.
22. Kelly-Ballweber D, Dobie RA: Binaural interaction measured behaviorally and electrophysiologically in young and old adults. *Audiology* 23:181–194, 1984.
23. Konkle DF, Beasley DS, Bess FH: Intelligibility of time-altered speech in relation to chronological aging. *J Speech Hear Res* 20:108–115, 1977.
24. Kryter KD: Presbycusis, sociocusis and nosocusis. *J Acoust Soc Am* 73:1897–1919, 1983.
25. Leski MC: Prevalence estimates of communicative disorders in the U.S.: language, hearing and vestibular disorders. *ASHA* 23:229–237, 1981.
26. Luterman D, Welsh O, Melrose J: Responses of aged males to time altered speech stimuli. *J Speech Hear Res* 9:226–230, 1966.
27. McCarthy P, Alpiner J: An assessment scale of hearing handicap for use in the family. *J Acad Rehab Audiol* 16:256–271, 1983.
28. McCroskey RL, Kasten RN: Temporal factors and the aging auditory system. *Ear Hear* 3:124–127, 1982.
29. Moscicki EK, Elkins EF, Baum HM, McNamara PM: Hearing loss in the elderly: an epidemiologic study of the Framingham heart study cohort. *Ear Hear* 6:184–190, 1985.
30. Mueller HG: Binaural amplification: attitudinal factors. *Hear J* 39:7–10, 1986.
31. Nabelek AK, Mason D: Effect of noise and reverberation on binaural and monaural word identification by subjects with various audiograms. *J Speech Hear Res* 24:375–383, 1981.
32. Nabelek AK, Robinson PK: Monaural and binaural speech perception in reverberation for listeners of various ages. *J Acoust Soc Am* 71:1242–1248, 1982.
33. National Center for Health Statistics: Prevalence of selected impairments, United States, 1977. *Vital Health Stat* [10], No. 134. DHEW Pub. no. (PHS) 81-1562, 1981.
34. Northern JL, Downs MP: *Hearing in Children,* ed. 2. Baltimore, Williams & Wilkins, 1978.
35. Otto WC, McCandless GA: Aging and auditory site of lesion. *Ear Hear* 3:110–117, 1982.
36. Palva A, Jokinen K: The role of the binaural test in filtered speech audiometry. *Acta Otolaryngol (Stockh)* 79:310–314, 1975.
37. Patterson RD, Nimmo-Smith I, Weber DL, Milroy R: The deterioration of hearing with age: frequency selectivity, the critical ratio, the audiogram, and speech threshold. *J Acoust Soc Am* 72:1788–1803, 1982.
38. Pestalozza G, Shore I: Clinical evaluation of presbycusis on the basis of different tests of auditory function. *Laryngoscope* 65:1136–1163, 1955.
39. Punch J, McConnell F: The speech discrimination of elderly adults. *J Aud Res* 9:159–166, 1969.
40. Roush J: Aging and binaural auditory processing. *Semin Hear* 6:135–146, 1985.

41. Runge CA, Hosford-Dunn H: Word recognition performance with modified CID W-22 word lists. *J Speech Hear Res* 28:355–362, 1985.

42. Rupp R, Higgins J, Maurer J: A feasibility scale for predicting hearing aid use (FSPHAU) with older individuals. *J Acad Rehab Audiol* 10:81–104, 1977.

43. Schmitt JF: The effects of time compression and time expansion on passage comprehension by elderly listeners. *J Speech Hear Res* 26:373–377, 1983.

44. Schmitt JF, Carroll MR: Older listeners' ability to comprehend speaker-generated rate alteration of passages. *J Speech Hear Res* 28:309–312, 1985.

45. Schow RL: Success of hearing aid fitting in nursing homes. *Ear Hear* 3:173–177, 1982.

46. Schow RL, Nerbonne MA: Communication screening profile: use with elderly clients. *Ear Hear* 3:135–148, 1982.

47. Shaw W, Newman E, Hirsh I: The difference between monaural and binaural thresholds. *J Exp Psychol* 37:229–242, 1947.

48. Siegenthaler B, Gruber V: Combining vision and audition for speech reception. *J Speech Hear Disord* 34:58–60, 1969.

49. Tillman T, Carhart R, Nicholls S: Release from multiple maskers in elderly persons. *J Speech Hear Res* 16:152–160, 1973.

50. United States Health Examination Survey: Hearing levels of adults by age and sex in the United States, 1960–1962, Publication 1000, Series 11, No. 11. U.S. Public Health Service, DHEW, Washington, DC, 1965.

51. Ventry I, Weinstein B: The hearing handicap inventory for the elderly: a new tool. *Ear Hear* 3:128–134, 1982.

52. Vertes DR, Newman CW, Dentino ML: Speech recognition-in-noise and perceived hearing handicap in geriatrics. Presented at the American Speech-Language-Hearing Association Convention, Detroit, 1986.

53. Walden B, Demorest M, Hepler E: Self-report approach to assessing benefit derived from amplification. *J Speech Hear Res* 27:49–56, 1984.

54. Weinstein B: Management of the hearing impaired elderly. In Jacobs-Condit L (ed): *Gerontology and Communication Disorders.* Rockville, MD, American Speech-Language-Hearing Association, 1984, p. 244.

55. Willeford J: The association of abnormalities in auditory adaptation to other auditory phenomena. Unpublished Ph.D. thesis, Evanston, IL, Northwestern University, 1960.

14 Treatment for the Hearing Impaired Older Individual: A Gerontological Perspective

CAROLYN A. RAIFORD

Editor's Note

Although most communication disorder professionals view assessment and intervention as being components of the same continuum of management services, the dichotomy between the two is particularly artificial when a hearing impairment is involved. This chapter, therefore, should be read as a direct companion piece to Chapter 13. Raiford begins Chapter 14 with some fairly challenging remarks concerning the efficacy of hearing management procedures with the older adult. A relative paucity of rehabilitation programs designed for the elderly is noted. Chapter 14 then continues with a discussion of management of the hearing impaired older adult by focusing on specific topics related to enhancing communicative functioning, including the selection and fitting of the personal hearing aid, the nature and potential value of assistive listening devices (ALDs), appropriate training in the use of the aid/ALD and in relistening strategies, auditory-visual communication training, and counseling for the hearing impaired older adult and family members or caregivers. As with the previous chapter, the intent is to provide practical suggestions based on an understanding of the needs and characteristics of the elderly and their environments. The final section of the chapter highlights other variables that must be addressed in the intervention process, including financial and environmental considerations.

Management of hearing impairment in the older adult is one of the most difficult, frustrating, and least successful areas of aural rehabilitation. The communication problems which accompany hearing loss in any individual are only exacerbated in the elderly. Not only must the unique age-related changes in auditory processing (discussed in Chapter 13) be addressed, but also the unique changes in life-style which accompany aging (24).

While these statements may sound pessimistic, they should not be taken to mean that rehabilitation should not be undertaken with the elderly. Rather, any audiologist working with this population should realistically be aware of the problems that will be faced. Many older adults will respond to and benefit from intervention programs, but a number will not (5).

Few studies have attempted to determine the efficacy of aural rehabilitation programs with older clients (36, 43). Generally, the measure of efficacy is the number of patients who follow through on audiological recommendations. Follow-through stages may include hearing aid evaluation or orientation, therapy/counseling sessions, and finally maintenance of continued use of personal hearing aids.

In the studies reported, follow-through rates may range from 4 to 86%, with the most common rate around 50% (18, 20, 38). Higher success rates are generally associated with those older adults who are active, independent, in good physical health, and with higher educational and socioeconomic levels (31). In addition, programs which include an "educational" component to the rehabilitation process show improved follow-through activity (19, 43).

While rehabilitation programs for hearing impaired adults have been developed over many years (cf. 2, 10, 23), only a few programs have been oriented toward the older adult (cf., 2, 3, 5, 11, 17, 24, 28). Even these programs remain very similar to the traditional adult rehabilitation management procedures. Programming typically consists of the evaluation and selection of a personal hearing aid, orientation to the hearing aid, therapy sessions to improve listening skills and lip reading skills, as well as sessions designed to provide information about hearing loss. The primary difference with respect to older clients seems to be the emphasis on motivational, informational, and family counseling (1, 24, 45).

Rehabilitation of hearing loss in the older person is most commonly directed toward a single goal: the selection and fitting of a personal hearing aid. This is a very limited approach to rehabilitation and will not, by itself, meet the real communication needs of most older patients. A more comprehensive approach to rehabilitation should incorporate at least three areas of training, based on the individual needs of each patient. The three areas of training include: (a) the selection and fitting of personal hearing aids and the consideration of possible alternative amplification systems such as assistive listening devices; (b) training in the use of any and all amplification systems and appropriate communication techniques; and (c) counseling the client and the client's family and friends on techniques or ways to minimize the problems in communication created by a hearing loss.

There are, of course, many drawbacks to the extensive programming proposed here. The first, and most serious, is the availability of appropriate services. Only an audiologist is adequately trained to carry out all three aspects of training, and in many areas of the country, no local audiologist is available. Consequently, the only recourse an older person may have is a hearing aid dealer who is not qualified to provide any rehabilitation service except the dispensing of the aid. A second problem involves the amount of time inherent in a comprehensive program of management of hearing loss in the elderly. Training and counseling sessions necessitate the addition of several return appointments to the audiologist. The transportation difficulties experienced by many older persons may become a major deterrent to utilization of these additional rehabilitation sessions.

The third problem may rest within the clients themselves. As indicated in the efficacy studies, the majority of older clients actively or passively resist the use of a hearing aid. Many, if not most, older persons have friends who have purchased hearing aids, only to find that they cannot get adequate benefit from the aid. As a result, they have given up. Another reason for resistance relates to the many misconceptions about the types of hearing aids and what hearing aids can and cannot do. Some older persons, for example, still believe that the only aid is the body aid with a totally unacceptable cord running from the body to the ear. This is the aid that, perhaps, a grandmother or grandfather used, and it remains the individual's only experience with such devices.

Both of these problems contribute to a lack of motivation, one of the barriers to management of hearing loss in the elderly that has been noted by audiologists (1, 24, 46). Support for this lack of motivation can be found indirectly in a study by Garstecki and Marrer (18). Free screening services were provided to elderly users of services at a senior center. About two-thirds of those who failed the screening elected to take advantage of further testing, and only half of the screening failures expressed interest in learning more about hearing loss and appropriate management options. Of those who received further testing, half elected to use a personal hearing aid. None purchased personal use assistive listening devices.

Sources of motivation to seek assistance with a hearing loss remain poorly understood. For example, Etienne and Naas (13) reported that peer reactions and beliefs did not adversely affect older clients' decisions to try amplification. However, use of a personal aid did appear to be related to whether or not the client felt that the ability to hear and better understand family members was important.

In addition to motivation problems, a more pervasive reason for failure to seek assistance with hearing impairment may result from the perception that admission that one needs a hearing aid is simply another admission of aging. Put more directly, many older persons simply refuse to acknowledge a hearing problem, despite constant evidence of hearing difficulties in daily communication situations (18).

Regardless of the reasons, if an older client is resisting rehabilitation, then no matter what type of training is instituted, successful use of amplification is doomed to failure. Information from self-reported attitude and perception scales can be particularly useful in identifying problems of motivation and denial. If resistance is present, counseling the patient before an aid is recommended is imperative (25). Until the individual is willing to attempt the use of an aid in an open, honest, accepting fashion, rehabilitative fitting of such a device should not be attempted.

SELECTION OF AN AMPLIFICATION SYSTEM

Rehabilitation of hearing loss is difficult even under the best of circumstances. When it is accompanied by the many complicating conditions surrounding old age, the process is further impeded. In addition, all of the management techniques available are designed to compensate for the hearing loss through the use of some type of amplification device. Unfortunately, no one amplification system can be effective in all communication situations, and there will be some situations in which no device will help.

Despite these qualifying comments, the first step in the rehabilitation process must be the selection of an appropriate amplification system or systems. The most common of these is the personal hearing aid. More recently another type of system, the assistive listening device, has been developed. Assistive listening devices are designed for use in those specific listening situations for which the personal hearing aid is ineffective.

Personal Hearing Aids

Much research has been devoted to developing audiological techniques for selecting the most appropriate aid for a given patient out of the vast array of makes and models of hearing aids. The basic premise is to compare or analyze how different aids influence the client's performance and select the most appropriate aid (7, 16, 21, 26, 34). Unfortunately, as suggested by Walden and colleagues (42), no technique has been found that distinguishes among homogeneous aids or predicts success in the real world.

There are probably two reasons for this failure. First, most manufacturers of hearing aids today produce aids of equal quality and choices in terms of type, input and output controls, gain settings, and frequency response. Thus any make of aid, appropriately set, will probably be equally effective for a wide range of patients. The second reason is one that cannot readily be measured—it is the way in which a given aid performs on a given patient. The unique physiological and anatomical characteristics of each client's loss, the presence of possible distortion effects in the auditory system, and other elusive variables all will affect the way the hearing aid will perform for a particular person.

One important point to be considered here is the effect of the earmold on the selection of an aid. Much of our recent research has indicated that the effectiveness of any hearing aid may be due primarily to the acoustic characteristics of the earmold, not the amplification instrument itself. There is much evidence to suggest that changing the type and/or characteristics of the earmold may turn an ineffective aid into an effective one (9).

The first decision regarding aids is the type of aid to be used: all-in-the-ear, behind-the-ear, eyeglass, or body aid. The latter two types, eyeglass and body aid, have all but disappeared.

The body aid is used in very limited situations, usually with young children in classroom amplification systems. The eyeglass aids are bulky, unsightly, and cause numerous problems in repair. With the improvement in miniaturization of hearing aid circuitry, most hearing problems can be met with either the in-the-ear or behind-the-ear aids.

Most patients prefer the smallest and most invisible aid possible, which is the all-in-the-ear aid. This little device, once considered only an advertising gimmick, has come into its own in recent years. Today it provides an effective amplification system and is the most popular aid among hearing aid users. The only limitations to this type of aid are the gain settings and the fact that the patient must have an ear canal large enough for the aid to be built into the earmold. There is an additional problem for some older patients. The in-the-ear aid is quite small, and the controls are often difficult to handle for patients with reduced tactile sensitivity or mobility in the hands or fingers. Those patients with reduced visual acuity also may have a problem with this type of aid. Its major advantage, in addition to its cosmetic appeal, is the fact that it places hearing at the level of the ear and can be very effective in establishing binaural hearing in a binaural fitting.

If the all-in-the-ear aid cannot be used, the next choice is the behind-the-ear aid. This type of hearing aid can be used with just about any type or degree of loss. It has the further advantage of being slightly larger than the all-in-the-ear, thus making it easier to handle. Several companies have introduced modifications in the design of the behind-the-ear aid to accommodate older persons, including enlarged volume control switches.

One of the major determining factors in selection of type of personal hearing aid should be the maximization of the individual's independent use of and functioning with the aid (45). Obviously, independence can be enhanced by consideration of the patient's sensory or motor restrictions, as outlined above. However, the simple fact of personal preference for or dislike of a particular type of aid may dictate whether or not that device is used effectively by a given client.

The next decision to be made is whether to fit monaurally or binaurally. Because of the significant advantages of binaural over monaural hearing (discussed in Chapter 13), the binaural fitting is preferable if at all possible. There are objections to this. First, the cost of two, versus one, aid may be prohibitive for some clients. Second, many clients may simply prefer to wear only one aid, perhaps perceiving it as more manageable or less noticeable (29). Third, there are little except subjective data to support an advantage of binaural over monaural aids except in the subjective reports of patients (12, 22, 29, 30).

The remainder of the decisions in hearing aid selection are audiological ones based on the hearing test results. These include amount of gain, frequency response, limiting system, and maximum power output levels. These adjustments or controls will determine the model of aid selected.

Finally, a choice must be made among the various makes of aids. This selection process may be accomplished in several ways. As indicated earlier, the traditional approach involves comparisons of the performances of three to four aids on a word discrimination test. Discrimination scores are obtained once each aid is fitted on the client. The aid yielding the best discrimination score would then theoretically be the aid of choice.

The disadvantages of such a procedure are many. The time required is extensive and may be fatiguing to older persons, as well as adding to the expense of the evaluation procedure. The test facilities needed to carry out this type of sound field testing effectively are also expensive and are not always available in the particular audiological practice. Most importantly, this procedure has not been shown to be effective in determining the "best" aid (42). Often, the patient will prefer the aid which yielded the poorest word discrimination score.

Because of the above limitations, most audiologists have adopted a more informal approach to hearing aid choice. In this case, an aid will be selected based on the acoustic characteristics needed and the client's subjective evaluation of performance and preference. The client is then allowed to take the aid home and try it out.

While this informal technique circumvents most of the disadvantages of more formal testing, it has one major drawback. An assumption made in this approach is that the client knows how to "try out" the hearing aid. In many instances, however, clients will have difficulty simply learning how to put on the aid, how to adjust the controls, and how and when to start using this amplification tool. For these reasons, a series of additional sessions are recommended in order to train the client to use the aid in a systematic and controlled manner (as described in "Hearing Aid Orientation").

While not commercially available at this time, the potential impact of the digital hearing aid on rehabilitation for the older adult should be mentioned (4, 32, 39). The application of computer technology to the hearing aid may have the potential to solve the major problems typical of older clients. Staab (39) points out that such problems as background noise and acoustic feedback can be eliminated. The digital aid can be programmed and reprogrammed any number of times (performed, perhaps, through a telephone linkup).

Assistive Listening Devices

Before describing procedures in training the patient to use a personal hearing aid, a discussion of the role of assistive listening devices is appropriate. This relatively new field of research and clinical applications involving assistive listening devices, or ALDs, has developed in response to the limitations of personal aids (27, 40). As stated earlier, ALDs are designed for use in those listening situations in which the hearing aid is not particularly effective (35). Examples of such situations include: using the telephone; watching television; listening to programs in large auditoriums (such as churches or theaters); and communicating with individuals in noisy environments. In addition, ALDs may be useful when a variety of factors (finances, psychosocial problems, other handicapping conditions) rule out fitting with a traditional personal aid. Other special sensory devices may also prove useful: captioned television; telecommunication devices for the deaf (TDD), light activators for doorbells; smoke alarms; weather alerts; and even hearing dogs. All can help in alleviating communication problems and encouraging independence for older clients (44).

Assistive listening devices have a number of major advantages, including favorable S/N ratio; high fidelity microphones; portability; durability; ease of manipulation; reasonable cost; situational specificity; and relative ease of orientation and immediacy of usage (27). All of the systems are commercially available, and a number can be made at home by the do-it-yourselfer.

Complete descriptions of the various types and variants of assistive listening devices are provided in a number of sources (27, 35, 40, 45). All ALDs share common characteristics. The system components involve a microphone held near or hooked into a sound source, an amplifier, and a transducer (headphone or coupling with a personal hearing aid). The various systems differ primarily in terms of the manner in which the acoustic signal is transmitted from the receiving microphone to the person's ear. There are three major variants of this transmission process: the hardwire, infrared, and frequency modulation (FM) systems.

Hardwired systems depend upon a hardwired connection between the microphone, amplifier, and receiver. Since the microphone can be used by a single speaker or passed from speaker to speaker in a small group or noisy environment, the hardwired system is useful for both personal/familial communications and for interactions with professionals. Hardwired systems can also be coupled directly with the television, radio, stereo, or phone. This type of ALD is the least expensive of all the systems, and components for system construction are readily available at commercial establishments.

In contrast, infrared systems rely upon infrared light waves as the carrier for acoustic information. Because of this more sophisticated mechanism of conversion of acoustic to infrared to acoustic signals, the costs of this form of assistive listening device are greater than for the hardwired system, although costs are also highly variable, depending upon the specific desired applications. Infrared listening systems are most useful for indoor transmission of sound in large areas, although modifications for home use (e.g., with the television) are available. Portability is limited somewhat by the system's demand for alternating current (AC) power.

The third, and most versatile, ALD system is the FM system. FM devices use radio frequencies as the carrier signal. While they are the most costly of the assistive listening devices, their advantages include: a high level of portability; a relatively unobtrusive physical structure; compatibility with a personal hearing aid; and (as noted above) applications in almost any listening situation.

In working with the hearing impaired older adult, a discussion of ALDs should be included as part of the hearing aid evaluation. (Chapter 13 has already noted the need to document situational communication needs.) Even when a personal aid is recommended, there is still an important place for the assistive listening device within the context of the total management picture. A current problem is the availability of these devices in clinics and hearing aid dispensing offices. However, ALD demonstration centers have been established since 1981 (14, 15), providing a way of demonstrating these devices. In addition, Vaughn and her associates at the Birmingham Veterans Administration Hospital have prepared an excellent videotape which demonstrates use of such devices (41).

The real value of the ALD, however, may be for the patient who is not a candidate for a personal aid. One of these groups, the non-ambulatory patient, was discussed in the last chapter. Any patient who resists use of a hearing aid may be more amenable to a telephone amplifying system or to a TV listening system. In fact, use of one of these systems may eventually break down resistance to the wearing of a personal aid.

TRAINING IN THE USE OF AMPLIFICATION AND OTHER COMMUNICATION STRATEGIES

At least three major problems must be addressed once a hearing aid has been selected if we are to be successful in maximizing the client's communicative performance. The first problem concerns the actual use and care of the personal hearing aid (or ALD). The second relates to the difficulties the client may experience in accepting and processing the modified acoustic signal provided by the aid. Both of these problems will be discussed in greater detail in immediately following sections of this chapter. The third rehabilitation difficulty stems from the client's patterns of emotional maladjustment to hearing loss (those already developed) and/or from an individual's general resistance to acknowledging hearing loss and working constructively at managing its consequences. These latter difficulties will be discussed later in the section on counseling.

Hearing Aid Orientation

While the term hearing aid orientation is used in a variety of different ways by different authors (2, 26, 28), it is intended here to refer only to the immediate process of preparing the client to *begin* utilizing the aid for listening purposes. Thus, the term encompasses four of the five topics or content areas identified by Weinstein (45), specifically:

1. Explanation of the purpose(s) of a hearing aid;
2. Discussion of the advantages and limitations of any hearing aid and of the specific aid that has been selected;
3. Clarification of the function or operation of the components of the aid and explanation of ways to manipulate the various controls;
4. Suggestions for care and maintenance of the hearing aid, earmold, and battery.

(The fifth topic area, suggestions for adjustment to amplification, is addressed in "Relistening Training.")

The importance of each of these topics in the hearing aid orientation must not be minimized. During training exercises designed to familiarize the older client with the operation and care of the hearing aid, special attention must be paid to particular age-related characteristics and deficits that may interfere with the learning process or with the actual utilization of the device. Problems with vision, motor functioning, memory, attention, and/or health may need to be addressed. Frequent practice, associated with high levels of reassurance and reinforcement, will be required. A detailed analysis of the requisite skills that must be taught during the hearing aid orientation is provided by Weinstein, along with a convenient chart describing hearing aid components, functions, and training strategies (45).

In most instances, at least one family member or daily caregiver should also attend the hearing aid orientation sessions. Not only will this ensure that information has been adequately communicated, but it will also guarantee that there is at least one other person in the client's environment who is knowledgeable about hearing aid operation and maintenance.

Relistening Training

Once a hearing aid has been selected and training in the appropriate use and maintenance of the aid has been provided, the real problems in hearing aid use begin. If a hearing aid is to be used successfully, the user must realize that signals amplified through an aid will not sound the same as they did through the natural ear. These new signals will neither be as clear nor as pleasant. The aid will sound noisy, and the quality of sound may be harsh and/or tinny. The point of these observations is that the hearing aid is not a perfect instrument. Unlike glasses, it will not perfectly compensate for a hearing loss.

This failure of the hearing aid to solve hearing problems immediately is one of the areas of greatest disappointment and frustration to both users of such aids and their families. The problems the client was experiencing before the hearing aid was selected will continue after the aid is fitted. The new user of a personal hearing aid must learn to listen all over again.

Relistening requires the hearing aid user to reacquaint himself with familiar environmental sounds and with the speech and vocal characteristics of the people around him. He must be able to redevelop the ability to discriminate among many sounds occurring simultaneously and/or in the presence of background noise.

Relistening skills are not easy to obtain and may require anywhere between 3 months to a year to acquire. Thus, the 30-day trial period provided with most new hearing aids is close to farcical, particularly with older clients. The audiologist's only hope is to provide the hearing impaired client with a clear understanding of the nature and length of the process of learning relistening skills, and with as many positive experiences as possible within the 30-day period. Hopefully, this combination of understanding of the process and success in early training will insure that the hearing aid user stays with the aid.

Some examples of relistening tasks are learning to identify sounds that are commonly heard in the home; listening to the voices of each family member and friend and learning to differentiate among them; and finally, learning to identify the message in various speech signals (37). It is important to systematically rebuild the auditory skills necessary for a variety of settings and background noise characteristics. Typically, tasks should be designed in a kind of hierarchy moving from the simple to the complex in various dimensions, including acoustic, linguistic, and situational. Recommendations should be made concerning optimum and maximum time limits for using the aid during the initial stages of adjustment. The client should also be counseled concerning selection of situations in which to use the hearing aid during the first days and weeks, as well as situations to avoid. Some older persons may require considerable assistance and structure in completing the process of relistening, and the support or direct participation of family members or caregivers may be necessary.

Auditory-Visual Communication Training

In addition to teaching the hearing aid user to relisten, it is also important to train the client in the use of visual cues in association with auditory information. Some authors have used the term auditory-visual communication to describe the fact that communication can always be enhanced by improving use of visual cues to supplement the speech message (17, 24, 45). Every one of us utilizes such cues on a daily basis. Visual cues are available from facial expressions, gestural movements and body postures, situational contexts, and articulatory movements. Communication efforts focused upon interpreting articulatory movements are commonly known as lip reading or speechreading.

Unfortunately, one of the greatest misconceptions individuals have about hearing loss pertains to the role of speechreading. Many believe that speechreading skills, if properly developed, can take the place of hearing in understanding speech. Certainly television shows and some theatrical productions have contributed to this myth. It is not uncommon for an older individual to spurn a hearing aid while expressing intense interest in enrolling in a lip reading class of some kind. In reality, such classes have been and continue to be offered with some regularity, although the focus of training procedures has shifted radically in recent years.

Before beginning any program of auditory-visual communication training, therefore, the client must be disabused of the notion that speechreading can substitute for hearing. This perception is simply not true; in fact, only about 13% of the movements associated with speech are actually visible on the lips. A few skillfully designed demonstrations or training activities may illustrate the point adequately.

This is not to say that speechreading cannot be a helpful adjunct to the hearing aid amplified listening skills of the older client. In fact, the combination of both visual and auditory cues of speech can greatly facilitate speech understanding in almost any listening situation. In this author's opinion, however, speechreading skills cannot be directly taught—at least not in the sense of teaching recognition of individual components of the speech message. In all probability, speechreading is a skill that all of us possess to some degree and frequently use, even if we are not hearing impaired. The hearing impaired individual, however, must rely more heavily on this skill than normal hearing persons. Thus speechreading (or visual communication) training should more appropriately be oriented to demonstrating to the hearing aid user the ways in which existing skills can be maximized.

This type of approach is more synthetic than analytic in nature (26). The synthetic approach to speechreading training emphasizes learning to utilize the redundancies available in both verbal and nonverbal messages and in the surrounding topical, personal, and environmental contexts. Use of redundancy allows the individual to predict the context and structure of new communications. Communication strategies and flexibility are emphasized. This type of approach has been shown to be effective in reducing perceptions of hearing handicap, increasing communicative effectiveness and self-assertiveness, and sometimes (but not always) increasing actual measured speechreading abilities (5).

COUNSELING

Pollack (33), among many others, has been a strong advocate for the inclusion of routine psychological counseling in the rehabilitation process for hearing impaired older adults. He emphasizes that counseling activities need to address both the provision of information and the production of affective or emotional change. The recent literature suggests that counseling preparation in graduate educational programs is less than adequate, at least with respect to the management of emotional responses (see Chapter 19 for more detail).

Nevertheless, the need for counseling with hearing impaired elderly clients and their significant others is evident. Hearing loss threatens the psychological integrity of the individual and demands some form of coping response, whether adaptive or maladaptive. Corso describes a typical ". . . chain of psychological reactions" (8, p 171) observed in older hearing impaired individuals. At first, there is a sense of personal frustration which creates stress and typically leads to a stress management strategy of social isolation. As the isolation continues, however, feelings of depression, insecurity, and suspiciousness develop. Paranoia, confusion, and loss of ego strength are described by others (2, 23, 37). Clearly, any developing patterns of emotional dysfunction, coupled with a worsening of daily communication patterns, will in turn create great stress for family members or caregivers in frequent contact with the hearing impaired older adult. A downwardly spiraling pattern of maladjustment may develop. The simple introduction of a hearing aid may not be sufficient to halt this process entirely.

Both hearing impaired older adults and their significant others typically have more than one of the following needs for:

1. Understanding of basic hearing processes and of the critical role hearing plays in daily communication;
2. Understanding of the ways in which age-related hearing loss affects both loudness and clarity;
3. Understanding of situations which create particular difficulty for the hearing impaired older adult;
4. Understanding of the emotional responses of the hearing impaired individual and of those in his/her immediate communication network;
5. Understanding of the proposed management program, its strengths and weaknesses, the demands that will be placed upon the client and significant other, and

the operation of amplification devices (noted above);

6. Understanding of appropriate environmental modifications;
7. Understanding of the role of nonauditory channels in communication (see above);
8. Understanding of communication strategies to facilitate interaction with the hearing impaired older adult;
9. Support and counseling with respect to emotional needs and frustrations;
10. Assistance in making necessary behavioral changes to improve or reestablish relationship patterns.

Many of these counseling needs have been addressed in other sections of this chapter. Throughout the period of training in use of the hearing aid, a great deal of counseling should be interjected into the process. The client must learn that no amplification system is going to solve all of his problems, although the majority can be solved or reduced if the amplification is used effectively. Setting up specific communication settings and having participants role play or problem solve solutions to the difficulties presented by such situations can be particularly helpful. The majority of my older clients have proved to be very clever in solving such problems. The fact that they can, in most situations, control a situation and improve their communication abilities may be the most important reality learned in the rehabilitation process.

If more intense or intractable emotional problems emerge throughout the course of early rehabilitation sessions, the audiologist should consider implementing more direct emotional counseling, either individually or in a group setting. The extent to which an outside professional (psychologist, family therapist, psychiatric social worker, etc.) is required must be determined by the audiologist based on his/her assessment of the individual's needs and situation and the audiologist's own skills.

Clients should also be made aware of the many consumer groups devoted to the hearing impaired. Groups such as Self-Help for Hard of Hearing People (Shhh) and Consumer Organization for the Hearing Impaired (COHI) were founded by hearing impaired individuals and work with various State and Federal agencies to help with the problems of the hearing impaired. Most publish a bulletin of some type which keeps hearing impaired individuals, their families, and professionals apprised of the latest improvements in amplification systems and in the laws protecting the hearing impaired. These organizations have reportedly been very

helpful to both older clients and to the audiologist working with this client base.

ADDITIONAL REHABILITATION CONSIDERATIONS

Some other factors related to hearing loss in general, or more specifically to hearing loss and the elderly, need to be considered in designing comprehensive rehabilitation programs. A few selected concerns are mentioned briefly in the following sections.

Public Education

Audiologists and speech-language pathologists must become more active in alerting the public-at-large as to the nature of hearing problems in the elderly and effective management strategies for coping with these problems. A particular target for public information efforts should be the older community. As with other age groups, older individuals tend to take hearing and communication for granted. The hearing impaired older person has not, however, been provided with the opportunities for adjustment to hearing impairment that are available to younger persons. Opportunities for discussing and adapting to the emotional and social problems created by hearing loss are limited. In fact, as noted earlier, hearing loss in the elderly tends to assume a highly negative associative connection with aging and senility. Thus, discussion of the subject may actually be taboo.

Since so much of the resistance to acknowledging hearing loss and using hearing aids on the part of older person is due to lack of information and/or misconceptions about hearing impairment and amplification, one approach to this problem would be to educate older adults *before* they need or seek help. While media specials and public service announcements may provide some information, a more comprehensive and systematic programming approach is needed. Such an approach, called Pre-Crisis Intervention, was developed by Shadden et al [37].

As described further in Chapter 19, Pre-Crisis Intervention proposes that information about the speech-language and hearing problems for which older persons are at risk be presented in a series of two to five workshops. In the sessions on hearing impairment, the types of hearing loss, problems created by the loss, hearing test procedures, and rehabilitative techniques and communication strategies are discussed. Hearing aids and assistive listening devices are available for participants to see and use. The myths and misconceptions associated with hearing loss are discussed and demonstrated. Information is provided through lecture, visual aids, and group training experiences. Printed materials summarizing workshop information are given to each participant.

The effectiveness of Pre-Crisis Intervention (PCI) workshops is evident in subsequent clinical interactions with workshop participants. All of the older clients who have come to our clinic after having attended a PCI workshop have become successful hearing aid users. They enter the clinical situation with good background information, realistic expectations regarding rehabilitation, and no resistance to the process. The information and attitudes they bring to the diagnostic and rehabilitative sessions makes counseling a joy. In fact, many of them begin to smile and nod their heads knowingly when material previously covered in a workshop is reviewed.

The workshops are also very helpful to those health care professionals working with older clients (see Chapter 22). Most of these individuals have had little or no background in hearing loss, yet they may be called on to help in the rehabilitation of their hearing impaired clients. The need for appropriate education is particularly true for those working in hospitals, nursing homes, convalescent centers, and retirement communities.

Financial Concerns

Many older persons are operating with considerably reduced and relatively fixed financial resources, compared to younger adults. Nevertheless, the cost of living continues to rise, and industry health care costs are escalating at an unbelievable rate. Thus, one factor limiting utilization of audiological services by the elderly may be financial. Older adults may be unwilling to undergo a full battery of tests, only to discover that the hearing aid being recommended is not within their budget.

Audiologists must be sensitive to these concerns and must be willing to become more active in exploring and spearheading alternate strategies for providing older community members with much-needed amplification. In particular, support from community agencies and institutions should be solicited. Possible sources for assistance include the various business service organizations, churches, youth groups, the American Association of Retired Persons (AARP) or similar organizations of retired individuals, Area Agencies on Aging, and a range of service agencies. Any or all of these may be willing to provide direct funds, purchase a hearing aid, or sponsor a client. Some organizations or individuals may also be willing to provide needed services, such as transportation, that will reduce the financial strain on an individual client. Hearing aid banks may be established, although mixed success has been reported with this strategy in the past. None of these resources can be tapped, however, without the audiologist's advocacy and commitment to provision of services to all interested older clients.

Environmental Issues

The best hearing aid and the finest program of aural rehabilitation will ultimately prove ineffective if the older client's environment presents sufficient barriers to communication interactions. The environment includes both the physical setting and the persons within those settings (10). While environmental issues are of concern in all settings, they warrant particular attention in institutional environments such as nursing homes. Physical barriers to listening and communication can be reduced by considering the following variables:

a. Lighting and visual cues—adequate and accessible windows, visual access to everyday activity areas, pleasing colors with appropriate contrasts, environmental color coding, adequate illumination without glare;

b. Acoustic treatment—of walls, floors, and ceilings, or consideration of assistive listening devices for particular rooms or favorite activities;

c. Furniture arrangements—moveable furniture, small conversational groupings for privacy or personal space, circular arrangements to maximize small group conversation;

d. Environmental props—making certain that personal items and assistive or orienting devices are readily accessible.

Speech-language pathologists and audiologists should be willing to assume an active role in identifying the communication opportunities available to our clients, determining communication barriers that may exist (whether they be physical or related to the attitudes and availability of conversational partners), and designing intervention plans that will systematically reduce these communication barriers. Input can be provided through other professionals working in a particular setting, through administrators, through family members, or through older clients themselves. While this type of consultation is not readily reimbursable, it is a critical ingredient in the rehabilitation process.

Miracle Cures

While the title of this section appears somewhat tongue-in-cheek, the topic to be considered is of serious concern. All individuals coping with disabling conditions of one form or another are prone to seek miracle solutions to their problems. Given the typical older person's lack of information about hearing loss and the media's unfortunate tendency to favor human interest stories featuring the dramatic resolution of a personal tragedy, it is not surprising that older adults can be surprisingly gullible concerning solutions to the problem of hearing impairment. Most audiologists have received numerous inquiries about new programs or technological advances reported in newspapers or on television. The majority of these reports are ill founded or, at best, relate to rehabilitation options not appropriate to the particular client's needs.

It is critical that the audiologist remain abreast of current professional developments (e.g., cochlear implants) as well as publicized stories and sales pitches related to hearing impairment. Most clients will accept an informed judgment (negative or positive) on the part of the professional. However, if they suspect that the "expert" knows little or nothing about the rehabilitation program or device of interest, they will remain unconvinced. More appropriate rehabilitation efforts will in turn be hampered by the client's unwillingness to give up the hope for that "miracle cure."

CONCLUSIONS

This chapter has reviewed some of the major problems in the rehabilitation of the hearing impaired elderly individual. Criteria for selection of an appropriate amplification system, whether a personal hearing aid or an assistive listening device, were discussed. The importance of follow-up training in the use of amplification was emphasized and procedures useful in this process were described. It was indicated that, to the extent possible, auditory-visual training should be introduced along with the amplification device(s). The importance of counseling was stressed, and some types of counseling activities were recommended.

The difficulty encountered in rehabilitating the older hearing impaired client makes it necessary to approach the management of this group with a realistic and informed point of view. Clearly, programming should be provided, and it should be as complete as possible, given the needs of the particular client. However, more clinical research is required in order to explore modifications of current intervention procedures that may better address the unique situation of the hearing impaired older person.

References

1. Alpiner JG: Audiologic problems of the aged. *Geriatrics* 18:19–26, 1963.
2. Alpiner JG: Rehabilitation of the geriatric patient. In Alpiner JG (ed): *Handbook of Adult Rehabilitative Audiology.* Baltimore, Williams & Wilkins, 1978, p 141.
3. Alpiner JG: Community aural rehabilitation programs. In Alpiner JG (ed): *Handbook of Adult Rehabilitative Audiology,* ed 2. Baltimore, Williams & Wilkins, 1982, p 238.
4. American Speech-Language-Hearing Association: Hearing aids: future prospects. *ASHA* 38:29–32, 1985.
5. Bate HL: Aural rehabilitation of the older adult. *Semin Hear* 6:193–204, 1985.
6. Berger KW, Millin JP: Hearing aids. In Rose DE (ed): *Audiological Assessment.* Englewood Cliffs, NJ, Prentice-Hall, 1971, p 471.
7. Carhart R: Tests for selection of hearing aids. *Laryngoscope* 56:780–794, 1946.
8. Corso JF: Auditory processes and aging: significant problems for research. *Exp Aging Res* 10:171–174, 1985.
9. Cox RM: Integrating the earmold in hearing aid selection. *Hear J* 35:7–10, 49, 1982.
10. Davis JM, Hardick EJ: Rehabilitation programs for adults. In Davis JM, Hardick EJ (eds): *Rehabilitative Audiology for Children and Adults.* New York, John Wiley, 1981, p 448.
11. Dodds E, Harford ER: A community hearing conservation program for senior citizens. *Ear Hear* 3:160–166, 1982.
12. Erdman SA, Sedge RK: Preferences for binaural amplification. *Hear J* 39:33–36, 1986.
13. Etienne JE, Naas JF: Factors influencing successful use of auditory amplification by the elderly. Presented at the American Speech-Language-Hearing Association Convention, Washington, DC, 1985.
14. Fellendorf GW: A model demonstration center of assistive devices for hearing-impaired people. *J Acad Rehab Audiol* 15:70–82, 1982.
15. Fellendorf GW: ALDS demonstration centers. *Hear Instr* 37:36–40, 1982.
16. Freeman BA, Sinclair S: Hearing aids for the elderly. In Beasley DS, Davis GA (eds): *Aging: Communication Processes and Disorders.* New York, Grune & Stratton, 1981, p 281.
17. Garstecki DC: Rehabilitation of hearing handicapped elderly adults. *Ear Hear* 3:167–172, 1982.

18. Garstecki DC, Marrer JL: Community/clinic management of hearing-impaired aging adults. Presented at the American Speech-Language-Hearing Association Convention, Washington, DC, 1985.

19. Hardick EJ: Aural rehabilitation programs for the aged can be successful. *J Acad Rehab Audiol* 10:51–67, 1977.

20. Hardick EJ, Lesner SA: The need for audiological rehabilitation. *J Acad Rehab Audiol* 12:21–29, 1979.

21. Harford ER: The use of a miniature microphone in the ear canal for the verification of hearing aid performance. *Ear Hear* 1:329–337, 1980.

22. Hawkins DB, Yacullo WS: Signal-to-noise ratio advantage of binaural hearing aids and directional microphones under different levels of reverberation. *J Speech Hear Disord* 49:278–286, 1984.

23. Hull RH: Assisting the elderly client. In Katz J (ed): *Handbook of Clinical Audiology*, ed 2. Baltimore, Williams & Wilkins, 1978, p 596.

24. Hull RH: Techniques of aural rehabilitation treatment for elderly clients. In Hull RH (ed): *Rehabilitative Audiology*. New York, Grune & Stratton, 1982, p 242.

25. Hull RH: Hearing aids for the older adult: considerations for fitting and dispensing. *Semin Hear* 6:181–191, 1985.

26. Jeffers J: Quality judgment in hearing aid selection. *J Speech Hear Disord* 25:259–266, 1960.

27. Mahan WJ: Assistive devices and systems: the market lifts off. *Hear J* 38:7–13, 1984.

28. Maurer JF, Rupp RR: *Hearing and Aging: Tactics for Intervention*. New York, Grune & Stratton, 1982.

29. Mueller HG: Binaural amplification: attitudinal factors. *Hear J* 39:7–10, 1986.

30. Nabelek AK, Pickett JM: Monaural and binaural speech perception through hearing aids under noise and reverberation with normal and hearing-impaired listeners. *J Speech Hear Res* 17:724–739, 1974.

31. Nelson RD: Providing hearing aid services to residents of nursing homes. *Hear Instr* 30:12–14, 1979.

32. Nunley J, Staab W, Steadman J, Wechsler P, Spenser B: A wearable digital hearing aid. *Hear J* 36:29–35, 1983.

33. Pollack MC: The remediation process: psychological and counseling aspects. In Alpiner JG (ed): *Handbook of Adult Rehabilitative Audiology*. Baltimore, Williams & Wilkins, 1978, p 121.

34. Rupp R, Higgins J, Maurer J: A feasibility scale for predicting hearing aid use (FSPHAU) with older individuals. *J Acad Rehabil Audiol* 10:81–104, 1977.

35. Rupp RR, Vaughn GR, Lightfoot RK: Nontraditional "aids" to hearing: assistive listening devices. *Geriatrics* 39:55, 1984.

36. Schwartz MS, Matsko TA: The need for audiological service in an urban population. Presented at the American Speech-Language-Hearing Association Convention, Los Angeles, 1981.

37. Shadden BB, Raiford CA, Shadden HS: *Coping with Communication Disorders in Aging*. Tigard, OR, C.C. Publications, 1983.

38. Smith CR, Fay TH: A program of auditory rehabilitation for aged persons in a chronic disease hospital. *ASHA* 19:417–420, 1977.

39. Staab WJ: Digital hearing aids. *Audiotone Tech Rep* 7:1–8, 1986.

40. Vaughn GR: Assistive listening devices and systems (ALDS) come of age. *Hear Instr* 37:12–16, 1986.

41. Vaughn GR: Now Hear This: a program about assistive listening devices and systems. Birmingham, AL, University of Alabama in Birmingham, School of Dentistry, 1982.

42. Walden BE, Schwartz DM, Williams DL, Holum-Hardegen LL, Crowley JM: Test of the assumptions underlying comparative hearing aid evaluations. *J Speech Hear Disord* 48:264–273, 1983.

43. Warren VG, Daily LB: Efficacy of aural rehabilitation with the geriatric hearing-impaired. *Hear J* 38:15–19, 1984.

44. Wayner DS: Assistive listening devices for improved communication and greater independence. *Hear Instr* 37:21–24, 1986.

45. Weinstein B: Management of the hearing impaired elderly. In Jacobs-Condit L (ed): *Gerontology and Communication Disorders*. Rockville, MD, American Speech-Language-Hearing Association, 1984, p 244.

46. Willeford JA: The geriatric patient. In Rose DE (ed): *Audiological Assessment*. Englewood Cliffs, NJ, Prentice-Hall, 1971, p 281.

15 Modifications in Speech-Language Assessment Procedures for the Older Adult

MICHAEL E. GROHER

Editor's Note

As with the preceding chapters on assessment and management of hearing impairment in the elderly, the next two chapters focus primarily on ways in which speech-language management procedures must be modified to accommodate to the special needs of the older population. Chapter 15 examines speech-language assessment techniques in some detail. Groher begins with the premise that a variety of medical and nonmedical contributing problems complicate the process of assessment and diagnosis in the older client. The importance of obtaining a thorough medical and social history is stressed, and specific data useful in evaluating communication disorders in elderly persons are identified. Techniques for gathering and utilizing history information are summarized. The remainder of Chapter 15 provides a step-by-step analysis of the assessment process as it must be adjusted to patterns of behavior and deficit in older clients. Consideration is given to the testing environment, procedures (e.g., response time variables), visual and auditory restrictions, fatigue, order of task presentation, and ethnic background. While formal speech-language tests are described briefly, Groher emphasizes assessment of functional communication through patient and family reports, completion of perceptual scales, and language sampling.

The goal in planned clinical assessment procedures is to obtain information that establishes a clear diagnosis. Ideally, the assessment delineates the causative factors, lending support to the validity of the diagnosis. From this diagnosis, prognostic statements are made, and a treatment plan is established. If the diagnosis is unclear or questionable, treatment can be delayed or misdirected. In the assessment of speech and language capacities of older persons, the communication specialist must be prepared to overcome obstacles particular to this population that often make it difficult to establish a definitive diagnosis. These obstacles include lengthy medical and social histories (often complicated by lack of information and misinformation); difficulty delineating the patient's complaint; and problems encountered in test selection, administration, and interpretation.

In general, older persons have multiple medical diagnoses that involve both sensory and motor systems, none of which may contribute directly to speech or language impairment. An example is the 75-year-old patient who presents with a history of multiple sub-cortical strokes, longstanding hypertension and diabetes, compromised vision, noise-induced hearing loss, use of multiple medications, and a family that complains he no longer remembers well. If impairment exists, the assessment may not uncover any one particular causative factor. In fact, there may not be one. Instead, these deficits can be explained as the result of the cumulative effects of motor and sensory loss that decompensate communication.

While the concept of cumulative effects leading to decompensation of communication competency is enticing, it can be equally misleading. The clinician often is biased by previous diagnoses that lead to the assumption that the patient's poor communication skills are a result of multiple past medical diagnoses when, in fact, the deficits are the product of new, as yet undiagnosed pathology. While attention to previous medical history is important, it should not be the sole guide to diagnosis, particularly if the previous history does not explain the patient's current complaints. Skillful test selection and interpretation will keep the clinician from overlooking undocumented pathology.

Nonmedical contributions to communication deficits also must be considered. Included are problems with psychosocial adjustment whose manifestations may include depression, social withdrawal and unwillingness to communicate, and a lack of interest in communicative interaction.

The clinician, therefore, will be faced with the task of preparing to uncover potential causes of deficit that emanate from a broad spectrum of medical and nonmedical factors. This suggests that the examiner must approach the evaluation prepared to assess the full range of behaviors that might impact on communication effectiveness. A comprehensive assessment plan must include a thorough review of the medical and social history; screening of end organ sensory and motor integrity for speech, vision, hearing, and respiration; a psychometric and pragmatic evaluation of language; attention to cognitive deficits such as perception and memory; and an analysis of the strength of the patient's psychosocial adjustments. The task for the examiner is to identify which elements contribute to communication deficits and to determine the strength of their impact.

PREPARATION FOR THE EVALUATION

The Medical History

Referrals for a communication evaluation come from a variety of sources such as family members, public health workers, physicians, nurses, social workers, dietitians, and program volunteers. Frequently, the accompanying reason for referral is vague. The clinician will be faced with statements like "The patient doesn't talk anymore" or "She has difficulty understanding what you say." Requests rarely come with a good medical and social history that is appropriate to communication. Contact by phone with the referring source can help clarify the need for evaluation.

When possible, the clinician should make an attempt to secure complete medical records before the evaluation. Ideally, if previously ordered consultations (particularly those involving the specialties of audiology, neurology, otolaryngology, and ophthalmology) are completed, the evaluation process will be facilitated. The written report of these consultations is preferable to anecdotal accounts, as the patient and/or family may not be able to summarize results in sufficient detail.

A complete history is important for two reasons. First, it should assist the communication specialist in deciding which psychometric or physiologic test(s) may be most appropriate initially to utilize in assessment. For instance, if the patient complains of difficulty understanding what he hears, and there is no apparent history of stroke, brain damage, or other mental changes, a thorough hearing evaluation may preclude the need for further testing. Second, a good medical and social history may provide the only data which the communication specialist is able to gather before planning a treatment program. The reality is that due to severe communication and/or behavior disabilities, some older persons are untestable by standardized procedures. In such instances, the history becomes vitally important in establishing a treatment plan. In geriatric medical clinics, the majority of clinical diagnoses are based solely on this history (45).

Many times the nature of a communication deficit will rule out taking a history from the elderly candidate for evaluation. However, if the clinician's early impressions suggest the patient will be able to provide background information, the interview should proceed in this direction. The clinician should be guided by listening not only to what the patient says but also to what he does not or may not be able to say (48).

The most important requirement in the initial interview with elderly persons is that it not be one-sided (40). The communication specialist should not begin by asking the patient a series of questions in an attempt to fill the blanks in the medical and social history. Instead, the examiner should initiate the process by explaining the need for evaluation and the importance of gathering more information in order to understand the nature of the problem. During the interview it is important to review and summarize the historical data as it is gathered as part of the clinician-patient interaction (40). Such give-and-take minimizes the anxiety which new people and situations may create, especially in elderly persons (2). Reducing anxiety will assist in obtaining an accurate history and will help make the transition into the formal assessment less threatening.

After the history is completed, an explanation of the plan for formal assessment should be reviewed with the patient. Ample time for questions should be allowed. If the clinician suspects distrust or anxiety from the patient, a review of the need for assessment, with the clinician proposing hypothetical questions, is appropriate. It is not uncommon for older patients to disagree about the severity of their problem or need for evaluation (11). Time for explanation and questions will establish the necessary rapport essential to assessment and treatment.

It is vital that the clinician attempt to delineate the patient's complaint. Evidence suggests that some elderly persons belittle illness and will not complain or give an accurate account of disability (6). Using a large sample, Hale and associates (20) found that elderly persons were willing to identify major complaints when provided with a questionnaire that listed common medical problems. This suggests that, when given choices of pathology, older persons may be better able to describe their complaints. We have found this method to be useful in our clinic in the patient interview. Rather than ask the patient about his hearing acuity or comprehension skills, we provide him with choices from familiar situations, such as "Is it more difficult to hear the news?" or "Is it harder to remember what you read in the newspaper?" or "Is it harder to follow a conversation with your friends?" In this way, the clinician can focus more on what the symptoms mean to the patient rather than on the cause of the problem.

The patient's complaint should always be compared with the referring person's need for evaluation. Noted discrepancies can help guide the evaluation. Sometimes the causative factor is the same, but the behavioral manifestations are interpreted differently by patient and family. However, differences between how the pathology affects the patient and how it impacts on the family provide useful information in planning assessment strategies.

In selected patients it is advisable for a friend or family member to be present to provide historical data. However, one should not always conclude that the family's description is more accurate than the patient's complaints. There is evidence to suggest that family members of aphasic patient's are reliable reporters of communication disability (21), although Gurland and co-workers did not feel that the evidence supported this reliability (19). Research controversy regarding the accuracy of family perceptions of speech-language disorders has yet to be resolved (16, 17, 32, 50, 54).

If a family member is providing historical data, it is preferable that this is done in the patient's presence to reduce any feelings of anxiety or rejection about being included. It is important that the clinician not allow the patient and the informant to engage in confrontational patterns such as the "You have a hearing loss"— "No, I don't" pattern. These confrontations only serve to raise anxiety levels, reducing the reliability of the assessment. If the clinician has a previous history suggesting the patient adamantly denies any communication difficulties, it may be most prudent to obtain background data from a friend or family member prior to the patient's clinic appointment.

A variety of preinterview history forms have been provided by clinicians (7, 15). Table 15.1 presents a summary of medical and social data appropriate for the evaluation of communication disorders in elderly persons. It is designed to assist the clinician in identifying important clues to etiology which will aid in designing the assessment protocol. The order in which the data are gathered will depend upon the patient and the examiner. One may choose to begin with Section II because it appears most relevant to the patient and may set a positive and nonthreatening tone for the entire assessment.

Most of the items contained in Table 15.1 are self-explanatory; however, a few portions require amplification. Determination of any behavioral changes (I.3) such as increased anxiety, excessive fatigue, poor self-care skills, or rapid mood changes, can provide helpful information in planning assessment strategies. In some cases, behavioral manifestations such as these may be early signs of neurologic disease (36) or of improper use of medications (25). History of arthritis (I.4) can interfere with formalized testing which may require pointing, arm raising, or the manipulation of test objects. Because diabetes (I.5) can affect the body's neurochemical balance, it may account for fluctuations in communication behavior if not properly controlled. Diabetes can also cause visual loss which may play a role in reducing communication effectiveness. The topic of surgical history (I.8) should particularly emphasize questions which pertain to any surgical procedures relating to the auditory, articulatory, phonatory, respiratory, and neurological systems.

The suspected presence of hearing loss (I.11) should be followed by questions related to history of noise exposure, family history of hearing disorders, tinnitus, and complaints of excessive cerumen or ear drainage. Ascertain if the hearing loss has been properly evaluated and what treatment was prescribed. If the patient wears a hearing aid, the examiner needs to know if the patient makes good use of the aid, if the earmold fits properly, and if the patient is able to successfully change batteries and manipulate the controls. Questions specific to vision (I.12) should include inquiries into glaucoma, cataracts, presbyopia, and any visual changes following stroke. Some problems such as glaucoma are not easily recognized by the patient. Behaviors such as increased need for isolation, more dependency, facing away from direct light, and avoidance of close work may be signs of static or progressive visual loss and need to be fully evaluated. Muscle weakness (I.13) and questions relating to ambulation (I.14) may serve

Table 15.1
Suggested Case History Format for Elderly Persons with Communication Deficits

Name:

Chief complaint

Onset of problem:

Date:

Informant:

Section I: Medical History

1. Stroke
2. Trauma
3. Behaviorial changes/
   characteristics
4. Arthritis
5. Diabetes
6. Memory loss
7. Respiratory disease
8. Surgical procedures
9. Vocal changes

10. Swallowing disorders
11. Hearing loss
12. Visual loss
13. Muscle weakness
14. Ambulation
15. Alcohol abuse
16. Medications
17. Nutrition
18. Other medical

Section II: Current Communication Status

1. Communicates basic needs
2. Word-finding difficulty in
   conversation
3. Loses thought/rambles/talks off
   the topic
4. No longer corresponds
5. No longer reads
6. Loss of vocabulary
7. Word-finding difficulty during
   specific verbal or written
   requests
8. Problems with orientation

9. Utilizes communicative
   strengths if deficits
   have been previously
   identified
10. Communication settings
    a. Phone
    b. In TV room
    c. Time of day
    d. Particular activity
    e. Particular people
    f. Shopping/ordering

Section III: Related Psychosocial

1. Verbal inclinations
2. Communication needs
3. Depression/withdrawal
4. Living arrangement
5. Family/friend interaction

6. Communication style of
   family/friend
7. Occupation
8. Education
9. Ethnic background
10. Special interests

to confirm previous central nervous system involvement, or may be a signal of undiagnosed pathology. History of alcohol abuse (I.15) may be an etiological factor in memory loss and behavioral changes (11), both of which can lead to a reduction of communication abilities. It is important that the clinician obtain a list of current medication and establish if they are being taken in the prescribed fashion (I.16), as noted in Chapter 7. Medication toxicity, especially from tranquilizers and sedatives frequently taken by elderly persons, can lead to mental confusion by altering autonomic nervous system functioning (35). Poor nutrition (I.17) can cause fluctuations in central nervous system function.

Section II is designed to explore behavioral and social communication deficits in situation-specific instances. The elderly person may not always recognize a specific communication disorder; however, one may surface if specific contexts, persons, or situations are offered. Felix (14) has developed the *Subjective Communication Report*, which is an attempt to obtain a communication history with a yes/no format. The patient can fill out the form, or the examiner can read it aloud. The patient answers items such as "I understand better when people speak slowly," "I must read information 2 or 3 times to get the gist of it," "I sometimes miss the jokes," "I am slower in math problems," "I used to be a good speller," and "I used to talk more." Such items are helpful for the clinician, especially when the patient denies or is unaware of any communication impairment. It is important to compare the patient's response to items II.2 (word-finding difficulty in conversation) and II.7 (word-finding difficulty during specific verbal or writing requests), since elderly persons with defective vocabulary skills will have more difficulty in situations involving specific requests or use of words (37). Simulating these conditions in assessment may uncover deficits that can be managed.

Section III is an outline of some psychosocial phenomena which may be related to the communicative process. Many of these behaviors can be probed informally during the interview, although a variety of checklists and questionnaires can be found in the clinical literature. Available instruments may examine patterns of family interaction (15), coping/compliance behaviors (15), and communicative status (7).

It is important to assess the patient's verbal inclinations (III.1). Was the patient always verbose and now does not talk much, or was he never a talker? Eisenson (13) points out that knowledge of the patient's verbal inclinations or his propensity for the use of words assists the clinician in understanding the patient's motivation for relearning language. Tied closely with verbal inclinations are the patient's communication needs (III.2), family or friend interactions (III.5), and current living arrangements (III.4). Some patients do not communicate because they have no one with whom to interact. Exploration of the communication style of family members or friends (III.6) should help to reveal the quality of interactions and whether or not others understand how to compensate for the patient's deficits. Asking about prior or present occupational status (III.7) and/or special interests or hobbies (III.10) often encourages the elderly patient to talk about himself, especially if the examiner is quick to show an interest. Linguistic analysis of this conversation may be used in the assessment. Sometimes the patient may report a loss of interest in stamp collecting or knitting, both of which could signal early visual loss. They may report that their attendance at club or group meetings has declined because it is difficult to hear or understand the speaker. The examiner should establish an educational history (III.8), especially when the assessment protocol includes interpretation of test results which measure reading and writing competence. And finally, the clinician should explore the possible effects on communication skills that arise from ethnic influences (III.9).

This history form only provides some direction concerning areas which are important in assessing the communication status of elderly persons. If the clinician is interested in broadening the scope of the medical and social history, it is suggested that the one proposed by Das and associates (10) be considered. It is specifically designed for the assessment, treatment, and follow-up of elderly persons who require medical intervention.

Summarizing the History

After the medical and social communication history has been obtained, it is important for the communication specialist to summarize the information obtained *with* the patient as a method of verification and as a tool for reducing testing anxiety. At this point, the examiner should be able to formulate an idea of what types of test measures might be utilized in the evaluation and how long the evaluation may take. Discussing the rudiments of the testing procedure and the approximate time of the evaluation process aids in the overall reduction of fear that anticipation of psychometric testing creates in many older persons (2, 3).

After the medical and social history is complete, the communication specialist may feel that the patient should be evaluated by other health disciplines before the communication evaluation continues. For instance, if the patient's primary complaint centers around vocal changes which are affecting communication, it would be appropriate to consult a laryngologist before the completion of the evaluation. If the initial impression of the examiner reveals that the patient's communication problems are related to changes in vision, an ophthalmology referral is appropriate. In other words, it is essential that the communication specialist rule out any end organ or peripheral disease before completing an extensive psychometric test battery. Comprehensive knowledge of the scope and nature of such diseases will assist the examiner in test selection and interpretation. Because the communication specialist may be the first one in the health care systems to evaluate the patient, it is necessary to have a thorough knowledge of these referral sources.

THE ASSESSMENT

The Preparation

Before the patient comes for the evaluation, it is necessary to make phone contact to remind the patient to bring any sensory aids such as glasses, magnifiers, dentures, or hearing aids. Trying to assess reading skills while the patient is complaining he cannot see the type defeats the purpose of the evaluation and may create enough frustration that the patient decides not to continue.

The cardinal rule in testing and treating elderly persons is to remember that each segment of the test battery should receive a short explanation relative to its intended purpose. After reviewing a number of studies, Botwinick (3) concluded that the older person's motivation to complete a task improves if he/she understands its meaningfulness.

Screening Peripheral Systems

The evaluation should begin by examining the primary peripheral speech and language input and output systems, including the oral speech mechanism, hearing, and vision. Knowledge that a sensorineural hearing loss may interfere with tests of language comprehension, or that muscle weakness in the oral mechanism may interfere with expressive language tasks, is important in interpreting test results.

All elderly persons who come to the communication specialist with complaints of communication deficits should receive a complete hearing evaluation, including speech audiometry and tympanometry. The audiometric evaluation should be preceded by an inspection of the external auditory meatus. Accumulation of cerumen is a frequent occurrence in older persons and should be removed before hearing is evaluated.

The oral peripheral speech mechanism evaluation is administered in the standard fashion with one exception. Frequently, elderly persons who wear dentures may prefer to remove them before the oral examination. If they are loose or become bothersome during the examination, the clinician should suggest that they be removed. Any embarrassment related to removal can be avoided with a matter-of-fact attitude on the clinician's part and a ready supply of sterile gauze for the patient's convenience.

If the medical or social history suggests that the patient may be experiencing difficulty with visual acuity that has not been corrected, an acuity screening before formal testing is necessary. Peripheral visual screening can be performed easily by the communication specialist, utilizing standardized materials at prescribed distances. If a problem exists, formalized testing by an eye specialist should be completed before continuing with the communication evaluation.

The Testing Environment

The communication specialist should choose a room that has proper acoustic damping characteristics to eliminate any ambient noise distraction. The room size should allow ample space for the clinician, patient, and test materials. Entry doors should be wide enough for wheelchairs. Lighting fixtures should include dimmer switches so that illumination adjustments can be made to accommodate visual loss.

A frequent accompaniment of aging, in addition to loss of visual accommodation, is the yellowing of the lens, acting to reduce light perception at the retina (9). Lens yellowing also may result in difficulty with blue/green discrimination because blues become absorbed by the yellow lens (9). Therefore, the testing table or table covering should be red, orange, or yellow, allowing test objects to be more easily perceived when placed on the table surface.

Strong lighting onto an absorbent surface reduces glare and helps to focus the light for better vision. Glare can further be reduced by ensuring that the patient is seated with his back toward any windows. Patients with cataracts will have difficulty with bright light because the cataract acts to diffuse illumination, creating a reduction in light perception and vision. Such patients will benefit most from dim, nondirect lighting during the evaluation. Use of the dimmer switch is invaluable in this circumstance.

Testing Procedure

Time Variables

The most prominent variable affecting test performance in older persons is time. The evidence suggests that reduction of presentation rates alone can have significant effects on the performance during testing (55).

Studies have shown that older persons perform better when there are no time constraints (3), respond more slowly under test conditions because they value accuracy over speed (28), reduce response speed when task uncertainty increases (3), perform more slowly as the number of response choices increases (3), take longer on tasks which demand rapid shifts of response behaviors (4), and have initial stimulus traces which persist long enough to blur the following stimulus, resulting in slower response times (1). On language-specific tasks, the elderly perform more accurately on auditory comprehension tasks if rate of presentation is reduced regardless of grammatical or semantic complexity (55). Older persons display a broader vocabulary in conditions of relaxation (38), and retrieve words more efficiently if the stimulus material deals with past events and objects more familiar to their generation (42).

There is physiological evidence to substantiate these observations. Older persons may take longer to respond because their brain at rest is not as attentive to incoming stimuli (31, 41). Additionally, restrictions in blood supply and poor cell absorption commonly seen in the elderly prolong recovery times (52), and a reduction of brain cells reduces the initial strength of the signal (27).

The behavioral and physiological evidence suggests that the clinician should consider adopting the following assessment modifications, when appropriate:

(1) Before each testing task, the clinician should allow ample time for instructions and time between the termination of instructions and the beginning of the task.
(2) The instructions should be given slowly, repeated or rephrased if necessary at a comfortable volume, and should be presented close enough to the patient so that he can take advantage of any visual cues.
(3) The clinician should directly relate the intent of the test to the importance of the evaluation.
(4) Ample time should be allowed between subtests to indicate that one portion has ended and a new one is now beginning.
(5) Time should be allowed for questions or comments before beginning a new subtest.
(6) Up to 10 seconds per response should be allowed before repeating test instructions.
(7) Demonstration and practice on some items should be permitted if instructions are not understood.

Because the older person's performance usually is improved if time is manipulated in his favor, it becomes an important variable for the communication specialist to control. Since effective communication depends heavily on the time it takes to decode a message and encode a response, slowing of this process may interfere with normal communicative exchanges. If this is the presenting complaint, it may be necessary to provide strict time restraints by eliminating redundancy of instructions, not allowing additional time between subtests, eliminating transitions within subtests, and curtailing repetition of test instructions. Comparison of performance with and without these time controls can yield critical assessment data.

It is important to strive to finish the majority of the evaluation in one session, as it may be difficult for the elderly person to return for immediate follow-up because of transportation and/or mobility difficulty. In fact, transportation and/or mobility problems may prohibit the elderly person with a communication disorder from coming to an outpatient clinic. The com-

munication specialist should therefore be prepared to make a home visit. A visit may require the use of a portable audiometer and some streamlining of psychometric testing materials for easy handling. Home visits can be very beneficial because the communication specialist can take note of special conditions in the environment that may provide clues to the patient's communication successes or failures.

Vision

Many psychometric tests commonly in use depend heavily on the use of visual input systems to assess auditory and graphic language skills. Because of the large prevalence of visual disorders among the elderly, it is essential to help the patient compensate maximally for any visual loss which may confound testing results. The importance of proper lighting already has been stressed. In addition, if the clinician is testing reading skills, she should be prepared to utilize materials with large print. Patients with specific left or right visual field defects should have objects placed in front of them on the side which will assist them in compensating for their visual loss. In patients with severe visual defects who report difficulty finding words in conversation, it will be necessary to assess naming skills by use of the tactile sensory system.

Fatigue

The problem of fatigue and its effect on the reliability of test results is a factor involved in testing all age groups, particularly elderly persons. Fatigue can come from a number of sources, many of which are not mutually exclusive. First, the total time spent sitting in one place creates a sense of boredom and fatigue. If the task is too hard or troublesome, motivation dwindles and fatigue approaches. Sleep disturbances and medications whose side effects create drowsiness, both of which are common in the elderly, can have adverse effects on test performance. Other common ailments such as arthritis preclude lengthy examination sessions.

Experience suggests that the length of time for the entire communication evaluation, including the interview and a hearing test, should not exceed 90 minutes. If more time is necessary, an explanation should be given to the patient, and another appointment should be scheduled. If the history so suggests, two 45-minute evaluations can be scheduled initially. However, patients with a history of noncooperation should be assessed in one visit.

If possible the communication evaluation

should be scheduled in the morning hours. Short rest breaks between tests may be appropriate with some patients, although they will lengthen the total testing time. Test tasks should be arranged so that there are noticeable differences between the objectives of each task. This arrangement will serve to maintain the patient's interest, minimizing the effects of fatigue. For instance, if the examiner is testing writing skills, it may be best to have the patient copy words in one portion of the testing session, to write phrases in another, and to construct a paragraph in another, rather than placing all of these tasks into one section.

Presentation

The optimum order of presentation of test items remains controversial. Should more difficult tasks come first or last in the assessment? If they are placed last in the session, fatigue and frustration might confound the test results. If they are first, the patient may become overwhelmed and have little motivation to complete the test battery. Experience testing older patients suggests that beginning with easier tasks helps build confidence in the examiner and raises motivational levels because of the chance for immediate success. Mixing harder tasks with easier tasks throughout the testing period allows for the greatest flexibility, keeping motivation high and fatigue low. If the patient becomes frustrated with a more difficult task, follow with one which predictably will bring success. Skill at test selection is based partly on the historical data and on the clinician's perception of the patient's ongoing performance.

Ethnic Background

If the clinician has ascertained from the medical and social history that ethnic background may affect the communication assessment, it will be necessary to present some test items in the patient's native tongue. Statistics suggest that this possibility in the current generation of elderly persons over 65 will be higher than in future generations (5).

SELECTING TEST MEASURES

The most productive assessment of communication in older persons is the one that samples a broad spectrum of information in a short period of time without putting undo pressure on the patient to perform quickly. While this approach suggests use of multiple screening materials that ideally are high in predictive

capability, some evaluations will focus on the administration of one or two test batteries that yield a more specific and detailed analysis of a particular aspect of communicative competence. Most often, the history will dictate the approach. Some patients come with previous data obtained from screening measures. Review of these results may suggest more detailed analyses of areas of deficit or verification of modality strengths. Patients with a history of left cortical pathology often are candidates for standardized aphasia batteries. Those with right hemisphere damage may benefit from specific measures of their perceptual skills together with a pragmatic analysis of linguistic performance. Patients suspected of diffuse involvement (cognitive and language) should receive shorter screening measures in an effort to determine the most salient features contributing to their deficits.

Preparation will be needed to select tests that have the flexibility to measure linguistic input and output through a variety of cognitive channels. For instance, some patients will comprehend single words or phrases better if accompanied by gesture rather than by audition alone. Others may have difficulty responding to confrontational tasks, but may do well in casual conversation on a familiar topic. Observed discrepancies in these two circumstances, however, can provide useful data in planning management strategies and in family counseling. Detecting the patient's input and output strengths by selecting appropriate measures before and during the evaluation will assist the clinician by providing the best estimate of communication efficiency.

Communication Efficiency

Communication efficiency is operationally defined as the success a patient has in solving life's everyday problems. Our success depends on the quality of the relationship between the person and their changing environment. This relationship might involve writing, pointing, emotional utterances or head nods, and single words and phrases, alone or in combination, depending on the context. The efficiency of the patient's communication interaction with the environment can be misperceived by patient and family. The clinician must strive to gather data that will clarify either over- or underestimation of the patient's communication skills. For these reasons, some investigators (8, 33) have argued for the need to gather data relative to communication efficiency from the patient's own environment, considering settings and situations that are part of their daily routine. If such an approach becomes the focus of the evaluation, the clinician may need to teach family members or other health care providers how to observe and record data pertinent to the patient's communication efficiency. As attractive as this concept seems, it can be time consuming and unwieldy unless the clinician is employed in the environment, such as in a long-term care facility. Further, the validity of the data collected by family members or inexperienced clinicians is questionable.

Therefore, the clinician must make an attempt to sample the patient's communication efficiency in the clinic. Most standardized adult language test batteries do not place the patient and clinician in situations that simulate "real world" communication changes, although the Communicative Abilities of Daily Living (22) is a test battery that attempts to fill this gap. While some protocols are available for analysis of observational data obtained in the clinical setting (7, 15), one of the best measures is an analysis of a language sample taken from communicative exchanges between patient and clinician or patient and family member.

The Language Sample

Obtaining the Language Sample

How one elicits the sample is crucial to the quality of response the patient is capable of or chooses to give. The patient must be motivated sufficiently in an exchange that is not one-sided. Experience suggests that asking the patient to describe or react to pictures or photographs (Fig. 15.1) that recall past historical events serves to motivate and relax the patient. While not all patients will recognize Wendell Willkie (which in itself serves to stimulate conversation), his name and novel political career immediately enlist their interest, recalling stories of the historical Roosevelt era and the calamity of World War II. Photographs can be

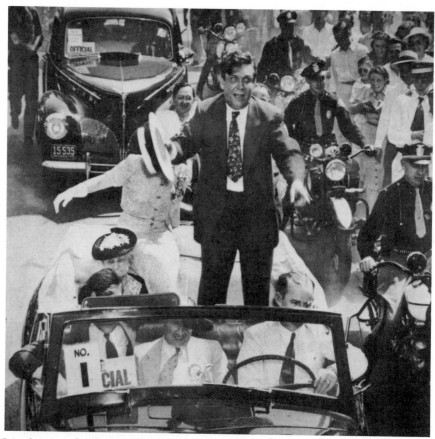

Figure 15.1 An example of a photograph used to elicit a language sample. The historical significance and the time in which it took place provide the interest needed to sustain conversation. From Scherman DE: *The Best of Life.* Time-Life Books, 1973, p 13. Reproduced with permission of Wide World Photos.)

preselected consistent with the patient's known interests or occupation. For instance, a picture of a 1940s Detroit assembly line worker will help elicit active conversation from a former auto worker. These stimuli can be used not only as elicitors of language but also as screening devices of visual perception (by asking the patient to attend to specific parts of the photograph), or as a confrontational naming or descriptive task (focusing the discussion on specific elements). Samples elicited from nonspecific naming or description tasks, and from more abstract requests for specificity, are compared for qualitative differences. Ideally the sample should contain a 10-minute conversation.

Analyzing the Language Sample

Traditionally, the communication specialist will focus on an analysis of the syntactic and semantic elements of language, the grammar and meaning in receptive and expressive linguistic tasks. While this approach is useful, it should be accompanied by an analysis of the pragmatic aspects in communicative exchange. In pragmatic analysis, the focus is away from the phrase or sentence toward communicative intentions and interactions. The analysis centers on how well the speaker and listener conveyed their intentions, the modalities used, the time taken, the redundancy, the number of utterances needed, emotional involvement, pause time, facial expressions, and body language. Even though there are limited normative data available on the pragmatic aspects of language in older persons, use of the pragmatic analysis is an excellent barometer of communication efficiency.

Hutchinson and Jensen (23) have suggested a systematic approach to pragmatic analysis. The analysis is completed in three parts: tabulation of utterances, analysis of the speech act, and topic control. The tabulation of utterances includes a numerical count of utterances, number of turns taken during the exchange, and the number of utterances per turn. The speech act, defined as the speaker's intent exclusive of syntax, is a tabulation of the number of representatives (assertions), directives (requests), expressives (how one feels), and commissives (commitments the speaker makes to a future course of action) contained within the sample. Topic control is a tabulation from the sample of the number of topics initiated, the number of utterances on the same topic, the number of times the patient continues on the clinician's topic, and the number of utterances not related to the topic. While there are no established norms for these tabulations, the categories represented reflect a sensitivity to the accumulation of experimental evidence that has begun to identify relevant parameters in the diagnosis of communication disorders in older persons, particularly in the differentiation between dementia and normal aging (39).

Formal Tests of Language

Since it is important to minimize the effects of fatigue and boredom in the assessment of older persons, shorter testing instruments with normative or predictive data are preferable. Two well-recognized standardized aphasia batteries have been shortened: the *Minnesota Test for the Differential Diagnosis of Aphasia* (MTDDA) (47) and the *Porch Index of Communicative Ability* (PICA) (43). Both shortened versions have been shown to have high correlations with their longer counterparts (12, 44). Subtests from the MTDDA are useful for their comprehensive approach, while the PICA possesses predictive data and norms for patients with bilateral disease. Holland (22) developed the *Communicative Activities in Daily Living* (CADL) battery in an attempt to provide a formal aphasia assessment tool that samples real-life communication situations. It contains normative data, accounting for aspects of institutionalization. Another useful measure that is administered easily and samples a wide range of linguistic behaviors is the *Aphasia Language Performance Scales* (ALPS) (26). Two measures of auditory comprehension particularly suited to the elderly because of administrative ease, novelty, and gestural response mode are the *Auditory Comprehension Test for Sentences* (49) and the *Functional Auditory Comprehension Task* (29). Most useful for a detailed analysis of reading skills is the *Reading Comprehension Battery for Aphasia* (30). Formal assessment of naming skills can be accomplished with the *Boston Naming Test* (24). Patients with persistent anomia often become frustrated on this test because of the length, and the clinician may find it more productive to assess naming in a less formal manner. Frustration can be minimized if the cues prescribed in the testing format are given promptly in an effort to reduce the patient's struggle behavior.

Because the evaluation of communication in older persons often is directed toward obtaining the best description of communicative ability rather than toward strict adherence to standardized measures and procedures, clinicians find it useful to select subtests from longer, standardized measures. Used in combination, they can be effective in sampling specific deficits noted during the evaluation. For instance, use of the repetition and complex ideation subtests of the Boston Diagnostic Aphasia Examination (BDAE) (18) and the paragraph reading and calculation subtests of the MTDDA (47) provides selective information. The "cookie theft" picture from the BDAE and items from the parietal lobe battery are used routinely as screening devices of language and perception.

Nonformal or Indirect Tests of Language

These measures are utilized in circumstances where the patient is either unwilling or unable to cooperate with standard psychometric test formats. The best known example of an informal assessment tool is the *Functional Communication Profile,* or *FCP* (46). Not requiring the patient's cooperation, the *FCP* rates the patient on 45 examples taken from daily communication situations. As an alternative instrument, Felix (14) has developed the *Subjective Communication Report.* Composed of a series of questions in yes/no format, the patient or family member can respond after hearing or reading each statement. Another informal measure of communication efficiency particularly suited for use with elderly persons was developed by Swindell and associates (53). Designed primarily as a prognostic tool, it also provides a systematic approach to gathering data about a person's communication skills without enlisting the patient's cooperation. Divided into three sections, background information, personal style (15 items), and communicative style (35 items), it asks the informant to rate personal style on a scale from 1 to 5. Rating communicative style requires either positive or negative responses to declarative sentences that sample functional communication skills such as "... can usually tell how *others* feel by *their* facial expressions," "... uses 'demonstrating gestures' to help explain something," and "... is a good joke and story teller." Section II, Personal Style, is an attempt to assess the patient's psychosocial and emotional behaviors as they might impact on communication. Examples include "is easily influenced," "expects the worst," "lacks confidence," and "can see only one solution to a problem."

CONCLUSIONS

The assessment of the communicative skills of older persons should be biased toward efficiency. Treatable and nontreatable causa-

tive factors that precipitate deficiency need to be identified. Clear identification can be difficult. Deficits may be the result of multiple factors contributing collectively to decompensate communicative efficiency. A thorough review of the patient's medical and psychosocial history and complete attention to the patient's and the family's explanation of the problem will facilitate diagnosis and will guide the approach and direction in assessment. Differentiation between specific communication disorders and communication deficits secondary to normal aging is essential.

Older persons benefit from an evaluation that begins with an explanation of its intended purpose and format. Instruction review of each subtest with liberal time allowance for questions or necessary demonstration will minimize fatigue and anxiety. The test environment should compensate for sensory or motor loss, because evaluation of cortical integrity might be invalidated due to peripheral disease. Test selection is predicated on the presenting complaint and/or prior historical data. Numerous test measures, both screening and formalized, are available for use, some of which do not require the patient's total cooperation. Elicitation of a language sample in an effort to establish the patient's level of communication efficiency is particularly valuable. Conventional analyses of syntactic and semantic content of the sample, as well as analyses of the pragmatic elements during conversational exchanges, are important.

Research efforts should be directed toward an understanding of those elements of language production and reception that are secondary to normal aging, in contrast with those that may be associated with a pathological process. Delineation of the specific aspects of syntax, semantics, and pragmatics during conversation that are validated as predictors of abnormality in communication efficiency is needed. Research data need to be adjusted for age, premorbid intelligence, and institutionalization. Assessment batteries specific to the communication evaluation of older persons must be developed. Some experimental protocols are already available commercially (34, 51). If these batteries provide a sufficiently high degree of sensitivity to deficiency, they could eventually prove useful in identifying early, abnormal changes in communication that may be amenable to treatment as part of a program of prevention of further deterioration.

References

1. Axelrod S, Eisdorfer C: Senescence and figural effects in two modalities. *J Genet Psychol* 100:85–91, 1962.

2. Blazer D: Techniques for communication with your elderly patient. *Geriatrics* 11:79–84, 1978.
3. Botwinick J: *Aging and Behavior*. New York, Springer, 1973.
4. Brinley JF: Cognitive sets and accuracy of performance in the elderly. In Welford AT, Birren JE (eds): *Behavior, Aging and the Nervous System*. Springfield, IL, Charles C Thomas, 1965.
5. Bureau of the Census, Washington, DC, March 1975.
6. Burnside IM: *Nursing and the Aged*. New York, McGraw-Hill, 1976.
7. Chapey R: The assessment of language disorders in adults. In Chapey R (ed): *Language Intervention Strategies in Adult Aphasia*, ed 2. Baltimore, Williams & Wilkins, 1986, p 81.
8. Chwat S, Gurland GB: Comparative family perspectives on aphasia: diagnostic, treatment, and counseling implications. In Brookshire R (ed): *Clinical Aphasiology Conference Proceedings*. Minneapolis, B.R.K. Publishers, 1981, p 212.
9. Corso JF: Sensory processes and age effects in normal adults. *J Gerontol* 26:90–103, 1971.
10. Das SK, Anderson J, Kataria MS: Geriatric medicine: model for computer oriented research analysis. *J Am Geriatr Soc* 27:27–33, 1979.
11. Davis GA, Holland AL: Age in understanding and treating aphasia. In Beasley DS, David GA (eds): *Aging: Communication Processes and Disorders*. New York, Grune & Stratton, 1981, p 207.
12. DiSimoni FG, Keith RL, Holt DL et al: Practicality of shortening the PICA. *J Speech Hear Res* 18:491–497, 1975.
13. Eisenson J: Rehabilitation of aphasic adults: a review of the issues as the state of the art. In *Rationale for Adult Aphasia Treatment* (conference proceedings). Lincoln, NE, University of Nebraska, 1976.
14. Felix N: *Subjective Communication Report*. Good Samaritan Hospital, Puyallup, Washington, 1977.
15. Florance CL, Conway WL: Transdisciplinary intervention: In Chapey R (ed): *Language Intervention Strategies in Adult Aphasia*, ed 2. Baltimore, Williams & Wilkins, 1986, p 162.
16. Flowers CR, Beukelman DR, Battorf LE, Kelley RA: Family members' predictions of aphasia test performance. *Aphasia-Apraxia-Agnosia* 1:18–26, 1979.
17. Furbacher EA, Wertz RT: Simulation of aphasia by wives of aphasic patients. In Brookshire R (ed): *Clinical Aphasiology Conference Proceedings*. Minneapolis, B.R.K. Publishers, 1978, p 227.
18. Goodglass H, Kaplan E: *The Assessment of Aphasia and Related Disorders*, ed 2. Philadelphia, Lea & Febiger, 1983.
19. Gurland GB, Chwat S, Wollner SG: Establishing a communication profile in adult aphasia: analysis of communicative acts and conversational sequences. In Brookshire R (ed): *Clinical Aphasiology Conference Proceedings*. Minneapolis, B.R.K. Publishers, 1982, p 18.
20. Hale WE, Perkins LL, May FE et al: Symptom prevalence in the elderly: an evalution of age, sex, disease, and medication use. *J Am Geriatr Soc* 34:333–340, 1986.
21. Helmick JW, Watamori TS, Palmer JM: Spouses' understanding of the communication disabilities of aphasic patients. *J Speech Hear Disord* 1:238–243, 1976.
22. Holland AL: *Communicative Abilities in Daily Living: A Test of Functional Communication for Aphasic Adults*. Baltimore, University Park Press, 1980.
23. Hutchinson JM, Jensen M: Evaluation of discourse in communication. In Obler LK, Albert ML (eds): *Language and Communication in the Elderly*. Lexington, MA, D.C. Heath, 1980, p 59.
24. Kaplan E, Goodglass H, Weintraub S: *Boston Naming Test*. Philadelphia, Lea & Febiger, 1983.
25. Kayne RC: Drugs and the aged. In Burnside IM (ed): *Nursing and the Aged*. New York: McGraw-Hill, 1976, p 436.
26. Keenan JS, Brassell EG: *Aphasia Language Performance Scales*. Murfreesboro, TN, Pinnacle Press, 1975.
27. Kent S: Structural changes in the brain may short-circuit transmission of information. *Geriatrics* 31:128–131, 1976.
28. Korchin SJ, Basowitz H: Age differences in verbal learning. *J Abnorm Soc Psychol* 54:64–69, 1957.
29. LaPointe L, Horner J: The FACT: protocol and test format. *Fla Speech Hear Assoc* 2:27–33, 1978.
30. LaPointe L, Horner J: *Reading Comprehension Battery for Aphasia*. Tigard, OR, C.C. Publications, 1979.
31. Lassen NA, Ingvar DH, Skinhoj E: Brain function and blood flow. *Sci Am* 239:62–73, October 1978.
32. Linebaugh CW, Young-Charles HY: The counseling needs of the families of aphasic patients. In Brookshire R (ed): *Clinical Aphasiology Conference Proceedings*. Minneapolis, B.R.K. Publishers, 1978, p 303.
33. Lubinski R: Environmental language intervention. In Chapey R (ed): *Language Intervention Strategies in Adult Aphasia*. Baltimore: Williams & Wilkins, 1981, p 223.
34. Matlock MC, Callaway EA: A language-based geriatric screening procedure. Presented at ASHA Convention, Washington, DC, 1985.
35. Mead BT: How to relate to the elderly patient. *Geriatrics* 32:73–77, 1977.
36. Merritt H: *Textbook of Neurology*. Philadelphia, Lea & Febiger, 1967.
37. Obler LK, Albert ML: *Language and Communication in the Elderly*. Lexington, MA, D.C. Heath, 1980.
38. Obler LK, Albert ML: Language and aging: a neurobehavioral analysis. In Beasley DS, Davis GS (eds): *Aging: Communication Process and Disorders*. New York, Grune & Stratton, 1981, p 107.
39. Obler LK, Albert ML: Language in aging. In Albert ML (ed): *Clinical Neurology of Aging*. New York, Oxford University Press, 1984, p 245.
40. Pfeiffer E: Handling the distressed older patient. *Geriatrics* 34:24–29, 1979.
41. Poitrenaud J, Hazemann P, Lille F: Spontaneous variations in level of arousal among aged individuals. *Gerontology* 24:241–249, 1978.
42. Poon LW, Fozard JL: Speed of retrieval from long-term memory in relation to age, familiarity, and datedness of information. *J Gerontol* 33:111–117, 1978.
43. Porch BE: *Porch Index of Communicative Abil-*

ity. Palo Alto, CA, Consulting Psychologist Press, 1967.

44. Powell GE, Bailey S, Clark E: A very short version of the Minnesota aphasia test. *Br J Soc Clin Psychol* 19:189–194, 1980.

45. Reiff TR: The essentials of geriatric evaluation. *Geriatrics* 35:59–68, 1980.

46. Sarno MT: *The Functional Communication Profile Manual of Directions* Rehabilitation Monograph 42. New York, New York University Press, 1969.

47. Schuell HM: *Minnesota Test for Differential Diagnosis of Aphasia,* rev. ed. Minneapolis, University of Minnesota Press, 1972.

48. Schwartz AN: Counseling: listening with the 3rd ear. *Geriatrics* 35:92–102, 1980.

49. Shewan C: *Auditory Comprehension Test for Sentences.* Chicago, Biolinguistics Clinical Institutes, 1979.

50. Shewan CM, Cameron H: Communication and related problems as perceived by aphasic individuals and their spouses. *J Commun Dis* 17:175–187, 1984.

51. Simon CS: *Communication Profile for the Elderly.* Tucson, AZ, Communication Skill Builders, 1986.

52. Smith BH, Sethi PK: Aging and the nervous system. *Geriatrics* 30:109–115, 1975.

53. Swindell CS, Pashek GV, Holland AL: A questionnaire for surveying personal and communicative style. In Brookshire R (ed): *Clinical Aphasiology Conference Proceedings.* Minneapolis, B.R.K. Publishers, 1982, p 50.

54. Vogel D, Costello RM: Relatives and aphasia clinicians—do they agree? In Brookshire R (ed): *Clinical Aphasiology Conference Proceedings.* Minneapolis, B.R.K. Publishers, 1985, p 237.

55. Wingfield A, Poor LW, Lombardi L et al: Speed of processing in normal aging: effects of speech rate, linguistic structure, and processing time. *J Gerontol* 40:579-585, 1985.

16 Treatment for the Speech-Language Impaired Older Individual: A Gerontological Perspective

BARBARANNE J. BENJAMIN

Editor's Note

Chapter 16 provides a logical extension to the preceding chapter on assessment of speech-language disorders in the elderly. Rather than providing a guide to common treatment approaches for specific disorders, Benjamin focuses on two broad topics: current trends in service delivery to the aged and therapeutic accommodations to the cumulative effects of aging. In both topic areas, her approach is holistic and communicative. The discussion of current trends in management includes consideration of client selection, therapeutic settings, and therapeutic emphases. In the latter category, she notes increasing involvement with pragmatic interventions, counseling and group treatment formats, and improved applications of technological advances. The discussion of therapeutic accommodations to typical age-related changes in function or status is comprehensive. The reader is provided with practical suggestions concerning ways to adjust treatment goals, tasks, and techniques to overcome or reduce the potential negative effects of specific socioeconomic, physiological, and psychological aspects of aging. Clinician and client strategies are emphasized.

Provision of speech-language pathology services for the elderly population has expanded in recent years. Increase in the proportion of elderly in our society (see refs. 108 and 178) and gradual expansion of the roles of speech-language pathologists[a] have contributed to an increased interest in provision of services to older adults. By the year 2050, an estimated 39% of individuals with speech-language impairments will be over the age of 65 (49). These older persons are likely to experience additional problems which affect their communication abilities and, consequently, the management of communication disorders. For instance, hearing loss, degenerative disease, and chronic health conditions are more prevalent in the older population than in other age groups; multiple disabilities are common (142, 175).

To provide effective service for the communicatively impaired elderly, speech-language pathologists must approach the task from a gerontological perspective. Professionals must be aware of current trends in service provision and the implications of those trends for client identification, modification of therapeutic setting, and alternative approaches to intervention. In addition, professionals must be familiar with changes which normally occur with aging in order to implement appropriate and necessary adaptations of intervention strategies. The first part of this chapter delineates current trends in service provision. The second section addresses modifications in intervention based upon current knowledge of the normal aging process.

This chapter attempts to provide a holistic orientation to service provision for speech-language impaired older adults. No attempt is made to survey specific existing treatment approaches. Instead, aspects of intervention that may be influenced by gerontological considerations are highlighted.

The basic premise of this chapter is that a communicative rather than linguistic approach is necessary for intervention with speech-language impaired individuals. With a communicative focus, therapeutic accommodation to the cumulative effects of aging becomes critical. This accommodation includes analysis and

From Committee on Communication Problems of the Aging, American Speech-Language-Hearing Association: The roles of speech-language pathologists and audiologists in working with older persons. A working draft of a position paper, 1986.

adaptation to preexisting communication abilities, effects of aging on speech production and language ability, age-associated changes in performance of certain linguistic and cognitive tasks, the environment, and the nature and severity of the communicative disorder. These factors and others must be considered in adapting current therapeutic approaches to the older individual.

CURRENT TRENDS IN MANAGEMENT

Traditionally, speech-language pathologists have provided services for older aphasic, dysarthric, and laryngectomized patients in individual or possibly group programs utilizing speech or linguistically based approaches. Current trends have expanded the role of speech-language pathologists to include prevention of communicative disorders as well as treatment of nontraditional disorders which affect communicative ability. The settings in which therapy occurs have also been expanded; involvement of family, friends, and caregivers in facilitating the older person's communication has increased. Finally, therapeutic intervention has evolved from a primary focus on the individual's linguistic abilities to greater emphasis on a pragmatic approach. This section of the chapter examines answers to the following questions: Who are appropriate clients? Where does therapy occur? How do therapeutic approaches address the comprehensive nature of communicative disorders?

Trends in Client Selection

One major trend in client selection pertains to the issue of preventive management. As noted in a recent report published by the American Speech-Language-Hearing Association, prevention of communication disorders is a legitimate concern of speech-language pathologists (35). Consequently, professionals are not restricted to working only with communicatively impaired individuals but also may work with those individuals who are at-risk for developing communication disorders (159, 185). Although the ASHA report was primarily concerned with development of speech and language in at-risk infants and children, the concept of prevention of communication problems is applicable to the older adult population.

For instance, a pre-crisis intervention program has been developed for older adults, their families, and caregivers (157). The program focuses on reducing negative attitudes toward communication disorders, provides basic information about common disorders, and develops constructive strategies for coping with communication breakdown (157–159). Although the program does not directly prevent communication disorders, it does prepare the individual with strategies to minimize the effects of speech and language disorders upon communication. Such a program is valuable for anyone who may interact with an older communicatively impaired person on a daily basis (see further discussion in Chapter 19).

Another trend in client selection reflects an expansion of the definition of those disorders and deficits which are considered appropriate for intervention by speech-language pathologists. Although aphasia, dysarthria, and laryngectomy have traditionally been treated through motor speech and/or linguistic approaches, Schuell set a precedent for considering nonlinguistic deficits within aphasic syndromes (163). Current therapeutic trends indicate a shift toward pragmatics; the impact of the disorder on the client's ability to communicate in normal, daily situations is of primary concern.

In addition to traditionally treated disorders, speech-language pathologists are involved in treatment of other disorders which affect the communicative abilities of older adults. Older patients with dysphagia, right hemisphere damage, closed head injury, and dementia may demonstrate deficits in their communicative abilities which necessitate intervention. Speech-language pathologists have not limited dysarthria therapy solely to speech production but have routinely included work with vegetative functions (103, 117, 141); provision of dysphagia therapy is a more recent instance of this type of management approach (97). The legitimacy of dysphagia therapy in relation to speech disorders is reflected in the 1986 Medicare regulations which provide reimbursement for dysphagia therapy in conjunction with other speech treatments. Patients with closed head injury and right hemisphere damage also demonstrate pragmatic language disorders which affect communicative interaction (57, 66, 113, 115, 116, 162, 186, 195). Finally, early and middle stage demented patients display pragmatic, communicative impairments due to deficits in memory and cognitive functioning (1, 7, 8, 129). Speech-language pathologists may work directly with these patients and may also work with the family and/or caregivers to provide a structured, facilitating environment for optimal communication (see Chapter 17).

Finally, speech-language pathologists must be active in identifying older clients for preventive or therapeutic intervention. Since involvement in gerontology is relatively new for the profession, administrators and other caregivers often are unaware of the types of services speech-language pathologists provide. As a result, speech-language pathologists must identify agencies and organizations which serve older adults, determine the need for preventive or therapeutic services, and, in most cases, convince administrators of the need for speech-language services through analysis of cost effectiveness, agency marketing strategies, quality of life, among others.

Trends in Therapeutic Settings

The traditional one-to-one therapeutic setting continues as a primary delivery system, but use of alternative settings is gaining increasing popularity. Alternative settings and alternative delivery systems have evolved as the natural result of constraints imposed by the physical limitations of older clients, needs of organizations serving the elderly, and modifications in third-party payment requirements.

The elderly comprise 23% of acute inpatient services (140), but therapy in an acute care hospital is often limited. With reduction of length of hospital stay, outpatient services have increased. The outpatient delivery system is cost-effective and convenient for the provider but it is inconvenient for the impaired individual who may depend upon others for transportation to therapy. Community speech and hearing clinics and rehabilitation centers may be equally inconvenient for the older adult client. Mental health centers, health maintenance organizations (HMOs), and otolaryngology (ENT) offices may provide speech-language services for elderly clients but may also be relatively inconvenient.

Therapy in long-term care facilities is provided at bedside or in available offices. Nursing homes and hospice facilities may also provide speech-language pathology services on an inpatient basis. Although these services are convenient for the impaired resident, other options are available. Provision of services at home through a home health agency is an alternative to institutionalization or protracted hospital stay for 5 to 10% of the older population (71). Senior citizen centers provide many services for older adults; in certain locations, adult day care is available for demented or physically impaired individuals. Since use of communication skills in the client's daily environment is a primary therapeutic goal, speech-language pathology services can be especially effective in these settings.

Trends in Therapeutic Intervention

In recent years, we have seen an evolution from speech disorders, to speech-language disorders, to communication disorders. Speech-language pathologists are interested in linguistic performance and/or competence insofar as it affects communication in daily life. Medical professionals now talk about quality of life rather than focusing solely on maintenance of life. Ethical considerations concerning the right to die and court cases such as "Baby Jane" reflect the American society's shift from quantity to quality.

This change in intervention goals is reflected in speech-language therapy trends affecting older adults. Therapeutic goals, objectives, and intervention strategies suggest the importance of language as a useful tool for effective communication. Focus upon communication in daily life situations has allowed for pragmatic language therapy with demented and closed head-injured patients. The pragmatic dimension of direct therapy has resulted in increased interest in indirect therapeutic techniques which involve significant others. Group sessions and related needs for counseling are also compatible with this communicative approach. Finally, the pragmatic approach encourages use of technological aids to communicate and focuses awareness on environmental impact.

Pragmatic Intervention

The pragmatic approach to intervention focuses attention on communicative effectiveness rather than linguistic form. Traditional therapy settings, however, tend to restrict the patient's role to that of responder. As a result, a limited number of speech acts are generally appropriate within the traditional therapeutic setting (189). A pragmatic approach seeks to expand acceptable speech acts within and beyond the therapeutic setting.

The change to a more pragmatic approach is reflected in current therapeutic programs designed to facilitate language use in social and everyday situations. For instance, PACE (Promoting Aphasic's Communicative Effectiveness) is a pragmatically based approach for aphasic adults which encourages successful communication rather than focus on the goal of correct production of linguistic form (42). Other therapeutic programs have been developed for use with both speech-language impaired older adults and older individuals without communicative impairment (93).

Programmed activities in the form of exercise have a positive influence on self-concept (128), and approaches which integrate movements and speech have resulted in improved orientation and increased socialization (154). Other programs have been designed to "exercise the brain" and involve the older person in meaningful communication.

Several programs designed to improve cognitive functioning and communicative abilities of older adults are based on the premise that active involvement of the individual is crucial. For instance, reminiscence has been used to review and clarify life experiences, improve cognitive functioning, and integrate intrapersonal and interpersonal abilities (see refs. 21, 78, 111). Active participation and discussion during multidisciplinary health seminars is thought to be the basis for program success (29). Coleman's education therapy, an approach involving discussion of literature and fine arts, provides a vehicle for older adults to support their ideas and disclose feelings within an interesting and challenging discussion (34). Schuetz's Lifelong Learning program provides older institutionalized adults with the opportunity for "significant conversation" (156, p 40). This program focuses upon communication education for the elderly and uses small-group settings to: enhance self-awareness; share cohort experiences; encourage disclosure of feelings; understand how others' perceptions influence self-perception; develop assertiveness; and participate in significant problem-solving discussions.

Feier and Leight's Communication-Cognition Program, based on the idea that learning is not only feasible but necessary for older institutionalized adults, involves active exchange of ideas and feelings, provides methods to help residents compensate for diminished abilities, and presents experiences which challenge the individual (48). Maximum benefit from this program was attained within 3 months, but continuation of the program was necessary for maintenance of skills. Active involvement and communication exchange is the central premise of this program and a critical component of each program described above.

Involving Significant Others

Significant others include the spouse, other family members, friends, neighbors, professionals, and others with whom the older speech-language impaired individual interacts daily. These significant others are called upon to provide emotional support during and after the precipitating crisis. They also must learn to alter their style of communication with the older impaired individual and may even participate actively in the rehabilitation process (118, 133, 155). During this time, family roles may change; additional stress is placed on the cohesiveness of the family (27, 83, 92, 127, 160). Chapter 19 addresses the impact and contribution of significant others in greater detail.

Professionals are particularly important as significant others in the lives of communicatively impaired individuals and may also benefit from suggestions concerning appropriate interaction strategies. Professionals and their related agencies provide a network of service for older adults. Chapter 21 describes agencies and programs serving the older population; Chapter 22 provides strategies for enhancing networking and interdisciplinary team participation.

Counseling and the Group Setting

The group setting, as an alternative to the traditional individual therapy format, is effective in providing service for older adults with communicative impairments. Within the group setting, the older adult receives support from other group members (48, 102) and learns that he/she is not the only person with a deficit. Expression of feelings leads to group discussion; solutions to communication and other problems are addressed. In fact, affective benefit may be the most valuable dimension of group therapy for older communicatively impaired adults.

With communicatively impaired older adults, care in selecting a quiet setting for group meetings is needed to compensate for changes in hearing ability due to aging. Seating arrangement and lighting may be modified to assure unobstructed view of group members; assistive listening systems may be utilized to enhance the auditory component of the environment. Special leadership skills are also required to direct attention, summarize, and organize information to enhance comprehension. Later sections of this chapter offer specific suggestions for adapting discourse to older listeners.

In the group setting, other group members may demonstrate strategies for coping with and compensating for communication disabilities (155). Within the group, the older impaired adult is able to practice communicative strategies in a sheltered situation (102). Creative dramatics and role playing may be used to create situations which parallel those encountered in daily life (41, 102, 173). The participants can explore situations, examine possible strategies and outcomes, and practice compensatory skills within the group setting. Chapter 20 examines general goals and techniques for group treatment in greater detail.

Group sessions are also appropriate for significant others. The family may need information concerning the cause, nature, and consequences of particular speech-language disorders. Information giving and receiving may occur efficiently with one professional giving information to a group, but discussion and confirmation of that information by other group members is extremely valuable for acceptance of the utility of the information by individual group members.

Group counseling is recommended for spouses and other family members (40, 95, 170, 184). Significant others have experienced extreme disruptions to their habitual life-styles; they experience intense emotions and face unique problems which create additional stress (27, 132, 174). Among other problems, these significant others may not know how to interact with a family member whose communication patterns have changed. Although individual counseling may be necessary in certain cases, group sessions have the advantage of peer support. It is important for the family to discuss, problem solve, and compare notes with others who are experiencing similar disruptions to their normal family life.

Technological Advances

Although recent advances have made technological marvels commonplace, a general prejudice exists against technological aids for communication. This prejudice is common in older adults who are likely to benefit from these advances. For instance, many older adults would rather blame speakers for mumbling than wearing a hearing aid. Wearing a hearing aid is perceived as a stigma, an admission of being old and infirm. Many older adults are unwilling to admit a problem exists. Perhaps President Reagan's acceptance of a hearing aid will reverse this tendency.

The technology used to alleviate communication disorders experienced by speech, language, or hearing impaired individuals has evolved rapidly in recent years. Advances in hearing aid amplification have improved the hearing ability of older adults with presbycusis. Assistive listening devices are useful in large, noisy rooms or group discussion sessions. Developments in prosthetic devices have provided certain laryngectomees with the ability to produce speech without reliance on electronic devices or esophageal speech. Electronic and computer-assisted communication aids are also undergoing rapid technological development. New computer programs are being developed to transcribe the spoken word into text and text into the spoken word. In addition, augmentative systems such as manual communication boards, electronic scanning devices, and direct-selection tools can be used by older adults in later stages of degenerative diseases (196).

Successful use of these technological aids depends upon the motivation of the older adult. Factors such as attitude, preference for an oral method and need to communicate can affect motivation. Usability (which includes speed and adaptation of input mode, visual display, and auditory output to limitations in motor and receptive abilities) also influences the older person's desire to use augmentative communication devices.

Environmental Concerns

A major trend in management reflects awareness of the impact of the environment on older adults' communication. The environment contains both opportunities and barriers to communication (98–101, 112, 150). For instance, the arrangement of furniture in a nursing home may facilitate or inhibit social interaction. Changes in lighting, acoustics, and even in the color of walls can also affect communicative interactions (98). These factors are, to some extent, determined by social-cultural preferences. These learned responses to the environment have a subtle impact on communication. In addition, the older individual's attitudes, values, and sensory abilities further affect perceptions of the actual environment.

The environment may be manipulated to facilitate communication through changes in the physical setting, but the total environment includes activities as well as inanimate objects. The quality of the environment is ultimately reflected in the array of activities and interactions which occur. A rich environment provides older adults with numerous communication partners and topics for communication. An impoverished environment decreases the need to communicate, opportunities to interact, and topics to share (44, 99, 101).

Summary

The pragmatic approach, which focuses upon communicative opportunity and intent rather than linguistic form, has far-reaching effects on therapeutic interactions. A communicative focus is compatible with trends toward treatment of nontraditional clients with impairments of communication abilities and toward expansion of traditional therapeutic settings to include those situations and settings which reflect daily life experiences.

Interest in communicative effectiveness supports the involvement of significant others and the use of group therapy to facilitate communication in normal daily activities. Concern with communicative effectiveness also supports the use of technology and nonoral methods of communication. Finally, the pragmatic approach calls attention to the impact of environmental factors on the quality and quantity of communication. Opportunities to communicate, interesting experiences which provide topics for communication, and barriers created by the physical setting must be analyzed and manipulated to create an appropriate, facilitating communication environment for older communicatively impaired adults.

GERONTOLOGICAL CONSIDERATIONS

Therapeutic intervention for the speech-language impaired older adult must be adapted to accommodate typical changes which occur with aging. Areas of particular concern include: changes in economic status and social networks; changes in sensory and motor abilities; and alterations in the psychological dimension which include changes in cognition and emotional behavior. This portion of the chapter addresses the impact of these gerontological considerations upon treatment strategies.

Economic and Social Impact on Intervention

Considerable changes occur in the social networks of older adults. Disengagement theory suggests a gradual reduction of social interaction (22) with the possibility that older adults may disengage *into* the family (176). Older adults often become more isolated from social contacts as they age (44, 60, 119, 162), with a number of factors contributing to this gradual isolation. Changes in available economic resources, environmental opportunities, attitudes and expectations of others, and personal interest and attitudes are important determiners of the quantity and quality of social interactions.

Changes in Economic Resources

Older adults are often restricted to a fixed income upon retirement; pension plans and supplemental Social Security benefits do not approach preretirement levels of financial income (69, 74, 161). Nearly one-fourth of older adults depend solely upon social security benefits upon retirement from the workforce (47, 182). As a result, maintenance of standard of living becomes increasingly more difficult, and dependence upon third party payment for speech-language services becomes more critical.

In addition, older adults are more susceptible to common illnesses (71, 177, 191) and often have chronic health-related problems (175, 191) which increase the financial burden at a time of limited income. Health care costs are not fully reimbursed by Medicare (30, 47, 138), and additional medical insurance is expensive. Older adults in need of assistive or augmentative devices may not be able to afford communication aids. It may be necessary for the speech-language pathologist to be involved in identifying funding sources and agency support to provide needed equipment and services (see refs. 18 and 51).

The Social Environment

Changes in the environment contribute to the number of communicative opportunities available to older adults. As the individual ages, the number of relatives, friends, and acquaintances is reduced (see refs. 27, 82, 119, 137, 191). Death claims some communication partners; other possible partners develop different interests and are not available for social interaction on a regular basis. With the advent of our mobile society, family and friends often move to distant locales (119). Limited economic resources can also restrict the frequency of telephone contacts initiated by older persons; changes in sensory and motor abilities may also limit the effectiveness and amount of oral and written correspondence.

Other environmental factors affecting social contact are more easily manipulated. Older adults may reside in age-segregated residences such as retirement communities or nursing homes. These environments affect the number and type of opportunities for communicative interaction (44, 45, 99, 101, 110).

Older adults often congregate in shopping malls, parks, or other public places; senior citizen centers also provide meeting places for socialization. Meals may be prepared and provided at or below cost to eligible older adults. These congregate meals not only provide balanced nutrition but also permit social interaction.

Generally, communicatively impaired older adults do not participate fully in these opportunities. Therapeutic intervention can have a significant impact on the quality of life if it encourages and facilitates increased social contact beyond the therapeutic setting.

Attitudes and Stereotypes

Expectations of age appropriate behavior are culturally determined; members of a society learn which behaviors are acceptable for certain roles and a societal stereotype of the older adult has developed (see 79, 82, 96, 181). Older adults are expected to take the role of kindly grandparent, garrulous oldster, crotchety recluse, or other typical roles. These stereotypical images have been fostered in the mass media and have, to some extent, shaped societal expectations of older adults (5, 43, 52, 183). These expectations in turn affect both partners in the communication interchange. The communication partner may interact with the older adult in such a way as to elicit the expected behaviors; the older adult may accept the "assigned" role and take on the expected characteristics. Thus, a self-fulfilling prophecy may affect the communication interchange.

When communicators' interactions are based on what they expect to hear rather than what actually occurs, communication barriers are erected. Awareness of personal attitudes and typical stereotypical images of the elderly is necessary for family members, professionals, and older adults themselves. For instance, older persons often hold a prejudicial attitude toward other older adults but do not consider the negative image as applicable to themselves (3, 46).

The attitudes of professionals who work with older adults are critical to effective communication interaction in these important situations. Health care professionals are not exempt from the influence of negative societal attitudes and expectations concerning older adults, and these attitudes may be expressed in subtle verbal and nonverbal ways (4, 14, 25, 64, 73, 87, 88, 123, 164, 168). Such attitudes can affect therapeutic success if the professional lowers goals in the belief that the older adult only has a few years remaining or because the older adult has limited needs and social contacts in a nursing home.

The advent of the movie "Cocoon" and the television series "The Golden Girls" may signal a change in societal perceptions of older adults. These programs have had wide distribution and have, to some extent, heightened awareness of the abilities of older adults and of the heterogeneity in this age group. It is hoped that older adults may no longer be perceived in terms of negative descriptors such as powerless, asexual, or frail (27, 83, 85, 166).

Physiological Impact on Intervention

Communicative interaction depends upon both sensory input and motoric ability. Although not all older adults experience sensory and motor reductions to the same degree, decreases in sensitivity to stimuli and reduction of fine motor ability are prevalent in the older population. The impact of these changes on communicative competence depends upon the individual and may not significantly disrupt older adults' daily lives (121). When older adults also experience communication disorders, however, these sensory and motoric changes may be more detrimental.

Sensory Changes

Although the majority of older adults do not have severe hearing losses, gradual loss of hearing begins during adulthood and progresses through old age (see refs. 58, 119, 124, 142, 188). A hearing loss which occurs by age 60 is likely to deteriorate with age (135). Typical presbycusic hearing loss increases with advancing age and affects understanding of speech due to loss of the high frequency component of the speech signal (36, 50, 106, 125). Surprisingly, in at least one study, hearing loss did not appear to cause social isolation or to greatly disrupt the social world of older subjects (120).

Typical age-related changes in hearing must be considered when selecting therapeutic activities, when counseling family members and caregivers, and when interacting with older clients. Auditory sensory loss, especially in an unfamiliar setting such as a hospital or rehabilitation center, is disorienting for the older person. The individual may respond inappropriately to a half-heard message and present an appearance of disorientation. Others may then label the older person as "confused," further isolating him/her from nursing staff and other professionals (86).

Clearly, speech-language pathologists working with older clients should take into account expected hearing losses with age. Raising the loudness of the voice without shouting can be effective, but speakers should make a conscious effort to have a pleasant facial expression while talking loudly to older hearing impaired adults (86). Lowering the pitch to accommodate typical high frequency hearing losses in older adults has been suggested, but the professional or caregiver should not abuse his/her vocal mechanism by talking loudly in an inappropriately low pitch.

A multisensory approach can be an effective method for facilitating information exchange with older adults. Persons talking with older adults can establish topic and reorient the older listener by using gestures and pointing to objects. A quiet, nondistracting environment is particularly useful since older adults experience difficulty in discriminating speech in noisy, adverse conditions (45, 124). Getting the older person's attention before speaking, using internal summaries, and paraphrasing rather than repeating can help the older adult follow the gist of a conversation. In addition, traditional speech reading techniques can be adapted for use with older hearing impaired adults. Facing the listener, focusing light onto the speaker's face rather than into the listener's eyes, and keeping a 3- to 6-foot distance from the older listener can facilitate ease of speech reading (45, 143).

Vision, critical for adaptation to the environment, is affected by changes in eye structure with age (84, 188). Due to deflection of light rays through thickened lens, visual acuity is diminished. Reduced adaptation to light/dark and increased sensitivity to glare (39, 75, 84, 86) dictate types of materials suitable for therapy with older individuals. In selection of therapy materials as in designing the environment, high contrast is desirable between figure and ground. Exaggerated contrast between floors and walls and between furniture and background (75) should be generalized to include pictures and other therapeutic materials for older adults. In addition, older adults need triple the amount of illumination that young adults use (75), and incandescent lighting is preferred.

Consideration of visual ability with aging affects selection of materials for speech-language therapy with the older adult. Materials must not only be appropriate to the individual's age and interests but must also be easily recognizable by older adults with sensory deficits. The speech-language pathologist must arrange therapeutic materials within the older adult's visual field (86) and develop strategies to encourage the older adult with visual deficits to scan neglected portions of the visual field. In addition, the older adult's visual requirements must also be considered when selecting and/or adapting augmentative communication systems or computer-assisted devices for the individual.

Although impact on communication and therapeutic intervention is minimal, changes in other senses also occur with age. The normally aging individual has diminished sensitivity to touch (39, 86); taste sensitivity is also slightly reduced, but wide individual differences occur in older age groups (58, 86). Overseasoning with sugars and salts is a nutritionally suspect compensatory strategy used by older adults (188). Lower olfactory sensitivity also contributes to reduced enjoyment of food (86, 188). Changes in these senses are most directly related to the quality and enjoyment of life but also may have long-term effects on the individual's health.

Motoric Changes

Changes in motoric ability affect speech production of older adults (80, 81). The general slowing associated with age is reflected in slower speech rates used by normal elderly speakers (146, 179); increased interjections and hesitations are also evident (61, 136, 179, 194). Articulatory characteristics of older speakers have been identified as a factor used in estimating age from voice samples (2, 10, 70, 89, 146), but these minor articulatory changes do not result in phonemic distortions. Although hoarseness may be perceptually associated with older speaking voices (2, 11, 70, 77, 89, 136), only 27% of older adult voices in one study were perceived as hoarse (179) (see Chapter 9 for a detailed examination of the speech characteristics of older adults).

These and other rather subtle changes in speech production combine to produce an array of vocal characteristics perceived as indicating old age. To naive listeners, perception of age in voice was most suggestive of speaker personality characteristics (6). Older female voices were judged as more reserved, passive, inflexible, and "out-of-it," and older male voices were perceived as less flexible (144). Thus, listeners attribute negative personality traits to older speakers, based on vocal characteristics alone. Even age peers associate negative characteristics with older sounding voices. For example, when listening to the voices of older female speakers, older female listeners attributed significantly reduced vitality and older male listeners attributed reduced intelligence and sincerity to these speakers (10). Such stereotypical reactions can influence social communication among older adults.

Negative reactions to older voices may unconsciously affect professionals working with older adults. Speech-language pathologists and other professionals must realize that vocal qualities are not necessarily correlated with personality characteristics (151). The professional must guard against normal tendencies to stereotype people based on their vocal production.

Psychological Considerations

The psychological domain, including both cognitive and emotional components, may be affected by aging. Subtle changes in central cognitive functioning and memory are reflected in language behaviors and discourse strategies. Older adults are also faced with many life changes which increase stress and require emotional adjustment. Optimal therapeutic intervention involves consideration of both cognitive and affective factors which affect the abilities of older adults.

Cognitive Influence

A general slowing of behavior has been consistently noted in older adults (see refs. 12, 148, 193) and has, in part, been attributed to a slowing of central processing (see refs. 9, 147, 192). Older adults are more susceptible to fatigue (171) and are more cautious and conservative in responding to unfamiliar tasks (see ref. 119). Finally, there is some indication that older adults encode new information less deeply and are less efficient at retrieving information stored in memory than are young adults (172). These subtle changes in basic cognitive functioning can influence learning, problem solving, and comprehension.

The combination of slowed response, susceptibility to fatigue, possible health-related problems, and cautious response activation suggests that older adults may benefit from a slower, less pressured environment. Professionals working with older clients must be sensitive to fatigue; length of session and scheduled time of day are variables which can be controlled to optimize therapeutic effectiveness (63, 190).

Differences between young and older adults have been shown to decrease when time demands are reduced, although differences in functioning remain. For instance, on a self-paced task in which subjects made notes to counteract any memory deficits, older adults remained less likely to solve the problem task (68). Those adults who did not solve the problem generally retained early formulated hypotheses and were less flexible in generating and considering alternative hypotheses. Speech-language pathologists must consider the impact of typical cognitive styles and select tasks and therapeutic goals with utilization and modification of communicative strategies in mind. Development of an array of potential strategies and flexibility in adjusting strategies to particular situations are possible goals.

To facilitate learning of, memory for, and recall of information, information must be encoded with sufficient depth. When working with older adults, professionals may use strategies to facilitate deeper encoding. Since older adults do not generate relevant elaborations as a strategy to encode memory (19, 53, 139), provision or facilitation of elaboration can be beneficial (139). Relevant elaboration focuses attention on the semantic features of the information to be remembered. Older adults are better able to remember meaningful than nonmeaningful information (23, 26, 28, 180).

Glynn and Muth have offered a number of suggestions for stimulating deep, elaborated memory traces in older adults (59). Priming strategies focus attention on key ideas and relevant information. Such techniques include provision of detailed instructions in testing situations, lists of objectives in educational settings, and introductory statements which announce the main proposition. These techniques help the older adult focus on key points, relate supplementary information to the main topic, and provide a framework by which the importance of supplementary information or major propositions can be assessed (72, 180).

Mediators can also be used to facilitate recall of certain types of information by older adults. Mediators such as imagery, pictures, and graphs have been shown to help older adults integrate information within an existing framework of related knowledge (19, 53, 165). Mnemonic devices using natural imagery also facilitated memory and recall in controlled tasks which ranged from paired-associates to name/face recall (67, 104, 134). In one investigation, older adults benefited from use of these strategies but, even with time pressures eliminated, they were not as likely to use them spontaneously as were younger adults (38). The professional working with the older adult can suggest and encourage use of such strategies.

A variety of investigations have established that older adults are sensitive to the organization of discourse when attention must be divided and material reorganized (31, 37, 59, 62, 109, 197). In recalling well-organized stories, older adults remembered information but included more additions and distortions (167). Professionals working with older adults can reorient the older listener to discourse organization by using internal summaries, orienting statements, and questions (38, 107, 169, 187). These techniques are suited to sustained discourse such as giving directions to a group of older adults during therapy/counseling meetings, addressing participants at a senior citizen center, or developing text or handouts for distribution to older adults. Repetition of instructions, demonstration, and incorporation of multisensory input may help orient and focus the older listener in group settings. Using attention-getting devices, announcing topic shifts, and eliciting both verbal and nonverbal feedback on message content can be used to help the older listener follow a conversation.

Prosodic features such as stress and intonation can also be used to highlight relevant segments of meaningful discourse (145). Focal stress on key words facilitated recall of relevant information (32) and may be useful in helping older adults organize incoming information. Focal stress on inference or integration has also been shown to benefit elderly listeners (9, 32). This accentuation may be particularly helpful in noisy situations or in group discussions in which older adults with presbycusic hearing losses are at a disadvantage (119, 124).

Since older adults may be slower in central processing tasks, rate of speech may affect older listeners' comprehension of oral material (see ref. 122). When speech was electronically compressed and/or expanded, older adult listeners retained more information than when speech was presented at normal rates (152, 153). Perhaps the novelty of the stimuli increased attention to and subsequent recall of information.

Intrasentence pausing, a method of slowing speech, has benefited certain aphasics (20, 94). The use of pausing allows listeners time to integrate and recapitulate information. Appropriate pauses following summary statements or rhetorical questions may facilitate organizational strategies in discourse comprehension. In addition, pausing also allows older listeners time to formulate responses and to enter into conversations (14, 17).

Suggestions to talk slowly to older adults and to simplify sentence structure (14, 20, 45, 55, 126) are supported by findings in the literature. Although the subject-verb-object structure is the easiest to comprehend, grammatical markers or semantic redundancy within discourse can be used to alert older listeners to modifications in the basic grammatical pattern (54, 130, 131). Confusions in listening to discourse may be partially alleviated by redundancy in the message, by effective use of prosodic features, or by redundant linguistic markers used to highlight semantic content or call attention to deviations from the basic syntactic pattern.

Another therapeutic consideration concerns the appropriateness of adapting speech and language styles to older listeners. Simplification of vocabulary and sentence structure may be interpreted as demeaning and may irritate older listeners (33). The degree to which such messages are negatively perceived is related, in part, to the level of functioning of the older client (24). Rather than offending the older listener, professionals must be sensitive to verbal and nonverbal feedback and must adapt their communication strategies to the individual person rather than to a stereotypical image of the older adult.

A final consideration concerns topic selection and maintenance. Older adults are not deficient in social language use and may rely on past experiences for topic integration and expansion (15, 16). This rich reserve of past personal experience is in direct opposition to the sparsity of interesting conversational topics available in the restricted communication environment experienced by older adults in many institutional settings. Topic selection depends upon individual concerns as well as daily experiences, so health and financial matters are frequent topics of conversation (58, 161). Lack of opportunity may deprive older adults of a wide variety of topics for conversational interaction (44, 82).

The pragmatic approach to intervention demands attention to daily experiences, partners for social interaction, and maintenance or development of communication skills. The professional may use a variety of topics within the therapy setting, but involvement cannot be limited to the therapy session. The professional must encourage changes and improvements in the environment which will result in an increase in topic availability as well as a better quality of life.

Emotional Adjustment

Older adults must cope with many stress-producing changes in their lives (76, 91, 174). Certain changes affecting the sensory channels, central processes, and motoric ability progress gradually. The older adult often adapts unconsciously to these changes until the deficits become severe enough to seriously affect communication. Other changes are abrupt and unexpected, thus creating life discontinuities. Such abrupt changes include loss of a spouse, death of friends or other peers, change of residence, altered life-style due to changes in financial status, loss of role identity with retirement, and excess leisure time (22, 76).

Older persons with any form of impairment may experience isolation. The speech-language disordered adult, in particular, may feel that the benefits of interaction are not worth the effort to communicate through an impaired system. Significant others in the environment may be neither proficient nor comfortable when interacting with a person with a communication impairment (27, 105). In addition, the impaired older individual may experience mobility reductions which limit chance social interactions. In effect, the older adult may be dependent upon others to initiate social contact (185).

Dependency of the older adult is not limited to dependency on others to initiate social contacts. Increased feelings of helplessness may result from the impaired individual's need to rely upon others for basic necessities (27, 56). Role reversals occur, with the spouse or children taking on responsibilities formerly assumed by the older impaired individual (83). Self-image and self-esteem can be affected. Extensive emotional adjustments must occur.

Depression, sleep disorders, anxiety, and other significant mental disorders may develop at any age and may affect older adults (13, 114, 119). Depressive symptoms increase with age (13) with 10 to 15% of the elderly population experiencing depression (65). Personality analysis shows increase in defensiveness and decrease in self-criticism with age; older adults are less like neurotic groups than are the general population (149). Of course, certain disorders such as Alzheimer type dementia and paraphrenia, a late onset paranoid disorder, primarily affect elderly persons (90).

These affective dimensions impact on the quantity and quality of social interaction (13, 56). For example, the depressed individual will not be motivated to communicate. Speech-language pathologists, interacting with other professionals on a multidisciplinary team, must coordinate efforts to help older clients. Since communication abilities are essential to emotional adjustment, speech-language pathologists must work closely with counselors to help the communicatively impaired older adult obtain needed services.

Summary

Therapeutic intervention for older adults with communication disorders must be modified to accommodate specific gerontological factors.

Social isolation is common in the older population. Reduction of earned income limits options for social activities, and older adults living in nursing homes or in restricted housing may be in a communication-diminished environment. Attitudes of others have a significant impact on interactions between the older person and peers, family members, professionals, and younger individuals. These factors restrict the generalization and effectiveness of therapeutic interventions by limiting opportunities for social interaction. Professionals cannot afford to limit management of communication disorders to the therapeutic setting; they must employ the daily environment in intervention approaches.

Physiological changes with advancing age are most obvious, but their effects on the daily lives of normal older adults are subtle. When these physiological changes accompany a speech-language disorder, the effects on communication become significant. The older adult may not elect to communicate if he/she experiences difficulty comprehending or participating in conversations. Use of assistive listening devices, hearing aids, augmentative communication devices, and computer-assisted aids can supplement the older person's sensory and motoric ability and facilitate ease of communication.

Changes in psychological adjustment and functioning must be taken into consideration in developing therapeutic strategies for use with older individuals. Self-paced tasks reduce the impact of slowed reaction time. Reduced memory function may be accommodated by providing relevant elaboration, using intonational stress to highlight key concepts, and aiding the older person in deeper encoding for memory.

Since meaningful material is most easily remembered, the speech-language pathologist can highlight relevant parts of messages through syntactic and semantic redundancy. Instructions, internal summaries, and reorienting statements can also help the older adult organize and relate new information to existing experience. A multisensory approach is effective since it provides supplementary, orienting and focusing markers in different modalities. Finally, the speech-language pathologist has access to nonverbal and verbal feedback to determine the older adult's understanding of the message.

CONCLUSIONS

Trends delineated in the first part of this chapter reflect the need for accommodating therapy to the characteristics and environments of older individuals. The expansion of traditional therapy settings and inclusion of nontraditional disorders in intervention approaches necessitate alterations in therapeutic strategies. The second part of this chapter provided general methods for adapting therapeutic techniques to the specific needs of older adults.

In reviewing the first section of this chapter, we find that client selection criteria have expanded to include programs designed to educate older persons, their families, and others to cope with typical communication disorders experienced by the elderly. Others have advocated provision of services to patients with dysphagia, dementia, and head injury who show an impairment of the ability to communicate. The role of the speech-language pathologist has expanded to include intervention with clients not previously considered eligible for therapeutic services.

Expansion of therapeutic setting has also been advocated. Older adults seek services in nontraditional settings such as long- and short-term medical care facilities, mental health centers, adult day care, home health organizations, and others. As a result, it is imperative that speech-language pathologists educate administrators to the need for speech-language services in nontraditional settings.

Current trends in therapeutic intervention further the evolution of speech-language services into communication services. The pragmatic approach to intervention has incorporated the premise that appropriate therapy must impact the client's daily use of language to communicate. Pragmatic intervention includes the active participation of the individual in relevant communication. Several programs incorporating such principles were briefly discussed in the text.

The holistic communication approach espoused in this chapter supports the inclusion of indirect therapy in the totality of service provision. Significant others with whom the older person interacts are important components in the success of therapeutic intervention. These partners can facilitate or impede progress in generalizing learned communication strategies into everyday communication experiences. Counseling and group sessions have been instrumental in helping both communicatively impaired older adults and significant others to explore their feelings, cope with problems, and receive emotional support.

Technological advances have often surpassed emotional acceptance of technological devices in everyday communication activities. Although advances in assistive listening devices,

prosthetic appliances, and augmentative communication systems have been phenomenal, speech-language pathologists must educate older adults concerning the usefulness and acceptability of such systems. Denial of the problem, embarrassment, and passive or active rejection of technological devices must be overcome before the older adult will use the assistive system. The use of alternative means of communication is compatible with the pragmatic approach, which focuses upon the use of language to communicate rather than upon the form of the linguistic production.

The pragmatic/holistic approach to speech-language therapy also calls attention to the environment in which communication occurs. The older adult's communication environment may be limited by sensory and/or motor deficits, by institutional procedures, or by physical barriers. Fewer communication partners may be available. Therapeutic intervention is no longer limited to the therapy setting; the speech-language pathologist has the responsibility to modify the daily communication environment to facilitate communication.

The second section of this chapter examined gerontological considerations used to adapt therapeutic intervention strategies to the abilities of older communicatively impaired adults. Reduced economic resources often restrict the number and type of opportunities available to the older individual while a reduction in the number of possible contacts restricts opportunities for social interaction. Within this restricted environment, older adults cope with societal expectations of appropriate age-dictated activities, behaviors, and roles. The attitudes of various communication partners also influence the quality and quantity of communication interchange.

Physiological changes of the sensory and motor systems impact communication interaction. Changes in vision, hearing, and other senses must be considered in designing educational, therapeutic, and recreational materials for older adults. Specific suggestions for enhancing interaction with older adults who have experienced age-related changes in sensory abilities were provided. In addition, changes in physical characteristics often associated with aging result in the typical older-sounding voice. Since listeners attribute personality characteristics to speakers based upon vocal characteristics, speech-language pathologists and other professionals must guard against stereotyping older adults based on images associated with their typical vocal productions.

Finally, psychological considerations included the impact of changes in central processing and emotional responses on therapeutic intervention. Specific suggestions to compensate for subtle cognitive changes which occur with advanced age were made in this section of the chapter. Strategies in scheduling, provision of organizing cues, and adaptation of speech styles may be useful in therapeutic, educational, and social settings. The need for emotional adjustment, feelings of dependency, and possible depression must also be considered in therapeutic design.

The principles of a communication-based intervention offer a viable approach to a comprehensive therapy program for older communicatively impaired adults. Observations and suggestions made throughout this chapter reflect considerations of the typical changes which occur with aging. Since groups of older adults are more heterogeneous than groups of other aged persons, each professional must utilize and adapt therapeutic techniques to the specific individual's abilities and needs.

References

1. Albert M: Language in normal and dementing elderly. In Obler L, Albert M (eds): *Language and Communication in the Elderly*. Lexington, MA, DC Heath, 1980, p 145.
2. Amerman JD, Parnell MM: Clinical impressions of the speech of normal elderly adults. Presented at the American Speech-Language-Hearing Association Convention, Washington, DC, 1985.
3. Atchley RC: *Aging: Continuity and Change*. Belmont, CA, Wadsworth, 1983.
4. Bader J: Attitudes towards aging, older age, and old people. *Aged Care Serv Rev* 2:1–14, 1980.
5. Barbato CA, Feezel JD: Cross generational connotations of language of aging. Presented at the Speech Communication Association Convention, Washington, DC, 1983.
6. Bassili JN, Reil JE: On the dominance of the old-age stereotype. *J Gerontol* 36:682–688, 1981.
7. Bayles KA: Language and dementia. In Holland A: *Language Disorders in Adults*. San Diego, College-Hill, 1984, p 208.
8. Bayles KA: Management of neurogenic communication disorders associated with dementia. In Chapey R (ed): *Language Intervention Strategies in Adult Aphasia*, ed 2. Baltimore, Williams & Wilkins, 1986, p 462.
9. Belmore SM: Age-related changes in processing explicit and implicit language. *J Gerontol* 36:316–322, 1981.
10. Benjamin BJ: Dimensions of the older female voice. *Lang Commun* 6:35–45, 1986.
11. Benjamin BJ: Phonological performance in gerontological speech. *J Psycholinguist Res* 11:159–167, 1982.
12. Birren J, Woods AM, Williams MV: Behavioural slowing with age: causes, organization, and consequences. In Poon LW (ed): *Aging in the 1980s: Psychological Issues*. Washington, DC,
American Psychological Association, 1980, p 293.
13. Blazer D: Depressive illness in late life. In Committee on an Aging Society, Institute of Medicine and National Research Council: *America's Aging: Health in an Older Society*. Washington, DC, National Academy Press, 1985, p 105.
14. Blazer D: Techniques for communication with your elderly patient. *Geriatrics* 33:79–84, 1978.
15. Boden D, Bielby DD: The past as resource: a conversational analysis of elderly talk. *Hum Dev* 26:308–319, 1983.
16. Boden D, Bielby DD: The way it was: topical organization in elderly conversation. *Lang Commun* 6:73–89, 1986.
17. Bollinger RL, Waugh PF, Zatz F: *Communication Management of the Geriatric Patient*. Danville, IL, Interstate Printers and Publishers, 1977.
18. Boone DR: Ageism: A negative view of the aged. *ASHA* 27:51–53, 1985.
19. Botwinick J: *Aging and Behavior: A Comprehensive Integration of Research Findings*, ed 2. New York, Springer, 1978.
20. Brookshire RH, Nicholas LE: Consistency of effects of slow rate and pauses on aphasic listeners' comprehension of spoken sentences. *J Speech Hear Res* 27:323–328, 1984.
21. Butler RN: The life review: an interpretation of reminiscence in the aged. *Psychiatry* 26:65–75, 1983.
22. Bulter R, Cumming E, Henry WE: *Growing Old*. New York, Basic Books, 1961.
23. Calhoun RO, Gounard BR: Meaningfulness, presentation rate, list length, and age in elderly adults' paired-associate learning. *Educat Gerontol* 4:49–56, 1979.
24. Caporael LR: The paralanguage of care giving: baby talk to institutionalized aged. *J Pers Soc Psychol* 40:876–884, 1981.
25. Carmichael CW: Research on nonverbal communication and the aged. Presented at the Speech Communication Association Convention, Chicago, 1986.
26. Cerella J, Paulshock D, Poon L: The effects of semantic processing on memory of subjects differing in age. *Educ Gerontol* 8:1–7, 1982.
27. Cicirelli VG: Adult children and their elderly parents. In Brubaker TH (ed): *Family Relationships in Later Life*. London, Sage, 1983, p 31.
28. Clark E: Semantic and episodic memory impairment in normal and cognitively impaired elderly adults. In Obler LK, Albert ML (eds): *Language and Communication in the Elderly*. Lexington, MA, DC Heath, 1980, pp 47–57.
29. Clark PG: Participatory health seminars for nursing home residents: a model for multidisciplinary education. *Gerontol Geriatr Educ* 4:75–84, 1984.
30. Clark RL, Maddox GL, Schrimper RA, Sumner DA: *Inflation and the Economic Well-Being of the Elderly*. Baltimore, Johns Hopkins University Press, 1984.
31. Cohen G: Language comprehension in old age. *Cogn Psychol* 1:412–429, 1979.
32. Cohen G, Faulkner D. Does elderspeak work? The effect of intonation and stress on compre-

hension and recall of spoken discourse in old age. *Lang Commun* 6:91–98, 1986.

33. Cohen G, Faulkner D: Memory for discourse in old age. *Discourse Processes* 4:253–365, 1981.

34. Coleman CA: Gymnasium for the mind. *Geriatrics* 33:97–100, 1978.

35. Committee on the Prevention of Speech, Language, and Hearing Problems: Definitions of the word "prevention" as it relates to communicative disorders. *ASHA* 24: 425, 431, 1982.

36. Corso J: *Aging Sensory Systems and Perception.* New York, Praeger, 1981.

37. Craik FIM: Age differences in human memory. In Birren JE, Schaie KW (eds): *Handbook of the Psychology of Aging.* New York, Van Nostrand Reinhold, 1977, p 384.

38. Craik FIM, Rabinowitz JC: The effects of presentation rate and encoding task on age-related memory deficits. *J Gerontol* 40:309–315, 1985.

39. Curtis AP, Fucci D: Sensory and motor changes during development and aging. In Lass N (ed): *Speech and Language: Advances in Basic Research and Practice,* vol. 9. New York, Academic Press, 1983, p 153.

40. Dancer J: General considerations in the management of older persons. In Jacobs-Condit L (ed): *Gerontology and Communication Disorders.* Rockville, MD, American Speech-Language-Hearing Association, 1984, p 172.

41. Davis BW: The impact of creative drama training on psychological states of older adults: an exploratory study. *Gerontologist* 25:316–332, 1985.

42. Davis GA: Pragmatics and treatment. In Chapey R (ed): *Language Intervention Strategies in Adult Aphasia,* ed 2. Baltimore, Williams & Wilkins, 1986, p 251.

43. Davis RH: *Television and the Aging Audience.* Los Angeles, University of Southern California Press, 1980.

44. Dean K: Self-care behaviour: implications for aging. In Dean K, Hickey T, Holstein BE (eds): *Self-Care and Health in Old Age.* London, Croom Helm, 1986, p 58.

45. Dreher B: *Communicating with the Elderly.* Dayton, OH, Wright State University, 1984.

46. Dunkel RE, Haug MR, Rosenberg M: *Communications Technology and the Elderly.* New York, Springer, 1984.

47. Estes CL, Newcomer RJ: *Fiscal Austerity and Aging.* London, Sage Publications, 1983.

48. Feier CD, Leight G: A communication-cognition program for elderly nursing home residents. *Gerontologist* 21:408–415, 1981.

49. Fein DJ: Projections of speech and hearing impairments to 2050. *ASHA* 25:11, 1983.

50. Fisch L: Special senses: the aging auditory system. In Brocklehurst JC (ed): *Textbook of Geriatric Medicine and Gerontology.* New York, Churchill Livingstone, 1978, p 276.

51. Flower RM: Economic consideration in implementing service delivery models. In Jacobs-Condit L (ed): *Gerontology and Communication Disorders.* Rockville, MD, American Speech-Language-Hearing Association, 1984, p 301.

52. Freimuth VS, Jamieson K: *Communicating with the Elderly: Shattering Stereotypes.* Urbanna,

IL, and Falls Church, VA, ERIC and Speech Communication Association, 1979.

53. Fullerton AM: Age differences in the use of imagery in integrating new and old information in memory. *J Gerontol* 38:326–332, 1983.

54. Fullerton AM, Smith AD: Age-related differences in the use of redundancy. *J Gerontol* 35:729–735, 1980.

55. Gardner H, Albert MC, Weintaub S: Comprehending a word: the influence of speed and redundancy on auditory comprehension in aphasia. *Cortex* 11:155–162, 1975.

56. Garland J: Prevention of dependency. In Muir Gray JA (ed): *Prevention of Disease in the Elderly.* London, Churchill Livingstone, 1985, p 18.

57. Gauwain J: Communication defects following right hemisphere damage: a pragmatic perspective. Presented at the American Speech-Language-Hearing Association Convention, Washington, DC, 1985.

58. Geist H: *The Psychological Aspects of the Aging Process with Sociological Implications.* Huntington, NY, Robert E. Krieger, 1981.

59. Glynn SM, Muth KD: Text-learning capabilities of older adults. *Educ Gerontol* 4:253–269, 1979.

60. Goldberg EM: The effectiveness of social care for the elderly. In Bronley DB (ed): *Gerontology: Social and Behavioral Perspectives.* London, Croom Helm, 1984, p 102.

61. Gordon, KC, Hutchinson JM, Allen CS: An evaluation of selected discourse characteristics in normal geriatric subjects. In *Laboratory Research Reports* Pocatello, ID, Department of Speech Pathology and Audiology, Idaho State University, 1976, vol 1, p 11.

62. Gordon SK: Organization and recall of related sentences by elderly and young adults. *Exp Aging Res* 1:71–80, 1975.

63. Gounard BR, Hulicka IM: Maximizing learning efficiency in later adulthood: a cognitive problem-solving approach. *Educ Gerontol* 2:417–427, 1977.

64. Greene MG, Adelman R, Charon R, Hoffman S: Ageism in the medical encounter: an exploratory study of the doctor-elderly patient relationship. *Lang Commun* 6:113–124, 1986.

65. Gurland BJ, Toner JA: Depression in the elderly: a review of recently published studies. In Eisdorfer C (ed): *Annual Review of Gerontology and Geriatrics,* New York, Springer, 1982, vol 3, p 228.

66. Hagen C: Language disorders in head trauma. In Holland A (ed): *Language Disorders in Adults.* San Diego, College-Hill, 1984, p 245.

67. Hanley-Dunn P, McIntosh JL: Meaningfuless and recall of names by young and old adults. *J Gerontol* 39:583–585, 1984.

68. Harley AA: Adult age differences in deductive reasoning processes. *J. Gerontol* 36:700–706, 1981.

69. Harris CS: Income adequacy in retirement. In Kolker A, Ahmed PI (eds): *Aging.* New York, Elsevier Biomedical, 1982, p 80.

70. Hartman DE, Danhauer JL: Perceptual features of speech for males in four perceived age decades. *J Acoust Soc Am* 59:713–715, 1976.

71. Havighurst RJ: Health problems in aging. In

Kolker A, Ahmed PI (eds): *Aging*. New York, Elsevier Biomedical, 1982, p 141.

72. Hess TM: Effects of semantically related and unrelated contexts on recognition memory of different-aged adults. *J Gerontol* 39:444–451, 1984.

73. Hickey T, Bragg S, Rakowski W, Hultsch D: Attitude instrument analysis: an examination of factor consistency across two samples. *Int J Aging Hum Dev* 10:359–375, 1979.

74. Hickey T, Cruise P: Social aspects of aging and health in late life. In Jacobs-Condit L (ed): *Gerontology and Communication Disorders*. Rockville, MD, American Speech-Language-Hearing Association, 1984, p 131.

75. Hiatt LG: Is poor lighting dimming the sight of nursing home patients? *Nurs Homes* 29:32–34 1980.

76. Holstein BJ: Health related behaviors and aging: conceptual issues. In Dean K, Hickey T, Holstein BE (eds): *Self-Care and Health in Old Age*. London, Croom Helm, 1986, p 35.

77. Honjo I, Isshiki N: Laryngoscopic and voice characteristics of aged persons. *Arch Otolaryngol* 106:149–150, 1980.

78. Hughston GA, Merriam SB: Reminiscence: a nonformal technique for improving cognitive functioning in the aged. *Int J Aging Hum Dev* 15:139–149, 1982.

79. Itzin C: The double jeopardy of ageism and sexism: media images of women. In Bromely DB (ed): *Gerontology: Social and Behavioral Perspectives*. London, Croom Helm, 1984, p 170.

80. Jacobs-Condit L, Ortenzo ML: Physical changes in aging. In Jacobs-Condit L (ed): *Gerontology and Communication Disorders*. Rockville, MD, American Speech-Language-Hearing Association, 1984, p 26.

81. Kahane JC: Anatomic and physiologic changes in the aging peripheral speech mechanism. In Beasley DS, Davis GA (eds): *Aging: Communication Processes and Disorders*. New York, Grune & Stratton, 1981, p 21.

82. Kaplan M: *Leisure: Lifestyle and Lifespan*. Philadelphia, WB Saunders, 1979.

83. Karp DA, Yoels WC: *Experiencing the Life Cycle: A Social Psychology of Aging*. Springfield, IL, Charles C Thomas, 1982.

84. Kline DW, Schieber F: Vision and aging. In Birren JE, Schaie WK (eds): *Handbook of the Psychology of Aging*, ed 2. New York, Van Nostrand Reinhold, 1985, p 296.

85. Kolker A, Ahmed PI: Aging and society. In Kolker A, Ahmed PI (eds): *Aging*. New York, Elsevier Biomedical, 1982, p 17.

86. Kopace CA: Sensory loss in the aged: the role of the nurse and the family. *Nurs Clin North Am* 18:373–384, 1983.

87. Kosberg JI: The importance of attitudes on the interaction between health care providers and geriatric populations. In Kleinman MB (ed): *Interdisciplinary Topics in Gerontology*, vol 17. Basel, A Karger, 1983, p 132.

88. Kreps GL: Health communication and the elderly. *World Commun* 15:15–70, 1986.

89. Kukol RJ: Perceptual speech and voice characteristics of aging male and female speakers.

Ph.D. thesis, Wichita, KS, Wichita State University, 1979.

90. La Rue A, Cessonville C, Jarvik LF: Aging and mental disorders. In Birren JE, Schaie KW (eds): *Handbook of the Psychology of Aging*, ed 2. New York, Van Nostrand Reinhold, 1985, p 664.

91. Lazarus R, Olbrich E: Problems of stress and coping in old age. In Bergener M, Lehr U, Lange E, Schmitz-Scherzer R (eds): *Aging in the Eighties and Beyond*. New York, Springer, 1983, p 272.

92. Levin J, Levin WC: *Ageism: Prejudice and Discrimination against the Elderly*. Belmont, CA, Wadsworth, 1980.

93. Lieb-Brillhart B: Lifelong learning: a challenge for communication education. *Commun Educ* 27:142–145, 1978.

94. Liles B, Brookshire R: The effects of pause time on auditory comprehension of aphasic subjects. *J Commun Disord* 8:221–235, 1975.

95. Linebaugh CW, Cryzer KM, Oden SE, Myers PS: Reapportionment of communicative burden in aphasia: a study of narrative interaction. In Brookshire RH: *Clinical Aphasiology Conference Proceedings*, Minneapolis, BRK Publishers, 1982, p 4.

96. Linville PW: The complexity-extremity effect and age-based stereotyping. *J Pers Soc Psychol* 42:193–211, 1982.

97. Logeman J: Neurogenic swallowing disorders: evaluation and treatment. In Chapey R (ed): *Language Intervention Strategies in Adult Aphasia*, ed 2. Baltimore, Williams & Wilkins, 1986, p 437.

98. Lubinski R: Environmental language intervention. In Chapey R (ed): *Language Intervention Strategies in Adult Aphasia*. Baltimore, Williams & Wilkins, 1981, p 223.

99. Lubinski R: The environmental role in communication skills and opportunities of older people. In Wilder CN, Weinstein BE (eds): *Aging and Communication Problems in Management*. New York, Haworth Press, 1984, p. 47.

100. Lubinski R: Language and aging: an environmental approach to intervention. *Topics Lang Disord* 1:89–97, 1981.

101. Lubinski R: Why so little interest in whether or not old people talk: a review of recent research on verbal communication among the elderly. *Int J Aging Hum Dev* 9:237–245, 1978–1979.

102. Luterman D: *Counseling the Communicatively Disordered and Their Families*. Boston, Little, Brown, 1984.

103. McDonald ET, Chance B: *Cerebral Palsy*. Englewood Cliffs, NJ, Prentice-Hall, 1964.

104. McFarland CE, Warren LR, Crockard J: Memory for self-generated stimuli in young and old adults. *J Gerontol* 40:205–207, 1985.

105. Marge M: The prevention of communication disorders. *ASHA* 26:29–33, 37, 1984.

106. Marshal L: Auditory processing in aging listeners. *J Speech Hear Dis* 46:226–240, 1981.

107. Martin AD: Language problems in the elderly. In Wilder CN, Weinstein BE (eds): *Aging and Communication Problems in Management*. New York, Haworth Press, 1984, p 31.

108. Maurer JF: Introduction. In Jacobs-Condit L (ed): *Gerontology and Communication Disorders*.

Rockville, MD, American Speech-Language-Hearing Association, 1984, p 9.

109. Meyer BJF, Rice GE: The amount, type, and organization of information recalled from prose by young, middle and old adult readers. *Exp Aging Res* 7:253–268, 1981.

110. Middleton L: Friendship and isolation: two sides of sheltered housing. In Jerrome D (ed): *Ageing in Modern Society*. London, Croom Helm, 1983, p 255.

111. Molinari V, Reichlin RE: Life review reminiscence in the elderly: a review of the literature. *Int J Aging Hum Dev* 20:81–92, 1984–1985.

112. Moos RH, Lemke S: Specialized living environments for older people. In Birren JE, Schaie KW (eds): *Handbook of the Psychology of Aging*, ed 2. New York, Van Nostrand Reinhold, 1985, p 864.

113. Moscovitch M: Right hemisphere language. *Top Lang Disord* 1:41–62, 1981.

114. Muir Gray JA: Prevention of family breakdown. In Muir Gray JA (ed): *Prevention of Disease in the Elderly*. London, Churchill Livingstone, 1985, p. 83.

115. Myers PS: Right hemisphere communication impairment. In Chapey R (ed): *Language Intervention Strategies in Adult Aphasia*, ed 2. Baltimore, Williams & Wilkins, 1986, p 444.

116. Myers PS: Right hemisphere impairment. In Holland A (ed): *Language Disorders in Adults*. San Diego, College-Hill, 1984, p. 177.

117. Mysak ED: Treatment of deviant phonological systems: cerebral palsy. In Perkins WH (ed): *Current Therapy of Communication Disorders: Dysarthria and Apraxia*. New York, Thieme-Stratton, 1983, pp 3–33.

118. Newhoff M, Bugbee JK, Ferriera A: A change of PACE: spouses as treatment targets. In Brookshire RH: *Proceedings of the Clinical Aphasiology Conference*. Minneapolis, BRK Publishers, 1977, p 234.

119. Norris JE, Rubin KH: Peer interaction and communication: a life span perspective. In Lass N (ed): *Life Span Development and Behavior*, vol 6. New York, Academic Press, 1984, p 355.

120. Norris ML, Cunningham DR: Social impact of hearing loss in the aged. *J Gerontol* 36:727–729, 1981.

121. North AL, Ulatowska HK: Competence in independently living older adults: assessment and correlates. *J Gerontol* 36:576–582, 1981.

122. Obler LK, Albert ML: Language and aging: a neurobehavioral analysis. In Beasley DS, Davis GA (eds): *Aging: Communication Processes and Disorders*. New York, Grune & Stratton, 1981, p 107.

123. O'Hair D, O'Hair MJ, Kontas G: An examination of relational communication during physician and patient interaction. Presented at the Speech Communication Association Convention, Denver, 1985.

124. Olsho LW, Harkins SW, Lenhardt ML: Aging and the auditory system. In Birren JE, Schaie KW (eds): *Handbook of the Psychology of Aging*, ed 2. New York, Van Nostrand Reinhold, 1985, p 332.

125. Orchik DJ: Peripheral auditory problems and the aging process. In Beasley DS, Davis GA (eds): *Aging: Communication Processes and Disorders*. New York, Grune & Stratton, 1981, p 243.

126. Pashek GV, Brookshire RH: Effects of rate of speech and linguistic stress on auditory paragraph comprehension. *J Speech Hear Res* 25:377–382, 1982.

127. Patterson JM, McCubbin HI: Chronic illness: family stress and coping. In Figley CR, McCubbin HI (eds): *Stress and the Family*, vol 2. New York, Brunner/Mazel, 1983, p 21.

128. Perri S, Templer DI: The effects of an aerobic exercise program on psychological variables in older adults. *Int J Aging Hum Dev* 20:167–172, 1984–1985.

129. Petit TL: Neuroanatomical and clinical neuropsychological changes in aging and senile dementia. In Craik FIM, Trehub S (eds): *Aging and Cognitive Processes: Advances in the Study of Communication and Affect*, vol 8. New York, Plenum Press, 1982, p 1.

130. Pierce RS: Facilitating the comprehension of syntax in aphasia. *J Speech Hear Res* 25:377–382, 1982.

131. Pierce RC: Facilitating the comprehension of tense related sentences in aphasia. *J Speech Hear Disord* 46:364–368, 1981.

132. Piggren GW, Schmidt LD: Counseling the elderly. *Counsel Hum Dev* 14:1–12, 1982.

133. Pinkston Em, Linsk NL: *Care of the Elderly: A Family Approach*. New York Pergamon Press, 1984.

134. Poon LW: Differences in human memory with aging: causes and clinical implications. In Birren JE, Schaie KW (eds): *Handbook of Psychology of Aging*, ed 2. New York, Van Nostrand Reinhold, 1985, p 427.

135. Powers JK, Powers EA: Hearing problems of elderly persons: social consequences and prevalence. *ASHA* 20:79–83, 1978.

136. Ptacek PH, Sander EK: Age recognition from voice. *J Speech Hear Res* 9:273–277, 1972.

137. Query JL, Deller DR, Bonaguro EW: An assessment of communicative strategies employed by an elderly support group. Presented at the Speech Communication Association Convention, Denver, 1985.

138. Rabin DL: Waxing of the gray, waning of the green. In Committee on an Aging Society, Institute of Medicine and National Research Council: *America's Aging: Health in an Older Society*. Washington, DC, National Academy Press, 1985, p 28.

139. Rankin JL, Collins M: Adult age differences in memory elaboration. *J Gerontol* 40:451–458, 1985.

140. Rocheleau B: *Hospitals and Community Oriented Programs for the Elderly*. Ann Arbor, MN, AUPHA Press, 1983.

141. Rosenbek JC, LaPointe LL: The dysarthrias: description, diagnosis and treatment. In Johns DF (ed): *Clinical Management of Neurogenic Communicative Disorders*. Boston, Little, Brown, 1985, p. 97.

142. Ruben R, Druger B: Hearing loss in the elderly. In Plum F (ed): *The Neurology of Aging*. Philadelphia, FA Davis, 1983, p 123.

143. Rupp RR: Speech input processing, hearing loss, and aural rehabilitation with the elderly. In Obler LK, Albert ML (eds): *Language and Communication in the Elderly.* Lexington, MA, DC Heath, 1980, p 159.

144. Ryan EB, Capadano HL: Age perceptions and evaluative reactions toward adult speakers. *J Gerontol* 33:98–102, 1978.

145. Ryan EB, Giles H, Bartolucii G, Henwood K: Psycholinguistic and social psychological components of communication by and with the elderly. *Lang Commun* 6:91–98, 1986.

146. Ryan WJ, Burk KW: Perceptual and acoustic correlates of aging in the speech of males. *J Commun Disord* 7:181–192, 1974.

147. Salthouse TA: *Adult Cognition: an Experimental Psychology of Human Aging.* New York, Springer, 1982.

148. Salthouse TA: Speed of behavior and its implications for cognition. In Birren JE, Schaie KW (eds): *Handbook of the Psychology and Aging,* ed 2. New York, Van Nostrand Reinhold, 1985, p 400.

149. Savage RD, Gaber LB, Britton PG, et al: *Personality and Adjustment in the Aged.* New York, Academic Press, 1977.

150. Schallenkamp K, Swisher W, Pistulka L, et al: The communicative environment in settings for elderly persons. Presented at the American Speech-Language-Hearing Association Convention, Detroit, 1986.

151. Scherer KR: Personality markers in speech. In Scherer KR, Giles H (eds): *Social Markers in Speech.* Cambridge, Cambridge University Press, 1979, p 147.

152. Schmitt JF, Carrol MR: Older listeners' ability to comprehend speaker-generated rate alteration of pauses. *J Speech Hear Res* 28:309–312, 1985.

153. Schmitt JF, McCroskey RL: Sentence comprehension in elderly listeners: the factor of rate. *J Gerontol* 36:441–445, 1981.

154. Schneider EG: Stimulating communication in the institutionalized female geriatric population. Presented at the American Speech-Language-Hearing Association Convention, Detroit, 1986.

155. Schow RL, Christensen JM, Hutchinson JM, et al: *Communication Disorders of the Aged: a Guide for Health Professionals.* Baltimore, University Park Press, 1978.

156. Schuetz J: Lifelong Learning: communication education for the elderly. *Commun Educ* 29:33–41, 1980.

157. Shadden BB: Pre-crisis intervention: a tool for reducing the impact of stroke-related personal and family crisis. *J Gerontol Soc Work* 6:61–74, 1983.

158. Shadden BB, Raiford CA, Shadden HS: *Coping with Communication Disorders in Aging.* Tigard, OR, CC Publications, 1983.

159. Shadden BB, Raiford CA, Shadden HS: Pre-crisis intervention: preparing older Americans to cope with communication disorders. A short course presented at the American Speech-Language-Hearing Association Convention, Toronto, 1982.

160. Shewan CM, Cameron H: Communication and related problems as perceived by aphasic individuals and their spouses. *J Commun Disord* 17:175–187, 1984.

161. Shomaker D: Financial dilemmas. In Furukawa C, Shomaker D (eds): *Community Health Services for the Aged: Promotion and Maintenance.* Rockville, Aspen, 1982, p 83.

162. Shomaker D, Furukawa C: Working with groups of elderly. In Furukawa C, Shomaker D (eds): *Community Health Services for the Aged: Promotion and Maintenance.* Rockville, MD, Aspen, 1982, p 225.

163. Sies LF: *Aphasia Theory and Therapy: Selected Lectures and Papers of Hildred Schuell.* Baltimore, University Park Press 1974.

164. Simpson JM: Assessing attitudes toward old people. In Bromely DB (ed): *Gerontology: Social and Behavioral Perspectives.* London, Croom Helm, 1984, p 206.

165. Smith AD: Adult age differences in cued recall. *Dev Psychol* 13:326–331, 1977.

166. Smith MC: Portrayal of the elderly in prescription drug advertising. *Gerontologist* 16:329–334, 1975.

167. Smith SW, Rebok BW, Smith WR, Hall SE, Alvin M: Adult age differences in the use of story structure in delayed free recall. *Exp Aging Res* 9:191–195, 1983.

168. Soloman K, Vicker J: Attitudes of health workers toward old people. *J Am Geriatr Soc* 27:186–191, 1979.

169. Spilich GJ: Implications of cognitive change for gerontological pedagogical practice. *Int J Aging Hum Dev* 18:31–37, 1983–1984.

170. Stevens N, Wimmers M: Encounter groups with elderly persons: a supplement to the familial support systems. In Dooghe G, Helander J (eds): *Family Life in Old Age.* The Hague, Martinus Nijhoff, 1979, p 179.

171. Tamir LM: *Communication and the Aging Process.* New York, Pergamon Press, 1979.

172. Taub HA: Comprehension and memory of prose materials by young and old adults. *Exp Aging Res* 5:3–13, 1979.

173. Taylor EJ: *Counseling with Parents of Handicapped Children: Guidelines for Improving Communication.* New York, Grune & Stratton, 1977.

174. Taylor R, Ford G: Life style and ageing: three traditions in lifestyle research. *Aging Soc* 1:329–345, 1981.

175. Thomas P: Experiences of two preventative clinics for the elderly. *Br Med J* 2:357–360, 1968.

176. Troll LE: The psycho-social problems of older women. In Lesnoff-Caravaglia G (ed): *The World of the Older Women.* New York, Human Sciences Press, 1984, p 21.

177. Troll LE, Stapley J: Elders and the extended family system: health, family, salience, and affect. In Munnichs JMA, Mussen P, Olbrich E, Coleman PG (eds): *Life-Span and Change in a Gerontological Perspective.* New York, Academic Press, 1985, p 211.

178. US Bureau of the Census. In: *America in Transition: an Aging Society.* Current Population Reports, Series p-23, No. 128, 1983.

179. Walker VG, Hardiman CJ, Hedrick DL, Holbrook A: Speech and language characteristics of an aging population. In Lass N (ed): *Speech and Language: Advances in Basic Research and Practice*, vol 6. New York, Academic Press, 1981, p 143.

180. Walsh DA, Baldwin M, Finkle TJ: Age differences in integrated semantic memory for abstract sentences. *Exp Aging Res* 6:431–443, 1980.

181. Waltman MS: Attitudes toward the elderly: a constructivist review of past problems with suggestions for the future. Presented at the Speech Communication Association Convention, Denver, 1985.

182. Wan TTH: *Well-Being for the Elderly: Primary Preventive Strategies*. Lexington, MA, DC Heath, 1985.

183. Webb L: Mediated images of elders: an exercise in the case study of prime time TV. Presented at the Florida Speech Communication Association, Tampa, 1983.

184. Webster EJ, Newhoff M. Intervention with families of communicatively impaired adults. In Beasley DS, Davis GA (eds): *Aging: Communication Processes and Disorders*. New York, Grune & Stratton, 1981, p 229.

185. Welford AT: Social skill and aging: principles and problems. *Int J Aging Hum Dev* 17:1–5, 1983.

186. Wertz RT: Language disorders in adults: state of the clinical art. In Holland A (ed): *Language Disorders in Adults*. San Diego, College-Hill, 1984, p 1.

187. West RL, Boatwright LK: Age differences in cued recall and recognition under varying encoding and retrieval conditions. *Exp Aging Res* 9:185–189, 1983.

188. Whitbourne SK: *The Aging Body: Physiological Changes and Psychological Consequences*. New York, Springer-Verlag, 1985.

189. Wilcox MJ, Davis GA: Speech act analysis of aphasic communication in individual and group settings. In Brookshire RH: *Proceedings of the Clinical Aphasiology Conference*. Minneapolis, BRK Publishers, 1977, p 166.

190. Wilder CN: Management of speech and language disorders in the elderly: some general considerations. In Wilder CN, Weinstein BE (eds): *Aging and Communication Problems in Management*. New York, Haworth Press, 1984, p 41.

191. Williams I: *The Care of the Elderly in the Community*. London, Croom Helm, 1979.

192. Wingfield A, Poon LW, Lombardi L, Lowe D: Speed of processing in normal aging: effects of speech rate, linguistic structure, and processing time. *J Gerontol* 40:579–585, 1985.

193. Woodruff DS: A review of aging and cognitive processes. *Res Aging* 5:139–153, 1983.

194. Yairi E, Clifton NF: Disfluent speech behavior of preschool children, high school seniors, and geriatric persons. *J Speech Hear Res* 15:714–719, 1972.

195. Ylvisaker MY, Szekeres SF: Management of the patient with closed head injury. In Chapey R (ed): *Language Intervention Strategies in Adult Aphasia*, ed 2. Baltimore, Williams & Wilkins, 1986, p 474.

196. Yorkston KM, Dowden PA: Nonspeech language and communication systems. In Holland A (ed): *Language Disorders in Adults*. San Diego, College-Hill, 1984, p 283.

197. Zelinski EM, Light LL, Gilewski MJ: Adult age differences in memory for prose: the question of sensitivity to passage structure. *Dev Psychol* 20:1181–1192, 1984.

17 Communication and Dementia: A Clinical Perspective

LEE ANN C. GOLPER

Editor's Note

While there is no question that communication impairment is a prominent characteristic of the dementias, speech-language pathologists were involved minimally in the assessment and management of these patients until very recently. In Chapter 17, Golper suggests that clinicians can and should play a critical role in the process of diagnosing dementia and assisting all concerned individuals to find ways to maximize the patient's functional communication at any given point in the course of the disease process. In order to perform these roles effectively, the clinician must understand the causes, characteristics, and typical prognoses of the different dementia types, as well as the nature of medical and geropsychological diagnostic procedures. Chapter 17 proceeds to provide detailed information on each of these topics. The coexistence of dementia with other communication disorders (as in Parkinson's disease) is noted whenever appropriate. The final section of this chapter addresses treatment decisions. Golper indicates that, in some instances, we may need to provide direct speech-language treatment to an older client, in spite of the dementia. In other words, we may work with some other communication pathology despite the problems created by mild cognitive decline. The use of diagnostic-prognostic therapy may be helpful in these situations. In general, it is suggested that management decisions concerning appropriate professional roles are dictated by the clinical phase of the dementia.

INTRODUCTION

Chapter Focus

Consultation with geropsychology and geriatric speech-language pathology is becoming increasingly necessary and demanded in the management of patients with suspected or known dementia. To meet this demand clinicians need to be prepared to assist in diagnosing dementia and guiding patients, staff and families to wrestle with the task of maintaining optimal functional status in the presence of cognitive losses. Clinicians need a broad understanding of the diseases that produce dementia, the cognitive problems associated with dementia and the array of communication deficits that can emerge both in parallel with or as a function of dementia. Toward this end, this chapter focuses on a clinical perspective on dementia with a review of diagnosis and assessment in medicine and geropsychology, as well as an examination of the role and practices of speech-language pathologists with dementia patients.

A Growing Demand For Clinical Services

Short of death, dementia is certainly the worst possible consequence of the various debilitating diseases frequenting old age. It is also among the most prevalent and costly problems for health care management. As society has begun to appreciate the prevalence of dementia and its costs to the public, trends in the management of patients with cognitive problems have turned away from widespread neglect toward widespread intervention (46). Alzheimer's disease accounts for approximately 50 to 60 percent of the dementias (45, 65). It is said to affect 1.5 million Americans (approximately 15% of people over the age of 65) with an annual cost of $20 billion (45) and may be the fourth most common cause of death in the United States (46). Thus, research and increased clinical services involving Alzheimer's disease and related disorders are motivated both by the growing incidence of dementia and by its costs (both financial and personal) to society.

The drive to better understand and eradicate

diseases that cause cognitive problems in older persons, supported in large part by the National Institute on Aging, has altered our clinical perspective concerning dementia. "Senile dementia," "organic brain syndrome," and "senile psychosis" were once commonly used broad diagnoses for what are now recognized to be different and, in some cases, treatable disease states. We are no longer resigned to think of dementia as an unfortunate but natural consequence of aging. Rather, dementia is seen as a behavioral finding indicative of neurologic dysfunction. Identifying the source of this dysfunction is recognized as crucial to appropriate intervention. Patients routinely undergo a variety of procedures in the "dementia workup" to identify treatable conditions, yet the clinical diagnosis of disorders such as Alzheimer's type dementia is currently arrived at largely by the process of exclusion of other causes of dementia. Although Alzheimer's type dementia is not yet considered reversible, substantial research efforts are underway to identify the cause, or causes, of the disorder with the hope of finding a rational means of therapeutic intervention for this prevalent and devastating disease (46).

The public attention given to the dementias, along with the increasing incidence of these disorders, has produced a demand for better clinical assessment and behavioral treatment. In many settings the "rehabilitation model," "geriatric assessment programs," (52), or "OARS" methodology (17) have replaced the traditional "medical model" in geriatric patient care. Although the medical management of dementia sits at the center of diagnosis, rehabilitation and long-term care for affected persons, the expertise of allied health professionals for assessment outside of the medical domain has achieved a level of prominence unknown in past decades (66).

Rationale for Services to Dementia Patients in Geriatric Speech-Language Pathology

Appreciating that there is a growing need, or *market*, for services to the cognitively impaired elderly, is there a corresponding *rationale* for such services? If we consider "epidemiologic probabilities," a substantial proportion of patients over age 65 with speech and language disorders could be predicted to have associated subclinical or clinically significant intellectual deficits. Speech-language pathologists have an accepted, long-standing history of working with patients who have certain types of motor speech disorders (for example, pro-

gressive supranuclear palsy and parkinsonism) known to have associated cognitive deficits. Some patients with a primary aphasia have sufficient additional cognitive deficits to be said, according to some definitions, to have dementia (15). Providing speech and language services to patients with some degree of dementia is not only rational but often unavoidable.

Speech-language pathologists have traditionally viewed themselves as the professionals best prepared to diagnose, assess, and treat speech and language behaviors and pathologies. In the past 20 years this role has become generalized, or perhaps more broadly defined, to "specialists in communication disorders." Even this broader definition fails to entirely encompass the breadth of practices by speech-language pathologists. For example, speech-language pathologists routinely address the communication problems of language and learning disabled children (including severely developmentally delayed children and autistic children). We have become specialists in the selection and application of augmentative communication systems (e.g., computerized speech synthesis devices). We examine many forms of breakdown in interpersonal communication and provide counseling therapies. We are taking tentative steps into cognitive reorganization programs for the head injured person. And we have generalized our knowledge about the vocal tract to the deglutition tract and have become consultants in the management of dysphagia.

Speech-language pathologists have consistently followed an inclination to participate in educational, medical, or rehabilitation decisions whenever specialized knowledge about *communication processes*, or the functions of cranial muscle groups, could contribute to better assessments, more accurate diagnoses, and more appropriate interventions. This inclination, coupled with the social, epidemiological and medical practice trends discussed earlier, has naturally led to a move toward expanding speech-language pathology services in geriatric health care programs and, accordingly, our contact with cognitively impaired older persons has increased.

GERIATRIC PRACTICE

As we attempt to place our traditional knowledge bases into the new context of geriatric practice, particularly if we are going to assess cognitive status, we need to be aware of factors that might influence communicative-cognitive performance. Most of these factors, as well as other important concerns, are reviewed in detail elsewhere in this text. To highlight the problems, however, it is useful to consider that many of the impaired elderly patients referred to us will have:

- sensory losses in all modalities;
- multiple medical problems with many of the chronic risk factors for central nervous system (CNS) damage;
- a need for more than three prescribed medications which may have direct or interaction effects on CNS functions;
- less than 8 years of formal education;
- limited financial and social supports;
- risk factors for affective disorders (depression);
- a subclinical or clinically significant dementia.

What this means is that *most* of the impaired elderly individuals referred for speech-language pathology services will present with disorders that are complicated by sensory losses, general health problems, medications, and dementia. Elderly patients with impaired speech or impaired language without these complicating factors are exceptional.

THE DEMENTIA SYNDROME: A HOLISTIC PERSPECTIVE

Wang (63) has illustrated the interaction of primary and secondary factors in the dementia syndrome and discussed dementia as a "bio-psycho-social disorder" that consists of many components. According to Wang's "holistic view of dementia," one needs to examine individuals for *primary components* within the context of *secondary components* of the syndrome. Primary components include: the structural changes in the brain; cognitive impairments; and clinical and behavioral manifestations associated with dementia. Secondary components include: functional or metabolic disorders of the brain; physical illnesses; depression, inactivity, social deprivation; and intrapsychic factors, interpersonal factors and environmental factors. Wang's model provides a comprehensive, multifaceted perspective on dementia that fits nicely with the interdisciplinary team approach to evaluation and management and the rehabilitation model for geriatric health care services. Management is an amalgam of various disciplines (medicine, psychology, nursing, social work, rehabilitation therapies, and/or speech-language pathology). Speech and language disorders, as behavioral manifestations, need to be appreciated in the contexts of struc-

tural changes in the brain, metabolic disorders, and physical illness as well as the underlying cognitive disorders. Thus, medical and psychological assessments are critical to an appreciation of the communication disorders of dementia.

Dementia Evaluation in Geriatric Medicine

"Dementia is a symptom complex of many causes and is not a disease" (20, p 232). In other words, dementia is the behavioral manifestation of disease processes. A crucial issue in the management of dementia is the identification of the disease culprit; consequently, dementia evaluation by the physician is pivotal to appropriate management.

Most patients with dementia will be seen initially by a physician (usually an internist or general practitioner). Sometimes patients go directly or are referred to specialists such as neurologists, geropsychiatrists, or geriatricians (who are usually internists with at least a one year subspeciality training in geriatric medicine). Some forms of dementia occur as a late-stage consequence of diseases that have been diagnosed; for instance patients with certain motor neuron diseases, such as amyotrophic lateral sclerosis (ALS), may eventually have cognitive losses. Such patients are not likely to undergo an extensive series of tests to determine the cause for their dementia.

However, when dementia is suspected and the etiology is not clear, the physician usually conducts a "dementia workup" the breadth of which will vary depending upon the signs, symptoms and indicators gathered from the history, physical examination and clinical neurologic examination. The description of the onset of problems will alert the physician to possible underlying diseases and disorders.

Physician's Examination

When the course of the illness is described as gradual or progressive ("We've noticed problems with dad's memory for about a year now" or, "My memory got so bad I finally had to give up playing bridge a few months ago"), the possibility of an Alzheimer's type dementia is considered. Typically these patients, or their families, complain of generic "memory problems" and cite impaired abilities to do some sort of routine task, such as balance the checkbook or find their way in a shopping mall. Often it is an observant relative who first notices a lack in initiative, reduced interest in work or neglect of routine tasks (67). Complaints of either a gradual or abrupt onset of fatigue, memory problems, impaired concentration, restlessness, decreased appetite, and changes in sleep patterns may be suggestive of metabolic or other illnesses or may indicate a psychiatric problem, such as depression. Depression is both a common cause of cognitive impairment in the elderly and a common symptom of early dementia (37). These complaints, therefore, need to be actively pursued to find treatable conditions.

Patients who show a reduced awareness of the environment and appear to have a "clouded state of consciousness" may have some form of delirium, rather than dementia. Misdiagnosis of delirium is a serious problem, because the conditions causing delirium can lead to permanent brain damage, dementia, or death (69). The diagnostic criteria for delirium according to the American Psychiatric Association (1) are summarized after Zisook and Braff (69) in Table 7.1.

An abrupt onset of signs and symptoms of a more focal nature can suggest the possibility of various cerebrovascular diseases, cardiovascular disease, or neoplasms ("Last Thursday I was sitting in my car and I noticed I was having a problem with my eyes, my vision went gray and then came back; ever since then I haven't been able to think straight"). The initial descriptions coupled with a general medical history give the physician some directions, or suspicions, to explore. As part of the medical history the physician will ask questions about: past neurologic problems; use of alcohol; treated cancer; any family history of neurologic or psychiatric illness; medications, use of nonprescription drugs, or ingestation of toxins; prior gastric surgery (predisposing the patient to vitamin B_{12} deficiency); and thyroid disease. Some of the treatable causes of dementia include:

(1) Depression;
(2) Medication toxicity;
(3) Endocrine/metabolic disorders;
(4) Systemic illness;
(5) Nutritional disorders;
(6) Sensory deprivation;
(7) Intracranial mass;
(8) Chronic CNS infection.

The physician's physical examination is directed toward ruling out any medical illness that might cause cognitive losses. Principal disorders that receive focus in the examination are: hypertension, anemia, liver disease, malignancies, infections, and uremia. The neurologic examination will be directed toward finding any evidence of focal motor or sensory losses as well as a cursory assessment of higher cortical functions. Physicians typically examine memory functions by testing: *immediate recall* of digits forward and backward; *recent memory* of the names of three objects recalled by the patient after 3 to 5 minutes of intervening distraction; and *remote memory* of previous personal or world events (e.g., "Who was the president before Carter?") Some physicians will also ask patients to name several common and less common objects (watch, stethoscope, watch crystal) and may examine concentration and calculation by asking the patient to count by serial sevens backward from 100 (93, 86, 79, 72, 65. . .). Other physicians, such as geriatricians or geropsychiatrists, however, might conduct more formal mental status examinations and screening tests.

Laboratory and Neuroradiologic Tests

At this point in the medical examination the physician will determine the need to order various laboratory tests. An extensive battery of

Table 17.1
Diagnostic Indicators for Delirium[a]

- Clouding of Consciousness
- At least one of the following:
    Perceptual disturbance (misinterpretations, illusions, or hallucinations)
    Incoherent speech
    Disturbed sleep-wake cycle
    Abnormal psychomotor activity (increased or decreased)
- Disorientation and memory impairment
- Clinical features developing over a short period of time (hours to days) and fluctuating over the course of the day
- Evidence from history, physical examination, or laboratory tests of specific organic etiologies

[a] Modified from Zisook S, Braff DL: Delirium: recognition and management in the older patient. *Geriatrics* 41: 67–68, 1986; APA: *Diagnostic and Statistical Manual of Mental Disorders*, ed. 3. Washington, DC, APA, 1980.

screening tests has been recommended by the Task Force on Aging (46). These tests include: blood and urine analyses; complete blood count (CBC); erythrocyte sedimentation rate (ESR); serum electrolytes (sodium, potassium, chloride, carbon dioxide); serum calcium and phosphate; renal function tests, blood urea nitrogen (BUN) or serum creatinine; serum thyroxine (T_4); serum lipids; serum vitamin B_{12}; and serologic tests for syphilis (STS). Patients also undergo chest and skull x-rays, electroencephalograms (EEGs), computed tomography of the brain (CT scans), and lumbar punctures. When indicated by the history or physical examination, the physician may order a metastatic survey, toxic screen of urine and/or blood, angiography, brain biopsy, and viral and fungal titers. CT scanning is a routine and valuable diagnostic procedure in the dementia workup. Tumors, infarctions, hydrocephalus, basal ganglia atrophy (e.g., caudate atrophy in Huntington's disease) and cortical atrophy (sulcal enlargement and ventricular dilation) can be readily identified by these scans. However, CT scans are less useful in the differential diagnosis of earlier stages of degenerative disorders, depression, or metabolic and toxic disorders (12, 13, 23).

This broad spectrum medical examination is *typical* for patients presenting with intellectual or cognitive problems of unknown etiologies. Physicians will make a brief assessment of cognitive impairments and behavioral manifestations, but will focus their diagnostic efforts primarily on the physical examination and laboratory tests looking for illness or brain dysfunction. In some cases (for example, normal pressure hydrocephalus, NPH) mental status may dramatically improve or the progression of cognitive declines may be arrested with medical or surgical therapies. However, the majority of patients ultimately diagnosed as having early dementia of the Alzheimer's type (DAT) are likely to have normal laboratory and neuroradiologic findings during their initial workup.

Clearly the use of an extensive battery of screening tests to rule out other causes and diagnose DAT by exclusion is not very cost effective. Consequently the search for biological markers to identify patients with DAT is economically important. Examples of such research include studies of: immunocytochemistry of paired helical filaments (30); fibroblast phosphofructokinase activity (55); erythrocyte lithium countertransport rates (16); platelet monoamine oxidase activity (3); and philothermal response (43). Until biological markers are found to reliably and unequivocably detect DAT, the diagnosis may best rest with clinicians trained and experienced in recognizing the cognitive/behavioral problems strongly suggestive of Alzheimer's type progressive degenerative dementia.

Dementia Evaluation in Geropsychology

Patients with early dementia usually come to the attention of clinicians such as geropsychologists (or neuropsychologists with a geriatric practice) because the physician, or the geriatric team, would like a broad behavioral assessment to confirm or rule out a suspicion of DAT versus some other dementing disease versus depression. Lezak (39) speculates that "probably the most common diagnostic request for neuropsychological assessment of elderly persons involves patients who appear to be demented" (39, p 3). Clinical diagnostic methods in geropsychology described in Teri and Lewinsohn (59), Reisberg et al (50), and by Houlihan (unpublished data from Geropsychological Assessment in Dementia. presented at the Western Regional Conference of the American Speech-Language-Hearing Association, Seattle, WA, 1986) are summarized here for the purposes of illustrating the breadth of testing dementia patients typically undergo and describing the features considered important in the geropsychologist's (or in some settings, psychiatrist's) differential diagnosis of dementia etiologies.

Geropsychology Screening

The clinical diagnostic assessment by geropsychology typically begins with a patient and family (or "significant other") interview. In addition to reviewing the medical history, the psychologist will ask questions to elicit descriptions of concerns, the functional decrements noticed, and the emotional impact of these problems on the patient and family. Information about the patient's and family's attitudes, activities, and expectations will be elicited at this time. The psychologist will attend to clues or subjective evidence of memory problems (such as whether or not the patient can answer questions or tends to defer to a family member, or problems such as distractibility).

A screening for dementia will usually be made at the time of the initial interview. The *Mini-Mental State* (22), for example, is administered to identify the presence of clinically significant dementia. Several behavioral rating scales are also available and allow for ratings of severity based on either behavioral observations and descriptions or task performance. Such scales include: *Dementia Behavioral Scale* (27); *Short Portable Mental Status Questionnaire* (48); *Brief Cognitive Rating Scale* (50); and *Dementia Rating Scale* (42). These screening tests and rating scales are usually a prelude to a more comprehensive battery of tests and assessments.

Geropsychological Assessment

The purpose of psychological assessments with dementia patients is principally to provide a diagnosis, along with a functional description and a base for treatment planning. The domains examined and some of the tests that may be used to examine those areas are outlined in Table 17.2.

Strub and Black (57) emphasize that dementia cannot be identified unless cognition, language, memory, visuospatial skills, and personality are assessed. Cummings *et al* (14) stipulate that the diagnosis of dementia requires

a *persistent* loss of intellectual activity in "at least three" of the following areas: language, memory, visuospatial abilities, emotion, personality, and cognition (mathematics, abstraction, judgment, executive planning, and so forth). Neuropsychological screening tests for dementia, such as the *Mini-Mental State* (22), and testing across various pertinent domains of intellectual functions are largely tests of *verbal functions* in that these tests contain a proportionately high number of items requiring verbal abilities (information, vocabulary, and memory tasks) (39). Although the Cummings *et al* (14) criteria for dementia require identification of multiple areas of deficit, patients with mild latent *aphasia* (affecting their comprehension of directions, verbal memory, verbal formulation, reading comprehension, and manipulation of numerical symbols) are not going to perform very well on several of the tasks and instruments listed below. Therefore, language testing by the speech-language pathologist may be necessary to help clarify the differential diagnosis.

Table 17.2
Geropsychological Assessment with Dementia Patients (59)[a]

Domains Examined	Tests
Memory	
Attention and concentration	Wechsler Memory Scale (64)
Storage and retrieval	Inglis Paired-Associates (31)
Working memory, recent memory, remote memory	Benton Visual Retention Test Multiple Choice Form (8)
Verbal, nonverbal, visuospatial	
Cognition	
Intelligence	WAIS-R (65)
Concept learning	Raven's Progression Matrices (49)
Arithmetic ability	
Abstract reasoning	
Language	
Naming	Boston Naming Test (33)
Comprehension	Western Aphasia Battery (35)
Reading	Boston Diagnostic Aphasia Examination (26)
Writing	
Visuospatial and Visuomotor	
Visuospatial memory	Rey Complex Figure (47)
Recognizing/copying shapes	Bender-Gestalt (7)
Personality	
Affect	Rorschach (51)
Mood	Beck Depression Inventory (6)
Thought content	
Activities of Daily Living	
Self-care activities	OARS (17)
Personal business and finances	Functional Assessment (38)
Ambulation/driving	
Job performance	

[a] Modified from Houlihan J: Geropsychological assessment in dementia. Presented at the Western Regional Conference of the American Speech-Language-Hearing Association, Seattle, WA, 1986.

DEMENTING DISEASES AND COMMUNICATION

Etiologies

Descriptions of the clinical features of diseases causing dementia are published elsewhere (cf. Chapter 11 of this text; 12, 24, 25, 67). Although the various diseases associated with dementia have characteristic neurologic, medical, cognitive, and behavioral manifestations, there is considerable evidence favoring both *pathologic differences* and *similarities* between syndromes (32, 34, 44, 56). Wells (65) provided frequency data for various dementing diseases based on a series of cases from three neurological centers. It is interesting to note that at least 1 in 20 patients in his review were ultimately found to have a reversible psychiatric disorder simulating dementia (depression or *pseudodementia*). The impact of a primary or secondary depression on cognitive functions in the elderly has received considerable attention in the psychiatric literature. Shraberg (54) challenged the concept in his discussion of the "myth of pseudodementia," while Feinberg and Goodman (19) argued that an association between depression and dementia is common. They suggested groups of patients may be found to have: (*a*) depression presenting as dementia; (*b*) dementia presenting as depression; (*c*) depression with secondary dementia; and (*d*) dementia with secondary depression.

Depending upon the disease culprit and the stage of progression, one can predict that dementing diseases produce a wide range of communication problems. Associated speech or language pathologies can include: dysfluencies; dysarthrias; mutism; jargon aphasia; anomia and word retrieval problems; and confused language. Bearing in mind also that some patients will have a "mixed bag" of communication deficits, we will briefly review here *dysarthria* occurring in association with dementia, speech and language problems with multifocal disease or *multi-infarct dementia* and, finally, the *semantocognitive* deficits associated with dementia of the Alzheimer's type (DAT).

Deficits in Parallel with Dementia

Dysarthria with Dementia

Earlier it was noted that speech-language pathologists routinely evaluate and treat *speech* pathologies associated with a number of movement disorders and motor neuron diseases known to have an increased frequency of associated dementia. In medical settings, commonly seen dysarthria-producing diseases include: parkinsonism; amyotrophic lateral sclerosis (ALS); progressive muscular atrophy (PMA); primary lateral sclerosis (PLS); progressive bulbar palsy (PBP); progressive supranuclear palsy (PSP); Huntington's disease; multiple sclerosis; olivopontinecerebellar degeneration; and cerebellar atrophy.

The dysarthric characteristics one finds with these diseases are well-known in speech-language pathology (see Tonkovich, Chapter 11 of this book). Describing speech characteristics, assessing levels of intelligibility, and helping patients make adjustments in rate, volume, phonation, articulation, respiration and resonance, as well as providing assistive augmentative devices when indicated, are standard practices for speech-language pathologists. However, except in cases where dementia is readily apparent (such that treatment cannot be achieved), the need for identification of a coexisting dementia is rarely discussed. Determining the presence of dementia in patients with motor neuron and extrapyramidal movement disorders can be difficult. One must circumvent gross motor deficits and decreased speech intelligibility as well as account for any mood, attention, or memory problems that result from drug toxicity. However, since the presence of dementia can influence the nature of and prognosis for speech rehabilitation, dementia screening should be a part of the diagnostic workup with these disorders.

Severe dementia is an inevitable finding in late-stage Huntington's disease and verbal memory disorders are early focal signs (9). Approximately 5% of patients with ALS will have severe dementia and another 5 to 10% will have language difficulties (62). Patients diagnosed to have parkinsonism have an even greater incidence, with 20 to 40% found to have severe dementia of the Alzheimer's type (56). This increased frequency of Alzheimer's disease in parkinsonism has caused some researchers to propose similar etiologic mechanisms for these two disorders (56). It should be noted here that *parkinsonism* is not always the result of *Parkinson's disease*. The cause of Parkinson's disease is not all that well understood but is broadly attributed to a premature aging process that affects the nerve cells of the substantia nigra. Clinically similar states mimicking Parkinson's disease can also be induced by neuroleptics, encephalitis, and atherosclerosis (18). When these causative factors are known, the patient is more accurately said to have parkinsonism (e.g. "drug-induced parkinsonism"). Thus, diagnoses based solely on clinical symptomatology need to be considered when examining research with parkinson's patients or planning treatment.

Bayles and her associates (5) found that groups of patients with mild Alzheimer's disease, moderate Parkinson's and Huntington's disease differed significantly from normals on judgments of sentence meaning, while groups of patients with mild Parkinson's disease and mild Huntington's disease did not differ significantly from normal performance (though their scores were lower than those of normals). Antiparkinson's medications are known to produce confusional states that are often mistaken for dementia (56). One ought not, of course, to presume the presence of dementia without performance testing. Matthews and Haalund (41) pointed out that the impoverished facial expression of parkinsonism belied the level of intellectual acuity, giving a false impression of apathy, depression, and dementia (53).

Multiple Infarctions and Dementia

Elderly patients with cerebrovascular disease make up a large proportion of the caseload in geriatric speech-language pathology. Patients with completed strokes producing dysarthria or aphasia often have a history of previous small strokes, transient ischemic attacks (TIAs), or resolved ischemic neurologic deficits (RINDs). A history of multiple strokes is usually, though not always, a negative factor in treatment prognosis. We sometimes characterize a communication problem as "aphasia plus" or "dysarthria plus," indicating that the patient appeared to have an underlying confusion or dementia deserving further analysis before proceeding with treatment. The source of these cognitive deficits will often, for want of a better explanation, be attributed to "multi-infarct dementia."

Multi-infarct dementia (MID) is a commonly used diagnosis denoting a cumulative loss of cognitive abilities as the result of multiple cerebrovascular insults. These patients are described as having a stepwise deterioration in mental abilities in association with a history of hypertension and strokes. Typically, these are multiple, bilateral lacunar infarcts in the internal capsule and deep gray structures. The diagnosis of MID is arrived at primarily from CT scan evidence of one or more old cerebral infarcts co-occuring with behavioral evidence of dementia. In his review, however, Kase pointed out that the "coexistence of cerebral infarcts and dementia does not imply a cause and effect relationship" (34, p 482). Kase (34) found limited pathologic support for the concept of MID, referring to studies by Tomlinson et al (60, 61) and Fisher (21) where nondemented patients had been found to have multiple lacunar infarcts in the internal capsule and basal ganglia. Kase suggested that dementia with multifocal infarctions may be due to one or more critical features: the total *volume* of brain lesions; the *location* of the lesions; and/or the underlying presence of Alzheimer's disease.

Tomlinson et al (61) found total lesion volumes of at least 150 to 200 ml to be correlated with dementia, while smaller lesion volumes were calculated in "nondemented" subjects (34). Relative to the location of a dementia-producing lesion, some theories of the etiology of Alzheimer's disease have implicated neurotransmitter reductions originating in subcortical nuclei degeneration, namely, the *nucleus basalis of Meynert* (11). Thus, the suggestion is that infarctions of brain substrate for cholinergic neurotransmitter activity might lead to an Alzheimer's type dementia. Such a notion does not entirely account for dementia with multiple infarctions. Judd and his co-workers (32) compared cognitive performances (using a brief cognitive status screening assessment) and cerebral blood flow (CBF) measures in patients with MID and AD. These authors found a loss of vasomotor responsiveness (reduced CBF) among MID patients but not AD patients, suggesting a vascular etiology for dementia with multiple infarction. Clearly, one finds within this controversy a need for better clinicopathologic analysis of MID, as Kase suggests, and better cognitive performance correlations.

These issues have an important bearing on speech and language analysis following multiple infarctions. Multifocal lesions do not necessarily produce a clinically significant dementia, but MID is a common finding in patients with multiple infarctions, accounting for about one quarter of dementia cases. Prominent speech and/or language deficits and "patchy" cognitive losses will also result from multifocal disease (24). One could predictably find upper motor neuron-type dysarthria, apraxia of speech, and/or aphasia within this population. Determining the primary deficits is both difficult and necessary, requiring knowledge of speech and language processes as well as an understanding of the broader impact of the dementia state itself on communication.

Before leaving this discussion of MID, one neurologic syndrome thought to be the result of a *single* lesion in the area of the angular gyrus of the dominant hemisphere, the so-called "angular gyrus syndrome" (15), deserves special attention. Cummings and his co-workers

(15) reported three cases of patients who had been diagnosed to have Alzheimer's disease but were later found to have focal lesions of the dominant hemisphere in the area of the angular gyrus. These cases had clinical features that the examining neurologists thought to be indistinguishable from DAT. The patients had fluent, paraphasic verbal output, notably lacking in content. All were agraphic; two had impaired language comprehension; and two had alexia. They all had acalculia, left-right disorientation, finger agnosia, and constructional impairments. All were said to have failed "most cognitive tasks" and complained of difficulty remembering. Presumably these features contributed to a misdiagnosis of DAT. Cummings et al (15) emphasized that determining "angular gyrus syndrome" from DAT is "difficult but of obvious significance for prognostic and therapeutic purposes" (15, p 618), stating further that the misdiagnosis of the angular gyrus syndrome as DAT is not uncommon and that "these individuals may represent an important portion of the dementia population" (15, p 619). Communicative behaviors may point to critical diagnostic differences between focal infarction syndromes and DAT (see Table 17.3).

Deficits Resulting from Dementia

Language in Alzheimer's Type Dementia

The preceding sections have emphasized the frequent associations between dementia-producing diseases and certain "primary" speech or language disorders. As examples, it was noted that aphasia can be a primary feature for some patients with MID and that dysarthria can be a primary finding in patients with certain movement disorders and dementia. It was also noted that Alzheimer's type neuropathologies can be found in association with other disorders. It is not at all clear whether or not Alzheimer' disease uniquely contributes to the cognitive deficits found in some patients with MID or Parkinson's disease, or whether the mechanisms of these latter disorders themselves produce clinicopathologies indistinguishable from DAT. Given this frequent relationship between DAT and other disease states, and the preponderance of DAT among dementia-producing states, specific attention to the language characteristics of DAT is warranted.

Table 17.4 summarizes the typical language findings in Alzheimer's patients at early, middle, and late stages of the disease process, after descriptions in Bayles and Kaszniak (4). In the absence of confounding problems (i.e., additional neurologic insults from other causes) Alzheimer's type dementia produces a gradual erosion of the *semantic* features of language and *pragmatic* features of interpersonal communication. Some authors have suggested that the relative preservation of phonologic, grammatical, and morphosyntactic features in the verbal expression of severely demented persons indicates that these language subsystems are more "tightly wired" neurolinguistic processes (2, 58, 68). Bayles (5) contends that since more mental operations are required to access semantic knowledge, one finds characteristic losses of lexical-semantic language subsystems in association with dementia. Semantic proc-

Table 17.3
Comparison of Findings with Alzheimer's Disease and "Angular Gyrus Syndrome"[a]

Alzheimer's Disease	Angular Gyrus Syndrome
Insidious, gradual onset with associated declines in memory functions and personality	Abrupt onset with deficits remaining static or remitting
Fluent aphasia in later stages (anomia and paraphasias)	Fluent aphasia (anomia and/or paraphasias in spontaneous speech)
Auditory comprehension, naming repetition, and reading are progressively impaired	Auditory comprehension, naming, repetition, reading abruptly impaired
Often unaware of their language problems	Apologetic and frustrated by their language problems
Semantic substitutions have less and less relation to the intended verbal production	Semantic paraphasias are usually related to the target word
Reading aloud may be retained	Reading aloud is seriously affected

[a] Modified from Cummings, JL, Benson DF, Tsai SY: Angular gyrus syndrome simulating Alzheimer's disease. Arch Neurol 39:616–620, 1982.

Table 17.4
Characteristics of Communicative Behavior in Early, Middle, and Late Stages of Alzheimer's Disease[a]

Stage	Phonology	Grammar	Words/Content	Usage
Early	Unimpaired	Generally correct	Omits meaningful word; reduced vocabulary; complains of problems thinking of the word	May have difficulty understanding humor or sarcasm
Middle	Unimpaired	Some sentence fragments and difficulty understanding complex sentences	Difficulty thinking of words within a category; impaired naming; reliance on automatisms	Rarely corrects a mistake; may be insensitive to conversational partners
Late	Generally correct; may have some phonologic paraphasias	Sentence fragments and deviations are common; fails to comprehend grammatical forms	Marked anomia; jargon; bizzare content	Unable to produce a sequence of related ideas; inappropriate repetitive utterances

[a] Modified from Bayles KA, Kaszniak A: *Communication and Cognition in Normal Aging and Dementia in the Elderly.* San Diego, College-Hill Press, 1987.

esses are particularly vulnerable in dementia because: "The associative matrices of words in the mental dictionary disintegrate and stimuli ultimately fail to elicit the appropriate target" (5, p 165). Similarly, pragmatic processes (knowledge about how, why and when to use various utterance forms) depend upon mental abstractions, awareness of context, and sensitivities to the intentions underlying utterance forms. These higher level language processes become gradually diminished as dementia progresses.

The "Aphasia" of Dementia. Physicians and psychologists may describe demented patients as aphasic if they have a notable difficulty talking and lack a prominent dysarthria. The demented patient who is mute as a function of generally decreased psychomotor activity brought on by diffuse bifrontal cortical degeneration will be described as aphasic. The patient who cannot follow directions or misnames common objects because he fails to recognize them, and the patient who fails to answer questions in a complete, coherent, and meaningful manner or shows a paucity of referential

nouns in verbal discourse, will be described as aphasic. Speech-language pathologists recognize that in many cases this label is not accurate, as it belies the source of the deficit.

Speech-language pathologists view "aphasia" as a psychological disruption in *primary language processes.* It is this language disruption, not a lack of initiation, attention, mental vigilance, or orientation, that "gets in the way" of the aphasic patient's communication efforts. Patients with aphasia have an intention to communicate, know what they want to say, and struggle with finding the form to say it. However, if one were to consider only *verbal test scores* (which, of course, one ought not to do) patients in the mid to late stages of DAT may not be easily distinguishable from patients with a primary aphasia without dementia (29). When dementia patients become mute or are found to have phonologic paraphasia and grammatical and morphosyntactic errors in their verbal output, "aphasia of dementia" joins the list of their cognitive deficits. At this point they are also likely to be incontinent, unable to walk, and entirely dependent upon others for their physical needs (50).

Evaluation in Speech-Language Pathology

Many impaired elderly patients have subclinical (not readily apparent) cognitive declines. Therefore, they may come to the attention of a speech-language pathologist without the diagnosis of dementia. Subtle indicators of cognitive problems emerging from the patient and family interview or the patient's test performance can be examined further with mental status tests, or a referral can be made for a full-scale geropsychological assessment.

Patients with mild dementia will complain of difficulty thinking of the words and names they want. During language testing these patients have particular difficulty with generative naming (naming within a specified class) and impaired verbal memory for grammatically complex sentences or paragraphs. They may have difficulty understanding written stories in reading tasks or generating written narratives. Since mildly aphasic persons can have similar problems, it is frequently quite difficult to distinguish language deficits due to early Alzheimer's disease from mild anomic aphasia due to focal damage. If early Alzheimer's disease versus mild aphasia cannot be determined from the initial clinical assessment coupled with the patient's history, then patterns of either improvement or declines in subsequent evaluations may be needed to establish the diagnosis.

Assessment Tasks for DAT

Bayles and Kaszniak (5) suggest that a language assessment battery for dementia patients focus on active, nonautomatic, generative and reasoning tasks. These tasks are found in the *Arizona Battery of Communication Disorders in Dementia* (5). Even with such a battery, diagnosis would necessarily rest with *interpretation* of performance on a wide range of verbal and nonverbal tasks. To capture verbal impairments with dementia, standard speech and language tests and assessments can be applied. Assessments of functional communication (like the CADL) (28) or tests examining for particular neurolinguistic or psycholinguistic deficits (like the ITPA) (36) can be useful. If there appears to be a prominent dysarthric component, then an oral motor and speech assessment should be made. Those areas that have been generally recommended for analysis of the language abilities of dementia patients include:

1) Orientation
2) Naming—confrontation, responsive, and generative
3) Analysis of written and oral discourse
4) Conversational style
5) Verbal memory and sentence comprehension
6) Verbal repetition
7) Interpretation of idioms and proverbs
8) Sentence construction and written discourse
9) Reading
10) Numerical functions
11) Drawing
12) Pantomime expression
13) Spatial recognition memory

Verbal testing with dementia patients is done for the purposes of arriving at an accurate diagnosis, appreciating the degree and characteristics of the verbal impairment, identifying concerns that need to be considered by either the staff or family in their interactions with the patient, and determining if there are any areas potentially remediable with speech-language pathology services. Some patients have undergone extensive medical and psychological testing before they are seen by a speech-language pathologist, while others come to speech-language pathology first with "speech problems" as the chief complaint. Clinicians should do as little and as much evaluation as is necessary to answer questions that affect diagnosis, staff and family education, and treatment options as well as to determine the need for further medical and/or psychological consultation. Any patient suspected of having dementia who has not been seen by a physician or not examined for this condition should be referred for a medical consultation.

DECISIONS IN TREATMENT

Decisions in appropriate management options for patients with communication problems in the context of dementia require a circumspect attitude from the clinician. When dementia is not a florid deterrent to treatment and it appears that some benefits can be gained, we are likely to make adjustments and allowances for the patient's decreased ability to learn a new skill. Hopefully, in such cases we are not treating dementia; we are treating speech and language disorders. We occasionally provide speech or language rehabilitation *in spite of* dementia, not *because of* dementia.

Clinical Phases of Dementia

The identification (from test performance) of very mild, mild, moderate, severe, or profound cognitive problems and observations of functional decrements are the primary indicators of the *clinical phases* of dementia—early, midstage, and late-stage dementia. Thus stages, or phases, of dementia are somewhat arbitrary, broad descriptions of severity. Usually stages of dementia are applied when describing patients with *progressive degenerative dementia* (PDD) (1), as in Alzheimer's disease. Patients with diseases such as Creutzfeldt-Jakob's disease may progress rapidly to late-stage dementia. Patients with MID may have cognitive deficits that remain static for some time or change dramatically from mild to profound impairment following a devastating stroke. The degree of cognitive losses and the functional declines, along with the etiology, have a major impact on decisions in treatment. These factors will direct the scope of the therapy and may weigh negatively in the prognosis for response to patient-directed therapy.

Mild Cognitive Decline

We acknowledged earlier that direct speech and language rehabilitation may be entirely appropriate in some cases with patients who have mild dementia. In cases where the speech or language impairments take prominence over a mild loss of intellectual abilities (at what Reisberg et al (50) called the "forgetfulness" and "early confusional" stages), treatment may be prudent, even if its effects are short-lived. For example, some parkinsonian patients can be taught to make use of delayed auditory feedback devices to slow down speech rate and increase intelligibility despite mild dementia. A laryngectomized person with mild or moderate cognitive declines would not, in most settings, be left without speech rehabilitation, even though he may require a longer than average course of instruction in the use of esophageal speech or an electrolarynx. A patient with a prominent aphasia who has other associated (and presumably static or remitting) cognitive deficits may be viewed as a treatment candidate with a "guarded" prognosis.

Golper and Rau (25) discussed the use of "diagnostic-prognostic therapy," the intent of which is to ascertain the efficacy of patient-directed treatment services. They suggest that patients with prominent speech or language deficits and a suspected associated dementia may require a *brief* treatment trial as part of the diagnostic assessment to determine the prognosis for an effective response to a more extended therapy. Treatment services to patients with bilateral, multiple infarctions, for example, ought to be undertaken with a diagnostic-prognostic intent. The purpose of this treatment trial should be carefully discussed with the family, staff, and patient. Although some patients are alert, attentive, and seem to be able to participate in the treatment milieu, frank evidence of general intellectual losses requires us to proceed cautiously in treatment.

Moderately Severe to Profound Cognitive Decline

When dementia is clearly recognized as the primary problem for management, *direct* speech and language treatment is neither indicated nor warranted. The patient's impaired vigilance and stimulability, along with an inability to learn new skills, will mitigate against speech and language rehabilitation strategies.

In such cases, speech-language pathologists become a source of information about communication and strategies to make the best of residual abilities. The environmental adjustments, aptly described by Lubinski (40, and this book), that promote communicative opportunities ought to be explored. Clinical strategies to maximize communication functioning by reducing the handicaps of attention and memory deficits may need to be explicitly described and demonstrated to staff and family members. Clinicians generally suggest that the staff or family:

1. Provide *orientation* to time, place, and person using verbal reminders as well as written signs, calendars, clocks, etc.
2. Provide *structure* and routine in all activities (meals, dressing, trips).
3. Provide *communication opportunities* at a time when the patient is not fatigued and in a manner that reduces distractions.

Staff and family members may need to be reminded to gain the patient's maximal attention before asking questions or making requests and to use redundancy, gestures, pointing to objects, paraphrases and repetitions to increase comprehension. Additional assistance to family members in the form of education, referral to local and national support groups, and counseling to increase their understanding and to develop problem solving and coping strategies is a crucial aspect of patient management with dementia patients (see Chapter 19, this text).

SUMMARY

In the foregoing discussion we have examined dementia and communication from a clinical perspective by appreciating a number of "clinical realities" in geriatric speech-language pathology. Due to the prevalent and rising incidence of dementia in geriatric practice, there exists a frequent and an increasing demand to extend services to patients with cognitive losses.

Communication pathologies associated with dementia are varied and complex. Like other neurogenic communication disorders, they must be understood as behavioral manifestations occuring in the context of structural changes in the brain and the resultant cognitive deficits. Consequently, the medical and psychological aspects of dementia have an important bearing on assessment and management of demented persons. Additionally, the speech-language pathologist's noninvasive behavioral tests can differentiate dementia from aphasia and help to diagnose clinical syndromes. Behavioral therapies for patients with known or suspected dementia should proceed cautiously. When patients have a prominent speech or language disorder and a mild underlying dementia, patient-directed treatment services may be indicated. With more severely impaired patients treatment should focus on the staff and family needs for education, counseling, and support services.

Most speech-language pathologists in hospital practice have extensive clinical experience with patients who have generalized intellectual deficits. In geriatric programs, such patients are the rule rather than the exception. Thus far, however, research in dementia from the perspective of the speech-language pathologist is extremely limited. An expanded knowledge base in communication pathologies associated with dementia is needed and, hopefully, forthcoming.

References

1. American Psychiatric Association: *Diagnostic and Statistical Manual of Mental Disorders*, ed 3. Washington, DC, American Psychiatric Association, 1980.
2. Appell F, Kertesz A, Fisman M: A study of language functioning in Alzheimer patients. *Brain Lang* 17:73–91, 1982.
3. Alexopoulos GS, Lieberman KW, Young RC, Shamoian CA: Monoamines and monoamine oxidase in primary degenerative dementia. In Shamoian CA (ed): *Biology and Treatment of Dementia in the Elderly*. Washington, DC, American Psychiatric Press, 1984, p 58.
4. Bayles KA, Kaszniak A: *Communication and Cognition in Normal Aging and Dementia*. San Diego, College-Hill Press, 1987.
5. Bayles KA: Communication in dementia. In Ulatowska H (ed): *The Aging Brain*. San Diego, College-Hill Press, 1985, p 157.
6. Beck SJ, Ward CH, Mendelson M, Mock J, Erbaugh JK: An inventory for measuring depression. *Arch Gen Psychiatry* 4:561–571, 1961.
7. Bender LA: A visual motor gestalt test and its clinical use. *Am Orthopsychiatr Assoc Res Monogr* 3:1938.
8. Benton AL: *The Revised Visual Retention Test*, ed 4. New York, Psychological Corporation, 1974.
9. Butters N, Sax D, Montgomery K, Tarlow S: Comparison of the neuropsychological deficits associated with early and advanced Huntington's disease. *Arch Neurol* 35:585–589, 1978.
10. Calkins E: OARS methodology and the "medical model." *J Am Geriatr Soc* 33:648–649, 1985.
11. Coyle JT, Price DL, DeLong MR: Alzheimer's disease: a disorder of cortical cholinergic innervation. *Science* 219:1184–1186, 1983.
12. Cummings JL: Dementia: neuropathological correlates of intellectual deterioration in the elderly. In Ulatowska H (ed): *The Aging Brain*. San Diego, College-Hill Press, 1985, p 53.
13. Cummings JL, Benson DF: *Dementia: A Clinical Approach*. Boston, Butterworths, 1983.
14. Cummings JL, Benson DF, LoVerme S Jr: Reversible dementia. *JAMA* 243:2434–2439, 1983.
15. Cummings JL, Benson DF, Tsai SY: Angular gyrus syndrome simulating Alzheimer's disease. *Arch Neurol* 39:616–620, 1982.
16. Diamond JM, Matsuyama SS, Meier K, Jarvik LF: Elevation of erythrocyte transport rates in Alzheimer's dementia. *N Engl J Med* 309:1061–1062, 1983.
17. Duke University Center for the Study of Aging and Human Development: *Multidimensional Functional Assessment: The OARS Methodology*, ed 2. Durham, NC, Duke University, 1978.
18. Duvoisin RC: *Parkinson's Disease: A Guide for Patient and Family*, ed 2. New York, Raven Press, 1984.
19. Feinberg T, Goodman B: Affective illness, dementia and pseudodementia. *J Clin Psychol* 45:99–103, 1984.
20. Fisher CM: Dementia and cerebrovascular disease. In Toole JF, Seikert RG, Whisnant JP (eds): *Cerebrovascular Disease: 6th Conference*. New York, Grune & Stratton, 1968, p 232.
21. Fisher CM: Lacunar strokes and infarcts: a review. *Neurology* 32:871–874, 1982.
22. Folstein MF, Folstein SE, McHugh PR: "Minimental state": a practical method for grading the cognitive state of patients for the clinician. *J Psychiatr Res* 12:189–198, 1975.
23. Fox J, Topel J, Huckman M: The use of computerized tomography in diagnosis of senile dementia. *J Neurol Neurosurg Psychiatry* 38:948–953, 1975.
24. Golper LAC, Binder LM: Communicative behavior in aging and dementia. In Darby JK (ed): *Speech Evaluation in Medicine*. New York, Grune & Stratton, 1981, p 225.
25. Golper LAC, Rau MT: Treatment of communication disorders associated with generalized intellectual deficits in adults. In Perkins WH (ed): *Current Therapies of Communication Disorders*. New York, Thieme-Stratton, 1983, p 119.

26. Goodglass H, Kaplan E: *Assessment of Aphasia and Related Disorders*. Philadelphia, Lea & Febiger, 1972.

27. Haycox FA: A behavioral scale for dementia. In Shamoian CA (ed): *Biology and Treatment of Dementia in the Elderly*. Washington, DC, American Psychiatric Press, 1984, p 2.

28. Holland AL: *Communicative Abilities in Daily Living*. Baltimore, University Park Press, 1980.

29. Horner J: Language disorder associated with Alzheimer's dementia, left hemisphere stroke and progressive illness of uncertain etiology. In Brookshire RH (ed): *Clinical Aphasiology: Vol. 15*, Minneapolis, BRK Publishers, 1985, p 149.

30. Ihara Y, Abraham C, Selkoe DJ: Antibodies to paired helical filaments in Alzheimer's disease do not recognize normal brain proteins. *Nature* 304:727–730, 1983.

31. Inglis J: An experimental study of learning and "memory function" in elderly psychiatric patients. *J Ment Sci* 103:796–803, 1957.

32. Judd BW, Meyer JS, Rogers RL, Gandhi S, Tanahashi N, Mortel KF, Tawaklna T: Cognitive performance correlates with cerebrovascular impairments in multi-infarct dementia. *J Am Geriatr Soc* 34:355–360, 1986.

33. Kaplan E, Goodglass H, Weintraub S: *The Boston Naming Test*. Boston, E Kaplan and H Goodglass, 1978.

34. Kase CS: "Multi-infarct" dementia: a real entity? *J Am Geriatr Soc* 34:482–484, 1986.

35. Kertesz A: *Western Aphasia Battery*. New York, Grune & Stratton, 1980.

36. Kirk SA, McCarthy JJ, Kirk WD: *The Illinois Test of Psycholinguistic Abilities*, revised ed. Urbana, IL, University of Illinois Press, 1968.

37. Larson EB, Reifler BV: Dementia in elderly outpatients: a prospective study. *Ann Intern Med* 100:417–423, 1984.

38. Lawton MP: The functional assessment of elderly people. *J Am Geriatr Soc* 19:465–481, 1971.

39. Lezak MD: Neuropsychological assessment. In Teri L, Lewinsohn PM (eds): *Geropsychological Assessment and Treatment: Selected Topics*. New York, Springer, 1986, p 3.

40. Lubinski R: Environmental language intervention. In Chapey R (ed): *Language Intervention Strategies in Adult Aphasia*, ed 1. Baltimore, Williams & Wilkins, 1981, p 223.

41. Matthews CG, Haalund KY: The effect of symptom deviation on cognitive and motor performance in Parkinsonism. *Neurology* 29:951–956, 1979.

42. Mattis S: Mental status examination for organic mental syndrome in the elderly patient. In Bellak L, Karasu TB (eds): *Geriatric Psychiatry*. New York, Grune & Stratton, 1976, p 77.

43. Matsuyama SS, Fu TK, Kessler JO, Jarvik LF: The philothermal response and the diagnosis of dementia of the Alzheimer's type. In Shamoian CA (ed): *Biology and Treatment of Dementia in the Elderly*. Washington, DC, American Psychiatric Press, 1984, p 49.

44. Meyer JS, Largen JW, Shaw T, Mortel KF, Rogers R: Interactions of normal aging, senile dementia, multi-infarct dementia and alcoholism in the elderly. In Hartford JT, Samorajski T (eds): *Aging and Alcoholism*. New York, Raven Press, 1984, p 227.

45. National Center for Health Statistics: *Vital Statistics of the United States, 1978, Vol. II, Section 5: Life Tables*. Department of Health and Human Services Publication No. (OHS) 81-1104. Washington, DC, US Government Printing Office, 1980.

46. National Institute on Aging: *A National Plan for Research on Aging: Report of the National Research on Aging Planning Panel*. NIH Publication No. 82-2453, 1982.

47. Osterrieth PA: Le test de copie d'une figure complexe. *Arch de Psychol* 30:206–356, 1944.

48. Pfeiffer EA: Short portable mental status questionnaire for the assessment of organic brain deficit in the elderly. *J Am Geriatr Soc* 23:433–441, 1975.

49. Raven JC: *Guide to Standard Progressive Matrices*. London, HK Lewis, 1960.

50. Reisberg B, Ferris S, Anand R, Buttinger C, Borenstein J, Sinaiko E, deLeon M: Clinical assessments of cognition in the aged. In Shamoian CA (ed): *Biology and Treatment of Dementia in the Elderly*. Washington, American Psychiatric Press, 1984, p 16.

51. Rorschach H: *Psychodiagnostics: A Diagnostic Test Based on Perception*. Berne, Huber, 1942.

52. Rubinstein LZ, Kane RL: Geriatric assessment programs: their time has come. *J Am Geriatr Soc* 33:646–647, 1985.

53. Scott S, Caird FI, Williams BO: *Communication in Parkinson's Disease*. Rockville, MD, Aspen Publication, 1985.

54. Shraberg D: The myth of pseudodementia: depression and the aging brain. *Am J Psychiatr* 135:601–603, 1978.

55. Sorbi S, Blass JP: Fibroblast phosphofructokinase in Alzheimer disease and Down syndrome. *Banbury Rep* 15:297–308, 1983.

56. Stern MB, Gur RC, Saykin AJ, Hurtig HI: Dementia of Parkinson's disease and Alzheimer's disease: is there a difference? *J Am Geriatr Soc* 34:475–478, 1986.

57. Strub RL, Black FW: *The Mental Status Examination in Neurology*. Philadelphia, F.A. Davis, 1977.

58. Swartz MF, Marin OSM, Saffran EM: Dissociations of language function in dementia: a case study. *Brain Lang* 7:277–306, 1979.

59. Teri L, Lewinsohn, PM: *Geropsychological Assessment and Treatment: Selected Topics*. New York, Springer, 1986.

60. Tomlinson BE, Blessed G, Roth M: Observations on the brains of non-demented old people. *J Neurol Sci* 7:331–336, 1968.

61. Tomlinson BE, Blessed B, Roth M: Observations on the brains of demented old people. *J Neurol Sci* 11:205–211, 1980.

62. Tyler HR: Nonfamilial amyotrophy with dementia or multisystem degeneration and other neurological disorders. In Rowland LP (ed): *Human Motor Neuron Diseases*. New York, Raven Press, 1982, p 173.

63. Wang HS: Dementia of old age. In Smith WL, Kinsbourne M (eds): *Aging and Dementia*. New York, Spectrum Publications, p 1.

64. Wechsler D: A standardized memory scale for clinical use. *J Psychol* 19:87–95, 1945.

65. Wechsler D: *WAIS-R Manual*. New York, Psychological Corporation, 1981.

66. Weiman HM: Rowing together: OARS and teamwork. *J Am Geriatr Soc* 34:485–486, 1986.

67. Wells CE (ed): *Dementia: Contemporary Neurology Series*, ed 2. Philadelphia, FA Davis, 1977.

68. Whitaker HA: A case of isolation of the language function. In Whitaker H, Whitaker HA (eds): *Studies in Neurolinguistics*, vol. 2. New York, Academic Press, 1976, p 1.

69. Zisook S, Braff DL: Delirium: recognition and management in the older patient. *Geriatrics* 41:67–78, 1986.

18 A Model for Intervention: Communication Skills, Effectiveness, and Opportunity

ROSEMARY LUBINSKI

Editor's Note

The preceding five chapters have addressed specific management considerations in clinical interventions emphasizing the older communicatively impaired client. The remaining chapters, grouped loosely under the subheading "Completing the Programming Cycle," explore ways to extend our outreach to communication environments, partners, and the community of older persons in general. Lubinski's comments in Chapter 18 provide an excellent starting point for this outreach. In this chapter, the problems involved in service provision in long-term care settings are identified. The communication needs of institutionalized elderly are described as including: communication skills; communication effectiveness; and communication opportunity. Each of these needs can be addressed through a different therapeutic approach. The Skills Approach is more traditional and familiar to speech-language pathologists and audiologists. Specific speech-language-hearing deficits are targeted, and the treatment program is designed to improve skills in the deficit areas. Lubinski argues that this type of approach may be minimally effective with a large number of older persons in institutional settings. In contrast, the Effectiveness Approach stresses improvement of the individual's communication through any channel and demands the involvement of one or more frequent communication partners. The Opportunity Approach focuses upon improving communication opportunities by enhancing the physical and social environment. Lubinski describes each of these approaches in detail and discusses factors influencing their implementation. A carefully conceived series of questions guides the clinician through the process of deciding which approach or combination of approaches is best suited to a particular client. Case history examples illustrate clinical applications.

Speech-language pathologists and audiologists working in long term care settings face a myriad of complex problems and frustrations in providing quality communication services to elderly patients and their care givers. The problems stem from the nature of the persons we serve and the institutional environment itself. This is compounded by rules and regulations which force us into a traditional and often stagnant model of providing communication services in this setting. The purpose of this chapter is to discuss; (a) the difficulties of working in a long term care setting; (b) the communication needs of the elderly in nursing home settings;

(c) options for providing service there; (d) factors affecting service delivery; (e) the decision-making process in best fitting service to patient/caregiver needs; and (f) case illustrations of alternative service delivery models. The basic philosophy permeating this chapter is that communication disorders specialists *do have* alternatives in providing services in nursing home settings.

PROBLEMS IN WORKING IN LONG-TERM CARE SETTINGS

Nursing home patients do not mirror the text book cases offered in our educational settings or the typical practicum placement. The patients screened, diagnosed, and seen for therapy are old or very old, have multiple physical, psychological, social, and emotional problems, and often have severe, longstanding communication problems. The average age of a nursing home patient is 78 years old (63), and average length of residence in that setting is about 2 years (63). Further, the average nursing home patient has 3.9 chronic illnesses requiring extended nursing care (63). These physical problems are multiplied by difficulties performing daily living activities, feelings of rejection, isolation, depression, anger, and frustration. Many nursing home patients also present cognitive disorders including dementia. Cummings and Benson (12) reviewed prevalence estimates of dementia and found that Alzheimer's disease accounted for 39% of dementias; at least 30% of nursing home patients had some form of severe dementia. Thus, the patients seen are likely to have a complex of problems of which the communication disorder is just one.

Further, it is difficult to differentially diagnose the basis of the communication disorder from effects of aging, physical and psychological problems, and effects of institutional life. For example, a patient may have Parkinson's disease, a profound hearing loss, a sometimes missing hearing aid, a broken arm from a fall, a "diagnosis of dementia" and a recent series of transient ischemic attacks. This is also a patient who has outlived most of her family and has few visitors. She is considered a "difficult patient" primarily because it is difficult to assess and meet her needs.

A second problem in working in this setting is that there may be a lack of or limited carryover of skills gained in traditional therapy to everyday life. This is a major frustration faced by communication disorders specialists. Several reasons exist for the lack of carryover. First,

the therapy targets designed for these patients may be unrealistic. For many of these severely multihandicapped persons, the goals must be framed in terms of "improved overall intelligibility" and "use of alternate communication means," rather than "perfection, normality and specificity of sound or word production." It is unreasonable to expect an 83-year-old woman who has dysarthria secondary to a stroke to produce perfect sibilant sounds when her dentures are loose, she is emotionally labile, hates being in a nursing home, worries about her home-bound cognitively impaired husband, and has very few visitors other than staff whom she perceives negatively. Traditional, sound correction therapy may result in little carryover for this person.

Carryover is also limited because patients may have few opportunities to use skills gained in therapy. Lubinski (41, 42, 45) stated that communicatively impaired nursing home patients are not viewed as viable communication partners by other patients. Patients want to talk to "normal" persons who are interesting, take the time to interact, and listen actively. Furthermore, many staff do not understand the value of communicating with elderly patients, perceive themselves as too busy to communicate, and limit their communication to care giving tasks. If the patient is to improve and maintain communication skills, there must be ample time to use them in meaningful contexts, ones which enhance the person's contributory role to that environment.

Unfortunately, many patients become "institutionalized" (1, 5, 6, 31) to this environment and expect very little from their caregivers in terms of socialization or communication (40, 42, 45). Communication attempts on the part of the patient with the staff may be extinguished through lack of response or curt, condescending replies. Further, as stated above, patients do not perceive each other as potential partners especially when the other patient is viewed as incompetent, disheveled, or communicatively impaired (40, 42, 45). Thus, there are few opportunities to communicate, and patients gradually but surely expect less communicative interaction from their environment. Motivation to improve or maintain communication skills may be meager and may deteriorate as the environment remains unreinforcing.

In addition to patient characteristics which reduce opportunities, the staff may present some negative attitudes toward the patients which reduce interaction. A number of studies (7, 9, 23, 61) indicate that nursing home staff may negatively view their positions in that setting and the patients they serve. In particular, a problem exists at the basic service level in the nursing home—that of the nursing assistant or aide. The nursing aide, while having the greatest work burden in the nursing home and the greatest potential face-to-face interaction time with the patients, is the least paid and perhaps the most poorly regarded by our culture. These individuals often have limited educational backgrounds and may be poorly motivated to work with the elderly. Nursing aides require meaningful, repeated inservice to educate them to their important communication role with the elderly (33).

Yet another major problem faces communication disorders specialists in nursing homes. Funding sources such as Medicare and Medicaid and other third party carriers view the role of the speech pathologist and audiologist from a medical model. The communication disorder specialist is expected to quickly specify the nature of the problem, provide therapy often for a regulated number of sessions, and document progress on standardized measures. Considering the multiplicity of chronic and severe problems these patients may have, specifying a diagnosis is a frequent difficulty, and one which cannot be overcome easily through use of existing standard tests. Differential diagnosis may take a number of sessions, including reviewing previous medical, psychological, and neurological testing, discussion with staff and family, and repeated interaction and observation of the patient in a natural context. Unfortunately, all too often there are few or no previous medical/psychological results to help form a diagnosis, and time constraints limit observation to the testing situation.

Further, the amount of therapy is scrutinized by review boards, and funding may be discontinued because of obvious lack of progress. Documenting progress with elderly multihandicapped individuals presents a host of problems, similar to those given above. For some of these persons, progress may be better indicated by the number of increased interactions regardless of performance perfection. For others, progress may be the increased willingness to use an alternate means of communication such as a communication board. For still others, progress may be maintaining present level of communicative competence in the face of progressive neurological disorders and deterioration. Thus, progress as measured by percentage of words gained in therapy or correct sound productions may be difficult to document.

The traditional rehabilitation model of individual therapy may not be the best model for many nursing home patients. Speech-language pathologists in this setting are developing a growing awareness that there is also a much larger population of potential clients than those with specific speech, language and hearing problems (40, 42, 45). Many of the patients have adequate communication skills but spend their days sitting, dozing, and interacting minimally with either fellow patients or staff members. When asked, however, these same patients say that they want to talk, enjoy talking, but do not find opportunities to interact in the nursing environment with meaningful partners. Lubinski (40, 42, 45) calls this a "communication impaired environment." Most funding sources, however, are not cognizant of this concept, and therefore will not pay for "therapy" other than in the traditional sense.

There is another problem which mitigates our role in long-term care settings: our own willingness to challenge what and how we can provide quality, meaningful communication services in this setting. For some speech-language pathologists, nursing homes are a quantity to be collected. Rather than become a visible participant in a nursing home, some provide infrequent services. Chapey et al (8) found that most nursing homes are served by part-time speech-language pathologists and have no on-site or regular audiologist. Weinstein and Lubinski (65), in a recent study of communication services in nursing homes in New York State, found a similar pattern with proprietary or for-profit nursing homes providing the least amount of both speech and audiological services. Some communication disorders specialists find it difficult to justify a visit to a nursing home for one or two patients, particularly when these are the difficult multihandicapped persons described above. It is easier to describe these individuals as "not a potential therapy candidate" than to face the frustrations of trying to meet their needs. This results in little visibility in the nursing home and thus fewer referrals, less interaction with administrators and staff, and of course, less therapy for patients.

The lack of communication services in long-term care settings has created a problem in New York State. In 1986 New York State began conducting a pilot project in conjunction with Medicaid for the funding of services to nursing home patients. RUGS (resource utilization groups) is a prospective rate payment method whereby patients are categorized upon admission to the setting according to the number and type of services they will require (similar to DRGs, or diagnostic related groups, in acute care hospitals) (16). Speech therapy and audiology were specifically excluded from the category of rehabilitation. While the exclusion of speech therapy from the rehabilitation category is being reconsidered, it still may present potential problems for communication disorders specialists. The initiation of RUGs in New York State highlights the fact that communication disorders specialists need visibility and viability in long-term care institutions. Speech-language pathologists and audiologists who wait for referrals and then discount many clients as too severe for rehabilitation may be perceived by administrators as the "norm." This satisfies the administrators' requirement that they have a consultant and eliminates paying for services and interacting more frequently with a communication disorders specialist.

COMMUNICATION NEEDS OF THE ELDERLY

One of the basic tenets of our profession is that diagnosis and therapy should be individualized for each patient or client, meeting their specific communication deficits and capitalizing on their particular communication strengths. This holds true for the elderly person in a long term care setting. Elderly individuals may have one or more of the following broad communication needs: communication skill, communication effectiveness, and communication opportunity.

Communication Skills

Communication skill is defined as the ability to receive, interpret, and send messages through verbal and nonverbal means. Communication skills include speaking, listening, reading, writing and nonverbal systems such as gesture. Skill is dependent on functional adequacy of the neurological system underlying communication, the adequacy and coordination of the individual components of the speech and hearing mechanisms, cognitive skills prerequisite for understanding and forming messages, and knowledge of the rules of interacting with others. Thus, communication skill results from a complex of internal mechanisms all of which require precision and coordination.

Communication skills may be affected by the normal process of aging and also the potential pathologies of aging. For example, hearing changes associated with aging for many individuals affect comprehension and eventually interaction opportunities for the older person (10, 26, 29, 46, 49, 50, 56). Visual changes also change receptive information which is a basis for communicative topics (22). Further, some researchers indicate that there may be normal cognitive changes with regard to memory (11,

64), problem solving, learning, and cognition (18, 19, 64), which in turn may alter the communication act. Something as common as loss of teeth or new or poorly fitting dentures may affect how the individual communicates and perceives him or herself as a communicator.

Furthermore, many elderly individuals incur one or more severe, usually nonreversible pathologies affecting the neurological or speech mechanism including stroke, trauma, dementia, cancer, and progressive diseases (63). These may directly affect speech, language and hearing skills resulting in specific communication problems.

Communication Effectiveness

A second communication need of the elderly is communication effectiveness. This is defined as the success a person has in receiving and sending communication messages irrespective of communication skill itself. Communication impairment does not mean that the individual cannot find alternate ways to send messages to meet daily personal needs. Some severely communication impaired persons effectively communicate with one or more members of their environment through intonation, gesture, pointing, and other nonverbal means. Some communication partners are able to decode sound and word errors in an effort to interact more successfully with the speech-language-hearing impaired older person. Communication effectiveness requires that the elderly person want to communicate and have a partner who is willing to work at understanding this new communication system. Having a desire to communicate forces individuals to be creative in finding ways to impart their messages.

Communication effectiveness balances the burden of communication between the communication impaired older person and those in his or her environment. Communication through any means possible becomes the goal rather than perfect production or reception. It requires the deliberate concerted effort and tolerance on the part of the communication partners to understand the messages produced, to decipher phonological and paraphasic distortions and errors, and to reinforce the use of alternate means of communication. At a time when an elderly individual may have a host of severe problems, it helps to have partners who share in the work of communicating and who do not expect normal communication. Further, the reinforcement received from being able to communicate effectively may encourage the individual to work to maximum to improve specific skills. Thus, communication effectiveness involves working with potential communication partners to understand speech and language breakdowns and to facilitate message adequacy. It may also involve making these persons aware of the usefulness and viability of alternate means of communication such as communication boards and electronic devices.

Communication Opportunity

The third communication need of the elderly is communication opportunity. Communication opportunity is defined as the presence of desired partners, meaningful activities, and an attitude which values the participation of the elderly person in a communicative event. It is insufficient to have adequate communication skills and a variety of means to communicate if the individual does not have a real need to communicate. Skills and effectiveness become more meaningful when the elderly person has a physical and social context in which to use them.

Opportunities to communicate stem from the person's external physical and psychosocial environment and from his or her internal need to communicate. The external environment creates the arena for ideas to arise and interaction to occur. The physical environment must be conducively arranged to facilitate communication. For example, the acoustic and visual properties of the environment must be such that elderly persons can see and hear potential partners within a reasonable distance. The physical environment must contain stimulating props, and ambulation within the environment must be easily accessible. Further, the environment must be a socially accepting and reinforcing one for the older person. Simply stated, they must have an environment which stimulates ideas and interaction, encourages communication attempts, and responds meaningfully to any type of message sent.

ALTERNATIVES IN INTERVENTION WITH THE ELDERLY

Alternatives in providing service to the elderly in long-term care settings flow from their communication needs. The three alternatives include the Skill Approach, Effectiveness Approach, and Opportunity Approach. These are not meant to be mutually exclusive, though particular emphasis may be placed on one approach with an elderly patient, depending on needs. These approaches are applicable to any type of communication disorder.

The Skill Approach

The Skill Approach focuses on improving the specific speech, language and/or hearing disorders of the elderly patient. This is our traditional approach to working with the communicatively impaired person. The schematic below outlines the sequence of events and the goal of this approach.

The Skill Approach begins with identifying the specific areas of need, usually through standardized tests which can be repeated for documentation of progress. For individuals with aphasia this may be administration of any of a number of standardized aphasia tests or batteries, including the Boston Diagnostic Aphasia Examination (25), the Minnesota Test for the Differential Diagnosis of Aphasia (57), the Porch Index of Communicative Ability (51) and the Western Aphasia Battery (32). In addition there are numerous other tests which focus on specific areas of evaluation such auditory comprehension (15, 47, 58) and reading (35). These tests which vary in focus and design provide a structured profile of comprehension and expression skills. Similarly, for the individual with dysarthria, administration of structured word and sentence articulation tests (20, 66, 67) or more informal but comprehensive assessment procedures (54) provides specific skill information. For the individual with voice problems a variety of speech science instruments contribute quantifiable data to describe areas of need (3). Peripheral, central and speech discrimination hearing evaluations also provide hard data describing the individual's hearing disorder (2).

Once the areas of need are defined, the clinician determines the goal and format of therapy in the Skill Approach. Activities tend to be highly structured and involve learning principles such as imitation, discrimination, problem solving and self-evaluation (e.g., 17, 48, 52, 53, 55). Therapy tasks also tend to be "acontextual," in that the individual practices drills or exercises outside of real-life situations in which the stimuli might be used. For example,

THE SKILL APPROACH

| Disordered individual | $\longrightarrow$ | Specific skill therapy | $\longrightarrow$ | Improvement documentation | $\longrightarrow$ | Perfection normality |

the individual listens to a clinician production of a target, imitates it, receives an evaluation or self-evaluates the production and continues on to the next set of similar targets. The patient is usually not included in the decision making regarding what skills to improve in therapy nor the stimuli for practice. These are clinician determined as is the sequence of therapy. The clinician may keep a daily log of number of trials and percentage of correct, improving or incorrect responses. The clinician usually provides homework and encourages the elderly person to practice daily.

While this approach may work for some cases, it has a number of inherent difficulties in it, especially for the older nursing home patient. The older person may not fully understand how the drills facilitate everyday comprehension and production. Practice of homework may be seen as child-like and demeaning. Others in the environment may expect the individual to be able to carryover skills immediately to conversation and when this is not possible, may consider therapy a waste of time. Thus, the individual patient and those in the environment may have different expectations from therapy; when these are not met, therapy becomes an exercise in futility. Funding agencies supporting therapy may consider a few percentage points of improvement either on a monthly basis or on repeated test measures as insufficient for continued financial reimbursement. Families paying for therapy may have even greater expectations for improvement when the cost of therapy is added onto expensive monthly charges for nursing home care.

Underlying this alternative to nursing home therapy is the fact that normal communication is the goal for all patients in this setting. Normal communication is defined as the type of communication skills the person had previous to severe chronic illness, institutionalization and perhaps changing cognitive skills. While this may be a reasonable goal for some, return to normal may be unrealistic, unfair, and futile for many of the most impaired persons in a long-term care setting. Placing an unrealistic burden on the older person to perfect his or her speech in the face of myriad other problems is poor judgment on the part of the speech pathologist or audiologist.

The Effectiveness Approach

In contrast, the Effectiveness Approach stresses improving the individual's ability to receive and transmit messages through any means possible with the aid of a trusted, facilitating communication partner. Thus, the burden for communicating and repairing any communication breakdowns is shared between the elderly patient and his or her partners (39, 44). Therapy involves both the communication impaired person and any significant communication partners who are available (21). In the nursing home setting this might include the individual's roommate, favorite communication partner, nurses from each shift when possible, and nursing assistants directly involved in daily care. Family members should also be included when possible. The schematic below outlines the principles and sequence of events in this approach.

The primary goal of this approach is that the patient communicate through any means possible. Thus, goals may involve improved speech intelligibility, gesture, pointing, writing, letter, picture or word communication boards, or electronic devices. Second, the message sent does not have to be structurally perfect. The message is evaluated on its transmission adequacy. Third, the primary communication partners must be involved in therapy. Their role is to work with the individual during communication breakdowns to facilitate better communication adequacy. For example, the partner might use a variety of repair strategies such as providing cues, hints, questions and corrections to help the elderly aphasic patient with word finding difficulties (44, 62). The communication partner becomes an integral component to the therapy process by learning a variety of techniques to facilitate communication adequacy and by reinforcing communication attempts through meaningful, appropriate and sincere responses. For the unintelligible patient, the communication partner may need to learn how to decode less intelligible responses, respond to intonation cues, and encourage the use of an alternate device.

Two examples of speech/language therapy programs illustrate this Effectiveness Approach.

THE EFFECTIVENESS APPROACH

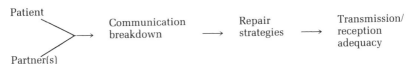

First, Davis and Wilcox's PACE therapy (Promoting Aphasic's Communicative Effectiveness) encourages each of these principles for the aphasic person and communication partner by capitalizing on the aphasic person's comunication strengths and equal participation between patient and partners (13, 14). Lubinski (43) also described a social communication approach to an elderly aphasic institutionalized woman which encouraged clinican modeling of facilitating communication strategies with staff and other patients in a naturalistic context. Any approach which stresses the functional use of language, speech and hearing may be included within the Effectiveness Approach.

The Opportunity Approach

The Opportunity Approach to communication therapy in nursing homes is the most encompassing of the three approaches presented in this chapter. This approach emanates from the philosophy that individuals must want to communicate and have an environment which stimulates and reinforces communication in order for communication to occur. This approach also focuses on nursing home patients who might not be the typical speech therapy client, in that any individual, regardless of communication skill, might be included in this program. Observation in most nursing homes reveals that there are many patients who have adequate communication skills but spend little time during their days talking in meaningful conversations. Lubinski (45) has noted that much of the communication in nursing homes focuses on food and social amenities other than when patients are asked direct questions about their needs and care. Both the physical and social environments may reduce communication opportunities for any patient in a nursing home setting. The schematic below describes the sequence and goal of this alternative to nursing home therapy.

Improving the external environment focuses on becoming more aware of the physical setting of a nursing home and the social mores which govern interaction within that institution. Components of the physical environment which might either facilitate or reduce communication opportunities include: (a) easy access to activities and communication partners of choice; (b) the acoustic environment particularly in areas where most communication occurs; (c) the vis-

ual environment in which communication occurs; (d) the comfort level of the patient regarding temperature and sitting; (e) a sensory and cognitively stimulating environment; and (f) private places to communicate. Communication disorders specialists need to be cognizant that the physical arena influences where and how older people will communicate.

The social environment is even more important but less tangible than the physical environment (30, 60). The social environment is composed of the generally unspoken but powerful rules staff and patients have for interacting with each other. Other writers such as Goffman (24), Bennett (5, 6), and Lawton (37, 38) have discussed the roles patients and staff have in long term care settings and their potency as a driving force in the socialization of nursing homes. Of particular interest are the role relationships between elderly patients and each other or nursing aides directly involved in most daily care routines. Patients and staff develop unspoken rules for living, working and communicating with each other. This forms the social environment of the nursing home.

Each elderly patient also contributes his or her own personal qualities (internal environment) to the nursing home setting. Elderly patients come with a variety of personal histories, skills, impairments and interaction styles (41). For some, institutionalization is imposed either directly by family members or social agencies or indirectly because of lack of alternative care possibilities in the community. Elderly persons must mesh their personal qualities with the expectations of the nursing home environment.

Implementing the Opportunity Approach forces the speech-language pathologist or audiologist into a new role in the nursing home setting. The goals now become people oriented rather than client oriented and communication focused rather than disorder focused. This approach requires that the communication disorders specialist become acutely aware of the physical and social context in which communication occurs and of the barriers present which may hinder interaction opportunities. This can be done through direct intervention entailing working with architects and nursing home operators in designing or remodeling a physical environment conducive to communication. It also involves careful monitoring of everyday activities in the nursing home to identify the places and activities where most communica-

THE OPPORTUNITY APPROACH

External Environment
                    ⟶ Increased   ⟶ Optimal
Internal Environment   Opportunities   Opportunity

tion occurs and hence making these available to patients. Furthermore, it involves working with staff, particularly those providing the most intimate and frequent care, to help them realize their important role in communicating with patients. This can be done through inservice or through clinician modeling with patients during daily interactions with patients and staff. It should be noted that more speech-language pathologists are incorporating these concepts into their therapeutic endeavors with a variety of patient types (e.g., 28) as well as with entire nursing home populations (40, 41).

FACTORS AFFECTING SERVICE DELIVERY

The communication therapy approaches outlined in this chapter require that the speech language pathologist or audiologist working in a nursing home setting carefully evaluate the communication needs of individual patients, the staff, and the larger physical and social environment. The three approaches taken together present a comprehensive approach to the communication life of an institutional setting. Communication specialists need to understand the factors affecting their service delivery in this setting. At least five factors influence what and how communication specialists provide service: (a) our understanding of the aging process; (b) our understanding of the communication needs of the elderly in long term care settings; (c) the commitment and understanding of employers, families and funding agencies; (d) the desire of the elderly to participate in therapy; and (e) our definition of progress.

How we approach nursing home patients stems in part from our knowledge of the aging process. In a society where many young people have minimal interaction with older family members in extended family situations, there is little opportunity to become aware of the characteristics of the elderly. Many graduating students from master's degree programs have had minimal educational coursework in adult and aging development and little direct contact with older patients other than an occasional aphasic, dysarthric, hearing impaired person or laryngectomy. These professionals may carry the same stereotypes of older people as much of our society (4, 38), in that the elderly are viewed as less competent, nearing death, senile, too impaired, difficult to get along with, etc. In a society which values youth and competence, working with multihandicapped elderly individuals in a nursing home setting may not be a life goal. While there is no direct evidence to substantiate this in our own field, there is little reason to doubt that this philosophy may affect at least some of the professionals working in nursing homes. The fact that many of the professionals in nursing homes assume this position only as "moonlighters" may indicate that this setting is only perceived as added income after the regular job is completed (8).

Communication disorders specialists working in long-term care settings should be well educated to the physical, psychological, cognitive, emotional, social, political and economic characteristics of the aging process and the particular needs of the elderly. Furthermore, these professionals should understand the impact of institutionalization on older persons and their families, since this directly affects service given and progress made in therapy. Similarly, they must understand the important role of staff members in complementing and supplementing our therapy efforts on a daily basis.

Communication professionals should also be aware that the traditional rehabilitation model for assessment and therapy may not fit all elderly patients in a nursing home. This chapter highlights the fact that some patients may need to improve skills while others improve their overall effectiveness, and yet others need increased opportunities to communicate. Expecting that all elderly patients will benefit similarly from traditional, didactic, drill-oriented therapy makes us less effective, stagnant, and boring.

In addition, nursing home administrators, funding sources, families, staff and even patients themselves must understand the important role of communication to elderly patients and the abilities of speech-language pathologists and audiologists to help facilitate this. Communication disorders specialists must take the lead in educating others to the variety of possible roles we can play in this setting and the potential benefits to patients and staff. Communication disorders specialists must be viewed as integral members of the nursing home team and not as a part-time, invisible, but expensive ancillary service. Continued documentation of the effectiveness of traditional skill oriented approaches is needed (59). Likewise, additional research is needed to document the effectiveness of alternative approaches such as those outlined in this chapter. Our role begins with dialogue and education of those in decision-making positions in government and nursing home administrations. This ultimately will provide the support needed to implement more nontraditional approaches with a greater variety of elderly patients in long-term care (see Chapter 22 for elaboration).

The elderly patients themselves also affect

the service we deliver. When possible, patients should be included in the decision making regarding the type of therapy approach employed, the topics and stimuli for therapy and the documentation of progress. Elderly patients must understand the rationale for therapy and their role in this process. A therapist appearing twice weekly and drilling words or sentences has little meaning to many patients. Given the opportunity, many elderly patients have the cognitive ability to understand the therapy process and contribute to its effectiveness. Patients can also be an excellent source of information regarding carryover of skills, techniques which facilitate effectiveness, and identification of barriers to communication opportunities.

Finally, the communication disorders specialist's definition of progress affects the approach chosen for therapy. The Skill Approach stresses documentation of progress through administration of standardized tests and daily percentage of improvement (e.g., LaPointe's Base Ten approach to daily documentation) (34). For the severely impaired, multihandicapped individual, this type of progress documentation may not demonstrate to the best advantage the actual utilization of skills in real-life situations. Thus, communication disorders specialists must find alternative ways to document progress, including structured observation of patients communicating in activities of daily living; questionnaires to staff, family, and patients themselves when possible; and new types of pragmatically based tests such as the CADL (Communicative Abilities in Daily Living) (27). Progress should be measured on the number of attempts patients make to communicate, the number and variety of communication partners they have, their communicative effectiveness in receiving and transmitting information, their willingness to initiate use of alternate systems, and the effectiveness of communication partners to facilitate communication adequacy (43).

DECISION MAKING PROCESS

In order to decide what approach or approaches to implement with a given individual in a nursing home setting, the communication disorders specialist can review a number of questions. When possible, the professional should try to remediate any specific communication skills prior to or in conjunction with the Effectiveness and Opportunity approaches.

The first set of questions focus on determining the nature, extent and effect of any specific communication problems.

1. Does the elderly individual have a specific difficulty in:
   a. Transmission of an intelligible verbal message of increasing phonemic and linguistic complexity?
   b. Comprehension of auditory or visual messages of varying phonemic and linguistic complexity?
   c. Receiving auditory or visual messages in a variety of acoustic and social environments?
   d. Receiving or transmitting meaningful nonverbal messages?
   e. Using a variety of communication functions such as questions, commands, etc.?
2. Do any of the above difficulties with particular receptive or expressive skills interfere with the functional adequacy of communication on a daily basis with:
   a. Familiar communication partners?
   b. Unfamiliar communication partners?
3. How does the individual compensate for transmission or reception difficulties?
   a. Does the individual have self-initiated strategies for communicating?
   b. Do communication partners have a variety of strategies for facilitating communication adequacy?
   c. How effective are the above strategies?
4. Does the individual's standardized test performance match functional use of communication in activities of daily living?
5. How does the individual perceive specific speech, language or hearing difficulties?
   a. As a major problem worthy of concerted rehabilitation efforts?
   b. As a minor problem but worthy of some rehabilitation efforts?
   c. As insignificant compared to other personal health, social or family problems?
   d. As a problem to be dealt with in the future when other personal concerns are under control?
6. How do significant others perceive specific speech, language, or hearing difficulties?
   a. As a major problem worthy of concerted effort by patient and family?
   b. As a major problem worthy of concerted effort by patient alone?
   c. As a minor problem but worthy of some rehabilitation efforts?
   d. As an insignificant problem not worthy of rehabilitation?
7. Will speech-language therapy or auditory rehabilitation result in objective, consistent, meaningful improvement of specific skills?
   a. Changes are likely to be easily demonstrated and consistent.
   b. Changes are likely to be moderate,

depending on major help from others in the environment for carryover.

c. Changes are likely to be minimal with little carryover even with major facilitation from others in the environment.

8. Will focus on specific communication skills change the individual's original diagnosis of severely, moderately, or mildly impaired within a reasonable time frame?
   a. Changes will be obvious and consistent in a reasonable time frame.
   b. Changes will be difficult to carryover and will require extensive therapy of an unknown time frame.
   c. Few obvious changes are likely to occur even with maximum extensive therapy.

If the answers to the above questions indicate that focus on specific skills is not likely to result in at least some improvement within a reasonable time frame and there is little support from the individual or the environment to help carry over skills, the speech-language pathologist or audiologist ought to reconsider the Skill approach as the major focus of therapy. At this point, the following set of questions focus on other areas which might become goals for therapy.

9. Regardless of the level of receptive or expressive skill demonstrated by a particular patient, how frustrated is the individual in the communication process?
   a. Extremely?
   b. Moderately?
   c. Minimally?
10. How frustrated do primary communication partners become in communicating with the elderly individual?
    a. Extremely?
    b. Moderately?
    c. Minimally?
11. Does the elderly individual limit interaction because of perceived communication difficulties?
    a. With familiar communication partners?
    b. With unfamiliar communication partners?
12. How willing and effective are primary communication partners to repair communication breakdowns in a variety of situations?
    a. Both willing and effective in all situations?
    b. Inconsistent in willingness and effectiveness?
    c. Not willing and not effective?
13. How knowledgeable are primary communication partners in the use of alternative means as a viable communication avenue for the elderly individual?

a. Understand rationale and viability of alternate means and encourage use.
b. Encourage use only on a limited basis.
c. Discourage use of alternate means.

Answers to the above question should provide a profile of the motivation level of both the elderly patient and primary communication partners to work toward greater communication effectiveness. The following set of questions focus on the communication opportunities and barriers to communication within the institutional environment.

14. Is the elderly individual perceived as a viable communication partner regardless of level of communication skill by a variety of partners?
    a. Always by a variety of persons.
    b. Sometimes by a few persons.
    c. Infrequently.
15. Does the elderly individual have a variety of meaningful activities which promote thinking, independence and communication commensurate with ability?
    a. Many and varied stimulating opportunities of choice.
    b. Opportunities are designed primarily by caregivers.
    c. Few opportunities for self-initiated or structured, staff-planned activities.
16. Does the elderly individual have a variety of trusted communication partners easily accessible on a daily basis?
    a. Yes, at least one person perceived as a primary confidant.
    b. Most interaction is with acquaintances.
    c. Few communication partners of choice.
17. Is access to activities and partners in the physical environment of the institution easily available?
    a. Access is readily available and encouraged.
    b. Access is dependent on caregivers' routine.
    c. Access is difficult to self-initiate and is discouraged by caregivers.
18. Is the physical environment conducive to receiving and transmitting verbal and nonverbal messages?
    a. Acoustics and lighting are appropriate and well designed to maximize communicative interaction.
    b. Acoustics and lighting are appropriate in some areas and poor in others.
    c. The acoustic and visual environment discourages interaction.
19. Are there private places readily accessible to elderly persons to communicate with staff, friends or family?
    a. Yes, within easy access to patient.

b. Requires special permission or arrangements.

c. Not available on any basis.

20. Will the administration and staff of the institution understand and encourage increasing communication opportunities for elderly patients?
    a. Yes, support is given for maximizing opportunities.
    b. This goal is viewed as a byproduct of a traditional approach to individual skill-oriented therapy.
    c. This goal is discouraged and not viewed as a role of the communication disorders specialist.

22. Can therapy, regardless of approach used, be offered frequently enough to reach desired goals?
    a. Number and length of sessions is unlimited.
    b. Therapy can only be offered on a once or twice per week basis.
    c. Therapy is infrequently offered in this setting.

This last set of questions should help the speech-language pathologist or audiologist become more sensitive to the physical and social environment of the nursing home and possible barriers to communication occurring there.

DIFFICULTIES IN IMPLEMENTING APPROACHES

Implementing any approach to communication therapy in a nursing home setting begins with a sensitive, knowledgeable speech-language pathologist or audiologist. As stated previously, the clinician must understand the aging process, the communication needs of the elderly person, and the relationship of institutionalization to aging and communication. The clinician must also have a commitment to working with older people who may not demonstrate quick, startling progress and carryover to activities of daily living.

One of the major problems faced in long term care settings by communication disorders specialists is that other professionals do not know the extent of our skills nor the variety of roles we may play in improving the communication atmosphere of that institution. Physicians may neglect to refer appropriate cases, believing that communication problems caused by stroke, cancer, and progressive neurological diseases have no hope of improvement. Few physicians realize that speech-language pathologists and audiologists can play an important role in diagnosing these disorders as well

as dementia. Similarly, other staff members may not realize the potential contributory role these professionals may have in helping them communicate more successfully with patients and their families. Many families have no idea of the availability of speech-language pathologists or audiologists nor the benefits that may be given to their loved ones by these professionals.

This problem of awareness and acceptance may be improved by increased visibility within the nursing home setting primarily during the two day time nursing shifts. Appearance in the nursing home only when there is a specific referral limits this visibility and accessibility. Medical, nursing, activities, social work and other rehabilitation specialists must be made aware of the variety of roles possible and how we can integrate our goals for individual patients and for the larger environment into their special areas of focus. Staff members need to think about the communicative life of their patients and realize that improved communication skills, effectiveness and opportunities enhance their job performance and the overall functioning of their patients.

A second method to improve our image and viability within this setting is through continuing education of staff members and availability to families. Continuing education, usually called "inservice" in nursing homes, is often done on a once or twice per year basis in 1-hour time periods. During these sessions, the speech-language pathologist or audiologist tries to tell everything about every disorder to an audience of nurses and aides. Koury and Lubinski (33) stated this is an area which needs high priority by communication disorder specialists. They suggest shorter, one half hour sessions which focus on improving the problem solving abilities of staff to meet the communication breakdowns they incur with patients. Rather than lecturing about specific disorders, assessment techniques and therapy procedures, inservice ought to stress the staff members' ability to identify communication problems among patients and strategies for communicating effectively with all patients. By conducting a series of shorter sessions, geared to the specific interests and needs of the staff, the speech-language pathologist or audiologist will have more opportunity to gain rapport with staff, understand the problems they are having communicating, and reinforce strategies they generate and use for effective communication.

In addition, communication disorders specialists have a special and continuing role in working with the families of the traditional type of communication impaired person as well as others who have dementias (see Chapter 19).

While some of these patients may not be on active caseloads, communication disorders specialists still have a responsibility to work with the staff and families of patients who have communication needs. Many families of patients with dementia do not understand the effects of this disorder on communication nor do they have strategies for maximizing the communication which does occur. Families must realize that there is a specialist in the nursing home who can be a resource for information and techniques to communicate more effectively. Ways to become more available to families include giving families of new admissions informative brochures outlining the role and scope of communication disorders specialists. Other strategies might focus on afternoon, evening, or weekend presentations and availability to families. A video presentation describing the importance of communication to elderly institutionalized persons, the role of the speech-language pathologist and audiologist, and some key strategies for effective communication with the elderly might also be made available. Further, communication disorders specialists need to inform social service professionals and nursing staff that families can and should be referred to us for information, counseling, and communication facilitating techniques. Referral from other professionals is often vital in linking families to our profession.

CASE ILLUSTRATIONS

The following cases are presented to illustrate how therapy was approached for three different nursing home patients. All names used are fictitious though the information presented is based on real individuals.

Mrs. L. is a 68-year-old woman who suffered a stroke several months prior to her admittance to the nursing home by her 72-year-old husband. Due to his own increasing health problems, Mrs. L.'s husband felt that nursing home care was the only alternative available to them. The stroke resulted in right side paralysis and moderately severe dysarthria. Mrs. L.'s dysarthria was compounded by a discernible Southern accent and rapid speech. Administration of a structured articulation test and the Minnesota Test for the Differential Diagnosis of Aphasia revealed that there was little or no aphasia but moderately severe dysarthria characterized by slurring of consonants, weak production of final consonants, particularly consonant blends, and rapid rate of speech. Discussion with Mrs. L. also revealed that she enjoyed talking to "anybody," she was not opposed to her admittance to the nursing home, and she was eager to become involved in some of the activities offered. Informal observation of her at the nurses' station corroborated that she actively initiated communication

with both patients and staff though they tended not to understand her entire message. Thus, therapy focused on: (a) improving her overall speech intelligibility particularly focusing on adequately producing all phonemes in a word; (b) reducing rate through the use of a pacing board; and (c) working with two nursing aides directly involved in her care and her roommate to monitor and cue Mrs. L. about the above goals in her daily conversations. The first two goals stressed particular speech skills in a traditional practice, discrimination and self-evaluation paradigm. The final goal centered on improving her overall communication effectiveness by working with primary communication partners to help her carryover skills worked on in direct therapy. While articulatory improvement was inconsistent, rate reduction had a major effect in improving her intelligibility. Staff and her roommate were integral in helping Mrs. L. remember to carry her pacing board with her and reinforcing its use.

Mr. A. is an 84-year-old male who had been institutionalized for four years at the time of referral for a speech evaluation. His Parkinson's disease had been compounded by a stroke, and his speech was relatively unintelligible. In addition, he had a moderately severe unaided hearing loss in both ears, poorly fitting dentures which wobbled in his mouth when talking, and was partially sighted in both eyes. He was not able to take a standardized aphasia test. Results of informal assessment of speech and language through conversational analysis revealed that his language skills were relatively intact though there were some periods of confusion. His major problem was his severe speech unintelligibility. Traditional articulation therapy was tried for a trial period and resulted in no observable gains at even the imitation word level. Mr. A. was obviously annoyed by speech therapy, frequently saying "What's this going to do? How much is this costing me?" Nurses continued to complain that they could not understand him and were frustrated by his "garbled talk." New goals were established: (a) initiation of a picture communication board with primary needs portrayed; (b) direct work with two aides most involved in Mr. A.'s care to understand the functions of the picture board; (c) referral for a dental consultation to remediate the poor-fitting dentures; (d) referral for an audiological evaluation to determine the feasibility of a hearing aid. This individual would not profit from Skill-oriented articulation therapy. Goals related to making him a more effective communicator through alternate means and insuring that primary communicators in his environment would facilitate and reinforce the use of the alternate device appeared more reasonable. Further, this could be accomplished in a relatively short period of time, thereby minimizing cost to the family and institution. Most importantly, Mr. A. was less frustrated by this approach than the traditional articulation therapy first tried. Although he needed to be reminded to use the communication board, he was successful in transmitting his needs through it.

Mr. J. is a 63-year-old male who entered the nursing home 6 weeks following a massive stroke. While medically stable at the time of admission, he had right side paralysis and what initially appeared to be global aphasia. Mr. J. was attended around the clock by private duty practical nurses in addition to the regular nursing home staff. The family stated that they would spare "no expense" for dad, though they refused to become involved in his care or rehabilitation themselves. Their visits were infrequent and brief, centered on their own financial concerns. Nursing and social services staff stated that the visits were unproductive. Consequently, Mr. J. had maximum care available but was extremely depressed and uncooperative in therapy. Initial therapy sessions were difficult because of his reluctance to participate. Three therapy alternatives were targeted for this patient. First, three time per week therapy focused on improving receptive and expressive skills in a traditional aphasia therapy approach. Second, therapy also focused on including two of the private duty nurses. They were encouraged to participate in the therapy sessions, and communication facilitating techniques were modeled during conversational portions of the sessions. Third, contact was made with each of the adult children and they were encouraged to visit the nursing home when therapy was occurring. Again, communication facilitating techniques were presented while the family observed and eventually participated. Fourth, Mr. J. was encouraged to participate in one activity in the nursing home, a Trivia Game. Although he could not verbally express himself, he did enjoy the activity and offered some nonverbal encouragement to the other members of the group. Fifth, the family was encouraged to come in to the nursing home for discussions with the speech pathologist. While somewhat demanding and condescending, some members of the family gradually assumed a more positive role in working with their father and a more realistic expectation of therapy progress. Finally, the family was asked to encourage one of Mr. J.'s special friends to visit in the nursing home several times per week and participate in some therapy sessions and the Trivia activity. After 8 weeks of this combined approach, Mr. J. had improved both receptive and expressive skills; he was a more active therapy participant; some family members had become more involved; and Mr. J was attempting interaction with a greater number of patients and staff. He agreed to eat his meals in the dining room and sit in the lounge on occasion. Future goals include helping other patients and staff communicate more often and effectively with him.

CONCLUDING REMARKS

This chapter challenges communication disorders specialists to consider a variety of approaches in providing service to elderly individuals in long-term care settings. Traditional skill therapy approaches which focus on improving specific speech, language, or hearing disorders may be appropriate for many of these patients. There are, however, others who would benefit from focusing on improving their overall communication effectiveness and providing significant communication partners with

a variety of strategies for facilitating interaction. Yet a third alternative considers the communication life of the vast majority of nursing home patients who exist in a communication deprived environment with few communication partners of choice, things to talk about, and activities which promote interaction. This third approach stresses identifying aspects of the physical and psychosocial environment which may limit opportunities for communication.

Some communication disorder specialists, funding agencies, administrators, other professionals, and even patients and their families may question the feasibility of approaches to communication improvment other than the traditional skill alternative. While continued quality research is needed to add statistical data to support some effectiveness approaches and the focus on the environment, close observation and sensitivity to the communication occurring in nursing homes must propel us to try new approaches. The elderly institutionalized individuals in our society deserve our creativity, our competence and our commitment to developing every avenue possible to maximize communication skill, effectiveness, and opportunity.

References

1. Ainsworth T: *Quality Assurance in Long Term Care.* Germantown, Pa., Aspen Systems Corporation, 1977.
2. Arnst J: Presbycusis. In Katz J (ed): *Handbook of Clinical Audiology.* Baltimore, Williams & Wilkins, 1985, p. 707.
3. Baken R: *Clinical Measurement of Speech and Voice.* San Diego, College Hill, 1987.
4. Baum M, Baum R: *Growing Old: A Societal Perspective.* Englewood Cliffs, NJ, Prentice-Hall, 1980.
5. Bennett R: Meaning of institutional life. *Gerontologist* 3:117–124, 1963.
6. Bennett R, Nahemow L: Institutional totality and criteria for social adjustment in residences for the aged. *J Soc Issues* 21:44–78, 1965.
7. Campbell M: Study of the attitudes of nursing personnel toward the geriatric patient. *Nurs Res* 2:147–151, 1971.
8. Chapey R, Lubinski R, Chapey G, Salzburg A: Survey of speech, language and hearing services in nursing home settings. *Long Term Care Health Serv Q* 4:307–316, 1979.
9. Coe R: Professional perspectives on the aged. *Gerontologist* 7:147–151, 1967.
10. Corso J: Auditory perception and communication. In Birren J, Schaie KW (eds): *Handbook of the Psychology of Aging.* New York, Van Nostrand Reinhold, 1977, p 535.
11. Craik F: Age differences in human memory. In Birren J, Schaie KW (eds): *Handbook of the Psychology of Aging.* New York, Van Nostrand Reinhold Company, 1977, p 384.

12. Cummings J, Benson, DF: *Dementia: A Clinical Approach.* Boston, Butterworth, 1983, p 4.
13. Davis GA: Pragmatics and treatment. In Chapey R (ed): *Language Intervention in Adult Aphasia*, ed 2. Baltimore, Williams & Wilkins, 1986, p 251.
14. Davis GA, Wilcox M: *Adult Aphasia Rehabilitation.* San Diego, College Hill Press, 1985.
15. DeRenzi E, Vignolo L: The token test: a sensitive test to detect receptive disturbances in aphasics. *Brain* 85: 665–678, 1962.
16. Downey M, White S: Nursing Home Facility Reimbursement, Current Problems and Future Issues. Presented at Rehabilitation and Reimbursement Issues in Nursing Homes Workshop. American Speech-Language-Hearing Association, Washington, D.C. September, 1986.
17. Duffy J: Schuell's stimulation approach to rehabilitation. In Chapey R (ed): *Language Intervention Strategies in Adult Aphasia*, ed 2. Baltimore, Williams & Wilkins, 1986, p 187.
18. Eisdorfer C: Intellectual and cognitive changes in the aged. In Busse E, Pfeiffer E (eds): *Behavior and Adaptation in Late Life*. Boston, Little, Brown, 1969, p 237.
19. Eisdorfer C: Stress, disease and cognitive change in the aged. In Eisdorfer C, Friedel R (eds): *Cognitive and Emotional Disturbance in the Elderly*. Chicago, Year Book Medical Publishers, 1977, p 27.
20. Enderby P: *Frenchay Dysarthria Assessment.* San
21. Diego, College Hill Press, 1983.
    Florance C: The aphasic's significant other: training and counseling. In Brookshire R (ed): *Clinical Aphasiology Conference Proceedings*. Minneapolis, 1979, p 295.
22. Fozard J, Wolf E, Bel B: Visual perception and communication. In Birren J, Schaie KW (eds): *Handbook of the Psychology of Aging*. New York, Van Nostrand Reinhold, 1977, p 497.
23. Ginzberg R: The negative attitudes toward the elderly. *Geriatrics* 7:297–302, 1952.
24. Goffman E: *Asylums.* Garden City, NY, Anchor Books, 1961.
25. Goodglass H, Kaplan E: The Boston Diagnostic Aphasia Examination. In Goodglass H, Kaplan E (eds): *The Assessment of Aphasia and Related Disorders*. Philadelphia, Lea & Febiger, 1983.
26. Hayes D: Central auditory problems and the aging process. In Beasley D, Davis GA (eds): *Aging: Communication Processes and Disorders*. New York, Grune & Stratton, 1981, p 257.
27. Holland A: *Communicative Abilities in Daily Living.* Baltimore, University Park Press, 1980.
28. Holland A, Swindell C, Fromm D: A model treatment approach for the acutely aphasic patient. In Brookshire R (ed): *Clinical Aphasiology Conference Proceedings*. Minneapolis, BRK Publishers, 1983, p 44.
29. Hull R: The impact of hearing impairment on aging persons: a dialogue. In Hull R (ed): *Rehabilitative Audiology*. New York, Grune & Stratton, 1982, p 215.
30. Insel P, Moos R: The social environment. In Insel P, Moos R (eds): *Health and the Social Environment*. Lexington, MA, Lexington Books, 1974, p 3.
31. Kahana E, Cole R: Self and staff conceptions of institutionalized aged. *Gerontologist* 9:264–277, 1969.
32. Kertesz A: *The Western Aphasia Battery.* New York, Grune & Stratton, 1982.
33. Koury LN, Lubinski R, Duchan J: Assessing nursing aides' strategies for communicating with institutionalized elderly. Presented at the American Speech and Hearing Association Convention, Detroit, 1986.
34. LaPointe L: Base 10 programmed stimulation: task specification, scoring, and plotting performance in aphasia therapy. *J Speech Hear Disord* 42:90–105, 1977.
35. LaPointe L, Horner J: *Reading Comprehension Battery for Aphasia.* Tigard, OR, CC Publications, 1979.
36. Lawton MP: *Environment and Aging.* Monterey, CA, Brooks Cole, 1980.
37. Lawton MP: Environment as a communication mode. *Bull Audiophonol* 16:17–31, 1983.
38. Lewis S: *Providing for the Older Adult.* Thorofare, NJ, Slack Inc., 1983.
39. Linebaugh C, Kryzer K, Oden S, Myers P: Reapportionment of communicative burden in aphasia: a study of narrative interactions. In Brookshire R (ed): *Clinical Aphasiology Conference Proceedings*. Minneapolis, BRK Publishers, 1979, p 4.
40. Lubinski R: Creating a positive communication environment for the elderly. In Wilder C, Weinstein B (eds): *Aging and Communication*. New York, Haworth Press, 1984, p 47.
41. Lubinski R: Environmental language intervention. In Chapey R (ed): *Language Intervention for Adult Aphasia*, ed 1. Baltimore, Williams & Wilkins, 1981, p 223.
42. Lubinski R: Language and hearing programs in home health care and nursing homes. In Beasley D, Davis GA (eds): *Aging: Communication Processes and Disorders*. New York, Grune & Stratton, p 339.
43. Lubinski R: A social communication approach to treatment of an aphasic in an institutional setting. In Marshall R (ed): *Case Studies in Aphasia Rehabilitation: for Clinicians by Clinicans*. Austin, TX, Pro-Ed Publishers, 1986, p 167.
44. Lubinski R, Duchan J, Weitzner-Lin B: An analysis of breakdowns and repairs in the communication of an aphasic adult. In Brookshire R (ed): *Clinical Aphasiology Conference Proceedings*. Minneapolis, BRK Publishers, 1980, p 111.
45. Lubinski R, Morrison E, Rigrodsky S: Perception of spoken communication by elderly chronically ill patients in an institutional setting. *J Speech Hear Disord* 46:405–412, 1981.
46. Maurer J: The psychosocial aspects of presbycusis. In Hull R (ed): *Rehabilitative Audiology*. New York, 1982, p 271.
47. McNeil M, Prescott T: *Revised Token Test.* Baltimore, University Park Press, 1978.
48. Mills R: Computerized management of aphasia. In Chapey R (ed): *Language Intervention Strategies in Adult Aphasia*, ed 2. Baltimore, Williams & Wilkins, 1986, p 333.
49. Orchik D: Peripheral auditory problems and the

aging process. In Beasley D, Davis GA (eds): *Aging Communication Process and Disorders.* New York, Grune & Stratton, 1981, p 243.

50. Oyer H, Oyer EJ: Social consequences of hearing loss for the elderly. *Allied Health Behav Sci* 2:123–138.

51. Porch B: *The Porch Index of Communicative Ability.* Palo Alto, CA, Consulting Psychologists Press, 1967.

52. Porch B: Therapy subsequent to the Porch Index of Communicative Ability. In Chapey R (ed): *Lanuage Intervention Strategies in Adult Aphasia,* ed 2. Baltimore, Williams & Wilkins, 1986, p. 295.

53. Rao P, Horner J: Gesture as a deblocking modality in a severe aphasic patient. In Brookshire R (ed): *Clinical Aphasiology Conference Proceedings.* Minneapolis, BRK Publishers, 1978, p 180.

54. Rosenbek J, LaPointe L: The dysarthrias: description, diagnosis and treatment. In Johns D (ed): *Clinical Management of Neurogenic Communicative Disorders,* ed 2. Boston, Little, Brown, 1985, p 97.

55. Rubow R: Role of feedback, reinforcement and compliance on training and transfer in biofeedback based rehabilitation of motor speech disorders. In McNeil M, Rosenbek J, Aronson A (eds): *The Dysarthrias, Physiology, Acoustics, Perception, Management.* San Diego, College Hill Press, 1984, p 207.

56. Schow R, Nerbonne M: Hearing levels among elderly nursing home residents. *J Speech Hear Disord* 45: 124–132, 1980.

57. Schuell H: *The Minnesota Test for the Differential Diagnosis of Aphasia.* Minneapolis, University of Minnesota Press, 1965.

58. Shewan C: *Auditory Comprehension Test for Sentences.* Chicago, Biolinguistics Clinical Institutes, 1979.

59. Shewan C: The history and efficacy of aphasia treatment. In Chapey R (ed): *Language Intervention in Adult Aphasia* ed 2. Baltimore, Williams & Wilkins, 1986, p 28.

60. Synder L: Environmental changes for socialization. *J Nurs Admin* January:44–50, 1978.

61. Spence D, Feigenbaum E, Fitzgerald F: Medical student attitudes toward the geriatric patient. *J Am Geriatr Soc* 16:976, 1968.

62. Towey M, Pettit J: Improving communication competence in global aphasia. In Brookshire R (ed): *Clinical Aphasiology Conference Proceedings.* Minneapolis, BRK Publishers, 1980, p 139.

63. U.S. Department of Health and Human Services: *Characteristics of Nursing Home Residents, Health Status, and Care Received: National Nursing Home Survey.* Bethesda, MD, National Center for Health Statistics, Series 13, No. 51, April 1981.

64. Walsh D: Age differences in learning and memory. In Woodruff D, Birren J (eds). *Aging: Scientific and Social Issues.* New York, Van Nostrand, 1975, p 125.

65. Weinstein B, Lubinski R: Utilization of communication disorders services in long term care facilities in New York State. *New York State Speech Language Hearing Association Communicator* 13: 1986, p 5.

66. Yorkston K, Beukelman D: *Assessments of Intelligibility of Dysarthric Speech.* Tigard, OR, CC Publications, 1982.

67. Yorkston K, Beukleman D, Flowers C: Efficiency of information exchange between aphasic speakers and communication partners. In Brookshire R (ed): *Clinical Aphasiology Conference Proceedings.* Minneapolis, BRK Publishers, 1980, p. 96.

19 Education, Counseling, and Support for Significant Others

BARBARA B. SHADDEN

Editor's Note

As suggested in the preceding chapter, completing the programming cycle requires attention to the needs and roles of significant others. In Chapter 19, a significant other is defined as any individual who contributes in an important manner to the physical, emotional, mental, and social well-being of a particular individual. For communicatively impaired older adults, at least two groups of significant others can be identified. The first group consists of those persons in primary interactive or caregiving roles with respect to a particular client. These are typically family members, although close friends and service providers in institutional settings may also belong in this category. The second group consists of members of the extended social support network. Chapter 19 begins with a discussion of the nature of and potential roles served by each of these groups of significant others as they involve older persons. The impact of a communication disorder upon significant others, particularly families, is described, and the needs of family members are summarized. Four basic avenues of intervention are suggested: (a) support groups; (b) individual or group counseling; (c) direct involvement in treatment procedures; and (d) educational programming for the extended community. Communication disorder professionals are encouraged to expand their efforts to meet the needs of the significant others of communicatively impaired older persons. In essence, all members of the communication network require assistance.

Communication disorders affect more than just the disordered individual since, by definition, communication is essentially an interactive process. This simple fact has far-reaching implications in designing interventions. If the communication interaction is impaired, then all members of that interactive process must receive assistance. The task of the speech-language pathologist or audiologist, therefore, becomes one of coordinating or facilitating services to the impaired communication network (70). Professionals must actively seek to identify significant others, their potential roles in relationships to the older client, their needs, and the mechanisms available to meet these needs.

There is a tendency to think of members of the communication network as being primarily of value in assisting a client to communicate more effectively and/or to cope with residual speech-language or hearing deficits. This philosophical approach is evident in Barlow's discussion of the importance of family relationships for disabled individuals.

Adults are powerfully influenced by their family relationships. Many times these relationships strengthen the individual and help him adjust to a disabling condition. . .Other times, an individual's adjustment to a disability is handicapped by the family's patterns of interacting. A practitioner would be wise to keep in mind the power of the family. . . (6, pp 68–69)

Unfortunately, this focus on the client's needs for familial support and involvement in treatment may prevent us from recognizing that those most closely involved with a communicatively disordered older adult also have basic needs that must be met. At the very least, the quality and quantity of social interactions have been impaired (12, 65, 112). More typically, there have been major assaults upon the preexisting life-styles of all concerned individuals. Thus interventions with significant others must consider the needs of both the older client and the family member, caregiver, or participant in the communication network.

This chapter begins with some basic definitions of the term significant other, subdividing this group into primary caregivers (typically, but not exclusively, family members) and members of the extended social support network. The nature of families and social supports in the older population is described briefly, and the potential roles of each group with respect to the communicatively disoriented client are summarized.

Consideration is next given to the needs of significant others, with particular emphasis upon families. Of necessity, this discussion includes an explanation of the effects of communication disorders upon family members and on patterns of behavior, as well as the types of coping responses typically observed.

Finally, four broad avenues of intervention involving significant others are described, including: support groups; individual or group counseling; direct involvement in treatment procedures; and education/information exchange. While these intervention approaches are not mutually exclusive, they do allow consideration of most of the existing literature on current management approaches.

DEFINING "SIGNIFICANT OTHERS"

The term significant other has gained increasing popularity in recent years. Although definitions vary, the term is used in the chapter to refer to those individuals who contribute in an important manner to the physical, emotional, mental, and social well-being of the communicatively disordered individual (33). Thus, "significant" is taken quite literally to mean "of marked importance."

The pool of significant others, however, will be further subdivided to allow consideration of two potentially important but distinct types of support persons. For purposes of direct intervention planning, one group of significant others can be defined as those individuals who play central interactive or caregiving roles in the life of a particular client. This could include, but is not limited to, spouses, children, close friends, and professionals (particularly caregivers in institutional settings). These individuals must be targeted because of the essential roles they may play in direct speech-language-hearing interventions. The second group of significant others includes members of the extended social support network—the community of friends, neighbors, and other social contacts that constitutes the total communication environment of a given client.

Both primary caregivers and the broader social network will be discussed in more detail in the following sections. Particular attention is focused upon: (a) the status of each group of significant others when older individuals are involved; and (b) the potential and actual roles served by each group.

Primary Caregivers
The Nature of Families

Most of the literature concerning significant others and the elderly has focused upon families—family structures, crises, and interventions. In the case of communication disorders, this attention to the family should not be surprising. In many instances, family members have or must assume primary caregiving roles and are with the client 24 hours per day (98). It is also most likely that contact with one or more family members will occur during the course of treatment. Finally, families have lived together and have developed powerful patterns of interaction and of role behavior over a number a years. The relatively fixed nature of these paterns is what may be threatened by a communication disorder.

Families are patterned entities or systems (75). Their structures, rituals, roles, and associated life-styles have been discussed by numerous authors (6, 75, 89, 111). One central theme is the recognition that the family functions "as a unique, cohesive, and delicatively balanced unit" (111, p 229). The popular term for this state of balance is family homeostasis.

The term homeostasis does not imply any judgment of the quality of the equilibrium, nor does it suggest that this equilibrium is fixed and permanent. In reality, a variety of stressors may threaten family homeostasis at all times, forcing constant readjustments to this balance. Norlin (75) describes family stress as falling into one of two categories. Vertical stress (intergenerational transmission) results from pressures emerging from the family's past history. These pressures are particularly evident in the form of proscriptions and/or expectations as to how to behave. Horizontal stress, in contrast, results from the effects of events that have occurred within the immediate family's life span. A communication disorder might fit into the latter category.

When family homeostasis is threatened, family members resort to a variety of strategies to restore interpersonal and emotional equilibrium (35). These strategies generally evolve out of what Barlow calls "systemic life-style," that pattern of roles, situations, and interactions that a family evolves over time in order to solve problems (6, p 61). Roles are particularly interesting. While they are generally assigned within the family, one person's roles may be perceived very differently by various members of that family unit. Roles may be knowledge based ("Dad understands how appliances work"), emotion based ("Grandma is the nurturing one in the family"), or action based. In the latter category, Norlin (75) defines four possible behavioral roles: (a) the mover or initiator of action; (b) the opposer, who challenges the mover's actions; (c) the follower, who accedes to and supports actions; and (d) the bystander, who maintains some distance in order to observe and provide feedback. Roles or life-styles are also interesting in that they may dictate the nature of a family's adjustment to the short- or long-term disability of a family member. If the disabled or increasingly dependent family member has a life-style history of "being helped," the adjustment to disability and associated dependency may be relatively smooth (although there is always the risk of fostering overdependence) (6). In contrast, if the disabled individual is one who has always been dominant and independent (a mover), the relationship between that individual and his spouse may evolve into what has been termed a "lethal dyad" (51). Neither member of this immediate family unit will have any history of roles or rituals to help them adjust to such a major life change.

This brief review of basic family dynamics has some rather profound implications when considering family systems and the elderly. The very fact of the aging of one or more members of the immediate or extended family may be sufficient to disrupt homeostasis and all of the roles, relationships, and behavioral patterns associated with that homeostasis.

Families and the Elderly

A rather bleak portrait of abandonment and unconcern has occasionally been presented with respect to extended families and their older members. Frankfather (38) suggests that this portrait is neither fair nor accurate, referring to families as one of the major decentralized systems of support available to older persons. This observation is also echoed in Auburn's emphasis on the need for improved community care systems for the elderly and the important role of families in this care process (3).

Nevertheless, there are a number of aspects of aging in today's society that must be considered in understanding extended family dynamics. Webster and Newhoff (111) refer to the different topics, priorities, and interests that may characterize members of two or more generations of an extended family. Oyer (77) expands this discussion by listing a number of aging influences, including:

1. The generation gap, as evidenced in patterns of accepted socialization;
2. Changes in residence, due to social mobility and dispersal;
3. Types of housing, including problems associated with privacy, lack of stability, and limited control over decisions to move;
4. Attitudes (intrafamily) and role shifts;
5. Schedule conflicts, including the overcommitted, overactive schedules of both older and younger family members;
6. Language differences, particularly semantic or vocabulary variants discrete to each generation;
7. Health-related factors (communication requires energy that the older person may not have or the younger person may be unwilling to expend in talking with a hearing impaired relative);
8. Values conflicts, particularly between the tendency of older generations towards conservatism and traditionalism and the tendency of younger generations towards more open and liberal approaches to life's problems;
9. Social mobility, particularly the fact the children of older parents may be on a different social scale than their parents (creating stresses in attempting to operate in both worlds).

In essence, both immediate and extended families involving older adults may be experiencing a variety of stresses that interfere with adustments and relationships on a daily basis. Dowd (28) discusses these stresses within the perspective of exchange theory. As older persons become disadvantaged with respect to the resources they can bring to bear upon any interpersonal exchange, there is a gradual erosion of power within the family structure, frequently associated with an increase in dependency. This is particularly damaging when older persons and their situations begin to be viewed as "problems." In one rather interesting study of these hypotheses (29), it was reported that the more contact elderly fathers had with their children, the lower their morale became. This finding was interpreted as indicative of alterations in status and role relationships that reflected a ceding of control to the younger generations.

In view of the may potential stresses acting upon families involving an older member, it is not surprising to find that the extended family, at least, may not be faring well in terms of the degree of emotional support an older person feels can be obtained from the family unit (15). While older adults may reveal greater expectations of support from families in the form of assistance, friends may contribute more to morale (66). Certainly, the older interviewees described in Chapter 2 of this volume were much less likely than children of older parents or professionals to target family members as primary communication interactants. Geographical proximity to children remains a reality for both rural and urban elderly (85). However, there is some evidence that the perceived value of family contacts is eroding over time. In one series of studies, although two-thirds of a sample of rural elderly in Iowa had at least one child within a half-hour drive, those who reported deriving greatest satisfaction from contacts with family members dropped from 65% in 1960 to 5% in 1970 (13, 14).

Roles of Primary Caregivers

Despite the concerns raised in the preceding section, the importance of families to older adults cannot be ignored, particularly when the adult acquires a handicapping condition such as a speech-language or hearing disorder. Among the many roles that can be served by families assisting in the rehabilitation process, the following are most salient:

1. To provide information, particularly with respect to interests, patterns of daily activity, and functional communication;
2. To provide emotional support and act as confidants;
3. To serve as primary caregivers;
4. To act as mediators between the client and others in social contexts, with particular emphasis upon training others as to effective communication strategies;
5. To assist in facilitating the goals and activities of direct therapy, whether in actual treatment sessions or in carryover to the home environment;
6. To act as the primary communication partner to the older client;
7. To assist in the physical use of various communication aids (hearing aid, communication board, assistive listening device, etc.);
8. To assume activities and responsibilities previously assigned to the client.

The Social Support Network

The Nature of Social Networks and the Elderly

The second group of significant others to be considered in this chapter is the social support network. According to Goodman (43), the importance of natural helping among older adults cannot be ignored. No one type of social relationship satisfies all of an individual's needs (98). Thus the professional should maximize use of the contributions of all possible members of the older client's support network.

While the literature in this area of support systems for the elderly is proliferating, problems in terminology and definition are common. It is clear that what is being described is a system of informal supports (62), generally available through friends and community acquaintances. These informal supports are described as emotionally nurturing and free to respond spontaneously to an individual's needs in ways not available to formal agencies or professional supports.

However, Rundell (86) cautions us to avoid equating the term social network with support network, since the actual number of persons considered as frequent or occasional contacts in the social network may not adequately reflect the degree of support (actual or perceived) received from these persons. In fact, Strain and Chappell (100) have reported that the confidant relationship is more important to quality of life than any measure of the number of family and friend interactions. Unfortunately, some of the earlier literature failed to make this distinction, resulting in artificially inflated estimates of the size of the support network available to the average older person.

Another research focus has been upon the comparison of familial and nonfamilial supports. In general, families (at least extended families) do not hold up well on measures of life satisfaction, at least when compared with friends and community involvement (45, 99). It has been suggested, however, that it might be more appropriate to consider peer/nonpeer (or intra versus intergenerational) support distinctions, rather than familial/nonfamilial (18).

Most of the research in the area of support networks for the elderly has focused upon their potential benefits, as well as the factors that may contribute to reaping these benefits. For example, as suggested above, quantity of contacts is less important than quality. It has become apparent that self-initiated social contacts and relationships provide more powerful supports than those imposed by external sources (80). The level (depth) of interaction is also critical, but only if the individual is satisfied with the interaction (21, 86). Thus, artificial attempts to provide older adults with intensive relationships may meet with failure if the individual does not desire or value that particular contact.

Roles of Support Networks

With these qualifying observations in mind, it is useful to examine the potential roles that can be played by an older person's support network, as documented in the literature. Possible roles include:

1. Emotional nurturing and companionship (62);
2. Flexibility and spontaneity in responses to needs (42, 62);
3. Improvement in happiness, life satisfaction, and measures of well-being (5, 45, 80, 99, 100, 105), although this is not fully documented in all sources (21);
4. Reduction of negative physical or emotional symptoms (22);
5. Improvement in perceived social control (80);
6. Enhanced abilities to meet needs (22);
7. Provision of a buffering response to stress and improvement of adaptation (22, 23);
8. Increased self-esteem (80);
9. Enhanced utilization of services (21, 86).

THE IMPACT OF COMMUNICATION DISORDERS ON SIGNIFICANT OTHERS

The preceding sections have identified two key groups of significant others of interest in working with older clients. Some of the roles that could be served by both primary caregivers and members of the broader social network have been specified. It is appropriate to turn next to consideration of the needs of these significant others, particularly family members. If these needs can be defined accurately and managed appropriately, all members of the communication network, including the client, will be served. The needs of significant others can only be understood by examining the impact of communication disorders.

The pattern of impact of a specific communication disorder varies depending upon the nature and severity of the communication impairment, its onset characteristics and prognosis, and the family's preexisting patterns of functioning. In all instances, however, a communication crisis can be said to exist (92). The major characteristics of this crisis are: (a) the disruption of previous modes of behavior and relating; and (b) the introduction of an awareness of loss—of skills, function, roles or relational characteristics (27).

Breakdown in Familial Homeostasis

It was stated earlier that families can be viewed as complete systemic units, with specific operating rules, tasks, roles, and histories. Any change disrupts the homeostasis implicit in this systemic structure. Among the many changes associated with aging, speech-langage

or hearing disorders potentially rank among the most powerful sources of breakdown in the equilibrium of the immediate or extended family unit. The reason for this is obvious. Communicative interactions provide the foundation for defining and confirming roles and behaviors, as well as dictating social and vocational activities.

Families must be helped to reestablish a new form of homeostasis on all levels and in all arenas (75). Specifically, families must be assisted to discover healthy and adaptive ways of redefining roles and interactions. For example, an older man with a progressive worsening hearing loss may adapt by withdrawing from social activities and avoiding interpersonal contacts. After a time, this behavior becomes the accepted norm. On the surface at least, his withdrawal reduces the strain imposed on other family members who have been trying to communicate despite the hearing handicap or who have shouldered the burden of his irritability and confusion in social settings. While a new form of family equilibrium may have been reached, however, it is essentially a maladaptive one.

Stages in Reaction to Loss and Disturbed Equilibrium

Some years back, Tanner (103) proposed that speech-language pathologists and audiologists must recognize that a communication disorder is experienced by individuals and their families as a form of loss—whether it be real loss (of object, person, or function) or symbolic loss (of self-esteem, stature, and role). The kind and degree of loss experienced relates to the nature of the disorder and its accompanying problems (90). Perceptions of loss are also dictated by the innate priority systems of the concerned individuals and of family members. Each of us operates with a built-in set of hierarchial values which dictate which of our skills, attributes, and daily activities we value most and least. A similar unconscious ranking applies to those we care about. As one spouse indicated, "I could take his being paralyzed, maybe, but not the loss of memory. His mind makes him what he is. How can I deal with someone who can't remember from one minute to the next."

Ironically, both real and symbolic forms of loss may already be a fact of life for many older persons prior to the onset of a specific communication disorder. Examples of common losses include: loss of friends and family through death and geographic dispersal; loss of physical abilities and health; loss of familiar environments and associated security in the move to retirement residences; loss of mobility, etc. (see Chapters 3 through 6). The list is endless.

The effects of loss, and the nature of the resulting grieving process, are most clearly defined in instances of catastrophic illness. However, there is no question that all forms of loss demand a reaction—from both the affected individual and significant others. Much has been written about the loss-related grieving process or, more broadly, about common stages in reaction to crisis. The seminal work in this area, of course, evolved out of Kubler-Ross' examination of stages in response to the death and dying process (56). These stages include a sequence of denial, followed by anger, bargaining, depression, and ultimately acceptance.

Kubler-Ross' work is certainly not the only attempt to define the grieving process. Tanner (103) describes at least four others, placing particular emphasis on Schneider's (90) efforts to incorporate all theories into a single model. Schneider suggests that there are three basic stages which are consistent with the available literature in the area of loss or grieving. These stages include: (a) attempts to overcome the loss through denial, rage, bargaining, or any other comparable defense; (b) awareness of loss; and (c) acceptance of loss.

While the simplicity of this model is intuitively appealing, other writers have formulated hypotheses about the more general nature of responses to crisis. Schontz (97), for example, has suggested that responses to crisis may be categorized into four sequential stages: shock, realization, retreat, and acknowledgment. Cohn (24) also postulates a continuum of adjustment to disability, from shock (and denial), to expectancy of recovery, followed by mourning, defenses (healthy or neurotic), and ultimately adjustment. In a somewhat different analysis of responses to stress, Falek and Britton (31) include the following: denial, anxiety and fear, anger and hostility, depression, and equilibrium. The latter approach may be particularly useful in understanding gradual onset communication disorders.

Not all individuals will go through all of the stages specified in any of the models described above. Regardless of the type of disorder, however, the speech-language pathologist and audiologist can be relatively certain that some type of mourning or grief will occur, whether it is reflected in depression, fear, anger, or a host of other behaviors. These reactions must be anticipated, recognized, and dealt with by the professional. Norlin (75) particularly warns professionals to be alert for delayed reactions in family members who appear to be coping well during the early stages of crisis.

It is probable that defense mechanisms will emerge at some point during the coping process. The most common defenses used in cases of disability are described as including withdrawal, denial and repression, projection, displacement, regression, and rationalization (30). However, Eisenburg (30) advises professionals to be aware of more obscure defensive stances, such as emerging beliefs that there is peace and/or meaning in the act of suffering, or disavowal of a defective component of the body. Defense mechanisms are not intrinsically undesirable. In fact, defenses can provide a form of healthy protection of personal, emotional territory. The professional must simply remain sensitive to the undue prolongation of dependence on a particular mechanism, or inappropriate and damaging consequences of a particular defensive posture.

The goal in working with a family with a communication impaired member is the reassertion of individual and familial homeostasis—redefined and renegotiated, but predicated in part upon acknowledgment, acceptance, or adjustment. This reestablished equilibrium will not be an all-or-none phenomenon. Even once a basic acceptance and readjustment has occurred, there will be moments of reversion to earlier stages. Also, one can accept the basic reality (e.g., that a stroke has occurred and things will never be the same) without necessarily recognizing and accepting all the day-to-day problems and changes implicit in that reality.

Flesh-and-Blood Human Beings

At this point in the chapter, it might be appropriate to remind the reader that we are discussing flesh-and-blood human beings. All of the theoretical descriptions of family structure, or of stages in the grieving process, cannot possibly capture the depth of suffering of persons for whom a whole lifetime of "knowns" has been eroded, sometimes gradually but often abruptly. In fact, the theories may act as a barrier between clinician and client, providing convenient labels for the devastation that is apparent. While we cannot afford to empathize so completely and intensely with our clients and families that we become dysfunctional, empathy is critical to the clinical interaction. We must remain sensitive and open to the feelings that are being revealed directly and indirectly.

We must recognize, for example, that a communication disorder may feed negatively into previous maladaptive patterns of family interaction and behavior. We must also be sensitive to the fact that, particularly within the elderly population, there is very limited experience with communication disorders and their precipitating conditions, and even less substantial information (93, 94). Yet this limited information is utilized in formulating expectations and strategies for coping with the present problem. In addition, prior experiences may have been unpleasant. For example, if the wife of a stroke patient spent 10 earlier years of her life in a caregiver relationship with a parent who was totally disabled by stroke, her fears and negative emotions may interfere with adjustment to the current crisis.

Finally, in viewing these older clients and families as flesh-and-blood individuals, we must recognize that the onset of a communication disorder may function as one more reminder of the unpleasant side of aging. For the older spouse, expectations of a blissful retirement in the "golden years" may suddenly be challenged. For the child of a communicatively impaired older adult, the disorder and its causes may constitute the first real moment of recognition of the parent's growing frailty, perhaps even his mortality. Inevitably, these realizations, coupled with the accompanying family disruptions and increased care demands, seem to come at a time when the child is most firmly caught up in the demands of his/her own familial, professional and social life. Conflict and stress are inevitable.

Specific Responses to Speech, Language, or Hearing Problems

As a final preface to examining needs of significant others, therefore, it is appropriate to look more closely at specific familial responses to some of the more common conditions precipitating a communication disorder in older adults. Of primary interest are the patterns of response to sudden versus gradual onset disorders.

Sudden Onset Disorders

Stroke-related communication problems are the most comon form of sudden onset communication disorder. Thurston (106) describes stroke as a catastrophic event, literally restructuring the world of the client and family members overnight. Patterns of adjustment and rehabilitation are often complicated by the fact that stroke rarely affects only one mental or physical system. In addition, there is frequently the threat of a second or third stroke episode occurring. As a result, few life patterns are left unaltered. The process of adjustment can be extremely long, extending for months and years past the precipitating event.

Problems in psychosocial adjustment have been described by numerous authors (9, 12, 26, 65); it is clear that client and family patterns of coping cannot be separated readily (64). Of particular interest is the shifting focus of concerns during the weeks and early months poststroke. At first, since stroke is an acute medical crisis, family members fear for the life and survival of the client. This is followed by a growing recognition of the nature and severity of various residual impairments and the beginning of awareness of the ways in which these impairments will affect daily activities. Typically, the more overt impairments receive greatest initial attention. Coping with the consequences of a right-sided hemiparesis, for example, may receive greater focus than the client's moderate receptive aphasia. Only gradually are the full extent and implications of the communication disorder absorbed by the family (92). Interestingly, following an extended period of rehabilitation and partial recovery of functions, family members may find it most difficult to cope with the "little things," minor but irritating residuals of neurological damage. In a recent stroke group session, for instance, one wife spoke at length and with great distress about her husband's failure to maintain previous levels of personal hygiene.

Several studies define more specifically the nature of familial responses to stroke and its associated speech-language problems. Linebaugh and Young-Charles (61) surveyed 21 spouses and 17 children of aphasic adults. Three-fourths of the spouses reported shifts in relationships and responsibilities, and close to 100% of the children reported changes in familial responsibilities. Over two-thirds in both the spouse and child groups also reported modifications in their social lives. Dominant emotional reactions included: anxiety; frustration; helplessness; depression; and pity. These feelings were expressed by more than half of all spouses. While fewer children acknowledged such emotional responses, close to half noted frustration and depression. All of the spouses and almost two-thirds of the children indicated that they felt a need for counseling immediately after the stroke, and 42% of the spouses reported a continued need for counseling many months postonset.

In a separate study, Chwat and his colleagues (19) examined the responses of children of aphasic parents more closely, using a 50-item questionnaire. The greatest role change reported was the partial assumption of the parent's role, associated with assumption of increased responsibility for other family members and for household chores. More than half of the respondents reported that they had become more protective of both parents. The dominant emotional response was described as irritability, with over one-third also indicating that contacts with the aphasic parent created anxiety. Guilt was a common response. Over one-half reported that their own emotional health had been affected, and more than one-third noted changes in their social lives.

These studies provide just a glimpse of the types of changes and responses experienced by family members of older aphasic persons. While patterns of reaction to sudden onset speech-language problems are highly individualistic, a common core of needs is evident.

Gradual-Onset Disorders

The gradual onset communication disorders provoke a relatively distinct set of patterned responses, in that the time frame for adjustment is considerably extended when compared with sudden onset disorders. Two examples of these types of disorders are hearing impairment and dementia (the most common form of which is Alzheimer's disease). While each is characterized by a slow, subtle deterioration in communication skills, the effects on family members and caregivers may be very different.

Hearing Loss. Presbycusic hearing loss associated with aging develops over a period of months, years, and decades. There is no sudden transition from normal to disordered functioning. Several points should be considered in evaluating the effects of hearing loss upon individuals and families (see also Chapter 14).

Hearing impairment in the elderly is frequently associated by the lay person with senility. Not surprisingly, denial of symptoms or difficulties and refusal to seek assistance are common behavioral patterns. The slow onset of the hearing loss also allows for the gradual development of compensations on the part of the individual and those in the environment. Often, these compensations are made without a person's awareness of the process. Since communicative interactions may continue to worsen, the strain on family members will escalate. Patterns of response include fatigue, growing irritation, increasing reluctance to engage in communicative exchanges, among others (1, 78, 79).

In addition, hearing loss (as with any sensory impairment) interferes with the homeostatic balance within the individual and between the individual and his environment (55, 81). While hearing impaired persons react in a variety of ways, Corso (25) has summarized a fairly common pattern of responses, as described in Chapter 14. Changes such as withdrawal, suspiciousness, and confusion in turn take their

toll on families. It is not surprising that a high proportion of the respondents described in Chapter 2 made relatively pejorative remarks about hearing loss and hearing impaired persons. Unfortunately, while hearing aids, assistive listening devices, and appropriate aural rehabilitation can improve this situation, they may not automatically resolve the relatively unhealthy communicative and social dynamics that are already established.

Dementia. In contrast to hearing impairment, the progression of the disease processes in the irreversible forms of dementia ultimately affects most, if not all, aspects of functioning. Frequently a spouse is the first to recognize that a problem is developing (76). Once the presence of dementia has been identified, there is considerable evidence that the burden of care can be overwhelming (7, 49, 52, 72, 114). The combination of mental decline and loss of the patient's assistive or collaborative role in a relationship may be insupportable for some, particularly when the patient resists the care being provided. Common family and caregiver problems noted include: depression, anxiety, other forms of psychological distress, and the development or aggravation of health problems (76). The real horror is that the family member who has been known and loved through the years really no longer exists, at least in the later stages of the disease process (104). Acknowledgment of this reality may create intolerable guilt for some.

THE NEEDS OF SIGNIFICANT OTHERS

The preceding pages have attempted to clarify the status of older persons in relationship to their significant others, with particular emphasis upon the ways in which a specific communication disorder disrupts family adjustment. It has been suggested that both primary caregivers and members of the extended social support network can play many critical roles in meeting the needs of communicatively impaired older adults. However, significant others will be relatively ineffective in these various roles unless their own needs can also be addressed through appropriate interventions.

Defining Basic Needs

The primary goal in any family intervention should be to help the family members regain stability in all aspects of functioning (75). This process of facilitating adjustment and reestablishing homeostasis can only be accomplished if four basic needs are met. While these needs may differ in strength and specifics depending upon the particular communicatively impaired client and significant other, they should be considered in designing all interventions.

1. Information. The majority of significant others require information about normal communication processes, about the specific communication disorder present and its precipitating causes, and about the consequences that may be anticipated (including prognosis). A variety of studies have examined spouse knowledge of communication disorders in general and of the specific nature and severity of a client's problems (36, 39, 50, 82, 95, 96, 108). While results have been somewhat contradictory, it appears that most spouses have little information about the nature of aphasia, for example, and less than accurate or objective perceptions of the client's difficulties (at least at the beginning of treatment). Information may also be required concerning available resources for assistance and specific strategies for communicating with the client.

2. Techniques for Management. While related to the information needs described in no. 1, significant others require training in strategies for managing a variety of problems, including: the client's communication problems; the client's emotional/social problems; their own feelings and altered roles; and the physical and social environment.

3. Counseling. Family members (particularly spouses) must be provided with counseling that will assist them in working through the grieving process and the associated adjustment to the communication disorder. The depth and form of counseling will probably be dictated by the clinician's assessment of the severity of the adjustment problems being experienced and of the degree to which premorbidly impaired family dynamics are interfering with the rehabilitation process.

4. Support and Sharing. Technically, support and sharing might be addressed under the counseling needs described in no. 3. However, even those significant others requiring minimal counseling services will probably need more basic forms of support from others who care and who understand their problems and burdens. If a person has a viable existing support network, the professional's only role may be to suggest ways to educate members of that network concerning the types of problems being experienced. However, if a significant other lacks adequate personal resources or is reluctant to take advantage of those resources available, involvement in a family support group may be helpful. Family members have frequently reported that it is sometimes easier to share openly with virtual strangers who are experiencing similar problems and emotions.

Meeting these four needs of significant others is an integral part of the process of meeting the needs of the communicatively impaired older adult. Appropriate management programs cannot be developed, however, without a thorough assessment of the unique situational characteristics of the individual client and his/her significant others.

Assessment of Needs

Assessment of the needs of significant others must include the following areas of interest: (a) real and reported needs for information; (b) real and reported emotional stresses; (c) premorbid and current patterns of interaction with the client; and (d) premorbid and current social support systems available to both client and significant others. Obviously, the systematic and thorough investigation of all of these variables would be immensely time-consuming. Much data can be obtained from informal interviews and ongoing clinical contacts.

A variety of clinical assessment tools and scales, however, can also be gleaned from the available literature on families and communication disorders. Most of the research in this area involves aphasic adults and their significant others. A sampling of procedures is provided in the following paragraphs.

Chapey (17) provides a "Preinterview Form for an Analysis of the Nonlinguistic and Linguistic Behaviors of an Adult Aphasic Patient from His Child's Perspective." In addition to probes concerning language comprehension and output, the form examines issues of role change, irritability, guilt, altered social life, financial pressures, job and school neglect, health, oversolicitousness, and rejection. The specific knowledge and needs of spouses and children as they relate to a client's language deficits are explored further in Chwat and Gurland's "Aphasia Impact Rating Scale" (20).

Chapey (17) also provides a sample of a "Preinterview Family History and Family Status Form," which, in addition to basic identifying information, elicits brief descriptions of the client's communication status and personality, as well as others' responses to his problems. Similar background information on styles of communication and interaction may be obtained by using the "Questionnaire for Surveying Personal and Communicative Style" (102). Florance and Conway's (35) "Coping and Compliance Assessment" tool explores three coping and three compliance dimensions. The coping dimensions include well-being, psychiatric disease, and emotional stability; the compliance dimensions are cognition and problem solving, behavior change style, and readiness for change. While designed primarily for use with rehabilitation clients, similar data could be helpful in designing interventions for significant others.

If the clinician is interested in examining interactional behaviors more closely, a wide variety of tools are available in the clinical and research literature. Florance (34) originally developed a "Family Interaction Analysis" form that could be used to record the presence or absence of 33 facilitative and nonfacilitative behaviors produced by significant others. The form has since been revised to include only the original 17 facilitative behaviors and three additional behaviors (guessing, interrupting, repeating) (35). The group process evaluation form developed by Loverso et al (63) can also be adapted for use in considering family patterns of interaction.

Other resources for examining communicative interactions have focused primarily on strategies for enhancing comprehension or obtaining information in discourse situations (37, 46, 58, 59, 60, 113). Formal or informal assessment of significant other strategies in communicating with speech-language or hearing impaired older adults is essential to subsequent efforts to involve the significant other in treatment or to provide the significant other with effective communication strategies.

While there is relatively less literature relevant to assessment of the needs of the significant others of hearing impaired older adults, the scales of attitude towards hearing loss and of self-perceptions of the handicapping effects of hearing loss can be of considerable value (see Chapter 13, refs. 40, 67, 91, 107). Walden and colleagues (109) particularly emphasize the need to assess attitudes towards hearing aid usage.

Finally, Biegel et al (8, p 31) provide some excellent suggestions for evaluating the support network of the older client and his/her significant others. Working from adaptations of a lengthy research questionnaire, they recommend that professionals probe:

1. Network persons the individual feels very close to and has a deep trust or confidence relationship with;
2. Network persons who, while not as close, are still important to the individual;
3. The age, relationship, proximity, manner of contact, satisfaction with contact, and types of support provided by these network persons (as well as types of support not provided and why);
4. The desire for any more people in the social network.

MANAGEMENT STRATEGIES INVOLVING SIGNIFICANT OTHERS

Assuming that a relatively clear picture has emerged of the needs of the significant others of a particular client, decisions concerning appropriate management strategies must be made. At least four approaches can be taken; none are mutually exclusive.

Support Groups

The value of self-help and support groups for the elderly has been documented in general terms in a variety of sources (8, 57). Such groups provide a major vehicle for marshaling the resources of the informal support system in order to supplement formal resources or fill in gaps in service provision. In fact, general family well-being has been shown to be enhanced in group meetings of older couples (101).

When we turn to the significant others of communicatively impaired adults, the most notable examples of support groups include those provided for stroke patients and families, for laryngectomized individuals and their families, and for the families of Alzheimer's patients. There is no real clinical model for support groups involving hearing impaired persons, although group sessions are often a part of the rehabilitation process.

One of the problems in discussing support groups for significant others is that many such organizations include both handicapped individuals and their families. A second problem relates to the blurring of the lines of distinction between counseling and support groups (54). In many instances, their goals are remarkably similar, although the facilitation techniques and depth of personal exploration may distinguish the two entities. In addition to confusions related to group composition and goals, a third difficulty stems from the fact that support groups vary considerably in structure and leadership.

Nevertheless, the following sections will touch briefly on each of the more common forms of support groups. Speech-language pathologists and audiologists must assume leadership roles in initiating and maintaining the operation of such groups. There is probably no other single resource of greater value in meeting the long-term needs of the families of communicatively impaired adults.

Stroke Support Groups

Although stroke support groups require no particular affiliation, many are sponsored under the auspices of the American Heart Association. In a very simple definition, Sanders et al describe the stroke support group or stroke club as a:

... community organization formed by and for people who have had a stroke, their family members, their friends or those dedicated to helping stroke people and their families. By meeting regularly, participants can help themselves and each other adjust to or overcome some of the problems that result from stroke. (88, p 3)

From a survey of stroke club objectives gathered from groups around the country, Sanders et al list 15 representative goals. These goals can be condensed into the following five broad categories: (a) to provide education and information concerning stroke and its consequences; (b) to enhance socialization; (c) to promote self-help skills and independence; (d) to provide support in all forms; and (e) to encourage mutual assistance among stroke group members. While some of these goals appear more relevant to the stroke patient than to significant others, all may be beneficial to family members.

McCormick and Williams (69) state that the level of suffering experienced by stroke patients and their families is typically greater than what is observed on the surface. They conclude that stroke support groups provide opportunities for expression of fears, hostilities, and needs. Participants learn that most problems can be resolved. Brookshire (11) indicates that spouse-oriented groups in particular can provide opportunities for family members to express their feelings about the effects of the stroke upon family cohesiveness and functioning.

Those interested in beginning or participating in a stroke support group should refer to the excellent manual *You Are Not Alone* published under the auspices of the American Heart Association (88). Virtually every topic related to the organization, structuring, and ongoing maintenance of a stroke club is discussed in a clear simple fashion; numerous forms and examples facilitate understanding and expedite operations. The appendices provide thorough listings of reference sources for further information, both in the form of readings and organizations.

One of the more interesting sections of this manual is the discussion of problems in organization and maintenance, possible solutions to those problems, and reported factors in the success and/or failure of a stroke club. The authors divide problems into those occurring among members, those related to organization and structure, and those involving attendance and maintenance of membership. Personal experience would suggest at least seven major areas of concern:

1. The diversity of needs presented by individual members of the group;
2. The disparity, at times, between stroke patient and family member needs;
3. The problems inherent in finding an environment adequate to the types of communication problems experienced by stroke patients, as well as the geographical needs and nonsectarian preferences of the members;
4. The competition between equally viable group goals—(e.g., education, socialization, counseling, and support);
5. The sometimes disastrous consequences of bringing in speakers who cannot or will not adjust their content and style to the needs of communicatively impaired members of the group;
6. The group's tendency to become overdependent upon the professional(s) who acts in an organizational or advisory capacity;
7. The constant turnover of group members as needs are met, and the consequent need for an ongoing public relations campaign.

The Sanders et al text (88) provides some excellent strategies for avoiding or eliminating some of these problems. Additional assistance may be obtained by writing to:

American Heart Association
44 East 23rd Street
New York, NY 10010

Lost Chord Clubs

The basic purpose of most Lost Chord Clubs (or laryngectomee clubs) is to provide support and encouragement for laryngectomized persons and their families through personal interaction. Ausherman (4) recently expressed concern, however, that support groups not lose sight of their original purpose, as service clubs with a mission to provide information and assistance to laryngectomees.

Lost Chord Clubs are typically organized under the auspices of the International Association of Laryngectomees (IAL), an affiliate of the American Cancer Society. The IAL began with 10 charter clubs in 1951 and has expanded to over 300 member clubs at the present time. The IAL provides a manual with suggestions concerning procedures in setting up and maintaining a Lost Chord Club. It is recommended that the officers of clubs be laryngectomees, with assistance and advice being offered by professionals in the fields of speech-language pathology and medicine. Local club members automatically become members of the IAL and receive a monthly newsletter.

While the main purpose of the Lost Chord Club is to assist laryngectomized individuals, the informational and emotional needs of spouses are addressed as well. Family members frequently find a way to channel their concerns and distress into club activities, and discover opportunities of sharing with other spouses at club meetings.

Further information can be obtained by writing to:

International Association of Laryngectomees
c/o American Cancer Society
90 Park Avenue
New York, NY 10016

Alzheimer's Support Groups

Alzheimer's support group are almost always designed to assist families and caregivers in coping with the burden of managing the patient with dementia, although a few examples of groups for mild to moderately impaired Alzheimer's patients are described in the literature (cf. 16). A number of writers have described in detail the needs of family members (7, 49, 72, 76). Invariably, reference is made to the family's need for assistance in managing the stresses of caring for an Alzheimer's patient at home or in accepting the decision to institutionalize the patient.

The degree of caregiver strain is predicted by the availability of social supports (72), and perception of caregiver burden has been shown to be influenced by participation in support group meetings (53). One of the key resources available to families is reported to be the Alzheimer's support group, particularly if the patient is kept at home (76). Support groups serve a variety of functions, including: reduction of isolation; provision of practical information designed to enhance coping skills; and provision of strategies for obtaining further information about and assistance from community resources (76).

At least three types of Alzheimer's support groups have been identified—the self-help or basic support group, the educational group, and the psychotherapeutic group (41). In most instances, all three sets of goals are addressed to some degree in a given group. Haley (47) also describes a family-behavioral approach to treating cognitively impaired older adults, emphasizing the family's need to learn appropriate behavioral management strategies. Two representative support groups are selected here for further discussion.

Glosser and Wexler (41) describe an 8-week family group led by a neuropsychologist and a geriatric social worker. The group goals included: (a) to provide accurate information about the dementias; (b) to teach skills in managing behavioral, legal/financial, social, and interpersonal problems; and (c) to offer opportunities for sharing of feelings and mutual support. Session time was equally divided between provision of information and discussion/sharing of individual problems. Participants were asked to rate the group process in terms of most and least helpful experiences. The general supportive aspects of the group process were evaluated highly, along with information provided about medical and behavioral management. Issues of resolution of intrafamilial conflict and information about legal/financial/social problems were felt to be less adequately resolved.

Of more direct interest to communication disorder professionals is the Alzheimer's Disease Support Group described by Tardelli and Bocage (104). This group was organized and is maintained jointly by a speech-language pathologist and a social worker. Group goals include: (a) to provide information; (b) to increase awareness of resources; (c) to provide support through peer interaction and professional input; (d) to resolve issues through problem solving; and (e) to reduce isolation. Four basic participant needs are identified by the authors. First, the group process must focus on ways of allowing members to acknowledge the impact of Alzheimer's disease on family equilibrium and to vent emotional responses to the perceived family disruption. Second, effective strategies for accepting and managing caregiver responsibility must be provided. Third, participants must be helped to accept the gradual decline in cognitive and communicative skills, and finally, the basic grieving process must be allowed to occur in as natural a fashion possible.

Further information about Alzheimer's support groups may be obtained by writing to:

Alzheimer's Disease and Related Disorders
Association, Inc.
360 N. Michigan Avenue
Chicago, IL 60601

Counseling

Goals and Dilemmas

The counseling needs of family members should be readily apparent from earlier discussions. The most commonly cited list of counseling objectives evolves from Webster's work with both children and adults (110).

Webster contends that the four basic purposes of counseling are: (a) to convey information to the family member; (b) to receive information the family wishes to share; (c) to help family members clarify their ideas, emotions, and attitudes relative to the communicative disorder and disordered individual; and (d) to provide family members with strategies for changing behavioral and communicative patterns. Pollack (83) and Sanders (87) reduce these objectives to the two domains of informational and affective (personal adjustment) counseling.

There is some controversy concerning the extent to which all four of Webster's goals should be addressed by speech-language pathologists and audiologists alone. For example, Norlin (75) suggests that goal c (clarification of ideas and emotions) may be overstepping our bounds slightly and goal d probably requires the collaborative assistance of a trained family counselor.

Others question the extent to which we are adequately trained to assume counseling functions in therapy (68). It has been suggested that, by personal preference and/or professional preparation, communication disorders professionals tend to emphasize informational counseling at the expense of personal, affective kinds of interventions. For example, Newhoff and Davis (74) indicate that clinicians may hide behind their focus upon information exchange, because it is more comfortable than other aspects of counseling. Flahive and White (32) noted that audiologists spent a much higher per cent of their counseling time in information provision and rated their skills in this area more highly than skills involving personal adjustment counseling. It appears that the majority of our graduate educational programs (76%) offer counseling courses, but they are typically elective courses with a focus on general counseling principles rather than on the specific problems presented by communication loss (68).

A reasonable approach to the counseling dilemma, therefore, would be for the individual speech-language pathologist or audiologist to determine his/her own readiness for and skills in meeting the four basic counseling goals. If one truly does not feel qualified to address certain counseling needs, every effort should be made both to obtain additional skills and to develop a team collaboration with a qualified counselor (e.g., a family therapist, psychiatric social worker, psychologist, psychotherapist, etc.). However, we must not lose sight of the fact that we are probably best qualified to understand the nature of both communicative deficits and of familial responses to those deficits. If we deny our expertise in these areas, we do our clients a major disservice.

Examples of Counseling Interventions

Webster and Newhoff (111) very appropriately subdivide counseling approaches into individual and group treatments. Both options are viable, and choice of one or both counseling avenues is dependent upon several factors, including: the needs of the significant other (and client); the goals for the counseling session(s) (e.g., the agenda of both the professional and the family member); and the situational constraints. The decision to work with the family member alone, or with the communicatively impaired client present, must be made early in the counseling process and must be continually reassessed throughout treatment.

Individual counseling is probably best suited to obtaining and providing information, as well as clarifying treatment goals, procedures, and prognosis (111). It has also been suggested that individual sessions early in the treatment process may be a useful prerequisite to group sessions. Individual counseling also allows the clinician to probe the significant other's motivation and availability for participation in the client's treatment program; barriers to participation can be identified.

Group counseling sessions for family members (frequently spouses) of aphasic individuals have been described for over 30 years. Excellent summaries of these programs can be found in Kearns (54), Norlin (75), and Webster and Newhoff (111). As noted earlier, the goals of group family counseling often overlap with those of support groups. A team approach to facilitating most counseling groups is evident. Usually a speech-language pathologist will co-lead the group with a psychologist/psychiatrist or social worker; there are also reports of involvement of psychiatric nurses, occupational therapists, and physical therapists. In some groups, facilitation tasks are divided between the leaders in order to make optimal use of the professional skills of each discipline.

There is considerable variability in the size of counseling groups, definitions of appropriate participants, duration of participation, frequency of meetings, and structure of sessions. Counseling approaches (when identified) also distinguish different groups. For example, Porter and Dabul (84) relied heavily on a transactional analysis approach, whereas Gordon (44) utilized nondirective counseling techniques. In most instances, counseling group goals include both provision of information and facilitation of coping or communication strategies. In one of the few well-documented investigations of the efficacy of a spouse intervention program for aphasics, Newhoff and Davis (74) reported that both sets of goals were met. Spouses demonstrated increases in information, enhanced understanding of feelings and attitudes, and positive behavioral changes.

As Kearns suggests, "The need for counseling aphasic patients and their families is unassailable" (54, p 308). Ideally, perhaps, every family member should be provided with an initial information packet (supplemented by films, if available), individual counseling, interdisciplinary group counseling, and access to a support group. Clinicians should be aware that family members may feel considerable anxiety about participating in a group counseling experience. Many older persons come from a generation in which a high value was placed upon keeping one's feelings to oneself; there is little or no tradition of seeking outside assistance for emotional and familial problems. Thus, attempts must be made to allay possible resistance to counseling in any form.

Throughout the course of any group counseling experience, information may need to be repeated frequently, and certain counseling themes will recur. Group leaders should be alert for and patient with these patterns. In addition, clinicians should be sensitive to the shifting needs and concerns of family members. Often, it may be more appropriate to abandon or substantially modify a planned agenda in order to be responsive to participant needs. Finally, every attempt should be made to ensure that no one group member dominates group activities inappropriately. No other factor can be as destructive to motivation to participate.

These same observations and cautions apply to group counseling sessions involving hearing impaired older adults. The need for psychosocial counseling for significant others is well accepted (112). Unfortunately, there are few models for such programs in the literature. Haspiel and colleagues (48) described an intensive counseling program for hearing impaired adults and their spouses. The two- to three-day sessions were facilitated by two audiologists with family therapy training. Emphasis was placed upon communication interactions and problems occurring between spouses, with consideration give to preexisting communication patterns as well as difficulties specifically related to hearing loss.

Significant Others in Treatment

One positive byproduct of significant other involvement in support groups and counseling is the enhancement of direct participation in the older client's rehabilitation program. It is axiomatic that speech-language-hearing interventions that occur within the therapy room or audiological suite do not necessarily guarantee transfer of new skills or communication-enhancing devices to real life situations. Thus, ways must be found to utilize significant others in the treatment process. Since this topic is covered in some detail in the various chapters on assessment and management of hearing and speech-language disorders (Chapters 13 through 16), only a cursory discussion is provided here.

Theoretical Considerations of Roles

There are three basic types of literature addressing the use of significant others in rehabilitation programs for communicatively impaired older adults. The first group of publications consists of theoretical and clinical discussions of the possible roles of significant others in the treatment process. For example, Weinstein (112) devotes several pages to description of the ways in which significant others may assist the hearing impaired individual in use of the personal hearing aid as well as in enhancement of daily communications. A distinction is made between family members and professional caregivers (e.g., in a nursing home setting), with their different degrees of emotional involvement and potentially diverse roles. Florance (33) also describes the problems encountered by the spouse of an aphasic client who attempts to assume the teacher role. Nevertheless, she suggests that use of a significant other as an intervention aide results in decreased time in therapy, improved generalization, and more durable behavioral change.

Significant Others as Direct Participants in Treatment

The second type of literature in this area includes specific studies of programs in which spouses were used as therapy aides or adjuncts. Most of the available publications pertain to aphasia. Goodkin et al (42) described a program in which spouses of aphasic patients were trained to act as supplemental speech clinicians. Client-spouse communication interventions were analyzed in order to determine behaviors in need of intervention. Principles of behavior modification were introduced to the spouses, and they were trained to use these principles to modify target verbal behaviors at home.

Florance (34) also describes a "family interaction therapy" approach in which significant others are involved with the client and clinician in each of seven phases of treatment, from baseline assessment and development of a treatment plan through transfer/generalization and postevaluation. The core of the program is the "family interaction analysis" described earlier. The use of spouses as direct facilitators of communication is also described by Newhoff et al (73). In their study, four female spouses of aphasic patients participated in eight treatment sessions in which they were trained in the procedures of PACE therapy. Statistically significant group differences were not observed. However, discourse changes were reported in the areas of increased interaction, increased communicative attempts by the aphasic member of the dyad, changes in verbal strategies of the spouse, and apparently fewer episodes of comprehension breakdown.

Examinations of Communicative Strategies Employed by Significant Others

The involvement of significant others in treatment is also examined indirectly through studies exploring communicative interactions between aphasic adults and their communication partners, in order to identify behaviors that should be facilitated or eliminated through therapeutic intervention. For example, Flowers and Peizer (37) studied spouses' strategies for obtaining information from aphasic clients, examining the manner, form, and purpose of the strategy as well as its success. Yorkston et al (113) also explored the efficiency of information exchange with aphasic speakers using a combined measure of time and accuracy in a "hidden" stimulus paradigm. Gurland and others (46) investigated conversational breakdowns, signals to repair, actual repairs or revisions, and communicative success in aphasic/nonaphasic conversational dyads. Their findings were used to illustrate possible intervention strategies.

Linebaugh and colleagues (59) examined the reapportionment of the communicative burden in aphasic dyads. Communicative burden was defined as the share of responsibility in a conversation that ensures adequate transfer of information. Linebaugh has also been involved in a number of other investigations of the nature and effectiveness of comprehension-enhancing strategies used by spouses of aphasic clients (58, 60).

In all of these studies, the emphasis is placed upon understanding spouse-client communicative interactions. It is assumed that the knowledge gained will contribute directly or indirectly to effective utilization of significant others as partners in the therapeutic process.

Information Exchange

At the beginning of this chapter, it was suggested that two groups can be considered to be significant others for the communicatively impaired older adult. The information needs of families and primary caregivers have been stressed in preceding sections. Information dissemination was described as being accomplished in informal patient/family contacts, individual and group counseling sessions, support groups, and treatment sessions involving family members. It is now time to turn to the community of friends, neighbors and service providers who constitute the broader social support network. Information dissemination to service providers is typically accomplished through inservice education programs, as highlighted in Chapter 22. The remainder of this section, therefore, will focus upon the availability of information resources within any given community.

Community Access to Information

Adequate information access and retrieval has been decribed as one of the primary needs of older adults (8). How can information needs related to communication disorders be met? Where does an individual go to obtain quick access to information about stroke, for example—its causes, consequences, and resources for management? How can an older person obtain clear, unbiased facts about hearing loss without having to make an appointment for an audiological evaluation?

One answer to these questions is that communication disorders professionals must make every effort to ensure that community agencies, hospitals, service organizations, and libraries are made aware of the many publications and filmstrips available concerning communication impairment. Lists of resources (including local, State, and national organizations) should be provided to these facilities and agencies; if possible, copies of relevant materials should be made available. Resource persons (speech-language pathologists and audiologists) in the area should also be identified. Excellent descriptions of resources can be found in a variety of sources (see refs. 2, 10, 88, 94, as well as Chapter 21 of this text).

Communication disorders professionals must also recognize that their close involvement with the families of older adults places them in a rather unique position. Family members will frequently ask for information and assistance in coping with a variety of social, medical, economic, and legal problems that are not within our professional jurisdiction. It is our responsibility to ensure that we are adequately informed about community resources, particularly as they relate to aging and the elderly.

Pre-Crisis Intervention

Another approach to educating the community of potential significant others is to adopt a more proactive stance by providing programs of preventive education concerning communication, aging, and communication disorders in the elderly. One such program has been called "Pre-Crisis Intervention" (PCI). Pre-Crisis Intervention assumes that most, if not all, older persons will eventually have to cope with one or more peers with a communication disorder. However as noted earlier, the average older individual is ill-prepared emotionally or informationally to provide adequate interpersonal and communicative support (93). PCI programs, therefore, attempt to enhance the effectiveness of the community resource of peers by providing educational experiences prior to the onset of the crisis provoked by a communication disorder.

There are four basic goals in Pre-Crisis Intervention:

1. Modification of attitudes towards communication disorders and towards individuals with such disorders;
2. Enhanced understanding of the problems encountered by such individuals and their families and friends;
3. Development of constructive strategies for coping with communication breakdown and its consequences;
4. Enhanced knowledge of community resources and improved participation in appropriate rehabilitative efforts.

The development and implementation of PCI programs has been described in some detail in several sources (92, 94). The basic program consists of a series of five workshop sessions covering the topics of communication and aging (one session), speech-language disorders (two sessions) and hearing impairment (two sessions). If desired, only sessions or sections related to a specific topic may be presented. Because the program emphasizes understanding of emotional reactions to communication disorders and exploration of coping strategies, three primary instructional techniques are utilized.

Core information is presented through *lectures*, supplemented by handouts and visual aids. The nature of deficits and the problems

which may result from communication breakdown are explored through *training experiences*. A training experience is any form of activity that requires the participation of workshop attendees. It may be a simulated hearing test, listening and reacting to speech presented through hearing aids, role playing of communication with an aphasic adult, or analysis of tape-recorded samples of the speech of communicatively impaired persons. These training experiences allow participants to engage emotionally with the feelings and deficits experienced by speech-language or hearing impaired individuals and their families. Finally, though less frequently utilized, *discussions* in a small group format provide opportunities for exploring reactions further and for problem solving community solutions to the difficulties created by a communication disorder.

Pre-Crisis Intervention programs target older community members and can be presented to groups of varying sizes. Initiating PCI programming may be simplified by working through an agency, retirement organization, residential complex, or community church. All lecture, training experience, handout, and visual materials necessary for providing PCI workshops are included in the *Coping with Communication Disorders in Aging* manual (94). This manual also contains detailed instructions for setting up workshops, as well as for describing program development and initial outcomes.

Some of the advantages of PCI reported by program users include: (a) its emphasis upon reducing the *impact* of communication disorders; (b) its broad outreach to the communication network of the older person; (c) its reliance on experiential learning techniques; and (d) its relative cost effectiveness. The program is also consistent with the concept of education as a lifelong process (71).

CONCLUSIONS

The families, caregivers, and members of the support network of communicatively impaired older adults play a major role in the success or failure of any rehabilitation program. While it is important to design interventions that maximize the contributions of these significant others, it is far too easy to forget that they too have needs that must be addressed. Family members in particular suffer emotional crises when a communication disorder disrupts the delicate homeostasis of the family unit. The degree of stress and loss experienced is often complicated by existing pressures and changes related to the aging process.

In this chapter, it has been suggested that there are two groups of significant others that must be considered in interventions. The first group consists of primary caregivers, typically members of the immediate family, who are either in relationships of social and emotional intimacy with the client or whose caregiving activities provide the most frequent source of interpersonal interactions for that individual. The second group encompasses the broader social support network of the older individual. The status of both groups in relationship to the elderly was discussed briefly, and the roles that can be served by each group were delineated.

The needs of significant others were addressed by considering the impact of a communication disorder upon family systems, including discussion of disruptions of homeostasis and stages in response to loss or crisis. It was suggested that four basic forms of intervention might be helpful in addressing significant other needs and enhancing the significant other's ability to assist the communicatively impaired client. These four forms of intervention, while not mutually exclusive, were defined as: support groups, counseling, direct participation in treatment programs, and information dissemination (particularly to the community of older adults). Each intervention approach was discussed briefly.

Speech-language pathologists and audiologists must continue to expand their efforts to meet the needs of the significant others of communicatively disordered older adults. Given the dwindling support systems of many elderly individuals, we canot afford to ignore the contributions of these individuals. Further, our commitment to enhancing communicative adequacy for all persons must extend to members of our clients' communication networks.

References

1. Alpiner JG: Rehabilitation of the geriatric client. In Alpiner JG (ed): *Handbook of Rehabilitative Audiology*. Baltimore, Williams & Wilkins, 1978, p 141.
2. American Speech-Language-Hearing Association: *Resource Materials for Communicative Problems of Older Persons*, revised ed. Rockville, MD, American Speech-Language-Hearing Association, 1980.
3. Auburn S: Community-based care: An achievable goal? *The Southwestern* 2:33–39, 1985.
4. Ausherman WD: Speaking out. *IAL News* 32:1, 1986.
5. Baldassare M, Rosenfield S, Rook K: The types of social relations predicting elderly well-being. *Res Aging* 6:549–559.
6. Barlow MS: Lifestyle and the family of the disabled. In Rule WR (ed): *Lifestyle Counseling for Adjustment to Disability*. Rockville, MD, Aspen, 1984, p 61.
7. Bartol MA: Nonverbal communication in patients with Alzheimer's disease. *J Gerontol Nurs* 5:21–31, 1979.
8. Biegel DE, Shore BK, Gordon E: *Building Support Networks for the Elderly: Theory and Applications*. Beverly Hills, CA, Sage, 1984.
9. Biorn-Hanson V: Social and emotional aspects of aphasia. *J Speech Hear Disord* 22:53–59, 1957.
10. Broida H: *Coping with Stroke*. Waltham, MA, Little Brown, 1979.
11. Brookshire RH: *An Introduction to Aphasia*, ed 2. Minneapolis, BRK Publishers, 1978.
12. Buck M: *Dysphasia: Professional Guidance for Family and Patient*. Englewood Cliffs, NJ, Prentice-Hall, 1978.
13. Bultena G: Rural-urban differences in the familial interaction of the aged. *Rural Sociol* 34:5–15, 1969.
14. Bultena G, Powers E, Falham P, Frederick D: Life after 70 in Iowa. In: *Sociology Report 95*. Ames, IA, Iowa State University, 1971.
15. Byerts TO, Howell SC, Pastalan LA: *Environmental Context of Aging: Life-Styles, Environmental Quality, and Living Arrangements*. New York, Garland STPM Press, 1979.
16. Carey B, Hansen SS: Social support groups with institutionalized Alzheimer's disease victims. *J Gerontol Soc Work* 9:15–26, 1985/86.
17. Chapey R: The assessment of language disorders in adults. In Chapey R (ed): *Language Intervention Strategies in Adult Aphasia*, ed 2. Baltimore, Williams & Wilkins, 1986, p 81.
18. Chappell NL: Informal support networks among the elderly. *Res Aging* 5:77–99, 1983.
19. Chwat S, Chapey R, Gurland G, Pieras G: Environmental impact of aphasia: The child's perspective. In Brookshire RH (ed): *Clinical Aphasiology Conference Proceedings*. Minneapolis, BRK Publishers, 1977, p 127.
20. Chwat S, Gurland GB: Comparative family perspectives on aphasia: Diagnostic, treatment, and counseling implications. In Brookshire RH (ed): *Clinical Aphasiology Conference Proceedings*. Minneapolis, BRK Publishers, 1981, p 212.
21. Coe RM, Wolinsky FD, Miller DK, Prendergast JM: Social network relationships and use of physician services. *Res Aging* 6:243–256, 1984.
22. Cohen CI, Rajkowski MPH: What's in a friend? Substantive and theoretical issues. *Gerontologist* 22:261–266, 1982.
23. Cohen CI, Teresi J, Holmes D: Social networks, stress, adaptation, and health. *Res Aging* 7:409–431, 1985.
24. Cohn NK: Understanding the process of adjustment to disability. *J Rehabil* 27:16–18, 1961.
25. Corso JF: Auditory processes and aging: significant problems for research. *Exp Aging Res* 10:171–174, 1984.
26. Czvik PS: Assessment of family attitudes toward aphasic patients with severe auditory processing disorders. In Brookshire RH (ed): *Clinical Aphasiology Conference Proceedings*. Minneapolis, BRK Publishers, 1977, p 160.
27. Davis GA, Baggs TW: Rehabilitation of speech and language disorders. In Jacobs-Condit L (ed):

Gerontology and Communication Disorders. Rockville, MD, American Speech-Language-Hearing Association, 1984, p 185.

28. Dowd JJ: *Stratification among the Aged.* Monterey, CA, Brooks/Cole, 1980.

29. Dowd JJ, LaRossa R: Primary group contact and elderly morale. Presented at the Annual Meeting of the Gerontological Society, Dallas, 1978.

30. Eisenburg M: *Psychological Aspects of Physical Disability: A Guide for the Health Care Worker.* New York, National League of Nursing, 1977.

31. Falek A, Britton S: Phases in coping. *Soc Biol* 21:1–7, 1974.

32. Flahive MJ, White SC: Audiologists and counseling. *J Acad Rehabil Audiol* 14:274–287, 1982.

33. Florance CL: The aphasic's significant other: Training and counseling. In Brookshire RH (ed): *Clinical Aphasiology Conference Proceedings.* Minneapolis, BRK Publishers, 1979, p 295.

34. Florance CL: Methods of communication analysis used in family interaction therapy. In Brookshire RH (ed): *Clinical Aphasiology Conference Proceedings.* Minneapolis, BRK Publishers, 1981, p 204.

35. Florance CL, Conway WF: Transdisciplinary intervention. In Chapey R (ed): *Language Intervention Strategies in Adult Aphasia*, ed 2. Baltimore, Williams & Wilkins, 1986, p 162.

36. Flowers DR, Beukelman DR, Bottorf LE, Kelley RA: Family members' predictions of aphasia test performance. *Aphasia-Apraxia-Agnosia* 1:18–26, 1979.

37. Flowers CR, Peizer ER: Strategies for obtaining information from aphasic persons. In Brookshire RH (ed): *Clinical Aphasiology Conference Proceedings.* Minneapolis, BRK Publishers, 1984, p 106.

38. Frankfather DL, Smith MJ, Caro FG: *Family Care of the Elderly: Public Initiative and Private Obligations.* Lexington, MA, Lexington Books, 1981.

39. Furbacher EA, Wertz RT: Simulation of aphasia by wives of aphasic patients. In Brookshire RH (ed): *Clinical Aphasiology Conference Proceedings.* Minneapolis, BRK Publishers, 1983, p 227.

40. Giolas T: *Hearing Handicapped Adults.* Englewood Cliffs, NJ, Prentice-Hall, 1982.

41. Glosser G, Wexler D: Participants evaluation of educational/support groups for families of patients with Alzheimer's disease and other dementias. *Gerontologist* 25:232–236, 1985.

42. Goodkin R, Diller L, Shah N: Training spouses to improve the functional speech of aphasic patients. In Lahey BB (ed): *The Modification of Language Behaviors.* Springfield, IL, Charles C Thomas, 1973, p 218.

43. Goodman CC: Natural helping among older adults. *Gerontologist* 24:138–143, 1984.

44. Gordon E: A bi-disciplinary approach to group therapy for wives of aphasics. Paper presented at the American Speech-Language-Hearing Association Convention, Houston, 1976.

45. Goudy WJ, Goudeau, JF Jr: Social ties and life satisfaction of older persons: Another evaluation. *J Gerontol Soc Work* 4:35–50, 1982.

46. Gurland GB, Chwat SE, Wollner SG: Establishing a communication profile in adult aphasia: Analysis of communicative acts and conversational sequences. In Brookshire RH (ed): *Clinical Aphasiology Conference Proceedings.* Minneapolis, BRK Publishers, 1982, p 18.

47. Haley WE: A family-behavioral approach to the treatment of the cognitively impaired elderly. *Gerontologist* 23:18–23, 1983.

48. Haspiel M, Clement JR, Haspiel GS: Aural rehabilitation for hard of hearing adults. San Francisco, Veterans Administration Hospital (unpublished manuscript for distribution), 1972.

49. Hayter J: Helping families of patients with Alzheimer's disease. *J Gerontol Nurs* 8:81–86, 1982.

50. Helmick JW, Watamori TS, Palmer JM: Spouses' understanding of the communication disabilities of aphasic patients. *J Speech Hear Disord* 41:238–243, 1976.

51. Jaffe DR: The role of family therapy in treating physical illness. *Hosp. Commun Psychiatry* 29:169–174, 1978.

52. Jarrett WH: Caregiving within kinship systems: Is affection really necessary? *Gerontologist* 25:5–10, 1985.

53. Jenkins TS, Parham IA, Jenkins T: Alzheimer's disease: caregivers' perceptions of burden. *J Appl Gerontol* 4:40–57, 1985.

54. Kearns KP: Group therapy for aphasia: Theoretical and practical considerations. In Chapey R (ed): *Language Intervention Strategies in Adult Aphasia*, ed 2. Baltimore, Williams & Wilkins, 1986, p 304.

55. Koncelik JA: Human factors and environmental design for the aging: Aspects of physiological change and sensory loss as design criteria. In Byerts TO, Howell SC, Pastalan LA (eds): *Environmental Context of Aging.* New York, Garland STPM Press, 1979, p 107.

56. Kubler-Ross E: *On Death and Dying.* New York, McMillan, 1969.

57. Lieberman MA, Tobin SS: *The Experience of Old Age: Stress, Coping, and Survival.* New York, Basic Books, 1983.

58. Linebaugh CW: Communicative interaction with aphasic adults: Recent findings and applications. Presented at the American Speech-Language-Hearing Association Convention, Washington, 1985.

59. Linebaugh CW, Kryzer KM, Oden SE, Myers P: Reapportionment of communicative burden in aphasia: A study of narrative interaction. In Brookshire RH (ed): *Clinical Aphasiology Conference Proceedings.* Minneapolis, BRK Publishers, 1982, p 4.

60. Linebaugh CW, Margulies CP, Mackisack-Morin EL: Contingent queries and revisions used by aphasic individuals and their most frequent communication partners. In Brookshire RH (ed): *Clinical Aphasiology Conference Proceedings.* Minneapolis, BRK Publishers, 1985, p 229.

61. Linebaugh CW, Young-Charles HY: The counseling needs of the families of aphasic patients. In Brookshire RH (ed): *Clinical Aphasiology Conference Proceedings.* Minneapolis, BRK Publishers, 1978, p 303.

62. Lipman A, Longino CF: Formal and informal support: a conceptual clarification. *J Appl Gerontol* 1:141–146, 1982.

63. Loverso FL, Young-Charles HY, Tonkovich JD: The application of a process evaluation form for aphasic individuals in a small group setting. In Brookshire RH (ed): *Clinical Aphasiology Conference Proceedings*. Minneapolis, BRK Publishers, 1982, p 10.

64. Lubinski RB: Why so little interest in whether or not old people talk? A review of recent research on verbal communication among the elderly. *Int J Aging Hum Dev* 9:237–245, 1978–1979.

65. Malone PE: Expressed attitudes of families of aphasics. *J Speech Hear Disord* 34:146–150, 1969.

66. Mancini JA, Simon J: Older adults' expectations of support from family and friends. *J Appl Gerontol* 3:150–160, 1984.

67. McCarthy P, Alpiner J: An assessment scale of hearing handicap for use in family. *J Acad Rehabil Audiol* 16:256–271, 1983.

68. McCarthy P, Culpepper NB, Lucks L: Variability in counseling experiences and training among ESB-Accredited programs. *ASHA* 28:49–52, 1986.

69. McCormick GP, Williams P: The Midwestern Pennsylvania Stroke Club: Conclusions following the first year's operation of a family-centered program. In Brookshire RH (ed): *Clinical Aphasiology Conference Proceedings*. Minneapolis, BRK Publishers, 1976, p 315.

70. McFarlane SC, Fujiki M, Brinton B: *Coping with Communicative Handicap: Resources for Practicing Clinicians*. Waltham, MA, Little Brown, 1984.

71. Moody HR: Education as a lifelong process. In Pifer A, Bronte L (eds): *Our Aging Society*. New York, WW Norton, 1986, p 199.

72. Morycz RK: Caregiving strain and the desire to institutionalize family members with Alzheimer's disease. *Res Aging* 7:329–361, 1985.

73. Newhoff M, Bugbee JK, Ferreira A: A change of PACE: Spouses as treatment targets. In Brookshire RH (ed): *Clinical Aphasiology Conference Proceedings*. Minneapolis, BRK Publishers, 1981, p 234.

74. Newhoff M, Davis GA: A spouse intervention program: Planning, implementation, and problems of evaluation. In Brookshire RH (ed): *Clinical Aphasiology Conference Proceedings*. Minneapolis, BRK Publishers, 1978, p 318.

75. Norlin PF: Familiar faces, sudden strangers: Helping families cope with the crisis of aphasia. In Chapey R (ed): *Language Intervention Strategies in Adult Aphasia*, ed 2. Baltimore, Williams & Wilkins, 1986, p 174.

76. Ory MG, Williams TF, Emr M, Lebowitz B, Rabins P, Salloway J, Sluss-Radbaugh T, Wolff E, Zarit S: Families, informal supports, and Alzheimer's disease. *Res Aging* 7:623–644, 1985.

77. Oyer EJ: Exchanging information within the older family. In Oyer HJ, Oyer EJ (eds): *Aging and Communication*. Baltimore, University Park Press, 1976, p 43.

78. Oyer HJ, Kapur VP, Deal LV: Hearing disorders in the aging: Effects upon communication. In Oyer HJ, Oyer EJ (eds): *Aging and Communication*. Baltimore, University Park Press, 1976, p 175.

79. Oyer EJ, Paolucci B: Homemakers' hearing losses and family integration. *J Home Econ* 65:227–262, 1970.

80. Parmelee PA: Social contacts, social instrumentality, and adjustment of institutionalized aged. *Res Aging* 4:269–280, 1982.

81. Pastalan LA: Sensory changes and environmental behaviors. In Byerts TO, Howell SC, Pastalan LA (eds): *Environmental Context of Aging*. New York, Garland STPM Press, 1979, p 118.

82. Plumridge TS, Lapointe LL, Lombardino LJ: Definitions and perceptions of aphasia by spouses of aphasic individuals. Presented at the American Speech-Language-Hearing Association Convention, Washington, DC, 1985.

83. Pollack M: The remediation process: Psychological and counseling aspects. In Alpiner JG (ed): *Handbook of Adult Rehabilitative Audiology*. Baltimore, Williams & Wilkins, 1978, p 121.

84. Porter JL, Dabul B: The application of transactional analysis to therapy with wives of adult aphasic patients. *ASHA* 19:244–248, 1977.

85. Powers EA, Keith P, Goudy WJ: Family relationships and friendships among the rural aged. In Byerts TO, Howell SC, Pastalan LA (eds): *Environmental Context of Aging*. New York, Garland STPM Press, 1979, p 80.

86. Rundall TG, Evashwick C: Social networks and help-seeking among the elderly. *Res Aging* 4:205–226, 1982.

87. Sanders DA: Hearing aid orientation and counseling. In Pollack M (ed): *Amplification for the Hearing-impaired*. New York, Grune & Stratton, 1975, p 323.

88. Sanders SB, Hamby EI, Nelson M: *You are Not Alone. . .Organizing Your Local Stroke Club*. Nashville, Tennessee Affiliate of American Heart Association, 1984.

89. Satir V: *Conjoint Family Therapy*. Palo Alto, Science and Behavior Books, 1967.

90. Schneider J: The stresses of living: Loss. Paper presented at Michigan State University, 1974.

91. Schow R, Nerbonne M: Communication screening profile: Use with elderly clients. *Ear Hear* 3:135–148, 1982.

92. Shadden BB: Pre-crisis intervention: A tool for reducing the impact of stroke-related crisis. *J Gerontol Soc Work* 6:61–74, 1983.

93. Shadden BB, Raiford CA: Communication education and the elderly: Perceptions of knowledge and interest in further learning. *Commun Educ* 35:23–31, 1986.

94. Shadden BB, Raiford CA, Shadden HS: *Coping wth Communication Disorders in Aging*. Tigard, OR, CC Publications, 1983.

95. Shaughnessy A, Trupe E, Linden P. Comparison between family ratings of language and standardized test scores. Presented at the American Speech-Language-Hearing Association Convention, Washington, DC, 1985.

96. Shewan CM, Cameron H: Communication and related problems as perceived by aphasic individuals and their spouses. *J Commun Dis* 17:175–187, 1984.

97. Shontz F: Reactions to crisis. *Volta Rev* 67:364–370, 1965.

98. Simons RL, West GE: Life changes, coping resources, and health among the elderly. *Int J Aging Hum Dev* 20:173–189, 1984–85.

99. Spakes PR: Family, friendship and community interaction as related to life satisfaction of the elderly. *J Gerontol Soc Work* 1:279–293, 1979.

100. Strain LA, Chappell NL: Confidants: Do they make a difference in quality of life? *Res Aging* 4:479–502, 1982.

101. Strow C, Mackreth R: Family group meetings—strengthening a partnership. *J Gerontol Nurs* 3:30–35, 1977.

102. Swindell CS, Pashek GV, Holland AH: A questionnaire for surveying personal and communicative style. In Brookshire RH (ed): *Clinical Aphasiology Conference Proceedings.* Minneapolis, BRK Publishers, 1982, p 50.

103. Tanner DC: Loss and grief: implications for speech-language pathologist and audiologist. *ASHA* 22:916–928. 1980.

104. Tardelli MM, Bocage M: A team approach to family support groups in Alzheimer's disease. Presented at the American Speech-Language-Hearing Association Convention, Washington, DC, 1985.

105. Tesch S, Whitbourne SK, Nehrke MF: Friendship, social interaction and subjective well-being of older men in an institutional setting. *Int J Aging Hum Dev* 13:317–327, 1981.

106. Thurston FD: Stroke: A catastrophic event. *J Gerontol Soc Work* 3:53–61, 1980.

107. Ventry I, Weinstein B: The hearing handicap inventory for the elderly: A new tool. *Ear Hear* 3:128–134, 1982.

108. Vogel D, Costello RM: Relatives and aphasia clinicians—Do they agree? In Brookshire RH (ed): *Clinical Aphasiology Conference Proceedings.* Minneapolis, BRK Publishers, 1985, p 237.

109. Walden B, Demorest M, Hepler E: Self-report approach to assessing benefit derived from amplification. *J Speech Hear Disord* 27:49–56, 1984.

110. Webster EJ: *Counseling with Parents of Handicapped Children: Guidelines for Improving Communication.* New York, Grune & Stratton, 1977.

111. Webster EJ, Newhoff M: Intervention with families of communicatively impaired adults. In Beasley DS, Davis GA (eds): *Aging: Communication Processes and Disorders.* New York, Grune & Stratton, 1981, p 229.

112. Weinstein BE: Management of the hearing impaired elderly. In Jacobs-Condit L (ed): *Gerontology and Communication Disorders.* Rockville, MD, American Speech-Language-Hearing Association, 1984, p 244.

113. Yorkston KM, Beukelman DR, Flowers DF: Efficiency of information exchange between aphasic speakers and communication partners. In Brookshire RH (ed): *Clinical Aphasiology Conference Proceedings.* Minneapolis, BRK Publishers, 1980, p 96.

114. Zarit SH, Reever KE, Bach-Peterson J: Relatives of the impaired elderly: Correlates of feelings of burden. *Gerontologist* 20:649–655, 1980.

20 Group Treatment: The Logical Choice

JANE A. BARR

Editor's Note

Group therapy programs or group counseling approaches have been alluded to in several earlier chapters. These forms of programming only begin to hint at the clinical opportunities provided by the group treatment paradigm. In Chapter 20, Barr suggests that speech-language pathologists and audiologists should become more aware of the treatment possibilities presented by groups. Most commonly, group objectives include relationship goals, content goals, or some combination of these two. Barr describes each of these types of goals in some detail and provides examples of common therapeutic groups for the elderly drawn from the literature. Included in this discussion are brief descriptions of groups concerned with support, reminiscence, resocialization, sensory training, mental and physical management, memory training, maintenance of cognitive functioning, behavioral family interventions, and reality orientation. Matching the group intervention to the client involves consideration of primary goals, the nature of the existing deficit(s), and the severity of overall impairment. The types of clients best suited to each type of group are discussed, with particular emphasis upon communicatively disordered individuals. Barr encourages the reader to become more active in developing group interventions or in participating as consultant or facilitator in the maintenance of existing groups designed to enhance the social, cognitive, or communicative effectiveness of the older client. Suggestions for further reading designed to improve counseling and group facilitation skills are provided.

INTRODUCTION

Whether a group is formal (like a sorority) or informal (like a cluster of friends), socially oriented or organized to perform a specific task, the essence of the group is the communication among its members. The depth and content of the communication which takes place indicates the purposes and the cohesiveness of the group. From this perspective, all group treatment programs may be thought of as using, teaching, and changing communication patterns. The communication problems, and strengths, of the members will influence the effectiveness of the group in producing change, whether the type of change desired is greater emotional closeness, less depression and self-pity, or more willingness to practice a new communication technique.

For practitioners concerned with speech, language, and hearing disorders, groups constitute additional treatment possibilities. The group can serve as a safe setting for the practice of new communication skills, thereby freeing the therapist from the responsibility of providing all interactions for the patient. The group can offer advice, consolation, and examples of success from others who have overcome the same difficulty, thereby accomplishing functions which are outside the scope of the therapist's role. As noted in Chapter 19, the latter functions are particularly important to the significant others of individuals with communication disorders.

Even therapists who are not planning to form treatment or support groups may find themselves in settings, such as nursing homes, in which groups are already being offered to their clients. The communication specialist who understands the structure and purpose of various kinds of groups will be able either to offer the group leader suggestions regarding certain clients in the context of the group, or to step in as group leader in order to accomplish treatment objectives.

The facilitation skills needed to run a group are beyond the scope of this text; suggested books on counseling and group work are listed at the end of the chapter. The purpose here is to provide an orientation to goals which can be implemented in group settings, descriptions of a number of common types of groups, and suggestions on which types of interventions are likely to be successful for various populations.

Background

Psychological and psychiatric treatment in groups, rather than individually, was developed during and after World War II, as the need for therapy for "shell-shocked" soldiers exceeded the capacity of the therapeutic community. The elderly were soon included in this movement, with the first report of group psychotherapy for the "senile" being presented in 1950 by Silver (46). In 1953, Kubie and Landau (26) presented a charming anecdotal narrative of their experiences working with groups in a senior center. To date, the great majority of publications on group work with the elderly continue to be of a clinically descriptive nature, and many techniques have not been empirically tested (2). While the literature on group work includes statements on psychological needs of the elderly, there is little empirical evidence that their basic needs differ from those of younger people. However, their situations do differ; they are more likely to be caring for an ill spouse, for example, or to have had a stroke. Thus, group treatment for the elderly tends to encompass both general group practice appropriate for other age groups and applications for special needs.

Therapist Attitudes

If the therapist is influenced by stereotypes of old people, rather than dealing with the realities of the individuals who make up the group, the effectiveness of treatment will be compromised. A therapist who "knows" that old people cannot learn anything new, or who "knows" that the elderly are too emotionally frail to face a conflict of opinions, will not challenge group members to solve their own problems. A therapist who "knows" that old people are inflexible will not expect group members to learn and change. Actually, as in any age group, some elderly people are less psychologically flexible, and others more so. Sadly, a therapist's belief in the impossibility of improvement may become a self-fulfilling prophecy. Being treated as if one is helpless and incompetent fosters helpless and incompetent behavior, while expectations of hard work and success increase the likelihood that a participant will profit from the group experience.

How can therapists overcome their stereotypes? One way is to stay grounded in observations of actual behavior, rather than in interpretations of the behavior. Certainly suppositions about a client (such as "Maybe he isn't working on his speech because he is depressed" or "It seems that she enjoys the attention she gets from being unable to care for herself") are a part of understanding the client's situation. However, the effective therapist keeps such suppositions tentative and open to modification. The second technique for preventing stereotypes from determining the outcome of therapy is to avoid placing faith in predictions, including one's own. Instead, work from the basis that the client is now able to do X, and that a small improvement would result in the ability to do Y; then work with the client on Y. If Y is achieved, Z can be the next goal. Only when a concerted effort to accomplish Y fails can it legitimately be declared that therapy will not benefit the client.

GOALS OF GROUP WORK

There are two general types of goals in group work which can be separated for the sake of discussion even though they overlap in reality. (For purposes of this chapter, other goals specific to intensive long-term group psychotherapy are not included.) One type of goal is based on relationships, and includes such processes as identifying with other group members and increasing self-esteem through positive feedback from the group. The second type of goal involves the acquistion of specific content, such as new knowledge or skills. Both sets of goals may be appropriate for communicatively-impaired clients.

Relationship Goals

Relationship goals include identification, fostering realistic optimism, modeling developing feelings of self-worth through helping others, reducing obsession with one's own problems, developing more effective social behavior, and filling of needed social roles by other group members. Each of these goals is described below.

Identification means that a group member recognizes a basic similarity between the self and other group members. This feeling may be expressed as "We are all in this together," He knows what it's like because he's been through it too, " or "She has earned the right to be frank with me." The simple knowledge that others are in the same situation, having some of the same feelings, is an enormous comfort to many clients. Social isolation can produce an uncomfortable sense of uniqueness, which in turn may increase guilt at "unworthy" sentiments or weakness.

Optimism is encouraged by identification, because the client can see that other group members with similar problems have been making progress. Similarly, individuals can model their attitudes after the attitudes of successful others in the group. In this way, the group can give "permission" to express feelings and to overcome beliefs which may be interfering with a successful resolution of the problem. For example, hearing another group member describe how she persisted at a task in the face of hopelessness and then succeeded may encourage a client to think about success as feasible after all.

Because a group member not only receives help but also gives it, there is another set of emotional benefits associated with group treatment. Being able to encourage and sympathize with others offers clients an experience of being useful. It also adds a value to their negative experience: at least they have learned from it, and that learning can benefit others. The concern which develops for other group members has the added benefit of interrupting self-absorption. Clients who only think of their own problems are in danger of seeing those problems as even more overwhelming and hopeless. In contrast, thinking of others can break the cycle of discouragement and depression.

For some groups, a major goal may be the development of more appropriate social interactions. Some people have never interacted effectively with others. Some functioned well enough previously but have not been able to adapt to a new problem, while for others the problem itself has interfered with their ability to interact in productive ways. The group can provide a setting for rehearsing assertiveness skills, expressing feelings, really listening to others, or asking for help.

The last relationship goal to be considered is the filling of social roles by group members. This function may best be understood by a simple example. If a woman had a close friend for many years, with whom she shared her thoughts and fears, the role the friend occupied may be referred to as that of confidante. If the friend dies, the confidante role is empty. Possibly a particular group member, or even the group as a whole, can fill the role. Other roles may be filled more loosely, as various group members act from week to week as father, mother, sister, brother, or friend to each other.

Content Goals

Content goals include the learning of factual information, receipt of direct advice, acquisition of specific skills, development of problem-solving abilities, and demonstration of control over the environment. While each of these goals is described separately, they are highly overlapping in practice. In particular, skills and information increase the possibility of control.

Factual information may come from the group leader in a lecture-type format, or may be shared among group members. Advice also may be offered by anyone in the group, but a group leader must be aware that advice can be resented. Advice-giving is not recommended as a major thrust of group interactions.

Specific skills may effectively be learned and practiced in a group. Individual skills, such as memory improvement, may be learned more successfully in a group setting because of relationship factors (including encouragement from others). Interactional skills, including verbal and nonverbal communication styles and the content of interpersonal exchanges, are much more likely to generalize to "real life" if they can be practiced with a variety of people in addition to the therapist.

Groups emphasizing problem-solving may or may not teach specific methods, but in either case impart the underlying assumption that alternatives are available and changes can be made. Feeling able to approach problematic situations creatively, and believing that changes in one's behavior will have an impact on the world, are closely related to having a feeling of control over one's life. The relationship of losing the feeling of control to depression has been documented by Seligman (45) and others (23, 40). Langer and her colleagues (e.g., 27–29, 39) and Schulz (43, 44) have investigated control issues both in and out of nursing homes, with results that generally support the importance of feelings of control in alleviating depression and maintaining higher functioning. Loss of control is a common issue for the elderly, who may be faced with sudden changes in their own health and abilities, death of loved ones, and loss of professional and social influence. A group concerned with control issues may emphasize increasing either external control (skills and knowledge to change the external situation) or internal control (altering one's own reactions, through stress management or deliberate attitude change).

COMMON TYPES OF THERAPEUTIC GROUPS

Every group will involve interaction among participants, and every group will have some sort of content. For that reason, every group has (at least to some extent) the potential to foster both relationship and content goals. However, most groups have either relationship or content goals as their principal focus.

In this section, those types of groups which are primarily intended to help members with relationship goals are described first, followed by those groups in which the content covered is the central concern. For some groups with highly specific prescribed structures (such as reality orientation), origins of the method are noted. Some examples of studies illustrating uses or effectiveness of the various group models are included. If a group method was developed for a particular population, that will be included in the group description. Rules for matching client needs and goals to these various group structures will be discussed more explicitly in the following section.

Groups Emphasizing Relationship Goals

Support Groups

Support groups may be for any specified set of people—caregivers for the chronically ill, stroke patients, families of Alzheimer's patients, widows, aging parents of retarded adults. Specific examples relevant to communicatively disordered individuals and their families were discussed in Chapter 19. Support groups differ in how much professional input they receive, and in how much they emphasize content in addition to relationship goals. A topic is chosen for each meeting, either by a leader or by the group as a whole. Outside speakers may provide talks, but the heart of the group is in the contacts among the members.

Effective support groups foster all the relationship goals discussed here. The last of the goals listed, which involves group members filling needed social roles for each other, has been illustrated in a number of studies (e.g., 5, 19, 21). While the stresses associated with aging (such as retirement and widowhood) do not necessarily precipitate emotional problems (31), support groups which provide confidants can aid in maintenance of good mental health and reduce the negative effects of stressful situations (32).

Schmidt and Keyes (41) describe an ongoing support group for caregivers of Alzheimer's patients in which overemphasis on content (such as discussing the behavior of the patient) was used by participants to avoid discussing feelings about their situations. The group leaders began to encourage expressions of despair or anger, allowing discussion which was more helpful to some participants. However, leaders must be cautious about pushing participants to discuss feelings if they are not ready. "Shallow" discussions of practical matters during the first sessions of a new group can enable members to feel safe about revealing themselves later (5).

Reminiscence Groups

Reminiscence groups, as the name implies, consist of discussions of the past. These discussions can range from factual reporting (members tell what flowers grew in their yard when they were children) to deep introspection (members talk about what it means to them to remember their grandmother's lilacs). As a rule, the lower functioning the participants are, the more the leader decides the topics, encourages silent members, and perhaps even provides props (such as a 1910 Sears catalog) to get the discussion going.

The theoretical framework for reminiscence groups was the "life review," which Butler (7) had conceptualized as a spontaneously occurring individual activity (13). The process of life review involves remembering past events, looking for patterns of meaning, recognizing successes and mistakes, and reaching some intrapsychic resolution of conflicts from the past. The more intense, introspective reminiscence groups provide an opportunity for life review, while more casual reminiscence groups may avoid the conflicted aspects of personal history. Ebersole (14) states that group reminiscence has value beyond individual reminiscing, in that it raises the value of one's peers and therefore of oneself, increases opportunities for socialization, and leads to appreciation of group members' individuality.

Reminiscence can be used with a wide range of people. Cook (11) found that confused nursing home residents who participated in a simple reminiscence group began attending more to each other's contributions, responding with more relevant comments, and socializing more outside the group. Community residents participating in reminiscence may enjoy the interactions, although significant internal change may only occur in participants who have already self-initiated a life review (18, 30). Following one 8-week "There and Then" group, participants identified "their new awareness that others had similar problems" (24, p 204) as the most important part of the experience.

Practitioners may encounter family members, or other professionals, who believe that reminiscing is negative, perhaps even a symptom of "senility." However, a positive relationship has been found between a tendency to reminisce and various measures of psychological health (9). The relationship is particularly evident when reminiscences are happy or pleasant (22).

Resocialization Groups

A number of authors suggest that social skills training is needed for the elderly, due to their isolation and role loss (33, 34, 51). Those adjusting to new barriers to social interaction, such as stroke patients with speech difficulties, may also need retraining. There is some evidence that relationship-oriented social skills groups are more acceptable to community-based older clients than are behavioral training groups, which are content-oriented (52).

Resocialization is a priority for institutionalized populations, who have comparatively greater debilities and less likelihood of spontaneously associating with their peers. As with other institutionalized populations, geriatric patients may interact only with staff (who have power and status in the setting) and isolate themselves from other residents. If staff members pay them little attention, the situation is even worse. Organic deficits, when combined with isolation, depression, and lack of reinforcement for social behavior, can create a vicious cycle of progressively more confused and inappropriate behavior. As a result, resocialization can produce significant improvements in social functioning even though it does not directly impact on any organic deficiencies.

Resocialization groups in institutions usually center around refreshments, which provide both reinforcement for attending and an activity appropriate for practicing new behaviors such as learning the names of other members, verbally requesting items, passing cookies, pouring drinks, and cleaning up afterwards (6, 20, 37). Games and activities may be used if they increase positive social behavior and foster the self-esteem of group members (37).

Sensory Training Groups

Sensory training was developed for regressed psychiatric patients unable to take part in occupational, recreational, and other therapies. Groups of five to seven patients meet with a leader, who introduces one stimulus for each sense, ending with a taste treat (53). The leader elicits some response to each stimulus from each patient, usually expanding on that response to the group. Depending on the abilities of the participants, the leader may ask very simple questions ("do you like this scent?") or more complex questions ("does this scent remind you of anything?").

The interaction among group members in this model is at a minimal level, and is intended as a steppingstone to fuller relationships (in a resocialization group, perhaps). The stimuli provide concrete, nonthreatening objects to focus on, but the interaction itself is far more important than the particular objects selected. However, as with most models described here, it would be possible to adapt this method to emphasize content. Recovering trauma victims, for example, could be brought together to relearn vocabulary with the help of sensory stimuli.

Groups Emphasizing Content Goals

Mental and Physical Health Management

Depression is the most common emotional problem in all age groups, including the elderly. Certainly there are situational factors, including death of friends and family, loss of physical capabilities, and reduced earning power, which contribute to some cases of depression. However, in surviving life stresses at any age, the emotional outcome is heavily dependent on individual coping skills. Training elderly people to control their depressed moods through mood monitoring, identifying pleasant and unpleasant events which affect mood, identifying concrete goals, and rewarding themselves for goal achievement has been shown to be effective in improving participant's self-assessed mental health (50), both immediately after completion of six group sessions and 2 months later.

Depression management training, which demonstrates to participants that they have the ability to cope with their situation, increases what Bandura (4) calls their "self-efficacy." Self-efficacy, which is essentially the opposite of learned helplessness, increases as a person learns ways to manage or change a situation. Treatment of phobics to increase self-efficacy, for example, has been very effective in reducing fear and avoidance behavior. Stop-smoking programs are now being developed, and a major public health education campaign has been based on the concept (36). The application of the self-efficacy concept to communicatively impaired clients might include teaching them to use specific devices or aids, helping them develop their own exercise program or practice schedule, teaching them relaxation techniques to counteract physical or psychological stress, or assisting them in gaining control of at least some aspect of their daily lives.

Memory Training

Memory loss is often assumed to be inevitable in aging, and one study found that two-thirds of psychiatric outpatients over 50 years of age complained of memory problems. However, complaints of memory loss are often tied to depression, and do not correlate with actual decrements in memory (25, 49).

In order to avoid confounding the effects of depression with memory complaints, one study (49) used only nondepressed elderly as subjects. Mnemonic training using the method of loci (an ancient memory method, in which the objects to be remembered are pictured as appearing at various points on a walk through a familiar setting) was compared to a more general approach using relaxation, visualization, and selective attention. For this population, the specific method of loci training was more effective.

In a study of both depressed and nondepressed community-based women (54), a mnemonic approach and a "growth" condition (intended to increase self-esteem and reduce depression through discussion of enjoyable activities, training in assertiveness, and practicing nondefensive reactions to criticism) were equally effective in improving memory improvement. The results of the two studies cited here suggest the following: for depressed subjects, memory complaints may be reduced with groups which increase self-esteem and feelings of self-efficacy; for nondepressed subjects, mnemonic training is more effective.

Alzheimer's patients suffer physical damage to the brain which permanently impairs cognitive abilities, including the ability to store new information in memory. If their functional memory could be increased at all, it could reduce problems for caretakers and postpone the transfer of patients to institutions. However, neither visual imagery nor problem-solving training has been shown to produce any difference (55).

Maintaining Cognitive Functioning

Nursing homes' activity programs may keep residents busy, but too often the activities are irrelevant, inconsequential, and leader-dominated. Participation in bingo does little to help the resident maintain a sense of individual importance. Coleman (10) points out the loss of identity suffered when previous life roles are abandoned for the new formless role of patient, and suggests intellectually challenging discussion groups as the vehicle for building a new identity and sustaining a sense of purpose to life. Discussion of literature or the arts has the advantage (when properly managed by the group leader) of having no right or wrong answers, but eliciting deep thought and excitement. Physical impairment is no obstacle, and people who have been seeing themselves as handicapped by chronic illness can gain confidence in their mental skills.

Another approach to counteracting the fragmented, busywork feeling of the typical nursing home program is the Communication-Cognition Program (CCP) (17). The philosophical base of CCP is that continued learning is necessary to prevent mental deterioration, and that this learning can be tied to daily life in the home. Along with such environmental changes as arranging comfortable spots for personal conversations and keeping the ambient noise level low, and such individual-contact changes as having residents select their clothes and provision of communication boards, changes in group activities result from adoption of CCP. Group discussions may be on any topic, but the emphasis is placed on the opinions and feelings of the residents, not on content taught by the staff. Topics grow out of the real world and interests of the participants, and meaningfulness is enhanced by maintaining them through several activities. For example, a volunteer's slide show of photographs from a particular part of the world can lead into discussions of customs there, foods (and eating some of the foods), and current events.

While the paucity of intellectual stimulation in nursing homes is evident, older people living in the community may face similar stagnation for less obvious reasons. Particularly after retirement removes a major source of intellectual stimulation, or after the death of those close friends or relatives who were relied on for companionship and stimulation, daily life can become empty and meaningless (3). Senior center participants can take part in intellectually challenging discussions on great books, current events, or music appreciation, and begin to develop new interests. Schuetz (42) describes a communication education group program for community elderly which deals with areas of personal and interpersonal concern: self-awareness (with group exercises which would increase self-esteem, such as "bragging sessions"), life cycle and role change, control issues (including assertiveness), and problem solving.

Behavioral Family Intervention

Behavioral interventions are based on the concept that people tend to repeat actions which have desirable results, and discontinue actions which have results they wish to avoid. Often problem behaviors of clients are being unintentionally rewarded by their families. The reward may be a sense of control resulting from making others do one's bidding, the relative lack of effort the behavior requires of the client, or simply the attention received. Perhaps the son waits on the stroke victim rather than encouraging her to become more self-reliant, or the wife tries to decode her husband's gestures rather than insisting that he learn to talk again following his laryngectomy. In both cases, the long-term outcome is detrimental to the client, but the short-term outcome is reinforcing.

Experienced behavior therapists could educate groups of families to become aware of such problems, and teach them to reinforce healthy and independent behaviors (e.g., 38). Group presentation of behavior management skills would not only conserve professional time, but would also allow families to share in developing effective application of the methods. Even Alzheimer's patients, who are characterized by an inability to acquire new information, may respond to a consistent program of reinforcement during the disease's earlier stages. For example, if hugs and food treats are provided often in the kitchen but never in the living room, the family may in effect teach the patient to spend more time in the kitchen.

Remotivation Therapy

Remotivation therapy (RT) was developed at a psychiatric hospital "to stimulate patients into thinking about and discussing topics associated with the real world (and) to assist patients to relate to and communicate with other people" (53, p 113). At a typical RT meeting, the leader brings in some objects upon which to base a discussion. Controversial and emotional topics are avoided, and any feelings expressed by participants are acknowledged but not pursued. The leader strives for a classroom atmosphere, and directs the group to consider vocations related to the object of discussion.

While Dennis (12) cites studies supporting the use of RT with chronic mental patients, it is unclear whether it is effective for other populations. Psychiatric patients generally can be thought of as retaining knowledge (such as vocational information) but having emotional problems which interfere with their using their cognitive abilities. Patients with brain damage (from stroke or Alzheimer's disease, for example) may have lost not only knowledge, but also the ability to absorb new information. Furthermore, RTs vocational emphasis is not appropriate for most older people. Dennis (12) recommends a truncated version of RT which eliminates vocational aspects. For the RT label to be meaningfully attached, however, the group would still have to maintain the emphasis on facts and the classroom atmosphere. (Otherwise, the group would probably be better conceptualized as a resocialization or reminiscence group.)

Reality Orientation

Reality orientation (RO) was developed at a Veterans Administration Hospital for disoriented patients who were unaware of their surroundings (48). These original patients may have had no particular mental deficit on admission to the hospital, but had deteriorated from the effects of institutionalization and had become increasingly confused. For the individually administered component of RO, all staff members, including janitors, were trained so that patients would be reminded of "reality" 24 hours per day, beginning with awakening when "nursing assistants called them by name and told them the time, the day, and what time breakfast would be served" (47, p 209).

The group treatment component of RO consisted of half-hour daily classes using clocks, calendars, bulletin boards, maps, and other materials to provide instruction at a grade school level. In the classes, as well as throughout the day, patients in the original experiment "were given verbal reinforcement for successes, and failures were given little consideration" (47, p 209). After a brief time, patients were reported to be more alert.

Two recent studies (35, 56) have noted the paucity of research on RO, the equivocal results in the few studies done, and the necessity for actual measures of effectiveness. Some of the methodological problems noted include failure to consider participants' varying diagnoses, confounding the effects of individual attention (which is central to the 24-hour aspects of the program) with whatever effects the classroom content may have, and lack of a control or comparison group.

In an effort to establish which diagnostic groups might benefit from RO, a comprehensive RO program was instituted in a nursing home for a full year (56). Participants had diagnoses of senile dementia or organic brain syndrome. Despite $11,000 for extra staff and over 500 hours of volunteer work, there was virtually no improvement over an untreated control group. The authors point out that "the findings here, as in other quantitative studies, indicate that impressionistic reports have exaggerated the effectiveness of RO, "at least for those with chronic brain syndromes" (56, p 76). In another study, a sheltered workshop program was shown to foster improvement in nursing home residents, while RO did not have any positive effect (35).

The use of RO classrooms with unsuitable diagnostic groups is of concern not only because of the time, effort, and expense involved. It is possible that the emphasis on performance of cognitive tasks could be harmful to the self-esteem of patients who are unable to learn or to remember.

MATCHING THE INTERVENTION TO THE CLIENT

A range of group models emphasizing either relationship or content goals was described in the previous section. In addition to the relationship/content dimension, there are two other dimensions to be considered in deciding what kind of group experience would be likely to benefit a particular client. One consideration is the type of deficit or problem experienced. Psychiatric problems such as schizophrenia respond best to different interventions than those effective for emotional problems such as depression, or physical problems such as partial paralysis. The third dimension which must be considered is the severity of the problem or problems, including the feasibility of recovery or rehabilitation.

In this section, each type of group is identified as suitable or unsuitable for various clients, depending on the type of problem or deficit(s), their severity, and whether goals are relationship or content oriented. The possible combinations of deficits and the permutations of group models are virtually infinite, so this is not an exhaustive list. However, major considerations are covered, and examples relevant to communications disorders are given.

Matching Clients with Relationship-Oriented Groups

Support Groups

Support groups constitute an appropriate intervention for clients and for families who need emotional support and/or practical advice for coping with a new or chronic situation. Group membership may be particularly important for clients with communications disorders, because the deficit itself can disrupt interactions with those friends who previously constituted the client's social network.

The use of support groups with particular communications disorders is discussed at length in Chapter 19. Clients with varying degrees of impairment can take part in support groups, but the less able the clients are to express themselves, the more active the leader must be. In general, progressive diseases (such as Parkinson's or Alzheimer's) or moderate chronic impairments (such as aphasia) indicate long-term support group attendance. Mild chronic problems (such as mild-to-moderate hearing impairment) and acute conditions followed by rehabilitation (such as temporary speech and language impairment following stroke) can be treated with a support group at first, followed by a move to a reminiscence group or one of the content oriented groups when the client feels ready.

Reminiscence Groups

Reminiscence groups are effective for clients who exhibit symptoms of depression or low self-esteem or who are isolated for any reason. For the hearing impaired, the difficulty of communication may lead to a withdrawal from social contacts which can be remedied through this group model. Participation can help reestablish a feeling of self-worth for mildly impaired aphasics as well. This type of group serves some of the same functions as a support group, but because the discussion is not centered on the deficit it may actually be more effective for some clients in helping them overcome feelings of hopelessness or depression.

Reminiscence groups can accommodate a range of deficits, but any given group should not include too wide a range of clients. As a rule, the least able client should reasonably be expected to eventually do approximately as well as the most able. Alzheimer's patients can participate, even after the disease has progressed, but will do best with similar others rather than in a heterogeneous group.

Resocialization Groups

Resocialization groups are appropriate for clients who have at least some communication skills, but are too limited (either in speech capability or in the cognitive or emotional realms) to handle the free discussions of reminiscence groups. At the lowest level of resocialization group, a client can participate simply by passing cookies or drinking coffee, and perhaps stating her name or agreeing with a nod of her head to the leader's comments. At a slightly higher level, a client who is gradually relearning some speech can practice social greetings and names for common items in the course of the games or refreshments.

Some client's communication disorders are not severe enough in themselves to preclude membership in another type of group, but concurrent emotional or psychiatric difficulties necessitate a resocialization group. Schizophrenic clients can benefit from the safe emotional distance of resocialization groups, while some clients with dementia are able to follow the structure of serving refreshments but would not be able to participate in a true discussion.

Sensory Training

Sensory training is most appropriate for psychiatric patients, particularly chronic schizophrenics, who are very withdrawn and regressed. Some patients who are being rehabilitated following head injuries might also benefit from sensory training as an early step in treatment.

Sensory training will not be the treatment chosen for most clients with communication disorders. However, some of the ideas of this group model could be utilized in an ongoing support group for the hearing impaired. An occasional session on "appreciating the sense of touch" or "appreciating the sense of sight" could be an enjoyable change from problem-oriented discussions and could encourage the full use of all the senses.

Matching Clients with Content-Oriented Groups

Mental and Physical Health Management

Communication disorders of all types are commonly accompanied by depression, for family members as well as for the client. For mild depression, participation in a support, reminiscence, or cognitive functioning group will be sufficient. However, when depression is not alleviated by that level of intervention, direct training for depression management is indicated. For severe depression, or depression which does not respond to group support or training, further treatment from a mental health professional is indicated. (All speech-language pathologists and audiologists should become familiar with signs of suicidal intentions, and promptly make referrals to the appropriate agency.)

Self-efficacy training is appropriate for all degrees of communication disorders, although for the most severely disabled clients training will be directed to the caregiver. Usually specific skills (such as hearing aid maintenance or laryngectomy care) can be learned in a brief series of frequent meetings (such as once or twice a week for 3 or 4 weeks), after which members can continue skill maintenance meetings or can become involved in other group models.

Memory Training

If depression has led a client to perceive memory deficits when, in actuality, none exist, then memory training will be less effective than a group targeted to other deficits or goals. For example, a hearing impaired client who has become isolated and begun to worry about memory loss may receive more benefit from an art appreciation group (which falls under the "maintaining cognitive functioning" category) than from memory training.

Memory training is indicated for clients actually suffering memory loss. It is also suited to those who could compensate for other deficits if they could rely on improved memory skills. Conversely, clients whose memories cannot be improved (particularly Alzheimer's patients) can be helped through environmental cues such as lists and posted notes while they can still read, or markers such as a rose on the door to identify their bedroom when they can no longer read labels.

Maintaining Cognitive Functioning

Cognitive functioning approaches can be modified to fit nearly any level or type of communication deficit. At higher levels, clients who have physical (but not cognitive) problems can discuss art, literature, music, or current events, thereby maintaining their intellectual abilities and their self-esteem. Clients who retain sufficient physical abilities to paint or draw but have moderate loss of speech and language can express themselves through creating their own art, and using that as a basis for discussion.

Clients with moderate language deficits may become frustrated if placed in discussion groups with fluent others, but in a more homogeneous group they can take the time they need to express themselves. A literature discussion group, for example, could provide the setting for practicing communications skills either for regaining function or for overcoming embarrassment at speaking in spite of new deficits.

Behavioral Family Intervention

Behavioral interventions are appropriate when the client is engaging in behavior which will be harmful because it prevents or limits recovery, or which disturbs family caregivers and makes it more difficult for them to maintain the client at home. Withdrawn or "giving up" behaviors can indicate depression and/or a lack of skills needed to cope with a deficit. In such cases, behavioral methods must not be used in isolation but must be combined with whatever skill training and depression intervention are indicated.

For disorders such as Alzheimer's, when mental impairment renders logic and persuasion useless, behavioral intervention may offer the only possibility of changing family interactions. Even in less global deficits, changes in the condition of one family member will have upset the family homeostasis and disrupted the pattern of relationships (see Chapter 19 for a discussion of communication disorders as family disorders). The new relationship patterns may be unhealthy if they are based on seeing the client as an invalid. Family intevention is essential in cases in which the behavior of other family members encourages the maladaptive behaviors of the client.

Remotivation Therapy

Remotivation therapy is indicated for psychiatric patients, such as chronic schizophrenics, who are being rehabilitated for release from institutions. It might also be helpful for clients with knowledge gaps secondary to head injuries, who are undergoing rehabilitation and hope to return to employment. In most cases, this group model will not be appropriate for clients with communication disorders. However, there may be an occasional client who does fall into the categories fitting this model who also has a hearing, speech, or language deficit.

Reality Orientation

Everything said above regarding remotivation therapy is also true for reality orientation, which is suited to clients in the same categories but with even more severe deficits. For both types of groups, if there are clients with communication disorders included, then appropriate accommodations must be made. For example, the hearing impaired client will require a small group to avoid being overwhelmed by ambient noise levels.

BOOKS ABOUT GROUP LEADERSHIP AND COUNSELING SKILLS

Training in treatment of communication disorders is unlikely to include much formal instruction in group or individual counseling skills. The following books are particularly recommended for practitioners who want to increase their effectiveness by incorporating group work into their treatment repertoire.

Robert Carkhuff (8) found evidence that empathy, respect, and genuineness are basic requirements if a counselor wants to promote positive personality and behavior change in clients. *Counseling the Older Adult: A Training Manual for Paraprofessionals and Beginning Counselors* (1) applies Carkhuff's theory to working with the elderly. The book is meant for classroom use, and includes practice exercises which could also be used by the independent reader.

Gerard Egan's *The Skilled Helper* (15) similarly leads the reader through examples demonstrating the development of a therapeutic relationship. While the emphasis is on individual encounters, the content applies equally to groups. Egans' volume on group work, *You and Me* (16), would be more difficult reading for someone without a counseling background. However, it has an excellent section on the productive confrontation of such maladaptive behaviors by group members as not contributing to discussions, not practicing "homework," monopolizing group time, or bossing other members.

SUMMARY

This chapter has described a variety of group treatment models which might be utilized in the treatment of clients encountered by practitioners concerned with speech, language, and hearing disorders. Group treatment has the advantage of conserving professional time and thereby limiting costs. Even more importantly, group interactions are the most effective setting for increasing self-esteem, offsetting social isolation, reducing obsession with problems, maintaining cognitive functioning, learning coping techniques, and practicing new skills.

All group interactions include social relationship aspects and some degree of content, but each group model emphasizes either relationship or content goals. In addition to the type of goal, the type of deficit and its severity must be considered in choosing an effective group intervention. Following descriptions of the various treatments, examples of clients suited to each group model were included. In addition, books were recommended which can provide an introduction to group dynamics and group leadership skills.

There are two principal reasons speech-language pathologists and audiologists need to be aware of group treatment possibilities. Clients may be receiving concurrent treatment from other professionals who are providing group therapy, or may reside in institutions where groups are part of the daily routine. Practitioners need an awareness of the variety of groups in order to make recommendations regarding their clients' inclusion in available treatment. Secondly, they may choose to initiate, lead, or co-lead groups specifically designed to meet their clients' goals, appropriate to the clients' deficits and abilities.

Group interventions constitute a logically and intuitively appealing approach for treatment of speech, language, and hearing disorders. Communication is inherently interactive, and therapeutic groups provide a natural and powerful setting for the acquisition and practice of communication-related skills.

References

1. Alpaugh P, Haney M: *Counseling the Older Adult: a Training Manual for Paraprofessionals and Beginning Counselors.* Los Angeles, University of Southern California Press, 1978.
2. Altholz JAS: Group psychotherapy with the elderly. In Burnside IM (ed): *Working with the Elderly: Group Process and Techniques.* North Scituate, MA, Duxbury Press, 1978, p 354.
3. Atchley RC: *The Social Forces in Later Life: An Introduction to Social Gerontology.* Belmont, CA, Wadsworth, 1972.
4. Bandura A: *Social Foundations of Thought and Action: a Social Cognitive Theory.* Englewood Cliffs, NJ, Prentice-Hall, 1986.
5. Beaulieu ES, Karpinski J: Group treatment of elderly with ill spouses. *Soc Casework* 62:551–557, 1981.
6. Boudreault M, Larue V, Metzelaar L: *To Live with Dignity: A Report of a Project with Frail and Withdrawn Elderly Persons.* Ann Arbor, MI, University of Michigan Institute of Gerontology, 1975.
7. Butler R: The life review: an interpretation of reminiscence in the aged. *Psychiatry* 26:65–76, 1953.
8. Carkhuff RR: *Helping and Human Relations,* vols 1 & 2. New York, Holt, Rinehart & Winston, 1969.
9. Carlson CM: Reminiscing: toward achieving ego integrity in old age. *Soc Casework* 65:81–89, 1984.
10. Coleman CA: Gymnasium for the mind. *Geriatrics* 33:97–100, 1978.
11. Cook JB: Reminiscing: how it can help confused nursing home residents. *Soc Casework* 65:90–93, 1984.
12. Dennis H: Remotivation therapy groups. In Burnside IM (ed): *Working with the Elderly: Group Process and Techniques.* North Scituate, MA, Duxbury Press, 1978, p 219.
13. Ebersole P: Reminiscing. *Am J Nurs* 76:1304–1305, 1976.
14. Ebersole PP: Establishing reminiscing groups. In Burnside IM (ed): *Working with the Elderly: Group Process and Techniques.* North Scituate, MA, Duxbury, 1978, p 236.
15. Egan G: *The Skilled Helper: a Model for Systematic Helping and Interpersonal Relating.* Belmont, CA, Wadsworth, 1975.
16. Egan G: *You & Me: the Skills of Communicating and Relating to Others.* Belmont, CA, Wadsworth, 1977.
17. Feier CD, Leight G: A communication-cognition program for elderly nursing home residents. *Gerontologist* 21:408–415, 1981.
18. Georgemiller R, Maloney HN: Group life review and denial of death. *Clin Gerontol* 2:37–49, 1984.
19. Getzel GS: Helping elderly couples in crisis. *Soc Casework* 63:515–521, 1982.
20. Gray P, Stevenson JS: Changes in verbal interaction among members of resocialization groups. *J Gerontol Nurs* 6:86–90, 1980.
21. Hartford ME, Parsons R: Groups with relatives of dependent older adults. *Gerontologist* 22:394–398, 1982.
22. Havighurst RJ, Glasser R: An exploratory study of reminiscence. *J Gerontol* 27:245–253, 1972.
23. Hiroto DS: Locus of control and learned helplessness. *J Exp Psychol* 102:187–193, 1974.
24. Ingersoll B, Silverman A: Comparative group psychotherapy for the aged. *Gerontologist* 18:201–206, 1978.
25. Kahn RL, Zarit SH, Hilbert NW, Niederehe G: Memory complaints and impairment in the aged: the effects of depression and altered brain function. *Arch Gen Psychiatry* 32:1569–1573, 1975.
26. Kubie SH, Landau G: *Group Work with the Aged.* New York, International Universities Press, 1953.
27. Langer EJ, Janis IL, Wolfer JA: Reduction of psychological stress in surgical patients. *J Exp Soc Psychol* 11:155–165, 1975.
28. Langer EJ, Rodin J: The effects of choice and enhanced personal responsibility for the aged: field experiment in an institutional setting. *J Pers Soc Psychol* 34:191–198, 1976.
29. Langer EJ, Saegert S: Crowding and cognitive control. *J Pers Soc Psychol* 35:175–182, 1977.
30. Lewis MI, Butler RN: Life-review therapy: putting memories to work in individual and group psychotherapy. *Geriatrics* 29:165–173, 1974.
31. Lowenthal MF: Antecedents of isolation and mental illness in old age. *Arch Gen Psychiatry* 12:245–254, 1965.
32. Lowenthal MF, Haven C: Interaction and adaptation: intimacy as a critical variable. *Am Sociological Rev* 33:20–30, 1968.
33. Lowy L: The group in social work with the aged. *Soc Work* 7:43–50, 1962.
34. Lowy L: Roadblocks in group work practice with

older people: a framework for analysis a *Gerontologist* 7:109–113, 1967.

35. MacDonald ML, Settin JM: Reality orientation versus sheltered workshops as treatment for the institutionalized aging. *J Gerontol* 33:416–421, 1978.

36. McLeod B: Rx for health: a dose of self-confidence. *Psychol Today* 20:46–50, 1986.

37. Metzelaar L: *Social Interaction Groups in a Therapeutic Community*. Ann Arbor, MI, University of Michigan Institute of Gerontology, 1973.

38. Pinkston EM, Linsk NL: Behavioral family intervention with the impaired elderly. *Gerontologist* 24:576–583, 1984.

39. Rodin J, Langer EJ: Long-term effects of a control—relevant intervention with the institutionalized aged. *J Pers Soc Psychol* 35:897–902, 1977.

40. Roth S, Kubal L: Effects of noncontingent reinforcement on tasks of differing importance: facilitation and learned helplessness. *J Pers Soc Psychol* 32:680–691, 1975.

41. Schmidt GL, Keyes B: Group psychotherapy with family caregivers of demented patients. *Gerontologist* 25:347–350, 1985.

42. Schuetz J: Lifelong learning: communication education for the elderly. *Communication Educ* 29:33–41, 1980.

43. Schulz R: Effects of control and predictability on the physical and psychological well-being of the institutionalized aged. *J Pers Soc Psychol* 33:563–573, 1976.

44. Schulz R, Hanusa BH: Long-term effects of control and predictability enhancing interventions: findings and ethical issues. *J Pers Soc Psychol* 36:1194–1201, 1978.

45. Seligman ME: *Helplessness: On Depression, Development, and Death*. San Francisco, W.H. Freeman, 1975.

46. Silver A: Group psychotherapy with senile psychiatric patients. *Geriatrics* 5:147–150, 1950.

47. Taulbee LR: Reality orientation: a therapeutic group activity for elderly persons. In Burnside IM (ed): *Working with the Elderly: Group Process and Techniques*. North Scituate, MA, Duxbury, 1978, p 206.

48. Taulbee LR, Folsom JC: Reality orientation for geriatric patients. *Hosp Commun Psychiatry* 17:133–135, 1966.

49. Taylor LL, Yesavage JA: Cognitive retraining programs for the elderly: a case study of cost/benefit issues. *Clin Gerontol* 2:51–63, 1984.

50. Thompson LW, Gallagher D, Nies G et al: Evaluation of the effectiveness of professionals and nonprofessionals as instructors of "coping with depression" classes for elders. *Gerontologist* 23:390–396, 1983.

51. Toseland R, Rose S: Evaluating social skills training for older adults in groups. *Soc Work Res Abstr* 14:25–33, 1978.

52. Toseland R, Sherman E, Bliven S: The comparative effectiveness of two group work approaches for the development of mutual support groups among the elderly. *Soc Work Groups* 4:137–153, 1981.

53. Weiner MB, Brok AJ, Snadowsky AM: *Working with the Aged*. Englewood Cliffs, NJ, Prentice-Hall, 1978.

54. Zarit SH, Gallagher D, Kramer N: Memory training in the community aged: effects on depression, memory complaint, and memory performance. *Educ Gerontol* 6:11–27, 1981.

55. Zarit SH, Zarit JM, Reever KE: Memory training for severe memory loss: effects on senile dementia patients and their families. *Gerontologist* 22:373–377, 1982.

56. Zepelin H, Wolfe CS, Kleinplatz F: Evaluation of a yearlong reality orientation program. *J Gerontol* 36:70–77, 1981.

21 Who's Who in Aging: An Introduction to Federal and State Agencies Providing Services and/or Funding

G. SANDRA FISHER

Editor's Note

In working with older clients, it is impossible to treat only the speech-language or hearing disorder and ignore all other problems. Frequently, social, economic, or psychological pressures interfere with effective management of the communication impairment, or exacerbate the problem. Thus, professionals must assume responsibility for understanding the various funding and service resources available to the elderly, and the agencies that administer those resources. In Chapter 21, Fisher provides an excellent foundation of information for working within the aging network of services and service providers. Beginning with a brief history of the 1965 Older Americans Act, the chapter proceeds to outline various community, state, Federal, and national organizations that act as resources for the elderly or those working with the elderly. Communication disorder professionals are urged to become more active in the aging network system, and specific recommendations for appropriate roles and avenues of involvement are provided. Some of these recommendations are pursued in greater depth in the final chapter of this text. Chapter 21 concludes with an invaluable series of appendices which provide the reader with listings of: additional source readings; programs of Federal assistance to the elderly; state agencies on aging (names and addresses); Federal governmental agencies or committees specializing in aging; national voluntary organizations serving older persons; and major information sources or data bases that can provide critical information about aging and the elderly.

There is a special professional challenge for individuals who choose to work with older persons. In many professions, it is sufficient to be well prepared in a single discipline. However, since aging is a multidisciplinary field, there is the need to be acquainted with several areas of knowledge and with a wide range of resources in order to meet the needs of an older person effectively. Increasingly, academic curricula in a range of professional areas include content related to aging—and for a very good reason. Individuals who graduate during the 1980s and 1990s will be charged with rebuilding cities, revamping health and social service systems, designing new modes of transportation, creating new living environments, and perhaps even forging new ways of living.

The environment in which many of these developments will take root can be expected to be far different in many respects from the recent past. In the next 2 decades, practicing professionals and graduates in the health and social fields in all likelihood will face special challenges in working with a much larger number of older clients, many of whom will be in advanced years. The best place and the best time to prepare is the here and now. The current reality is that what the older person needs is not always available, and even when it is, putting the resource together with older persons and their families may require training by Scotland Yard!

Take the case of Mrs. X, who is 78 years old, and who was doing quite well before she began to lose her hearing. Mrs. X moved in with two

*The opinions presented are those of the author and do not represent the policy of the Department of Health and Human Services or the United States Government.

of her sisters after her husband died. She had always been more the follower than leader, and as one of her sisters became quite ill, Mrs. X started to withdraw from conversation and family activity. While she still did some household chores, she was uncommunicative and became increasingly dependent. Because she did little to help with household tasks and rarely communicated, friction developed between Mrs. X and her sisters. The one healthy sister now had two of her sisters to care for. At the insistence of a family member, Mrs. X was taken to an audiologist for a hearing test, and was found to have a profound loss of hearing. By this time, the relationship between Mrs. X and her sisters had deteriorated to a serious degree, and the behavior of Mrs. X made others afraid of her. A hearing aid was ordered, which she did not want to wear and wore only on rare occasions. Mrs. X's behavior became increasingly bizarre and threatening to the other family members. A social worker with the office on aging intervened at the request of the caregiving sister, and the family physician arranged for Mrs. X to live in a nursing home. She later moved to a group home with supervision. The story of Mrs. X is not complete, but actions taken (or not taken) have set a definite trend in motion for Mrs. X and members of her family, who now have a member living apart from the family in a group home. Let's look now at who was involved, who might have been helpful, what actions were taken, and what might have been done differently, if anything.

To begin, there were two physicians involved. How should they have communicated with each other?

Was there any possibility of arresting the trend in this family before the "inevitable"?

Was there a role for an aggressive communication disorders specialist with Mrs. X and her family, and if so, how could this specialist have been introduced into the situation?

How appropriate was the role of the social worker, and what did that person need to understand in order to work effectively with Mrs. X and her family?

In what ways might the caregiving sister have gotten some relief?

What outlets could have been introduced, and by whom (e.g. involving Mrs. X in a senior center activity, or the Retired Senior Volunteer Program) in order to lessen Mrs. X's isolation?

Of the three professionals involved, which one took the lead with Mrs. X and her family? Which one should have?

Are there supports which might have been available to this family long before the point of crisis? If so, what kinds of supports might have been useful, and

how would the family have known about them? How would they have accessed them?

Who in the community might have been able to see the trend developing?

What would you have done, as: the audiologist?
the family physician?
the social worker?

Among other things, this case illustrates the isolation of the health and social delivery systems as they have evolved over the years, and the extent to which funding mechanisms often dictate the solution (Mrs. X is on Medicaid).

For the foreseeable future, older persons, their families, their neighbors and friends, and the variety of professionals with whom they interact will have difficulty figuring out "the system." In fact, there are so many "systems" that in the eyes of an older person—Mrs. X and her family, for example—there may appear to be no system of help at all. This state of affairs brings us to a consideration of how things got to be this way, and what might be done about it.

THE OLDER AMERICANS ACT

Before 1965, governmental assistance available to older persons was mainly in the area of income support provided by the Social Security Act, which was enacted in 1935. Amendments to the Social Security Act which created Medicare for the population age 65 and over and the Older Americans Act were not enacted until 1965. However, the evolution of the field of aging in the United States has a much earlier history, the origins of which are found in a number of prominent voluntary agencies which date to the latter part of the 19th century. While an interest in aging (gerontology) can be found in early literature of various countries of the world, the field of "social gerontology," which encompasses broad social issues concerned with aging, was developed in the United States in the mid-1960s, and the term was coined here (see Additional Readings in Appendix A for readings from Binstock and Tibbitts).

In 1965, the Congress and the Executive Branch of the Federal government acted to establish what came to be called a "comprehensive and coordinated system" of services for older persons. The Older Americans Act of 1965 was the first Federal legislation to recognize the diverse service needs of the older population, the need for adjustments by major social institutions, and the need for new knowledge concerned with the total circumstances of the older person. The study of the evolution of the field of aging and services for older persons through various governmental and private avenues is a fascinating endeavor, for it is through that process that one develops an understanding of the plethora of services, systems, and professional approaches which abound (or are absent) in the 1980s. Knowing why "the system" is the way it is may not immediately help in solving the specific circumstances of Mrs. X, but it may help one to understand the system well enough to begin to *change the system itself* so that it is more responsive, efficient and humane.

Funding for State Agencies on Aging was authorized in 1965, and many local services for older persons were organized under State auspices after that time. At the same time, the Administration on Aging was created at the Federal level to administer the program of State and community services as well as programs to expand knowledge through research and development, and through education and training of persons to work in the field of aging. The position of Commissioner on Aging also was created with a broad mandate concerned with the needs of older persons in the present as well as future generations.

The provisions of the Older Americans Act are as follows:

Title I DECLARATION OF OBJECTIVES/DEFINITIONS
(1) An adequate income in retirement in accordance with the American standard of living.
(2) The best possible physical and mental health which science can make available and without regard to economic status.
(3) Suitable housing, independently selected, designed and located with reference to special needs and available at costs which older citizens can afford.
(4) Full restorative services for those who require institutional care, and a comprehensive array of community-based, long-term care services adequate to appropriately sustain older people in their communities and in their homes.
(5) Opportunity for employment with no discriminatory personnel practices because of age.
(6) Retirement in health, honor, dignity—after years of contribution to the economy.
(7) Pursuit of meaningful activity within the widest range of civic, cultural, education and training and recreational opportunities.

(8) Efficient community services, including access to low-cost transportation, which provide a choice in supported living arrangements and social assistance in a coordinated manner and which are readily available when needed, with emphasis on maintaining a continuum of care for the vulnerable elderly.
(9) Immediate benefit from proven research knowledge which can sustain and improve health and happiness.
(10) Freedom, independence, and the free exercise of individual initiative in planning and managing their own lives and full participation in the planning and operation of community-based services and programs provided for their benefit (1).

Title II ADMINISTRATION ON AGING
Title III GRANTS FOR STATE AND COMMUNITY PROGRAMS ON AGING
Part A General Provisions
Part B Supportive Services and Senior Centers
Part C Nutrition Services
Title IV TRAINING, RESEARCH, AND DISCRETIONARY PROJECTS AND PROGRAMS
Title V COMMUNITY SERVICE EMPLOYMENT FOR OLDER AMERICANS
Title VI GRANTS FOR INDIAN TRIBES
Title VII OLDER AMERICANS PERSONAL HEALTH EDUCATION AND TRAINING PROGRAM

Appendix A contains additional information on the aging service system as authorized under the Older Americans Act, and selected reading sources dealing with the Older Americans Act, aging policy, and the service system. Specific examples of programs providing Federal assistance to older persons are also provided in Appendix B.

THE COMMUNITY AND THE OLDER AMERICANS ACT

In 1971, the Older Americans Act was amended to provide for the establishment of Area Agencies on Aging for the purpose of creating a "comprehensive and coordinated service system" for older persons and their families in their community. These agencies are charged with coordinating existing services, planning for future needs of older persons in the community, discovering needs which are not being met, and working through a range of private, public, and voluntary resources to make sure that the needs of the individual older person and their family are met. This is a major challenge.

In fact, the community focus of the Older Americans Act is to create community-wide response to the situation of older residents. Thus, the role of the Area Agency on Aging is considerably different from the role of the traditional service agency. What is involved goes beyond the traditional modes of delivering service, to include: governance within the community (housing developments/ordinances); educational and cultural opportunities; opportunities for employment and volunteer service; active participation of older individuals in the full range of community activities; community-wide planning for the near and long term to meet the full range of interests and needs of residents with respect to aging; and comprehensive services, including health, social, and related areas (Fig. 21.1). Figure 21.1 provides an overview of the administrative structure involving Area Agencies on Aging.

In practice, one is confronted with situations in which there are waiting lists for services; the service required may be nonexistent; or the available service may not be exactly suited to the needs of the older person and the family. The daily reality faced by professionals on the

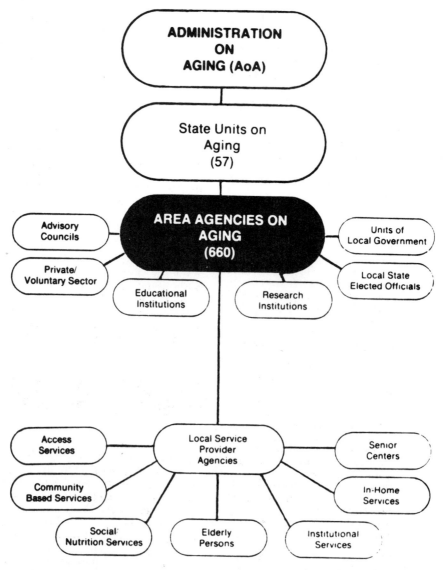

Figure 21.1. The administrative structures of the Area Agencies on Aging. Reproduced with permission from the National Association of Area Agencies on Aging, Washington, DC.

front line of service to older persons and their families is that the home-delivered meal must reach the home of the older person at just the right time, or more intensive services may be needed, perhaps institutionalization.

The communication disorder specialist, while treating one aspect of the older person's situation, is nevertheless dependent on a whole host of other supportive services, over which the specialist has no direct control. To further complicate the issue, the speech-language pathologist or audiologist may be dealing with other organizations and professionals in the community who are not sufficiently acquainted with communication to comprehend fully the interrelatedness of services and supports which may be required in total to respond effectively to the older person's situation. Thus, the practicing professional in communications—as in many other fields—must educate as well as draw on available resources when the client is an older person. Practice must include teaching, and the teaching will often occur outside one's professional area.

WHEN THE CLIENT IS AN OLDER PERSON

Let's take the case of Mrs. X again. Had the audiologist gone beyond the hearing test to find out more about the total family situation, various courses of action might have been instituted at that point. A specialist in communication behavior might have joined with a case manager of the local office on aging to evaluate the total family circumstances. Together, they might have introduced an individualized program of professional assistance for Mrs. X in coping with the hearing and psychological problems. They might have educated the family over a period of time as to the behaviors involved and as to how to deal with them effectively. They might also have lessened the social isolation for all three sisters by working with them individually to engage them in social activity suited to each, either outside the home or by bringing volunteer visitors or some social contact inside the home on a regular basis. Mrs. X's situation might actually have been handled by her sisters, had one not become ill. Therefore, to relieve the total family situation and make coping with Mrs. X's special situation a possibility, respite for the caregiving sister and attention to the medical and psychological needs of the sister who was quite ill also needed careful attention.

To complete the story, Mrs. X blossomed at the group home. She wore her hearing aid, talked with other residents of the home, began to draw and paint again (which she had not done since she was a young woman), went to church each Sunday with the help of church members—in short, Mrs. X improved socially rather dramatically. Although she developed a serious medical problem and was hospitalized, she recovered sufficiently to return to a group home with 24-hour maximum supervision for ambulatory individuals, rather than enter a nursing home. Mrs. X was still dependent on others for daily direction. It also became clear during her visits with the family that she was less socially interactive with them than she was at the group home.

In the end, it appears that a reasonable solution to the family situation had been worked out. Attention must now turn to the proper care of Mrs. X in the group home. There is no one to work with her on her developing interest in art; she misses her family despite her reasonable adjustment to the home; and she developed a major ear infection because of irritation from the earmold. While her occasional visits with her family are nice outings, she seems to have less social contact than she would like, and her sisters are concerned about her welfare away from the family.

What seems clear from this case is that effective management of Mrs. X's life circumstances requires attention to a whole host of other issues and needs over a long period of time. This is often the case when the client is an older person. Knowledge of how the Area Agency on Aging and other community organizations function, and of what their resources are, is essential if the totality of the situation is to be dealt with effectively. The time which the patient spends in the doctor's office may not even reveal the tip of the iceberg. For this reason, although competency in one's specialty is essential, one must also be an expert and persistent investigator—when the client is an older person.

ORGANIZATIONAL RESOURCES

Community

Start with the Area Agency on Aging. There are about 700 of these organizations in the country, and there should be one close by. The Area Agency on Aging does not usually manage direct services—it is an organization concerned principally with planning, development, and coordination. It should be able to direct you to the right organization or individual who is knowledgeable to work with you, and this is part of its job. Part of the job of the communication disorders specialist, in turn, is to inform the Area Agency on Aging of the service needs of older persons in the community, so that those needs may be taken into consideration as future programmatic plans are made. Professionals working in the area of communications behavior need to be seen and heard. Given estimates concerning the extent of expected hearing impairments in the older population in the future, the expert involvement of the communication disorders specialist is a must in charting proper plans for the community.

The Area Agency on Aging coordinates a complex array of organizational and financial resources for older people and their families, and the agency funds many community agencies for this purpose (see Fig. 21.1). Find out what these community services are, who manages them, and if there are any eligibility requirements to receive service. (Note: Under Older Americans Act-funded programs, there are no income eligibility requirements, although major efforts are made to ensure that services are available and are used by those older persons who are in greatest economic and social need, or who are considered to be "at risk" because of their health and/or social status). Ask the Area Agency on Aging about the best information-and-referral system for older persons in the community—for the clients' use and your own.

Find out whether there are any specialized programs for older persons with communication difficulties in the community, and who manages them. Be aware that there are many services and programs for older persons which, although not specifically oriented to communicatively impaired older persons, may be of importance in treating the total needs of the older client. Your local Area Agency on Aging probably manages senior centers, a sizeable congregate nutrition program, home delivered meals, some services in the home, as well as educational and physical fitness activities. If certain equipment or other arrangements are required in order for your clientele to use a service, bring this to the attention of the Area Agency on Aging or provider of the service and work on a solution—jointly. If necessary, go together to public officials or others in the community to seek help with the problem, and remember to bring the issue to the attention of older persons—older persons often have deep roots in the community and can help when addressing a community situation which needs attention.

The financial circumstances of older individuals vary widely, as do community-based funding sources for services for older individ-

uals. The average older person receives a monthly Social Security benefit, is eligible for Medicare if over age 65, and probably owns his/her own home. Assets in the home do not contribute, of course, to monthly cash flow, and it is the Social Security benefit that usually pays for food, upkeep of the house (or the rent payment if the house is not owned), doctor bills not covered by Medicare or by insurance, drugs, taxes, transportation, fuel, utilities, and other expenses of daily living. While the economic status of older persons has gradually improved over the last 20 years, the cost of medical care and insurance costs have risen as well. Devices or special treatments and services in the home which are not reimbursed by Medicare or the person's insurance (if available) may well create serious financial strains. If the older person's financial resources are quite limited and they qualify for Medicaid, that resource should be explored to determine whether there is coverage for any anticipated treatment, device, or specialized service in the home.

A small percentage of older individuals have pensions in addition to Social Security. The financial resources available to these persons to pay for services not reimbursed under various programs should be greater. The important word here is "should," however, because one must bear in mind that some pensions are quite limited. It cannot automatically be assumed that this additional resource is, in fact, a great help. Each older person's financial condition is different, and it is best to approach each situation accordingly.

Beyond individual resources or individual benefits under Medicare, Medicaid, or the Veterans Administration, there are often programs in the community especially organized for older persons which may be of enormous value. Such programs vary from community to community; however, the following list gives an idea of what programmatic resources may be available or accessed through the Area Agency on Aging:

- Advocacy, including legal services
- Case management
- Home services, such as home health, homemaker, and chore
- Information and Referral, for older persons, their families, and professional people who need to know community resources for older persons
- Nutrition services, including congregate and home-delivered meals
- Senior Centers, usually including a variety of social, educational, health, and recreational programs
- Older adult day care
- Protective services

- Counseling services
- Escort services, such as transportation and assistance in getting to medical appointments
- Ombudsman and other services for older persons who live in long-term care institutions, including group homes and nursing homes
- Mental health services
- Housing information and assistance
- Health information and medical treatment sources
- Cultural and recreational programs
- Employment counseling and referral
- Emergency services, i.e., fire, police, victims services, or specially organized emergency services for older persons
- Consumer information and local business discounts
- Volunteer opportunities through the Retired Senior Volunteer Program and other community volunteer programs
- Alzheimer's disease: resources and services for older persons and caregivers
- Financial management services for older persons who have difficulty managing their own money

Financial resources supporting community programs for older persons usually involve a mixture of public and private sources. In the community, local government (either county or city), is often important to the organization of services and their financing. General purpose government at the local level increasingly funds aging services and is also instrumental in securing funds from an array of outside sources. Community foundations are a particularly good resource for experimental programs for which no governmental support is available. These foundations vary in size, mission, and requirements, and are often created by families with strong roots in the community. Frequently, the chamber of commerce can provide useful information about all types of community resources, including business and foundation support. To create comprehensive, high quality, and fully responsive community supports for older persons, one needs to know "Who's Who in Voluntary Agencies," "Who's Who in Business," and "Who's Who in Government," in addition to "Who's Who in Aging." After all, the growth in the older population impacts on the total community environment.

State Government Resources

There were several State Agencies on Aging in existence before the Older Americans Act was enacted into law in 1965, and even prior to that time, there was considerable State governmental interest in matters concerning older individuals. For the communication disorder specialist, it is important to know that State government oversees many programs and regulatory activities which affect the daily life of the older person. State government sometimes leads the way in program development and can be instrumental in influencing Federal legislation. State licensure of facilities, accrediting of professionals, and regulation of certain equipment and devices are all of interest to the field of communications. While there may be several State departments and agencies of interest to the communication disorders professional, the State Agency on Aging is the one agency which concentrates on aging. State Agencies on Aging are listed in Appendix C.

State government has historically provided assistance to older persons through State appropriations, property tax relief, and a host of other avenues, depending on the interest of a particular State. It is important for all professionals to stay informed about developments statewide, especially those of an experimental nature. Staff of the State Agency on Aging possess a broad range of information and knowledge about aging programs and resources within the State and are there to help further developments which can better serve the interest of older persons. Just as one would contact the Area Agency on Aging in the community about aging resources, the State Agency on Aging is the focal point for aging information at the State level. The State Agency on Aging staff will be knowledgeable about resources available in other State departments, private resources which operate statewide, and professional associations related to aging within the State.

Under the Older Americans Act, each State Agency on Aging is charged with planning, development, and coordination of efforts to meet the current and future needs of older persons within the particular State. In this regard, the State Agency on Aging coordinates its activities with many State agencies and departments, the State legislature, and the Governor's office. There is a State advisory body concerned with aging, which advises State officials, depending on how the advisory body is constituted in a particular State. The advisory body often includes lay as well as professional and political representatives, and older persons. In addition to State-appropriated funds and personnel resources, the State Agency on Aging administers the Older Americans Act programs in the State and allocates funds to all of the Area Agencies on Aging within the State, based on an Area Plan and a statistical formula.

Federal Government Resources

There are many Federal departments and agencies which provide assistance to older individuals through regular programs, and some have specialized resources available in aging. The principal Federal department concerned with aging is the Department of Health and Human Services, which manages the Social Security Administration, the Health Care Financing Administration (Medicare and Medicaid), the Administration on Aging (Older Americans Act), and the National Institute on Aging of the National Institutes of Health (the principal research organization concerned with aging in the Federal government). Other departments and agencies which have special resources available related to aging include the Department of Agriculture (food and nutrition); the Older Americans Volunteer Programs administered by ACTION (Retired Senior Volunteer Program, the Foster Grandparent Program, and the Senior Companion Program); the Department of Labor (Employment: Title V of the Older Americans Act); the National Institute of Mental Health's Bureau on Aging; the Department of Housing and Urban Development (congregate housing and other forms of housing assistance); and the Veterans Administration. In addition to benefits and services, many of these agencies support research and demonstration efforts, have excellent publications available, and have staff who are knowledgeable about aging developments nationwide.

The Committees of the United States Congress have been of enormous importance in the development of the field of aging and services for older persons. Authorizing Committees as well as Committees which specialize in aging in the United States House of Representatives and in the United States Senate are listed in Appendix D. In addition to Committee staff, who are expert on aging developments on a national scale, the Congressional Committees produce publications reporting on important surveys, descriptive information on various Federal programs for older persons, and compilations of testimony and legislation concerned with aging. Federal agencies and programs concerned with aging are listed in Appendix D.

National Voluntary Organizations

Private nonprofit organizations which operate nationally have been at the forefront of developments in the aging area in the United States. There are many national organizations which offer information and assistance in a wide range of disciplines and subjects in the field of aging. Until 1970 there were only about five major national private organizations concerned with aging. Following the White House Conference on Aging of 1971, additional national organizations concerned with aging developed, some in very specialized areas (see Appendix E for partial listing). One such organization of interest to the communication disorders professional is the Gerontological Society of America, with a professional membership spanning the entire spectrum of disciplines involved in the study and practice of gerontology. The membership includes individuals in research, practice, and teaching in medicine, health, the social professions and related fields.

The American Association of Retired Persons (AARP), widely known as the largest membership organization of older persons in the United States, should be known to the communication disorders professional for its innovative training modules and other forms of assistance to local AARP Chapters which enable older persons to carry out educational programs themselves. AARP has a local, State, and national organizational structure, and supports a wide range of programs and services to its membership, as well as experimental activities.

The National Council on Aging (NCOA) is the home of several major national institutes concerned with senior centers, older adult day care, and the arts and humanities, among others. NCOA has a large membership of individuals and organizations which provide direct services to older persons. It often conducts national experiments with new and different approaches to service development and operation. NCOA publications can be useful as guides for actual program development and operation. Historically, NCOA has championed the cause of the older poor.

The National Association of State Units on Aging and the National Association of Area Agencies on Aging have available considerable information on the operations of State and Area Agencies on Aging. In addition, they work with many other national organizations to enhance the capabilities of the State and Area Agencies on Aging, and undertake efforts to ensure that older persons and their families know where to turn for help when help is needed.

Finally, national foundations can be a most important resource, particularly when a research or demonstration effort is desired and government funding is unlikely. There are several national foundations which make substantial investments in aging research, and others provide support for specific areas of interest. Appendix F provides data sources which can be useful in identifying foundations or other organizations which support developmental work in the aging field.

WHO's WHO IN AGING IN THE FUTURE

While there are many resources in the aging field, it is important to keep one's perspective as the future unfolds into what appears to be a much older society. Aging is quite new when compared to many other academic fields. Regardless of one's perspective—as a student, a researcher, a provider of services to older persons, and/or an older recipient of services, one is able to perceive that the system of policies and services for older persons and their families is far from perfect. As the number of older persons increases and the average age of the older population escalates, American society faces a new challenge. Graduates and practicing professionals in the 1980s and 1990s are particularly challenged. The preponderance of older clients in future years will require specialized knowledge of aging and assumption of leadership roles in serving an older community.

Communication disorder specialists are in a unique position to know firsthand the difficulties older persons face in coping with diminishing functioning. In particular, the speech-language pathologist and the audiologist are in a unique position to recognize the central role of adequate communication in meeting the needs of older persons and in enhancing quality of life. Unusual opportunities are available to exert leadership as an individual practitioner, member of a group practice, professor, or administrator. Aging is like a many-sided cube, with multiple possible approaches to creating a system of *real* help for older persons and their families that is responsive, resilient, efficient, and humane.

NEXT STEPS

What practical steps might be taken to bridge the communications gap among the various disciplines which are important to the older person in order to make "the system" more responsive? The following recommendations are meant to stimulate only, for the opportunities are truly boundless (additional suggestions are made in Chapter 22).

- As a specialist in communication behavior, concentrate on early detection. Take the initiative to organize ongoing seminars for physicians and other professionals in the community about communication disorders, and build a tight referral network among the various practicing professionals. Initiate joint evaluation and joint treatment.
- As a specialist in communication behavior, join with the Area Agency on Aging in approaching utilities companies and others which bill older persons monthly, so that early detection information can be included regularly in the mailings—not just once, but on a regular timetable.
- As a specialist in communication behavior, initiate training in the community on a variety of subjects related to aging so that individuals with diverse professional backgrounds will receive training *together* to enhance knowledge and a closer network.
- As a specialist in communication behavior, arrange for graduate students in communication disorders to be assigned to work for the Area Agency on Aging or major service providers in the community to study and implement improved approaches for the detection and delivery of services and treatment to older persons with diminishing functioning in communications. Build in university faculty supervision in communications, so that the project has knowledgeable guidance and the resources of the university community available.
- As a specialist in communication behavior, work for the inclusion of aging content in college and university communications curricula statewide. Likewise, work for the inclusion of communications curricula in gerontology.
- As a specialist in communication behavior concerned with aging, take steps to be a member of community committees and work alongside other professionals and older persons to tackle both immediate and long-range problems in the total service system.

Developments concerned with communications and aging are long-term in nature, and long-term professional commitment will be required to make a "whole," rather than a patchwork system. Students and professionals in the 1980s and 1990s have a system on which to build, but it is also a system which is in need of major repairs. Leadership exerted now can affect the current older population in positive ways and pave the way for a more rational and humane system of services for older persons in the future. The challenge to leadership is considerable—it involves retooling or remaking a major social system for several generations to come.

References

1. Committee on Education and Labor, United States Congress, *Older Americans Act of 1965 as Amended*: 1985, pp 1–2.

Appendix A

Additional Readings

1. *Aging America: Trends and Projections*, U.S. Senate Special Committee on Aging with the American Association of Retired Persons, 1985.
2. Binstock RH, Shanas E (eds): *Handbook of Aging and the Social Sciences*. Van Nostrand Reinhold, 1976.
3. Butler RN: *Why Survive? Being Old in America*. New York, Harper & Row, 1975.
4. *Developments in Aging*: A Report of the Special Committee on Aging, vols I and II. United States Senate, 1985.
5. Estes CL: *The Aging Enterprise*. San Francisco, Jossey-Bass, 1979.
6. Hudson R (ed): *Aging in Politics: Process and Policy*. Springfield, IL., Charles C Thomas, 1981.
7. Norman WJ: The Older Americans Act: Meeting the Changing Needs of the Elderly. *Aging Magazine*, Administration on Aging, Department of Health and Human Services, 1982.
8. National Association of State Agencies on Aging, *An Orientation to the Older Americans Act*, 1982.
9. Rich BM, Baum M: *The Aging: A Guide to Public Policy*. University of Pittsburgh Press, 1984.
10. Siegel JS, Davidson M: *Demographic and Socioeconomic Aspects of Aging in the United States*, Bureau of the Census, U.S. Department of Commerce, 1984.
11. Special Committee on Aging: *Older Americans and the Federal Budget: Past, Present, and Future*, United States Senate, 1984.
12. Tibbitts C (ed): *Handbook of Social Gerontology: Societal Aspects of Aging*. New York, Columbia University Press, 1960.

Appendix B

FEDERAL ASSISTANCE TO OLDER PEOPLE

Income Security

Social Security
Supplemental Security Income
Federal Civilian Retirement and Disability
Military Retirement System
Railroad Retirement
Veterans Pensions
Veterans Disability Compensation
Food Stamps Program
Energy Assistance
Coal Miners Affected by Black Lung Disease

Health

Medicare
Medicaid
Veterans Health

Housing

Public housing
Housing construction for older persons and people with physical limitations
Assistance to rural families: loans and home repair

Social Services

Food Commodities Program
Community service opportunities for older people
Employment opportunities
Transportation
Assistance with age discrimination complaints
Nutrition, including home-delivered meals
Legal services
Ombudsman services for nursing home and group home residents
Research and training to increase knowledge about the aging process
Volunteer opportunities
Weatherization assistance
Coordination of services through State and community organizations

Appendix C

STATE AGENCIES ON AGING

Alabama
Alabama Commission on Aging
502 Washington Avenue
Second Floor
Montgomery, Alabama 36130
Phone (205) 261-5743

Alaska
Older Alaskans Commission
P.O. Box C, MS-0209
Juneau, Alaska 99811
Phone (907) 465-3250

American Samoa
American Samoa Territorial
Administration on Aging
Government of American Samoa
Pago Pago, American Samoa 96799
Phone (684) 633-1252

Arizona
Arizona Dept. of Economic Security
Aging & Adult Admin.
1400 W. Washington St., 2nd Floor
P.O. Box 6123-950A
Phoenix, Arizona 85007
Phone (602) 255-4446

Arkansas
Division of Aging and Adult Services
Arkansas Department of Human Services
Main & 7th Streets
Donaghey Building, Suite 1417
Little Rock, Arkansas 72201
Phone (501) 371-2441

California
California Dept. of Aging
1020 19th Street
Sacramento, California 95814
Phone (916) 322-5290

Colorado
Colorado Aging & Adult Services Division
Department of Social Services
717 17th Street
Denver, Colorado 80218-0899
Phone (303) 294-5905

**Commonwealth of the Northern Mariana
  Islands**
State Agency on Aging
Department of Community and Cultural Affairs
  Civic Center
Saipan, Mariana Islands 96950
Phone 9-011-670-6011

Connecticut
Connecticut Department on Aging
175 Main Street
Hartford, Connecticut 06106
Phone (203) 566-3238

Delaware
Delaware Division of Aging
Department of Health and Social Services
1901 North Dupont Highway, 2nd Floor
New Castle, Delaware 19720
Phone (302) 421-6791

District of Columbia
District of Columbia Office on Aging
Executive Office of the Mayor
1424 K Street, N.W., Second Floor
Washington, D.C. 20005
Phone (202) 724-5622

Florida
Aging and Adult Services
Department of Health and Rehabilitative
  Services
Building 2, Rm. 328
1323 Winewood Blvd.
Tallahassee, Florida 32301
Phone (904) 488-8922

Georgia
Office of Aging
Department of Human Resources
6th Floor
878 Peachtree Street, NE
Atlanta, Georgia 30309
Phone (404) 894-5333

Guam
Public Health and Social Services
Government of Guam
Agana, Guam 96910
Phone (671) 734-2942

Hawaii
Hawaii Executive Office on Aging
335 Merchant Street, Rm. 241
Honolulu, Hawaii 96813
Phone (808) 548-2593

Idaho
Idaho Office on Aging
Statehouse, Rm. 114
Boise, Idaho 83720
Phone (208) 334-3833

Illinois
Illinois Department on Aging
421 East Capitol Avenue
Springfield, Illinois 62701
Phone (217) 785-2870

Indiana
Indiana Department on Aging and Community
  Services
251 North Illinois
P.O. Box 7083
Indianapolis, Indiana 46207-7083
Phone (317) 232-1139

Iowa
Iowa Department of Elder Affairs
236 Jewett Building
914 Grand Avenue
Des Moines, Iowa 50319
Phone (515) 281-5187

Kansas
Kansas Department on Aging
610 West 10th Street
Topeka, Kansas 66612
Phone (913) 296-4986

Kentucky
Division for Aging Services
Department for Social Services
Cabinet for Human Resources
275 East Main Street
Frankfort, Kentucky 40621
Phone (502) 564-6930

Louisiana
Governor's Office of Elderly Affairs
P.O. Box 80374
Baton Rouge, Louisiana 70898-0374
Phone (504) 925-1700

Maine
Bureau of Maine's Elderly
Department of Human Services
State House-Station 11
Augusta, Maine 04333
Phone (207) 289-2561

Maryland
Maryland Office on Aging
301 West Preston Street, Rm. 1004
Baltimore, Maryland 21201
Phone (301) 225-1100

Massachusetts
Massachusetts Executive Office of Elder Affairs
38 Chauncy Street
Boston, Massachusetts 02111
Phone (617) 727-7750

Michigan
Office of Services to the Aging
P.O. Box 30026
Lansing, Michigan 48909
Phone (517) 373-8230

Minnesota
Minnesota Board on Aging
Metro Square Building, Suite 204
121 East 7th Street
St. Paul, Minnesota 55101
Phone (612) 296-2770

Mississippi
Mississippi Council on Aging
301 West Pearl Street
Jackson, Mississippi 39203-3092
Phone (601) 949-2013

Missouri
Missouri Division of Aging
Department of Social Services
505 Missouri Boulevard
P.O. Box 1337
Jefferson City, Missouri 65102
Phone (314) 751-3082

Montana
Community Services Division
P.O. Box 4210
Helena, Montana 59604
Phone (406) 444-3865

Nebraska
Nebraska Department on Aging
301 Centennial Mall South
P.O. Box 95044
Lincoln, Nebraska 68509
Phone (402) 471-2307

Nevada
Nevada Division for Aging Services
Department of Human Resources
505 East King Street, Rm. 101
Carson City, Nevada 89710
Phone (702) 885-4210

New Hampshire
New Hampshire State Council on Aging
105 Loudon Road, Prescott Park
Building 3
Concord, New Hampshire 03301
Phone (603) 271-2751

New Jersey
New Jersey Division on Aging
Department of Community Affairs
363 W. State Street
CN 807
Trenton, New Jersey 08625-0807
Phone (609) 292-3765

New Mexico
224 East Palace Avenue
La Villa Rivera Bldg., 4th Floor
Santa Fe, New Mexico 87501
Phone (505) 827-7640

New York
New York State Office for the Aging
Agency Building 2
Empire State Plaza
Albany, New York 12223-0001
Phone (518) 474-4425

North Carolina
Division of Aging
Department of Human Resources
1985 Umstead Drive
Kirby Building
Raleigh, North Carolina 27603
Phone (919) 733-3983

North Dakota
Aging Services Division
North Dakota Dept. of Human Services
State Capitol Building
Bismarck, North Dakota 58505
Phone (701) 224-2577

Ohio
Ohio Department on Aging
50 West Broad Street
Columbus, Ohio 43215
Phone (614) 466-5500

Oklahoma
Division of Services for the Aging
Special Unit on Aging
Department of Human Services
P.O. Box 25352
Oklahoma City, Oklahoma 73125
Phone (405) 521-2281

Oregon
Senior Services Division
Department of Human Resources
313 Public Service Building
Salem, Oregon 97310
Phone (503) 378-4728

Pennsylvania
Pennsylvania Department of Aging
231 State Street (Barton Building)
Harrisburg, Pennsylvania 17101
Phone (717) 783-1550

Puerto Rico
Puerto Rico Gericulture Commission
Department of Social Services
Box 11398
Santurce, Puerto Rico 00910
Phone (809) 724-1039 or 722-2429

Rhode Island
Department of Elderly Affairs
79 Washington Street
Providence, Rhode Island 02903
Phone (401) 277-2858

South Carolina
South Carolina Commission on Aging
915 Main Street
Columbia, South Carolina 29201
Phone (803) 734-3203

South Dakota
Office of Adult Services and Aging
Richard F. Kneip Building
700 North Illinois Street
Pierre, South Dakota 57501
Phone (605) 773-3656

Tennessee
Tennessee Commission on Aging
715 Tennessee Building
535 Church Street
Nashville, Tennessee 37219
Phone (615) 741-2056

Texas
Texas Department on Aging
P.O. Box 12786
Capitol Station
Austin, Texas 78711
Phone (512) 444-6890

Trust Territory of the Pacific Islands
State Agency on Aging
Community Development Division
Trust Territory of Pacific Islands
Saipan, Mariana Islands 96950
Phone 9-011-670-9328

Utah
Utah Division of Aging & Adult Services
150 West North Temple, 4th Floor
P.O. Box 2500
Salt Lake City, Utah 84103
Phone (801) 533-6422

Vermont
Vermont Office on Aging
Waterbury Complex
103 S. Main Street
Waterbury, Vermont 05676
Phone (802) 241-2400

Virgin Islands
Virgin Islands Commission on Aging
6F Havensight Mall
Charlotte Amalie
St. Thomas, Virgin Islands 00801
Phone (809) 774-5884 or 6930

Virginia
Virginia Department for the Aging
101 North 14th Street, 18th Floor
Richmond, Virginia 23219
Phone (804) 225-2271

Washington
Aging and Adult Services Administration
Department of Social and Health Services
Mail Stop OB-44-A
Olympia, Washington 98504
Phone (206) 586-3768

West Virginia
West Virginia Commission on Aging
State Capitol Complex-Holly Grove
1710 Kanawha Boulevard
Charleston, West Virginia 25305
Phone (304) 348-3317

Wisconsin
Bureau on Aging
Dept. of Health and Social Services
One West Wilson Street
P.O. Box 7851
Madison, Wisconsin 53707-7851
Phone (608) 266-2536

Wyoming
Wyoming Commission on Aging
Hathaway Building, 1st Floor
Cheyenne, Wyoming 82002
Phone (307) 777-7986

Appendix D

FEDERAL GOVERNMENT AGENCIES WHICH SPECIALIZE IN AGING

Executive Departments

Administration on Aging
Department of Health and Human Services
330 Independence Avenue, S.W.
Washington, D.C. 20201
(Social, nutrition and supportive services under
the Older Americans Act)

Health Care Financing Administration
Department of Health and Human Services
200 Independence Avenue, S.W.
Washington, D.C. 20201
(Medicare/Medicaid)

National Institute on Aging
National Institutes of Health
Department of Health and Human Services
9000 Rockville Pike
Bethesda, Maryland 20505
(Biomedical, social, and general research in
aging)

Older Americans Volunteer Programs
ACTION
806 Connecticut Avenue, N.W.
Washington, D.C. 20525
(Volunteer activities for older people)

Social Security Administration
Altmeyer Building
6401 Security Boulevard
Baltimore, Maryland 21235
(Income Security)

United States Congress

House Education and Labor Committee
Subcommittee on Human Resources
U.S. House of Representatives
Rayburn House Office Building
Washington, D.C.

House Select Committee on Aging
U.S. House of Representatives
House Office Building Annex No. 1
Washington, D.C.

Senate Labor and Human Resources Committee
Subcommittee on Aging, Family and Human
Resources
U.S. Senate
Washington, D.C.

Special Committee on Aging
U.S. Senate
Dirksen Building
Washington, D.C.

Appendix E

NATIONAL VOLUNTARY ORGANIZATIONS WHICH SPECIALIZE IN AGING

American Association of Homes for the Aging
1050 17th Street, N.W., Suite 770
Washington, D.C. 20036

American Association for International Aging
1511 K Street, N.W.
Washington, D.C. 20005

American Association of Retired Persons
1909 K Street, N.W.
Washington, D.C. 20049

American Society on Aging
333 Market Street
San Francisco, California 94103

Asociacion Nacional Pro Personas Mayores
2727 West 6th Street
Los Angeles, California 90057

Association for Gerontology in Higher
Education
600 Maryland Avenue, S.W.
Washington, D.C. 20024

The Gerontological Society of America
1411 K Street, N.W.
Washington, D.C. 20005

Gray Panthers
311 South Juniper Street
Philadelphia, Pennsylvania 19107

International Federation on Ageing
Publications Division
1909 K Street, N.W.
Washington, D.C. 20049

National Association of Area Agencies on Aging
600 Maryland Avenue, S.W.
Washington, D.C. 20024

National Association of Retired Federal
Employees
1533 New Hampshire Avenue, N.W.
Washington, D.C. 20036

National Caucus and Center on the Black Aged
1424 K Street, N.W.
Washington, D.C. 20005

National Council of Senior Citizens
925 15th Street, N.W.
Washington, D.C. 20005

National Council on the Aging
600 Maryland Avenue, S.W.
Washington, D.C. 20024

National Indian Council on Aging
P.O. Box 2088
Albuquerque, New Mexico 87103

National Interfaith Coalition on Aging
9201 West Broward Boulevard
Plantation, Florida 33324

National Association of State Units on Aging
600 Maryland Avenue, S.W.
Washington, D.C. 20024

National Senior Citizens Law Center
2025 M Street, N.W.
Washington, D.C. 20036

Older Women's League
415 Madison Avenue
New York, New York 10017

National Pacific Asian Resource Center on Aging
1341 G Street, N.W.
Washington, D.C. 20005

The Villers Foundation
1334 G Street, N.W.
Washington, D.C. 20005

Appendix F

RESOURCE INFORMATION ABOUT AGING

The following information sources and data bases specialize in information about aging, or have substantial holdings related to aging as part of a larger data base. These organizations may be queried about other data bases which specialize in certain fields, and have holdings in the area of aging.

AGELINE
BRS Customer Service
1200 Route 7
Latham, New York 12110

Ageline is an online bibliographic database covering all aspects of social gerontology. The data system is operated by the American Association of Retired Persons. The database includes a large collection of information on aging which was transferred from the Administration on Aging's National Clearinghouse on Aging, including research and training reports and publications.

GOVERNMENT PRINTING OFFICE
Library Programs Service
Micrographics Unit
5236 Eisenhower Avenue
Alexandria, Virginia 22304

The Government Printing Office uses depository libraries throughout the country for permanent storage of government-supported publications. There are some 1400 libraries which have been designated as depository libraries. Current Federal publications are included in "Monthly Catalog," published by GPO.

PROJECT SHARE
P.O. Box 2309
Rockville, Maryland 20852

Project SHARE is a clearinghouse of information in human services supported by the Department of Health and Human Services. Its focus is improved management of human services. Publications and reports supported by the Department of Health and Human Services in research, training, and evaluation, as well as other types of studies, are available. Project SHARE publishes a newsletter quarterly, *Journal of Human Service Abstracts*.

National Archive of Computerized Data on Aging
Box 1248
Ann Arbor, Michigan 48106

The National Archive acquires, processes, and disseminates data sets on all aspects of aging with a concentration on economic, attitudinal and health related information. The data system is operated by the University of Michigan.

NATIONAL TECHNICAL INFORMATION SERVICE
5285 Port Royal Road
Springfield, Virginia 22161

NTIS is a central, permanent source of information generated by Federal departments and agencies directly, or through grants and contracts. Current summaries are published in "Government Reports Announcements and Index."

22 Networking Strategies for Enhancing Interdisciplinary Service Provision

BARBARA B. SHADDEN

JANE A. BARR

Editor's Note

Throughout this textbook, frequent mention has been made of the need for professionals to work collaboratively to address the communication needs of the elderly. It is fitting, therefore, that the concluding chapter should focus on strategies for networking professional and community resources. The term networking is used loosely to refer to the process of sharing of knowledge, skills, or services to enhance responsiveness to the needs of individual clients or groups of individuals with common problems or characteristics. Chapter 22 begins with a brief review of various developments that have led historically to a concern with networking. It is suggested that two primary arenas for change exist, including: modifications or alterations in existing programs to meet the demand for adequate networking of resources, and redefinition of professional roles to enhance interdisciplinary interactions. Four major interdisciplinary strategies for improving services to the elderly are then described: (a) informal networking organizations of service providers; (b) development and implementation of a community action plan; (c) formal interprofessional teams for service delivery; and (d) improved inservice education. Hopefully the reader will be able to use the information provided here to develop constructive personal strategies for participation in the networking process.

The terms network and networking have recently become buzzwords in various professional literatures. While terms as popular as these tend to be applied overenthusiastically, the networking concept is truly relevant to the planning and implementation of service delivery to the elderly and will remain important without regard to fashion. It is the thesis of this chapter that older persons need coordinated services and support, and that the adequacy, breadth, and comprehensiveness of those services depends on appropriate networking of the professionals involved. Speech-language pathologists and audiologists working with older clients cannot afford to distance themselves from such interdisciplinary involvements.

Barnes depicts a network as "a set of points which are joined by lines; the points of the image are people or sometimes groups and the lines indicate which people interact with each other" (5, p 43). This definition can accommodate any sharing of knowledge, skills, or services by a combination of individuals, agencies, and formal or informal groups. In health and social service delivery, the network col-laborates in responding to the needs of an identified client or group of clients.

This chapter will provide background information on the networking concept, describe the establishment of a representative informal aging network, and discuss professional issues which arise when networking is attempted. There are problems of territoriality and the lack of norms to define cooperation when service providers from a number of disciplines and agencies work together, and these must be addressed if the collaboration is to be effective. Ways in which speech-language pathologists and audiologists can personally facilitate networking by providing cross-disciplinary education are discussed.

ORIGINS OF THE CONCERN WITH NETWORKS

Historically, there have been at least three major service-related areas of development which influenced the interest in networks and networking for health and social services provision to the elderly. The first of these is an increased awareness of the importance of social support networks. The second, the development of interdisciplinary team practice models, represents a particular form of highly structured network whose principles can be applied to a broader range of collaborations. The third factor was the establishment of the Administration on Aging, one purpose of which was service coordination.

Social Support Networks

Research concerning the nature, structure, and roles of social networks in general and support networks for the elderly in particular began with the work of Barnes and Bott in the 1950s (5, 9), and its volume has progressively increased over the past 20 years. Biegel et al (7) have suggested that the elderly may have weaker social networks than other age groups, despite their apparently greater need for the socialization, assistance in daily living activities, and support in times of crisis provided by such networks. There is growing concern that diminished viability of an older adult's social network may play an important role in reducing utilization of services (7, 12, 14, 33). (The importance of social support networks is further discussed in Chapter 19.)

The recent expansion in self-help and mutual aid groups, many of which are grass roots developments, is evidence of growing public awareness of the need for supplementing or replacing naturally occurring support networks. Some self-help groups with goals of mutual support and guidance form in response to a common concern or problem (4) such as stroke or Alzheimer's disease. A second type of mutual aid group is the barter club, or formalized service exchange program, in which services are traded through a central record-keeping agency. Other support systems consist of artificial networks which attempt to compensate for specific gaps in existing networks. For example, a service club may organize to provide transportation to medical appointments for elderly community residents.

The needs of older individuals cannot be met currently, and may never be totally addressed, by agencies and professionals alone. Instead, we must look to the role of informal groups and support systems as mediators and supplementers of formal services (4, 13, 15, 39) and find ways of working with, organizing, and harnessing these informal networks (7, 8, 26). Some of these issues will be addressed in the discussion of strategies for networking.

Interprofessional Teamwork

Paralleling the development of concern with social support networks from the 1950s to the present, there has been an interest in the implementation of interprofessional service delivery models. The interdisciplinary team approach to service delivery can be conceptualized as a highly specialized form of networking, as in Bartlett's definition of this process as

the organized, continuous, coordinated activity of a small group of individuals from two or more of the health professions working together under the auspices of a single agency to further common objectives such as patient care or program development (6, p 226).

Certainly, no other client population demands greater interdisciplinary attention than the elderly, in view of the essentially hybrid nature of the knowledge base of geriatrics (10) and the interconnectedness of older clients' problems (25).

Unfortunately, team provision of services has been and continues to be fraught with difficulties. Too often, agencies and professionals pay lip service to the concept of multidisciplinary input in planning and intervention with relatively little practical attention to the structuring of the team mechanism. In addition, as services in aging expand it becomes more difficult to include all relevant professionals in an active management team. The decentralization of services inherent in the trend away from institutional delivery and toward home interventions can also undermine the cohesion of teamwork which traditionally has been agency-based. Strategies which speech-language pathologists and audiologists can implement to enhance interprofessional teamwork will be discussed later in this chapter.

The Administration on Aging as a Network

With the passage of the Older Americans Act (OAA) in 1965 (see Chapter 21) and its subsequent amendments, States were to be provided funds through the Administration on Aging (AoA) to be used for services, training, and research to assist the elderly (20). The term "aging network" was coined to "denote the arrangement of state units, area agencies, nutrition programs, senior centers, and other Older Americans Act agencies throughout the nation" (17, p 147). As early as 1978, there were at least 80 programs involving older persons listed in the Federal Register and more than 3000 heterogeneous agencies funded through OAA under AoA auspices.

Everyday use of the term "aging network" has also come to include services which are not affiliated with AoA. In both its specific and its broader applications, there are problems with the term's implication of unity and organization. Estes (17) warns professionals against assuming programatic cohesion, and Peters (31) notes that even under the AoA umbrella, each agency must be considered separately before patterns of action and interaction can be understood and utilized.

Problems in the Aging Network

On a practical level, it appears that the aging network suffers from a lack of networking. At least five major problem areas can be identified.

Fragmentation. The proliferation of services, both within and outside of Federally mandated program guidelines, has led to an unmanageable number of organizations and programs. The result appears to be extremely poor coordination of effort, inadequate interagency communication, a lack of mutual knowledge concerning what each agency and individual is doing, unclear role definitions, and a resulting tendency toward unnecessary jurisdictional disputes. This confusion constitutes a critical problem, exacerbating the need for information and referral programs (7, 17, 20, 31).

Accessibility. Ironically, as services proliferate, problems of accessibility become more apparent. Two aspects of accessibility must be considered. The first, and more obvious, is physical access: transportation to services, adequate mobility to leave the residential environment, etc. The second accessibility issue relates to information about the nature and availability of, as well as entitlement to, existing resources. Current research suggests that older persons make less use of community services than do other groups (7, 20), perhaps as a result of these two access problems.

Accountability. Estes (17) argues that the OAA has created massive problems of multiple accountability for the programs and services under its jurisdiction. These problems are aggravated by the difficulty of disseminating and retrieving information through the network, and the need for clarification of ambiguous policy statements.

Funding. The last 20 years has seen a sharp increase in social and professional awareness of the needs of the elderly. Ironically, just as concerted efforts began to meet these needs, the 1980s have brought major funding cutbacks affecting almost all levels of programming (7). It is clear that, at least for the present, Federal and state government sources can no longer be expected to provide adequate financial assistance. While this situation may suggest a need for professionals to consider increasing their legislative and social advocacy for the older American, it also implies that alternate resources and programming strategies must be explored.

Service Provider Preparation. The rapid proliferation of agencies and programs serving the elderly has led to a near-crisis state of underpreparation on the part of individual service providers. In Peters' (31) study of the State Unit on Aging and the Area Agencies on Aging in Kansas, personnel complained of lack of job introduction, orientation, and definition. The lack of on-the-job training was accompanied by limited qualifications, training, and gerontological experience prior to hiring. Peters found that rapid expansion of the aging network "meant that persons were hired without adequate guidelines detailing a desirable fit between professional qualifications and experience and the job demands" (31, p. 116).

THE FUTURE OF NETWORKING: MAKING IT WORK

The preceding discussion of the networking concept's historical origins describes the growth of professional interest in working together in providing services to the elderly, and a concurrent increase in problems related to doing so. Clearly, before networking can be fully effective the obstacles inherent in the current system must be recognized, and approaches must be designed to overcome them.

There are two arenas for change. The first is development of or alterations in programs in order to fill the networking needs identified below. The second arena is the redefinition and expansion of professional roles which is essential to the ultimate success of interdisciplinary cooperation. Following this section, four major types of networking approaches are described. Each of those approaches addresses the central needs listed here, and each requires that, at least to some degree, professionals adopt nontraditional roles.

Programmatic Needs

There were a number of problem areas mentioned in the discussion of the origins of networking. The principal needs identified include:

1. Comprehensive descriptions of community resources and targeted services for the elderly. Over the last 20 years both service entitlements and local community programs for older persons have proliferated. Rapidly changing Federal and state eligibility and procedural guidelines have made it difficult for professionals, as well as potential program participants, to keep up with available programs.
2. Methods of identifying unmet community needs and developing remedies for them.
3. Mechanisms for interfacing formal (agency or bureaucratic) and informal support and service systems.
4. Provisions for informal networking among professionals at the local level, both for information exchange and for cross-disciplinary psychological support in managing the frustrations of inadequate resources and overwhelming client needs.
5. Improved management of individual client needs through interdisciplinary teamwork or alternate case management strategies.
6. Access to education and training for service providers, in both discipline-specific and broader aspects of gerontology.

Redefining Professional Roles

Biegel et al (7) define 11 potential professional roles in building support networks for the elderly. These roles are equally useful in redefining possible approaches to older clients' needs and the structure of the service delivery system. As defined in Table 22.1, the roles which are most comfortable and familiar for speech-language pathologists and audiologists are direct service provider and (less commonly) consultant and supervisor/teacher.

It is possible to contribute to improvement of services to older clients through networking without adopting an unfamiliar role. For example, serving on an interdisciplinary appraisal team or attending meetings of an informal network of service providers may allow the professional to remain within the familiar confines of the direct service role. However, the service provider who is willing to forsake passive participation for a more active, creative stance may choose to become instrumental in developing new linkages between systems in advocating to other agencies or service providers, or in initiating innovative model programs.

The remaining sections of this chapter describe four interdisciplinary approaches to improving services for communicatively impaired older persons: informal networking organizations, community action plan development and implementation, formal service provision teams, and improved inservice education. Each of these strategic approaches requires that professionals from the relevant disciplines abandon their rigid adherence to traditional functions, and accept a wider range of roles as not only inappropriate but also necessary.

Table 22.1
Categories of Professional Roles[a]

Role	Definition
Advocate	Organizes activities to obtain desired resources
Consultant	Provides assistance to primary caregivers or to service providers
Coordinator	Brings together formal services to maximize the breadth and cohesion of service provision
Direct service provider	Provides all direct services to client
Facilitator	Expedites service or activity mobilization to improve accessibility and utilization
Initiator/developer	Creator of new services and programs
Linker: intrasystem	Links service components within a particular service delivery system
Linker: intersystem	Links service components across systems (particularly informal and formal supports)
Manager-Administrator	Oversees and manages the organizational aspects of provision of services
Resource provider	Actively brings resources to the community or creates resources to facilitate interventions
Supervisor/teacher	Trains and/or oversees providers of services

[a] Modified from Biegel DE, Shore, BK, Gordon E: *Building Support Networks for the Elderly: Theory and Applications.* Beverly Hills, CA, Sage, 1984.

STRATEGY ONE: INFORMAL NETWORKING OF SERVICE PROVIDERS

The expansion of services for the elderly over the past 20 years has made it difficult, if not impossible, for the individual service provider to keep abreast of new regulations, agencies, professions, and more general gerontological information. A service provider's inadequate knowledge of community, state, and Federal programs can mean that a client is not referred to needed auxiliary services; his general well-being and ability to respond to services is thereby impaired; and as a result he does not benefit fully from the disciplinary intervention which is provided.

This lack of knowledge about services is just one aspect of professionals' isolation from each other. It is also easy to feel overwhelmed by the complex needs of elderly clients when there are no colleagues with whom to trade encouragement and support. One possible vehicle for promoting both information exchange and social support for professionals is an informal networking organization for community service providers. An example of the development of one such organization is provided in the following paragraphs. While the Providers of Services to the Elderly organization in Northwest Arkansas is not intended to represent a model program, the story of its organization and maintenance reveals the strengths and weaknesses of such networks, and the problems likely to be encountered in implementation.

Organizational Origins

Early in 1983 three professionals (the chapter authors, whose disciplines are speech-language pathology and social work, and a registered nurse) from three unrelated agencies (a university, a community mental health center, and a home health program) met informally to discuss the possibility of initiating a gerontological workshop for service providers in the local community. Over a series of conversations, the initial idea of presenting one content-based workshop was abandoned as three themes kept recurring.

First, we found ourselves unable to select a workshop topic because we realized that in doing so we would have to impose our own ideas of what other providers needed, without having solid information concerning what they actually wanted to know. We became progressively more aware, as discussions of possible topics continued, of ways in which the unique perspectives of each profession shape perceptions of client needs, potentially blinding service providers to needs outside their areas of expertise.

A second, equally serious problem was the lack of knowledge of all the services available locally to older community members. As each of us realized that the others shared this lack of information, and at the same time each had information which was useful to the others, we recognized that the same situation was likely to be mirrored in the service community as a whole. Any one provider would know about only a limited part of the pie, but in combination they would be able to assemble a full picture of both client needs and available services.

The third factor which we found ourselves noticing was the way our discussions seemed to be meeting our previously unrecognized need for support. We speculated that other service providers might also find value in the combination of obtaining concrete information about services and sharing the difficulties and frustrations encountered in attempting to provide comprehensive and effective services to their own clients.

The First Workshop

Recognition of the above-described factors led to a major revision of our original plans. Instead of organizing an educational seminar, we decided to hold a workshop which would provide a forum for service providers to learn about community resources. We also wanted to obtain more information from attendees about their needs for information and support. Those invited to the first workshop included representatives of agencies serving the elderly, "gatekeepers" (clergy, physicians, pharmacists, and others who refer clients to the service system), and informal helpers, including older individuals themselves (7). Because the first meeting succeeded in attracting participants, eliciting their contributions, and developing their interest in continuing to meet as Providers of Services to the Elderly (PSE, the name which attendees chose for their group), it may be helpful to describe the format and content in some detail.

The workshop was organized around three case histories developed to reflect a range of typical problems and financial situations found in the older population (see the Appendix, for one example). After each case history had been read aloud and printed copies had been distributed, participants were divided into small groups of six to eight persons. The small group tasks were: (a) to define all the needs of the individual or family described; (b) to prioritize the needs; and (c) to describe, to the best of the group members' knowledge, community resources available for meeting those needs. After approximately 15 minutes, each group reported in turn to the entire workshop audience. Needs and priorities from all of the small groups were compared, compiled, and discussed. Needs which could not be met by the existing services were listed, thus identifying gaps in community resources. The audience was encouraged to problem solve ways of providing for the unmet needs, including using existing agency programs in unorthodox ways or soliciting help from informal groups.

The process of need identification, prioritization, and service identification was repeated for each case. During the subsequent 1-hour discussion of overall issues raised during the individual case discussions, participants were urged to identify future directions—for individual service providers, for the participating group, and for the community. An extensive written evaluation form supplemented this discussion by providing participants with an opportunity to describe their current needs as service providers, what could be done to meet those needs in the future, and what needs had been met by the workshop. In addition, the evaluation form explored willingness to help organize future events and interest in particular topics for additional workshops.

The success of the workshop was evident in that the needs which participants reported to have been met by the gathering matched the intentions of the organizers. Participants said they had been lacking, and had obtained in this gathering, information about other agencies and services, clarification of community needs, development of contacts and networking resources, and support and reinforcement (from the discovery of shared concerns and frustrations.)

Subsequent Developments

The Providers of Services to the Elderly group has continued to be informal in structure and leadership, with no dues, no formal membership applications, and no designated leaders. The stated mission of the group was agreed to be:

... to promote dissemination of information and facilitate networking among individuals and agencies offering services to the elderly population of our areas ... [and] ... to provide a support group for

problem solving among concerned professionals of northwest Arkansas.

A committee of five has assumed responsibility for designing and planning subsequent workshops, in response to stated needs of the service providers participating. Structured workshop topics have included Diagnostically Related Groups, Alternatives to Acute Hospital Care, The Legislature and the Elderly, Residential Alternatives, Elder Abuse, and The Psychology of Aging. These formal events have been interspersed with more casual social get-togethers designed to promote information exchange, professional sharing, and support in a relaxed atmosphere.

The PSE remains an infrequently activated but ongoing resource for professionals and agencies within a four-county region. For those who participate, it is a source of current, relevant information about gerontological services. Most important, attendees no longer feel isolated and overwhelmed when they work with clients who have a range of needs. There are now names, with faces, of others who can be called upon for assistance or referral.

Problems Encountered

Although the preliminary organization of PSE went smoothly, and initial reception was enthusiastic, this informal network is not without its problems. If similar programs were implemented in other communities, difficulties might arise in the same four areas described below.

Organizational Structure and Leadership

The informal organizational model selected for PSE has worked well on most occasions, and has kept participants from being overwhelmed by the prospect of an additional formal commitment to serve the community. Nevertheless, the number of service providers in the Northwest Arkansas area is relatively small compared to those in urban communities. Greater structure might be required in more heavily-populated areas. Within the PSE group, it has sometimes been difficult to balance and coordinate the contributions of the brainstormers with those of the workers. Finally, there is the question of who motivates and energizes the informal leaders (who make up the program committee), and how new leaders can be found when members of the original core group leave or burn out.

Finances

Two levels of financial problems may be encountered in maintaining an informal network of service providers. The first pertains to the relatively small but ongoing expenses of mailings, telephone calls, xeroxing of programs, and similar operations. These expenses have been handled in PSE by utilizing the resources of the agencies where planning committee members were employed, a solution which might not be acceptable to some agencies or which may become unacceptable if funding cutbacks continue. The second group of financial problems centers on the meetings themselves, including speaker fees or expenses and refreshments for workshops and social meetings. In this area as well, the PSE has managed to avoid any cost to participants. Speakers have graciously contributed their time and covered their own travel expenses, and refreshments have generously been provided by medical rentals companies. Some provider networks might find it more feasible to charge a small membership or workshop fee in order to cover expenses in either or both of these categories.

Topic Selection and Scheduling of Meetings

The PSE experience with topic selection by participant input has been highly successful. The difficulties encountered have been in balancing formal meetings with informal gatherings, to meet both information and support needs without deluging busy service providers with too many sessions to attend. A related question, the answer to which continues to elude the group, is how often meetings would ideally be held to provide continuity without demanding too much time. Experimentation within each community appears to be the best way to determine local preferences and needs.

Acting on Major Projects

Because of the loose-knit structure of the PSE, it is difficult to move the group to action. Participants may favor a project, yet protest (justifiably) that they don't have time to work on it personally. For example, PSE sessions frequently included discussion of the need for a computerized resource directory that could be accessed by service providers and older persons in the area (this concept is discussed below in greater detail as part of the community planning strategy). No action was taken by PSE to develop such a network because of the lack of a structured mechanism for initiating and pursuing cross-agency projects.

Despite these four areas of concern, networking by service providers is a viable strategy which can address many of the problems identified earlier in the chapter. The current status of the computerized resource directory, which PSE participants were unable to initiate, illustrates the kind of alternative approach that is possible once the flexibility characteristic of networking is accepted.

Cooperation among Networks

During the same year that the PSE program was beginning, another completely unrelated network was also in its early stages of development in a neighboring community. There had been an unusually high number of adolescent suicides and attempts, and parents, professionals, and community leaders began to discuss ways to approach the problem. The outcome of that informal networking was the establishment of a telephone Crisis Line which would both offer supportive listening and provide callers with referrals to other agencies.

When one of the authors became aware of the Crisis Line project, she approached that group to request that the needs of other age groups, in addition to those of adolescents, be considered in assembling referral information. The computerized resource directory is still being developed, but when it is operational, it will provide specific help for elderly community members, adolescents, and "latchkey kids," as well as information of interest to the community as a whole.

This chapter discusses networking among those providing services to the elderly, but the current example illustrates that such a network does not have to become self-sufficient and isolated. There are needs which various age groups have in common, and cooperation between two networks can solve problems for both. In addition, the example involves an individual member of PSE acting independently, without calling meetings of other PSE members. Once the goals and concerns of the network have been defined, single participants can operate from their agency positions to improve identified situations without the constant involvement of the network as a whole.

STRATEGY TWO: COMMUNITY PLANNING AND COORDINATION OF SERVICES

As noted earlier, one of the major purposes of attempting to network service providers is to find ways to identify community resources and needs. This section describes another approach to assessing the needs of the community and developing an action plan. Some of the strategies suggested here for carrying out an action plan require active participation in the less familiar professional roles shown in Table 22.1.

Assessing Community Needs

Biegel et al (7) refer to "the community as client," a concept which suggests that community needs must be assessed and planned for in much the same fashion as the needs of the individual older member of that community. Although it is appropriate for speech-language pathologists and audiologists to be aware of and concerned with the total needs of the older individual, this discussion will focus upon the communicatively impaired segment of the older community. Major assessment questions relevant to support networks can be adapted to consider the needs of this communicatively impaired subgroup:

1. What are the major problems or needs of communicatively impaired older persons?
2. What informal resources currently address these needs, and what limitations do those resources have?
3. What formal resources currently address these needs, and what limitations do those resources have?
4. What relationships exist between formal and informal resources, and how could these linkages be enhanced?
5. What problems or needs are not currently being met by existing resources?

Needs can be assessed in a variety of ways. Local, state, and national demographic profiles may be helpful in defining the current and projected size and characteristics of particular groups of older persons. Data may be gathered from agency records and from the records of key professionals. Public meetings may provide a forum for input from older residents similar to the forum which informal networks provide for professionals. A community survey of elderly residents may also clarify needs, resources, and barriers to service utilization from the perspective of the target client group. Surveys may involve a variety of sampling procedures and instruments, from lengthy open-ended interviews to brief questionnaires. Similar surveys may be performed with service providers as informants.

Regardless of the tools used in gathering information, assessment goals always involve clarification of the nature of available resources, access to and coordination of such resources,

and unmet needs. To insure that future program planning in the community incorporates a clear image of the status and requirements of speech-language-hearing impaired citizens, assessment data and conclusions must be shared with major planning agencies such as the Area Agency on Aging. In addition, assessment results can be employed in developing a community action plan.

A community action plan specifically defines and prioritizes the broad-based needs of a particular segment of the community, then suggests solutions for identified gaps in available programming. For the communicatively disordered, these needs extend beyond direct speech-language-hearing professional services to include: (a) environmental adaptions to insure physical access, promote auditory reception, and enhance communication opportunities; (b) public and professional knowledge of the nature of communication disorders, their consequences, and strategies for communicating with speech-language-hearing impaired persons; (c) psychological support and services (including counseling and support groups) for communicatively impaired older individuals and their families and friends; (d) social agency coordination of service delivery to maximize utilization of entitled services; (e) financial resources to fund needed communication interventions and devices; (f) recreational and vocational training and opportunities; (g) caregiver respite services; (h) remedies to any other identified barriers to service access (e.g., transportation problems) and communicative functioning; and (i) services parallel to those listed above for those who are also physically handicapped, visually impaired, or hearing impaired.

Meeting Some Common Community Needs

Issues of environmental interventions have been addressed in Chapter 18, and the needs of significant others (including education of the older community) were discussed in Chapter 19. Additional needs and approaches which are likely to be identified and addressed in a community action plan include the development of adequate information and referral systems (41), the tapping of alternate or nontraditional funding sources (35), and the use of volunteers as adjuncts to services (3, 35, see also Chapter 21).

Developing an Information System

It is arguable that the most central need is for an adequate information-and-referral system. As Gelfand (20) suggests, no network of services is of value unless potential users are aware of the availability of services and of the ways to access them. Forming a central clearinghouse for all the relevant data requires comprehensive identification and updated descriptions of all community resources, along with mechanisms for disseminating this information to service providers and directly to older individuals. Effective dissemination mechanisms include:

1. Annual publication of a services directory, with either a general focus on the elderly or a more specific focus on needs of communicatively impaired older persons;
2. Development of a community "helpline" or "hotline" which individuals can telephone for referral assistance concerning a specific problem;
3. Implementation of a computerized directory of services which can be updated constantly, and which can serve as the basis for a publication or helpline;
4. Presentation of a series of neighborhood workshops at which older persons can obtain information about community resources.

The first problem encountered in setting up and maintaining an information-and-referral system is getting organized. If there is already an organization serving the needs of one of the target groups (e.g., a stroke support group), it may be possible to work through that organization to develop the initial plans. Formal agencies or informal network organizations of service providers may provide the forum to explore preliminary ideas. It is also possible that a few professionals and community members may be able to link resources and begin an information-and-referral system without recourse to existing agencies or groups.

A second problem is developing an accurate and comprehensive listing of services while assuring that only reputable agencies, professionals, and vendors are included. As part of this concern, it should be noted that a clear definition of the target population to be served by the system must be developed, to serve as a guide in choosing which services to include.

The third problem is funding the information-and-referral system. Often, seed money is available (under the auspices of governmental agencies, or from local businesses or foundations), but funding for ongoing maintenance may require creative exploration of community financial resources. Affiliation with a particular agency which in turn receives funds earmarked for this purpose (e.g., from United Fund) may help resolve long-term funding problems.

The issue of affiliation is related to a fourth dilemma: Who will oversee and manage the system once it is established? If the project is the brainchild of a group of professionals from different agencies, which agency will physically house the directory sources or helpline? How will input from all concerned service providers and system users be ensured? Will one agency or some group of individuals from various agencies govern the ongoing operations?

Despite this list of problems, careful planning and coordination by community participants will insure development of an information-and-referral system that may prove to be the single greatest resource for meeting the needs of the target segment of the population. If such a system is to be effective in serving the older population, and particularly those persons who are communicatively impaired, the input of speech-language pathologists and audiologists is essential.

Funding Alternatives

Exploration of alternate or nontraditional funding sources may be necessary to supplement sparse resources, particularly when Federal support of agencies is being curtailed. For the communication disorders professional, alternate funding sources may be required to meet one of a number of needs: (a) to pay for direct service delivery; (b) to finance the costs of communication-enhancing devices (e.g., hearing aids, assistive listening devices, alternate or augmentative communication mechanisms, portable amplification devices); (c) to provide transportation to needed services; (d) to underwrite community screening programs; (e) to support innovative intervention programs not typically covered by third party reimbursement sources; and (f) to provide financial assistance for research efforts.

Most speech-language pathologists and audiologists recognize the need for exploration of alternate resources to cover the costs of communication-enhancing devices or research efforts. We are less comfortable with assuming an active role in seeking outside funding sources for some of the other needs described above, and may (understandably) see such efforts as consuming valuable time which might be spent in direct service delivery. The irony is that the value of professional efforts can be dependent on tapping financial resources to provide essential related services which will impact on the effectiveness of the direct service itself.

There are a large number of potential national, state, and local funding sources in addition to the availability of payment through Medicare, Medicaid, and other insurance carriers. National sources include the Administration on Aging, National Institute on Aging, other Federal agencies funding research and model programs in human services (see Chapter 21), national voluntary organizations (see Chapter 21), and nationally based private foundations with specific interests in aging, the elderly, or problems which touch the elderly. State sources include the State Unit on Aging, agencies and departments with concerns related to aging, State-based private foundations and professional associations, organizations overseeing coalitions of professionals or agencies, and branches of national voluntary organizations (particularly the American Association of Retired Persons).

The availability of local sources which can offer financial support differs across communities. Some of the following would be available in most areas: local chapters of organizations with older members, Area Agencies on Aging, area coalitions of service organizations or professionals who provide human services, community service organizations (e.g., Kiwanis, Sertoma, Lions, Rotary), local businesses, community-based private foundations, churches, community mental health centers, local universities, and nearby retirement communities.

Volunteers

Ashby (3) notes that, despite an extensive tradition of voluntarism in this country, speech-language pathology and audiology professionals and programs often appear reluctant to incorporate the services of volunteers into their interventions. Volunteers could be tapped for a variety of critical support functions, including transportation of clients to and from direct service sites, provision of relief to primary caregivers in the home, ongoing organizational maintenance of support groups, enhanced social communication opportunities for homebound or nursing home clients, advocacy for community changes in line with needs described elsewhere in the chapter, and fundraising. These functions do not impinge on the professional territory of the speech-language pathologist or audiologist but do address the broad-based needs of our communicatively impaired clients.

STRATEGY THREE: FORMAL INTERPROFESSIONAL TEAMWORK

Whitehouse (40) defines teamwork as "a close, democratic, multiprofessional union devoted to a common purpose—the best treat-

ment for the fundamental need of the individual" (19, p 79). The undesirable alternative to team planning occurs when the patient is viewed as the "sum of subspecialty parts . . . [and we] shuffle the patient from specialist to specialist" (19, p 160). The basic argument for interdisciplinary teamwork is that a team can deal with more complex problems than any number of professionals working independently, primarily because it allows consideration of the whole individual in his full complexity and with all of the interdependence implicit in his needs and problems. Thus teams are believed to provide the most efficient allocation of resources at any point in the treatment process. The advantages and disadvantages of such teams are summarized succinctly in Kane's (24) monograph on this subject. The thesis of this section of the chapter is that the advantages far outweigh the disadvantages, making interprofessional teamwork the preferred model for working with elderly clients.

Utilization of Interprofessional Teams

Many work settings routinely utilize some version of the interdisciplinary team as a component of the health care process. This practice is most common in rehabilitation-oriented settings or agencies, and decreases in frequency in acute care hospitals or custodial-oriented care facilities such as nursing homes. In addition to the lack of availability of a team practice model in some settings, it is clear that not all professionals have the opportunity to participate in the teams which do exist. Speech-language pathologists and audiologists, in particular, frequently provide services on a case-by-case basis, rather than being employed full time by the facility being served. In addition, many communication disorders professionals are employed at speech and hearing clinics where no other disciplines are represented.

There is a need for speech-language pathologists and audiologists to provide input as members of existing teams, and to encourage and participate in special staffings of clients being served by more than one agency. In a 1975 survey of 229 teams described in the literature, Kane (24) notes that only 65 of them included a physical therapist, occupational therapist, or speech-language pathologist. It seems likely that physical therapy was the most commonly represented of those three disciplines, indicating that the participation of speech-language pathologists was not at all common. Yet the interconnectedness of problems presented by older clients calls for the input of all relevant professions.

Making Interdisciplinary Teamwork Succeed

In order to function effectively on an interprofessional team, the service provider must first understand the dynamics of group and team interactions and be aware of common barriers to successful team communication and patient management. Areas to consider include professional territoriality and the lack of clearly defined roles, group norms for leadership and decision making, and communication channels and patterns.

Professional Territoriality and Role Definition

According to some of the earlier definitions (27), professions develop in order to: (a) unite competent individuals for a particular task; (b) advance knowledge through research; and (c) protect members. The latter goal has become a major source of breakdown in interprofessional interactions. Protection implies the definition of domain and is frequently exclusionary, leading to the professional territoriality which Kane describes as "a zealous guarding of function on the part of professions which extends to the use of space, equipment, tests or procedures, and, most absurdly, even to the use of certain language" (24, p 15).

A major concern in interprofessional teamwork, therefore, is the determination of ways of preserving professional autonomy while participating as a caring, collaborative member of the group. This is of particular concern for speech-language pathologists and audiologists, because we appear to be engaged in an ongoing battle to define for other professions and for third party reimbursement providers the nature of our professional roles and responsibilities. One of our greatest difficulties is that the behavior which we evaluate and treat, communication, embraces all human endeavors. A second problem is that the roles of the communication disorders professional do not fit tidily into the "multidisciplinary" paradigm proposed by Christopholos (11) and accepted as a model by many. According to this paradigm, three distinct orientations and contributions characterize different professions. The medical emphasis dominates definition of causal factors; the behavioral or psychometric emphasis dominates descriptions of current behaviors; and the educational or curriculum emphasis governs treatment planning. Because speech-language pathology and audiology incorporate all three orientations in addressing communi-

cation disorders, our role on the interprofessional team is frequently misunderstood or poorly defined.

While there are no simple and immediate solutions to these problems for the profession as a whole, individuals can be prepared to recognize and deal with problems of territoriality and role confusion when they arise. Some possible strategies useful in addressing these problems include:

1. Define one's professional roles and responsibilities, in terms of both client management and team participation, at the time of entering the team. If there appear to be problems with this definition, negotiate solutions with the entire group. While one should not undermine one's own professional standards regarding client management, team roles can and should be defined and accepted by the entire group.
2. Obtain a clear statement of the team leader's perceptions of one's professional role, responsibilities, and team contributions. Attempt to resolve conflicting views prior to actually staffing clients. Be prepared to offer a compromise proposal concerning team-based roles which allows the opportunity to establish professional credentials and expertise.
3. If territorial conflicts appear most likely to arise with only one or two of the team members, meet with them separately and work out an acceptable division of responsibilities.
4. Avoid defensive, territorial stances during actual team staffings; a reputation of being "difficult to work with" is hard to live down. Courteous disagreement over professional issues concerning patient assessment and management, on the other hand, is reasonable and appropriate.

Group Norms for Leadership and Decision-Making

The strategies above for avoiding problems about role definition emphasize the development of group norms. One of the greatest difficulties encountered in interprofessional teamwork results from the failure to develop group norms for leadership and decision-making. Often a decision is made to have an interprofessional team, which then attempts to begin functioning immediately without devoting any time or effort to defining its own operational guidelines.

Communication disorders professionals who have the opportunity to participate in planning for implementing a team approach to client management should advocate for systematic analysis of the proposed mechanisms of group functioning. Factors to consider include: team goals, responsibilities of individual members, group size, composition (fixed team, or variable team based on service needs of each client), procedures for choosing team leaders, rules governing decision-making (e.g., who participates, what degree of consensus is required), and steps for conflict resolution. In entering an existing team, it is essential that a new member obtain clarification of these same factors.

Norms for selection of the leader are of particular concern, because it is all too common to find that leadership automatically falls to the participating physician or team member with the most seniority in the facility without consideration of system needs. Other teams operate ostensibly without leadership, although one member typically convenes and manages the group. Neither of these approaches is intrinsically wrong, but neither should be passively adopted without consideration of the team's purposes (e.g., if the team leader will prepare important reports, writing ability will be a choice factor) and the qualities needed in a leader (e.g., interpersonal skills, breadth of cross-disciplinary knowledge, degree of professional involvement).

Communication Channels and Patterns

Implicit in the preceding discussion is the issue of communication patterns within the interprofessional team. In addition, there must be a definition of communication channels between the team and clients, other professionals, and administrators. If interdisciplinary teamwork is to be real rather than perfunctory, time must be allowed for communications that are two-way, informal as well as formal, and spoken as well as written. At the same time, communication efficiency can be improved by a deliberate analysis of patterns and efforts to increase productive exchanges while eliminating nonproductive behaviors and mechanisms.

Other Formal Networking Models

This section on interprofessional teamwork has emphasized the interdisciplinary team approach. In addition, there are two other formal networking models which will be mentioned briefly here: transdisciplinary intervention and case management.

The term transdisciplinary intervention has emerged recently in the literature. As used by Florance and Conway (19), the term refers to a process in which "professional disciplines have been intertwined" (19, p 166) in a team united by the single goal of patient autonomy and functioning for independent living. The definition of a single goal is believed to result in the patient receiving a single service, which is based on contributions of multiple professions. To facilitate participation in transdisciplinary intervention teams, as well as interdisciplinary efforts, professionals at the postgraduate level should receive training in cross-disciplinary content (see Strategy Four: Cross-Disciplinary Education below).

Case management also requires interprofessional interaction, but strategies for serving the client differ considerably. In this approach, "the case manager, a professional agency worker, attempts to coordinate a variety of public and private services for the maximum benefit of the client, and in so doing makes the impact of the service both more efficient and more effective" (7, p 87). Case management approaches are particularly common in social service agencies. Speech-language pathologists and audiologists can locate such services in their communities, identify clients who are in need of case management and refer them, and make case managers aware of the speech-language-hearing needs of the older population and the resources available for meeting those needs.

STRATEGY FOUR: CROSS-DISCIPLINARY EDUCATION

One major theme underlying the preceding strategies for networking and interprofessional cooperation is the need of professionals who work with older clients for information and education beyond the confines of any single discipline. It is impossible to provide the elderly with comprehensive services without an adequate understanding of aging, the characteristics of older persons, problems common in later years, and resources for managing those problems.

Educational Needs and Implementation Barriers

The need for improved gerontological education exists at the preservice level (for students receiving their initial disciplinary training), at the continuing education level (for practicing professionals), and at the target population level (see Chapter 19 for a discussion of educational programming for the elderly). Several surveys have established that graduate programs in speech-language pathology and audiology provide limited coursework options emphasizing gerontological aspects of communication behavior (29, 32); the same situation can be surmised to exist in other professional training programs. As a result, a student can graduate with too little knowledge of gerontological aspects of her own specialty area, and with even less knowledge of broader gerontological concerns. Professionals working with older clients report that their expertise *primarily* has been developed through on-the-job training and continuing education (18).

There are two ways in which speech-language pathologists and audiologists can take responsibility for filling these educational needs. First, it is the responsibility of each professional who works with the elderly to seek out additional educational opportunities. Gerontological knowledge can be obtained from books and journals, lectures, workshops, and university courses, as well as from sources recommended by colleagues in other disciplines.

The second responsibility is to provide inservice education to other professionals, with the combined goals of improving services to older clients and furthering recognition of the importance of speech, language, and audiological interventions. Service providers from other disciplines cannot be expected to refer clients for services, work collaboratively in service provision, or fully respect the contributions of speech-language pathology and audiology if they are unaware of the pervasiveness and importance of communication disorders, and the possibilities for effective intervention.

While the term inservice education is often used to indicate programs provided within an agency, it can also be more generally defined as training which follows the attainment of a formal degree and is concurrent with professional employment. Provision of inservice education in the broader sense, then, involves not only in-house efforts but also workshops for the larger community of service providers. In addition, there is a need for more presentations, papers, and workshops at local, State, and national meetings of professional organizations other than ASHA. The conference programs of the Gerontological Society of America, for example, reveal that communication problems and disorders are terribly underrepresented.

While there is a great need for cross-disciplinary gerontological knowledge, there are also obstacles to be encountered by those who accept the mission of providing inservice education.

Training sessions within an agency may be poorly attended, particularly if many of the staff are not interested in working with older clients, yet programs must be repeated at intervals due to staff turnover. If interest in outreach to other disciplines has not been aroused among local professionals (perhaps through development of an informal network of service providers), community response to workshop offers may also be less enthusiastic than the presenter would wish. The amount of time which is involved in developing and offering a program is a second obstacle, particularly if such time actually has to be taken away from direct service delivery. Third, the time spent in providing inservice education often does not directly produce revenues. Presenting papers and programs at state and national conventions does not even offer the possibility of indirect revenue production through resultant referrals, yet requires expenditures for registration and travel.

Despite these obstacles, it is the responsibility of those who provide services to older populations to broaden the base of knowledge shared across the professional community. Because a final obstacle to participation is the hesitation which stems from being unfamiliar with educational program design, the following paragraphs describe the steps involved in producing an effective inservice program.

Developing Successful Inservice Programs

Ashby (3) has provided an excellent and succinct description of the process of inservice or interdisciplinary education as it pertains to communication disorders and aging. His six stages in developing and implementing programming are expanded upon below.

Targeting the Participant Group

Any inservice program must begin with a series of decisions concerning who needs and would most benefit from an educational program. One priority involves the ability of the target audience to impact upon older communicatively impaired individuals. The presenter will also want to consider which participants are most likely to be offering complementary services, such that mutual referrals would result which would improve the treatment provided to clients. The presenter must further take into account her own knowledge and resources, to consider who might benefit from the knowledge she has to offer.

Securing Agreement of the Target Group

Once a target audience has been selected, appropriate administrators or professional leaders must be contacted in order to negotiate arrangements for presenting the inservice training. Mutual agreements must be reached regarding the time and place, fees (if any), and general content. If there is no local history of cross-disciplinary training, a major part of the negotiations may consist of convincing key persons that the program is needed. The following step both allows the content to be determined more specifically, and provides evidence to persuade target group leaders that the training will be worthwhile. A conditional agreement may be reached initially, with the understanding that planning will proceed only if the needs assessment suggests that the program will be useful.

Needs Assessment

A needs assessment may be formal, based on questionnaires, structured interviews, or journal research, or may consist of informal, nonstructured conversations with a sample of the target group. Regardless of the mechanism, an adequate assessment will insure audience interest in training goals and satisfaction with the content. In addition, as mentioned above, results of the needs assessment can be used to convince target group leaders of the need for a particular program.

Ashby (3) makes the strong point that speakers frequently assume that they know what an audience needs, rather than bothering to find out what the audience wants. If a beautifully designed program is "disrupted" by questions on "inappropriate" topics raised by participants, chances are the content was chosen without consideration of the needs of the target audience. With a preliminary needs assessment, there is the opportunity for creative planning to mesh the goals and interests of the potential participants with the objectives of the presenter.

Designing the Program

The three major variables in program design are content, time, and training methods. Selection of program content should be strongly influenced by a combination of data from the needs assessment and the presenter's own professional experience regarding the level of information needs within a target group. Content must also be limited by time constraints.

Workshops with a topic too broad to be covered in the time allotted are frustrating for both the presenter and the audience. There is a tendency to think of a program as the only opportunity there will be to influence and educate a particular audience, rather than as one step in an ongoing information exchange. Presenters should carefully consider program objectives and agenda times, and modify the schedule or the content as needed.

The selection of training methods is the single most important variable in program design, because the way in which content is presented determines what the audience will absorb, and what they will later incorporate into their professional procedures. It is well documented that behavioral and attitudinal change is primarily a product of participatory learning (28). The traditional methods of instruction, including lecture, passive demonstration, and observation, are among the least effective in modifying participant behavior. In contrast, interactive and experiential learning techniques such as brainstorming, gaming (e.g., role playing, simulations, and pseudotests), group discussions, and participatory demonstrations are highly successful (30).

Resource Availability

Although some facilitators will wish to develop training materials from scratch, in many cases existing materials can be modified to meet the chosen objectives at the level of the target audience. Ashby (3) has described some of the more valuable resources providing either strategies or content regarding general gerontology (see refs. 16, 22, 23, 37, 38). The American Speech-Language-Hearing Association has also published several training modules and resource guides useful in implementing programs related to communication disorders and aging. The training module "Breaking the Silence Barrier"(2) is designed to facilitate inservice programming for nursing home staff working with communicatively handicapped geriatric patients. The text, training manual, and materials for "Communication Problems and Behaviors of the Older American" (34) also provide extensive direction in developing workshops for professionals, and these materials can be supplemented by filmstrips, tapes, and handouts selected from ASHA's "Resource Materials for Communication Problems of Older Persons (1)."

The Shadden-Raiford-Shadden (36) workshop manual *Coping with Communication Disorders in Aging* was described in Chapter 19. In addition to a complete presenter's text for lecture content pertaining to communication and aging, speech-language disorders, and hearing impairment, the manual also provides materials for handouts and visual aids. Extensive use of experiential training exercises within this program makes it ideally suited for presentation to relatively uninformed audiences.

Evaluation and Feedback

The final component of successful inservice education consists of eliciting participant reactions to the program. While the perfunctory distribution of evaluation forms is sometimes resented, a serious request for criticisms and reactions indicates to the participants that their responses are valued, and leaves those who do wish to make comments with a sense of closure.

Both written and verbal evaluation processes can be employed. Written evaluation forms provide more precise record-keeping, and can be effective in convincing other groups of the value of training, but many participants' comments are brief to the point of opacity. Verbal evaluations, usually solicited at the end of the workshop, tend to provide a more accurate and complete impression of what participants learned and did not learn, which techniques they perceived as most effective or engaging, and which objectives were and were not accomplished.

SUMMARY

The concept of networking among health care and social service disciplines began in the 1950s and has continued to grow, as widespread recognition of the importance of social support networks has combined with professional interest in interdisciplinary team approaches for various groups of clients. The Older Americans Act promised to encourage networking among service providers to the elderly, but the rapid proliferation of agencies and programs has instead led to greater fragmentation of services, degradation of service quality, and problems with access to the services which are theoretically available. The interventions which are necessary to remedy current problems, and make networking viable, require that members of disciplines which serve elderly clients become more flexible in their definition of appropriate professional roles. Four strategies for improving interdisciplinary service delivery were discussed in this chapter: informal provider networks; community planning; formal teamwork; and continuing education. The ideal professional community would probably utilize aspects of all four approaches.

This entire text has been devoted to informing the reader of the broad and complex changes which make up the aging process, of the characteristics which distinguish older persons from the general population, and of the needs of communicatively impaired older clients. It is appropriate that this final chapter addresses issues of interprofessional networking, collaboration, and information dissemination, because meeting the current and future communication needs of older individuals will require a commitment on the part of all professionals to working together to ensure quality of life for the elderly. Professional roles and responsibilities can and must extend beyond the restrictive confines of the therapy room or audiological suite.

References

1. American Speech-Language-Hearing Association: *Resource Materials for Communicative Problems of Older Persons*, rev. ed. Rockville, MD, American Speech-Language-Hearing Association, 1980.
2. American Speech-Language-Hearing Association: *Breaking the Silence Barrier: Inservice Training Module*. Rockville, MD, American Speech-Language-Hearing Association, 1977.
3. Ashby JK: Professional/interdisciplinary considerations for implementing service delivery models. In Jacobs-Condit L (ed): *Gerontology and Communication Disorders*. Rockville, MD, American Speech-Language-Hearing Association, 1984, p 323.
4. Auburn S: Community-based care: an achievable goal? *The Southwestern* 2:33–39, 1985.
5. Barnes JA: *Social Networks*. Reading, MA, Addison-Wesley, 1972.
6. Bartlett H: *Social Work Practice in the Health Field*. New York, National Association of Social Workers, 1961.
7. Biegel DE, Shore BK, Gordon E: *Building Support Networks for the Elderly: Theory and Applications*. Beverly Hills, CA, Sage, 1984.
8. Boetscher EG: Linking the aged to support systems. *J Gerontol Nurs* 11:27–33, 1985.
9. Bott E: *Family and Social Network*. London, Tavistock, 1957.
10. Brody E, Cole C, Moss M: Individualizing therapy for the mentally impaired adult. *Soc Casework* 54:453–461, 1973.
11. Christopholos F: Multidisciplinary paradigm. *J Learn Dis* 3:167–168, 1970.
12. Coe RM, Wolinsky FD, Miller DK, Prendergast JM: Social network relationships and use of physician services. *Res Aging* 6:243–256, 1984.
13. Cohen CI, Teresi J, Holmes D: Social networks, stress, adaptation, and health. *Res Aging* 7:409–431, 1985.
14. Deimling GT, Harel Z: Social integration and mental health of the aged. *Res Aging* 6:515–527, 1984.
15. Dono JE, Falbe CM, Kail BL, Litwak E, Sherman

RH, Siegel D: Primary groups in old age: structure and function. Res Aging 1:403–433, 1979.

16. Ernst M, Shore H: Sensitizing People to the Process of Aging: the In-service Educator's Guide. Denton, TX, North Texas State University, 1975.

17. Estes CL: The Aging Enterprise. San Francisco, Jossey-Bass, 1979.

18. Fein DJ: The prevalence of speech and language impairments. ASHA 25(2):37, 1983.

19. Florance CL, Conway WF: Transdisciplinary intervention. In Chapey R (ed): Language Intervention Strategies in Adult Aphasia, ed 2. Baltimore, Williams & Wilkins, 1986, p 162.

20. Gelfand DE: The Aging Network: Programs and Services, ed 2. New York, Springer, 1984.

21. Goodman CC: Natural helping among older adults. Gerontologist 24:138–143, 1984.

22. Hickey T: Simulating age-related sensory impairments for practitioner education. Gerontologist 15:457–463, 1975.

23. Hubbard RW, Santos JF: Empathy training as an instructional tool for geriatric health professionals. Educ Gerontol 6:191–194, 1981.

24. Kane R: Interprofessional Teamwork, Manpower Monograph No. 8. Syracuse, NY, Syracuse University School of Social Work, 1975.

25. Kastenbaum R: Can the clinical milieu be therapeutic? In Rowles GD, Ohta RJ (eds): Aging and Milieu: Environmental Perspectives on Growing Old. New York, Academic Press, 1983, p 3.

26. Lipman A, Longino CF: Formal and informal support: a conceptual clarification. J Appl Gerontol 1:141–146, 1982.

27. McGlothlin WJ: The Professional Schools. New York, Center for Applied Research in Education, 1964.

28. Moore W, Campbell R: A pilot training program, and evaluation of training for an area agency on aging. Presented at the Gerontological Society Convention, Houston, 1978.

29. Nerbonne MA, Schow RL, Hutchinson JM: Gerontologic training in communication. ASHA 22(6):404–410, 1980.

30. Ohio State Department of Education: Focus on Inservice Education. Columbus, OH, Ohio State Department of Education, 1978.

31. Peters GR: Interagency relations and the aging network: the state unit on aging and AAA's in Kansas. In Streib GF (ed): Programs for Older Americans, Research Series, vol 1. Gainesville, FL, University of Florida Center for Gerontological Studies, 1981, p 96.

32. Raiford CA, Shadden BB: Graduate education in gerontology. ASHA 27:37–43, 1985.

33. Rundall TG, Evashwick C: Social networks and help-seeking among the elderly. Res Aging 4:205–226, 1982.

34. Sayles AH, Adams JK: Communication Problems and Behaviors of Older Americans. Rockville, MD, American Speech-Language-Hearing Association, 1979.

35. Shadden BB: Communication process and aging. Workshop presented at the Oklahoma Speech-Language-Hearing Association Convention, Oklahoma City, OK, 1986.

36. Shadden BB, Raiford CA, Shadden HS: Coping with Communication Disorders in Aging. Tigard, OR, CC Publications, 1983.

37. Slover D, Greco CM: Analysis and Selection of Training Resources in Aging. Syracuse, NY, Syracuse University Gerontology Center, 1975.

38. Spear M: Guide for Inservice Training for Developing Services for Older People. Washington, DC, U.S. Department of Health Education and Welfare, 1970.

39. Wagner DL, Keast F: Informal groups and the elderly. Res Aging 3:325–331, 1981.

40. Whitehouse F: Professional Teamwork, Proceedings of the 84th National Conference on Social Welfare. New York, Columbia University Press, 1957.

41. Yancey E: Aging connection: a coordinated information and referral system. Panel presentation at the Southern Gerontological Society 3rd Annual Meeting, Orlando, FL, 1982.

APPENDIX

A Case History Example for Workshop Use

I've been married to George for more than 50 years. He's retired now, but he was a school teacher so we get a small pension as well as Social Security. We've always felt lucky, with enough to live on and our own little house. Our three children are all living (although two of them live in New Mexico), and they have nice families. And we always said how lucky we were to have kept our health.

Then last month George had a stroke. The doctor said we were lucky then too, because it was only a moderate stroke. But I don't feel so lucky, so safe, anymore. The doctor says he'll probably be "almost as good as new" someday, but that's hard to believe. He's like a different person. He was always such an easy-going man, but now when he tries to tell me things and I don't understand, he gets so angry. Yesterday he tried to get something and dropped it, and when I tried to help, he looked like he wanted to hit me. I cried and cried.

Maybe I could cope better if I weren't so tired all the time. But George was in the hospital almost a month, because he had bladder problems and pneumonia after his stroke. I tried to be there all the time, but last week I got the flu and they made me go home. I really don't think I'm well yet, but I'll manage. I don't know what I would do without George's brother Vince. I can't drive, and I wouldn't dare leave George alone anyway, but Vince brings us groceries. I hate for him to come all the way out here, but there's no one else I could ask except our daughter Bernice.

I can't stand to talk to Bernice, because all she says is "Put him in the nursing home." She sounds just like those people in the hospital. They said George should go in the nursing home because he could get therapy there! Ha! Show me one person who has gone in a nursing home and gotten better and come home! It would be like sending George off to die. I could tell he felt the same way, so I just got Vince to help me bring him home.

But now Bernice says it's ridiculous to have George sleeping in the living room, because the bedrooms are all upstairs. And she says I'm depriving him of therapy. She says she can tell that he does know what I'm saying to him, he just might be that spiteful. And I try so hard to do everything right. I try to understand him, but I just can't. Then this morning I was helping him get from his wheelchair to the commode. They said he'll be able to do it himself someday, but for now I have to help him. I managed all right yesterday. But this morning when I was trying to help, I just couldn't lift him anymore. He wet in the chair. I was afraid he would get angry, but it was worse—he sat there in his wheelchair and cried.

Index

⟨Page numbers in *italics* denote figures; those followed by "t" denote tables.⟩